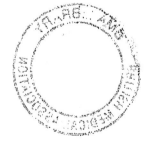

ANATOMY & PHYSIOLOGY
FOR SPEECH, LANGUAGE, AND HEARING

Fifth Edition

J. Anthony Seikel, Ph.D., Idaho State University

David G. Drumright, Computer Programmer

Douglas W. King, Ph. D. (deceased)

Photography by Sarah Moore and Susan Duncan

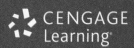
CENGAGE
Learning®

Australia • Brazil • Japan • Korea • Mexico • Singapore • Spain • United Kingdom • United States

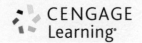
CENGAGE
Learning·

Anatomy & Physiology for Speech, Language, and Hearing, Fifth Edition
J. Anthony Seikel, David G. Drumright, Douglas W. King

SVP, GM Skills & Global Product Management: Dawn Gerrain

Product Director: Matthew Seeley

Product Manager: Laura Stewart

Senior Director, Development: Marah Bellegarde

Product Development Manager: Juliet Steiner

Senior Content Developer: Elisabeth F. Williams

Product Assistant: Hannah Kinisky

Vice President, Marketing Services: Jennifer Ann Baker

Marketing Manager: Jonathan Sheehan

Senior Production Director: Wendy Troeger

Production Director: Andrew Crouth

Content Project Manager: Thomas Heffernan

Senior Art Director: Jack Pendleton

Technology Project Manager: Patricia Allen

Cover image(s): © Hein Nouwens/Shutterstock.com

For product information and technology assistance, contact us at
Cengage Learning Customer & Sales Support, 1-800-354-9706

For permission to use material from this text or product, submit all requests online at **www.cengage.com/permissions.**
Further permissions questions can be e-mailed to
permissionrequest@cengage.com

Library of Congress Control Number: 2014956442

PKG ISBN: 978-1-285-19824-8
Book only ISBN: 978-1-285-19834-7

Cengage Learning
5 Maxwell Drive
Clifton Park, NY 12065
USA

Cengage Learning is a leading provider of customized learning solutions with office locations around the globe, including Singapore, the United Kingdom, Australia, Mexico, Brazil, and Japan. Locate your local office at: **www.cengage.com/global**

Cengage Learning products are represented in Canada by Nelson Education, Ltd.

To learn more about Cengage Learning, visit **www.cengage.com**

Purchase any of our products at your local college store or at our preferred online store **www.cengagebrain.com**

Printed in Canada
Print Number: 01   Print Year: 2014

DEDICATION

We wish to dedicate this text to the memory of Sarah Moore. Sarah was an extraordinarily talented artist who was internationally known for her renderings of archaeological artifacts. Sarah was also a dear friend and colleague. During the preparation of the first edition of this text and of ANATESSE, Sarah happily took on the task of developing the hundreds of illustrations and photographs that would help students learn anatomy. She was perhaps the most determined and focused individual we have ever known, and her line drawings and photos reveal her desire for perfection. We shared many cups of coffee at our kitchen table while poring over rough drafts of drawings and photos. She was undaunted by photo sessions in the cadaver lab and welcomed my suggestions for changes in figures that would emphasize the material being illustrated. In the end, Sarah's art was emblematic of the goal of the text: To give students the best possible learning tool to prepare them for their profession. Her drawings persisted into the third edition of this text and within ANATESSE, and her photos remain a tribute to her skill. The world has lost an amazing person.

(JAS & DD)

The programmer (DD) also dedicates this software to Professor Merle Phillips, who taught him something about audiology and a lot about life.

The narrative author (JAS) wishes also to dedicate the text to speech-language pathologists, audiologists, and learners in training, for their dedication to the betterment of the lives of their clients. He especially wishes to acknowledge the amazing instructors who have taught within the field, and who have given such inspiration over the years. You and your students represent that which is the best of the society.

CONTENTS

Chapter 3   PHYSIOLOGY OF RESPIRATION   143

Chapter 4   ANATOMY OF PHONATION   183

Chapter 5   PHYSIOLOGY OF PHONATION   245

Chapter 8   PHYSIOLOGY OF MASTICATION AND DEGLUTITION   447

Chapter 9   ANATOMY OF HEARING   499

Chapter 10   AUDITORY PHYSIOLOGY   531

Chapter 11   NEUROANATOMY   577

Chapter 12   NEUROPHYSIOLOGY   705

Appendix A   ANATOMICAL TERMS   761

Appendix B   USEFUL COMBINING FORMS   763

PREFACE

Anatomy & Physiology for Speech, Language, and Hearing, fifth edition, provides a sequential tour of the anatomy and physiology associated with speech, language, and hearing. It has been developed keeping today's students in mind and provides ancillary materials that greatly enhance learning. This fifth edition refines the presentation of the anatomy and physiology of the relevant topics under discussion, as well as acknowledges the advances that have occurred in the different fields of study.

This text and its support materials have been designed to serve the upper division undergraduate or graduate student in the fields of speech-language pathology and audiology; it can also serve as a learning tool and resource for the developing as well as the accomplished clinician. We, the authors of this text, are committed to the students within our professions, and to the instructors who have made it their life work to teach them. Learning is a life-long process, and our goal is to give instructors the tools to start students on that life-long professional path. Learning is not a spectator sport, and the degree to which we engage ourselves actively in the learning process determines our level of success. Our goal is to make the text and its ancillary materials as useful to twenty-first-century students as possible. This revision not only provides students with great interactive study tools in the revised ANATESSE study software, but also makes available a wealth of student and instructor resources to facilitate learning. We want you to be the best therapist you can be and sincerely hope that these materials move you along the path of your chosen career.

ORGANIZATION

The text is organized around the four "classic" systems of speech: the respiratory, phonatory, articulatory/resonatory, and nervous systems. The respiratory system (involving the lungs) provides the "energy source" for speech, whereas the phonatory system (involving the larynx) provides voicing. The articulatory/resonatory system modifies the acoustic source provided by voicing (or other gestures) to produce the sounds we acknowledge as speech. The articulatory system is responsible for the mastication (chewing) and deglutition (swallowing) function, an increasingly important area within the field of speech-language pathology. The nervous system lets us control musculature, receive information, and make sense of the information. Finally, the auditory mechanism processes speech and nonspeech acoustic signals received by the listener who is trying to make sense of her or his world.

There are few areas of study where the potential for overwhelming detail is greater than in the discipline of anatomy. Our desire with this text and the accompanying software lessons is to provide a stable foundation upon which detail may be learned. In the text, we have tried to provide you with an introductory section that sets the stage for the detail to follow, and we try to bring you back to a more global picture with summaries. We have also provided derivations of words to help you remember technical terms.

NEW TO THE FIFTH EDITION

This new edition of *Anatomy & Physiology for Speech, Language, and Hearing* includes many exciting enhancements:

- Completely revised physiology of swallowing now includes updated views of infant development, the stages of swallowing, and neurophysiological underpinnings of the process.
- A broadened discussion of the instrumentation associated with all the systems of communication conveys the richness of the research within the fields.
- New research covering the very latest industry trends and technology is highlighted through revised sections covering articulatory and auditory physiology, along with new and expanded content on the effects of aging, neuroimaging, and the DIVA model.
- Many new images have been added, with a focus on a clear and accurate understanding of the classical framework of the speech, language, and hearing systems.
- Clinical Notes boxes link anatomy and physiology with disorders seen by speech-language pathologists and audiologists to provide real-world applications for students.
- Fully revised ANATESSE software is now platform neutral and internet-based, providing on-the-go learning, with new labs, simulations, and updates to content. Experience the classic systems three dimensionally with animations that explore the important processes of hearing, phonation, respiration, swallowing, and more.

TEACHING PACKAGE FOR THE INSTRUCTOR

The *Instructor Companion Website to Accompany Anatomy & Physiology for Speech, Language, and Hearing,* fifth edition, contains a variety of tools to help instructors successfully prepare lectures and teach within this subject area. This comprehensive package provides something for all instructors, from those teaching anatomy and physiology for the first time to seasoned instructors who want something new. The following components in the website are free to adopters of the text:

- A downloadable and customizable *Instructor's Manual* containing materials and suggested activities for the lecture; and lab guides to facilitate learning outside of the classroom.
- A *Computerized Test Bank* with approximately 1,000 questions and answers, for use in instructor-created quizzes and tests.
- Chapter slides created in PowerPoint® to use as in-class lecture material and as handouts for students.

LEARNING PACKAGE FOR THE STUDENT

ANATESSE software is available to purchasers of the text and can be accessed through the Premium Website at www.CengageBrain.com. Enter your passcode, found in the front of the book, and the Premium Website will be added to your bookshelf.

ANATESSE software is your true partner in learning. These labs give you the opportunity to examine structures and functions of the speech mechanism in the more flexible environment of your personal computer. The ANATESSE software is keyed to the text, reinforcing identification of the structures presented during lecture, but more importantly illustrating the function of those structures. An icon in the margin of the text indicates that you'll find a related lesson on ANATESSE, where you can examine speech physiology through the interactive manipulation of the structures under study, and learn the relationship of the body parts and how they function together.

Reviewers

On behalf of the authors, Cengage Learning would like to thank the following reviewers for their insightful comments and suggestions throughout the development process:

Stefan A. Frisch, PhD
Associate Professor, University of South Florida
Tampa, Florida

Kate Krival, PhD, CCC-SLP
Assistant Professor, Kent State University
Kent, Ohio

Shawn L. Nissen, PhD, CCC-SLP
Associate Professor, Brigham Young University
Provo, Utah

ABOUT THE AUTHORS

J. Anthony (Tony) Seikel is part of the faculty at the Idaho State University in Pocatello, Idaho. His research interests center on the relationship of pathology with acoustics and perception, but extend as well to the improvement of pedagogy through technology.

David G. Drumright is a programmer and teacher in Spokane, Washington. He has taught electronics at numerous schools and has a background in speech-language pathology and audiology. His software includes the original ANIMA programs of this text; the ANATESSE application that you see in this fifth edition; AUDIN, which is software for instruction in audiology; and numerous smaller instructional tools.

Douglas W. King was a professor in the Basic Medical program at Washington State University until the time of his death in 2001. He was greatly loved by his students and fellow members of the faculty and had set up a scholarship program for anatomy for students with diabetes.

J. Anthony (Tony) Seikel
David G. Drumright

ACKNOWLEDGMENTS

We want to express our deepest appreciation to the dedicated members of the Cengage Learning team who were so instrumental in making this fifth edition a reality; it has been a pleasure to work with them on this project.

We would like to acknowledge the effort that reviewers put into their examination of our material and hope we have done justice to their work. Reviewers are the unsung heroes of textbook preparation. They put in long and often tedious hours, examining our work with an unflinching eye. We are very deeply indebted to them for their careful review, keen insight, and willingness to call our attention to areas that need refinement and improvement. This textbook is written, quite literally, on their shoulders.

We also wish to acknowledge all those who have, over the course of the past few years, given us corrections and suggestions for improving the text. Among those we remember are Margaret Rudelich Hoppe (University of Nevada at Las Vegas), Christina Bronson-Lowe, Lucy Kellogg and Allison Early. We appreciate the comments from Don Cooper, who informed our discussion of the root of the tongue. I have lost track of the many other instructors and students who have offered feedback on the text. Please know that we appreciate every one of you.

As speech-language pathologists and audiologists, we must acknowledge the tremendous debt we owe to the great researchers and teachers who have formed the profession, our colleagues with whom we consult and work, and, always, our clients, who have taught us more than any textbook could.

As authors, we must also acknowledge the source of our inspiration. We have been actively involved in teaching students in speech-language pathology and audiology for some time, and not a semester goes by that we don't realize how very dedicated our students are. There is something special about our field that attracts not just the brightest, but the most compassionate. You, students, keep us as teachers alive and vital.

Thank you.

INTRODUCTION TO THE LEARNER

We continue to be impressed with the complexity and beauty of the systems of human communication. Humans use an extremely complex system for communication, requiring extraordinary coordination and control of an intensely interconnected sensorimotor system. It is our heartfelt desire that the study of the physical system will lead you to an appreciation of the importance of your future work as a speech-language pathologist or audiologist.

We also know that the intensity of your study will work to the benefit of your future clients and that the knowledge you gain through your effort will be applied throughout your career. We appreciate the fact that the study of anatomy is challenging, but we also recognize that the effort you put forth now will provide you with the background for work with the medical community.

A deep understanding of the structure and function of the human body is critical to the individual who is charged with the diagnosis and treatment of speech and language disorders. As beginning clinicians, you are already aware of the awesome responsibility you bear in clinical management. It is our firm belief that knowledge of the human body and how it works will provide you with the background you need to make informed and wise decisions. We welcome you on your journey into the world of anatomy.

USING THIS TEXT

Use the elements found in the text to help guide you as you move along the path of your chosen career.

- **Margin notes** identify important terminology, root words, and definitions, which are highlighted in color throughout each chapter. Other important terms are boldfaced in text to indicate that a corresponding definition can be found in the Glossary. Use these terms to study and prepare for tests and quizzes.

- **Clinical Notes** relate a topic directly to clinical experience to emphasize the importance of anatomy in your clinical practice. Gain insight into your chosen profession by using the topics discussed for research papers, to facilitate in-class discussion, and to complete homework assignments.

- **Photographs** provide a real-life look at the body parts and functions you are studying. Use these pieces as reference for accuracy in describing body systems, parts, and processes. Allow yourself to be amazed by the intricacies of human anatomy!

- **Illustrations, graphs, and charts** provide visual examples of the anatomy, processes, and body systems discussed. Refer to the figures as you read the text to enhance your understanding of the specific idea or anatomical component being discussed. When reviewing for quizzes and tests, refer back to the figures for an important visual recap of the topics discussed.

- **Tables** highlight the various components, functions, structures, and pathologies of anatomical concepts related to what you might encounter in actual practice. Use these tables for quick reference to study and learn to relate your new anatomical knowledge to clinical experience.

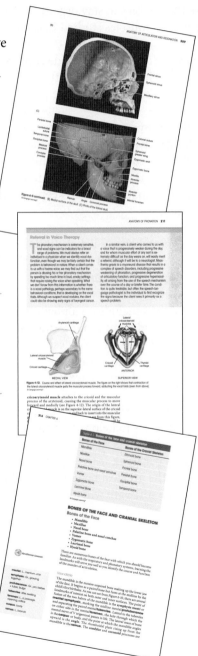

- **"To Summarize" lists** provide a succinct listing of the major topics covered in a chapter or chapter section. These summaries provide a great recap of the general areas where you should focus your time while reviewing for examinations.

- **Muscle tables** describe the origin, course, insertion, innervation, and function of key muscles and muscle groups. Use these tables to stay organized and keep track of the numerous muscles studied in each chapter.

- **Chapter Summaries** provide comprehensive reviews of content. The summary is offset from the running text to make it easily identifiable for quick review.

- **Study Questions and Answers** can be completed after reading a chapter to help you identify areas you may need to re-read or focus on while studying. Complete the questions again as you review for a midterm or final examination to help keep the content fresh in your memory.

- The comprehensive list of **Bibliography** provided at the end of each chapter offers great sources to start your research for a paper or class project.

- **Appendices** include an alphabetical listing of anatomical terms, useful combining forms, and listings of sensors, cranial nerves, and pathologies that affect speech production. You will also find a complete **Glossary** of all key terms found throughout the text.

- The **ANATESSE** software labs are self-paced, with frequent quizzes to help you examine the effectiveness of your study habits. If you spend two or three half-hour sessions per week with the ANATESSE software, you will get the greatest benefit from your classes and readings. The software will also prove a great refresher in preparing for quizzes and examinations.

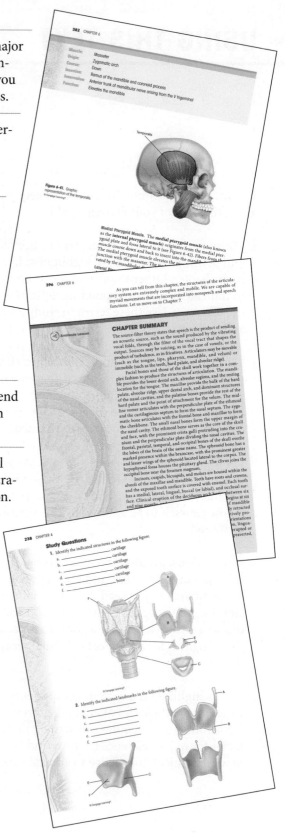

Chapter 1

BASIC ELEMENTS OF ANATOMY

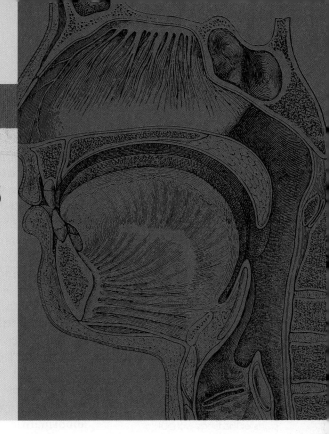

The study of the human body and its parts has a long and rich tradition. Although students of anatomy must still rely on their powers of observation, the task faced by the first anatomists was even more daunting. The modern study of anatomy and physiology is performed with myriad instruments and techniques, but our colleagues from earlier times were not so blessed. If you listen closely, you will hear the echoes of the early anatomists' voices as you, at times, struggle with terminology that seems foreign and confusing. It is then that you should open your medical dictionary to see for yourself the roots of the words that seem confusing. The fact that the terminology remains in our lexicon indicates the accuracy with which our academic ancestors studied their field, despite extraordinarily limited resources.

In this chapter, we will provide some basic elements to prepare you for your study of the anatomy and physiology of speech, language, and hearing. To do this, we will provide a broad picture of the field of anatomy and then introduce you to the basic tissues that make up the human body. When tissues combine to form structures, those structures must bind together to form a functioning whole; therefore, we will discuss the means of connecting those parts. This chapter sets the stage for your understanding of the new and foreign anatomical terminologies.

Anatesse Lesson

ANATOMY AND PHYSIOLOGY

The term **anatomy** refers to the study of the structure of an organism. At one time, it referred to the actual **dissection** or cutting of parts of the organism, but over time has evolved to encompass

anatomy: Gr., anatome, dissection

dissection: L., dissecare, the process of cutting up

1

physiology: Gr., physis, nature + logos, study

applied anatomy: application of anatomical study for the diagnosis and treatment of disease, particularly as it relates to surgical procedures

clinical anatomy: application of anatomical study for the diagnosis and treatment of disease, particularly as it relates to surgical procedures

descriptive anatomy: anatomical specialty involving the description of individual parts of the body without reference to disease conditions

systemic anatomy: a.k.a. descriptive anatomy, involving the description of individual parts of the body without reference to disease conditions

gross anatomy: study of the body and its parts as visible without the aid of microscopy

microscopic anatomy: study of the structure of the body by means of microscopy

surface anatomy or **superficial anatomy:** study of the body and its surface markings as related to underlying structures

developmental anatomy: study of anatomy with reference to growth and development from conception to adulthood

pathological anatomy: study of parts of the body with respect to the pathological entity

comparative anatomy: study of homologous structures of different animals

electrophysiological techniques: those techniques that measure the electrical activity of single cells or groups of cells, including muscle and nervous system tissues

a field of study that involves much more than gross separation of body parts. **Physiology** is the study of the function of the living organism and its parts, as well as the chemical processes involved. As science and technology advanced, subspecializations of both anatomy and physiology arose. **Applied anatomy**, also known as **clinical anatomy**, entails the application of anatomical study for the diagnosis and treatment of disease, particularly as it relates to surgical procedures. **Descriptive anatomy**, also known as **systemic anatomy**, involves the description of individual parts of the body without reference to disease conditions. Descriptive anatomy views the body as a composite of systems that function together.

Gross anatomy studies structures visible without the aid of microscopy, while **microscopic anatomy** examines structures not visible to the unaided eye. **Surface anatomy** (also known as **superficial anatomy**) is the study of the form and structure of the surface of the body, especially with reference to the organs beneath the surface. **Developmental anatomy** deals with the development of the organism from conception, continuing through the life-span.

When your study turns to disease conditions or structural abnormalities, you will have entered the domain of **pathological anatomy**. Quite often in anatomy and physiology, comparisons are made across species boundaries, because, among other things, knowledge of similarities and differences across the animal kingdom gives insight into the utility of different animal models of research. This study, **comparative anatomy**, provides that information.

Physiology has undergone similar changes as technology has been refined. Examination of physiological processes may entail the use of a range of methods, from fairly simple methodologies, such as those measuring forces exerted by muscles, to the highly refined **electrophysiological techniques** that measure the electrical activity of single cells or groups of cells, including muscle and nervous system tissues. Indeed, the audiologist will be particularly interested in auditory electrophysiological procedures that measure the electrical activity of the brain caused by auditory stimuli (**evoked auditory potentials**). You will sample the fruits of many of these areas during your study of anatomy. We rely heavily on descriptive anatomy to guide our understanding of the physical mechanisms of speech and to aid our discussion of its physiology as well. You will call on pathological anatomy as you deal with the results of conditions that change how systems work. Even as we discuss these changes in the text, we will call on microscopic anatomy to reveal the impact of diseases on structures invisible to the unaided eye.

You must also call on knowledge from related fields to support your understanding of anatomy and physiology. **Cytology** is the discipline that examines structure and function of cells; **histology** is the microscopic study of cells and tissues. **Osteology** is the study of structure and function of bones, while **myology** examines muscle

Teratogens

Ateratogen or teratogenic agent is anything causing teratogenesis, the development of a severely malformed fetus. For an agent to be teratogenic, its effect must occur during prenatal development.

Because the development of the fetus involves the proliferation and differentiation of tissues, the timing of the teratogen is particularly critical. The heart undergoes its most critical period of development from the third embryonic week to the eighth, while the critical period for the palate begins around the fifth week and ends around the 12th week. The critical period for neural development stretches from the third embryonic week until birth. These critical periods for development mark the points at which the developing human is most susceptible to insult. An agent destined to have an effect on the development of an organ or system will have its greatest impact during that critical period.

Many teratogens have been identified, including organic mercury (which causes cerebral palsy, mental retardation, blindness, cerebral atrophy, and seizures), heroin and morphine (causing neonatal convulsions, tremors, and death), alcohol (fetal alcohol syndrome, mental retardation, microcephaly, joint anomalies, and maxillary anomalies), and tobacco (growth retardation), to name just a few.

form and function. **Arthrology** studies the joints that unite the bones, and **angiology** is the study of blood vessels and the lymphatic system. **Neurology** is the study of diseases of the nervous system. You will capitalize on all of these disciplines to explain the mechanisms involved in speech production.

✔ *To summarize:*

- **Anatomy** is the study of the structure of an organism; **physiology** is the study of function.
- Several subspecializations of anatomy interact to provide the detail required for understanding the anatomy and physiology of speech, language, and hearing.
- **Descriptive anatomy** relates the individual parts of the body to functional systems.
- **Pathological anatomy** refers to changes in structure as they relate to disease.
- **Gross** and **microscopic anatomy** refer to levels of visibility of structures under study.
- **Developmental anatomy** studies the growth and development of the organism.
- Disciplines such as **cytology** and **histology** study cells and tissues, respectively, and **myology** examines muscle form and function.
- **Arthrology** refers to the study of the joint system for bones, while **osteology** is the study of form and function of bones.
- **Neurology** refers to the study of diseases of the nervous system.

cytology: Gr., kytos, cell + logos, study

histology: Gr., histos, web; tissue + logos, study

osteology: Gr., osteon, bone + logos, study

myology: Gr., mys, muscle + logos, study

arthrology: Gr., arthron, joint + logos, study

angiology: Gr., angio, blood vessels + logos, study

neurology: Gr., neuron, sinew; nerve + logos, study

TERMINOLOGY OF ANATOMY

Terminology in anatomy is very important, as it lets us communicate relevant information concerning the location and orientation of various body parts and organs. Clarity of terminology lets us accurately represent structures and is of the utmost importance in the study of anatomy. Terminology also links us to the roots of this field of study. To the budding scholar of Latin or Greek, learning the terms of anatomy will be an exciting reminder of our linguistic history. To the rest of us, the terms we are about to discuss may be less easily digested but are nonetheless important.

As you prepare for your study of anatomy, please realize that this body of knowledge is extremely hierarchical. What you learn today will be the basis for what you learn tomorrow. Not only are the terms the bedrock for understanding anatomical structures, mastery of their usage will let you gain the maximum benefit from new material presented.

Terms of Orientation

In the **anatomical position**, the body is erect and the palms, arms, and hands face forward, as shown in Figure 1-1. Discussion of terms of direction assumes this position. Intrinsic to this discussion is the concept of axis. The body and brain (and many other structures) are seen to have axes (plural of "axis") or midlines from which other structures arise. The **axial skeleton** is the head and trunk, with the spinal column being the axis, while the **appendicular skeleton** includes the lower and upper limbs. The **neuraxis**, or the axis of the brain, is slightly less straightforward, due to morphological changes of the brain during development. The embryonic nervous system is essentially tubular, but as the cerebral cortex develops, a flexure occurs and the telencephalon (the region that will become the cerebrum) folds forward. As a result, the neuraxis takes a T-formation. The spinal cord and brain stem have dorsal (back) and ventral (front) surfaces corresponding to those of the surface of the body. Because the cerebrum folds forward, the dorsal surface is also the superior surface, and the ventral surface is the inferior surface. Most anatomists avoid this confusing state by referring to the ventral and dorsal surfaces of the embryonic brain as "inferior" and "superior" surfaces, respectively.

Some terms are sensitive to the physical orientation of the body (such as *vertical* or *horizontal*). Other terms (such as *frontal, coronal,* and *longitudinal*) refer to planes or axes of the body and are therefore insensitive to the position of the body.

With the anatomical position in mind, let us turn to planes of reference. You may think of the following planes as referring to sections of a standing body, but they are actually defined relative to imaginary axes of the body. If you were to divide the body into front and back sections, you would have produced a **frontal section** or **frontal view**. However, if you cut the body into left and right halves this would be along the median plane and it would produce **midsagittal sections**. A **sagittal section** is any cut that is parallel to the median plane and divides the

---

frontal section or **frontal view:** divides body into front and back halves

midsagittal section: an anatomical section that divides the body into left and right halves in the median plane

sagittal: L., sagittalis, arrow-like

sagittal section: divides body or body part into right and left

body into left and right portions: The cut is in the sagittal plane. The transverse plane is that divides the body into upper and lower portions (this plane is often referred to by radiologists as transaxial or axial, and the radiological orientation is always referred to as if you were looking from the feet toward the head). Figure 1-1 illustrates these sections.

A **frontal** or **coronal section** results in front and back portions of a body and is so called because the plane is parallel to the coronal suture of the skull, which roughly divides the body in half along that axis. Armed with these basic planes of reference, you could rotate a structure in space and still discuss the orientation of its parts.

The term **anterior** refers to the front surface of a body. **Ventral** and *anterior* are synonymous for the standing human but have different meanings for a quadruped. The ventral aspect of a standing dog includes its abdominal wall, which happens to be directed toward the ground. The anterior of the same dog would be the portion including the face.

frontal or **coronal section:** divides body into front and back halves

anterior: L., front

ventral: pertaining to the belly or anterior surface

Those of you who play cards may remember "ante up," meaning, "put your money up front!" You may remember the term antebellum, meaning "before the war."

(A)

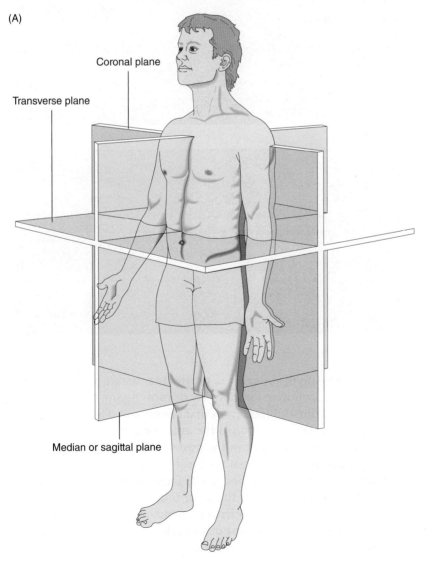

Coronal plane

Transverse plane

Median or sagittal plane

Figure 1-1. Terms of orientation. (A) Planes of orientation. (continues).
© Cengage Learning®.

(B)

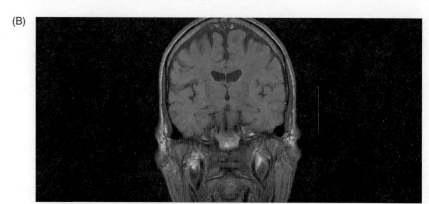

Figure 1-1 continued. (B) Coronal
section through brain and skull
using magnetic resonance
imaging (MRI).
© Cengage Learning®.

(C)

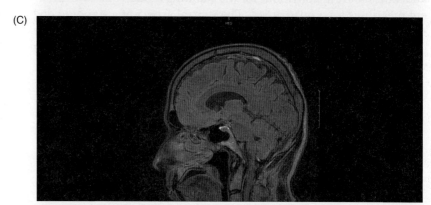

Figure 1-1. (C) Sagittal or median
section through brain and skull
using MRI.
© Cengage Learning®.

(D)

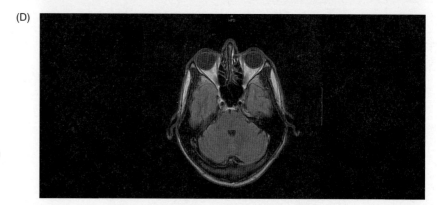

Figure 1-1. (D) Transverse section
through brain and skull using MRI.
(continues).
© Cengage Learning®.

*The term "quadruped" refers
to four-footed animals. The
term "biped" refers to two-
footed animals.*

posterior: toward the rear

dorsal: pertaining to the
back of the body or distal

rostral: L., rostralis, beak-like

The opposite of anterior is **posterior**, meaning "toward the
back," and the synonym for bipeds is **dorsal**. Again, the posterior of
a four-footed animal differs from that of humans. Thus, you may refer to a muscle running toward the anterior surface, or a structure
having a specific landmark in the posterior aspect. These terms are
body-specific: No matter what the position of the body is, anterior is
"toward the front" of that body. The term **rostral** is often used to
mean "toward the head." If the term is used to refer to structures
within the cranium, *rostral* refers to a structure anterior to another.

When discussing the course of a muscle, we often need to clarify its
orientation with reference to the surface or level within the body. Thus,

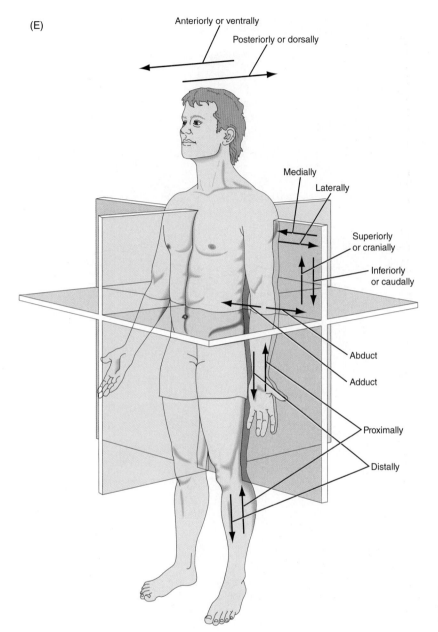

(E)

Figure 1-1 continued. (E) Terms of movement. (continues).
© Cengage Learning®.

a structure may be referred to as **peripheral** (away from the center) to another. A structure is **superficial** if it is confined to the surface.

When we say one organ is "**deep** to another," we mean it is closer to the axis of the body. A structure may also be referred to as being **external** or **internal**, but these terms are generally reserved for cavities within the body. Likewise, you may refer to an aspect of an appendicular structure (such as arms and legs) as being **distal** (away from the midline) or **proximal** (toward the root or attachment point of the structure).

A few terms refer to the actual present position of the body rather than a description based on the anatomical position. **Superior** (above, farther

peripheral: relative to the periphery or away from

superficial: on or near the surface

deep: further from the surface

external: L., externus, outside

internal: within the body

distal: away from the midline

proximal: L., proximus, next

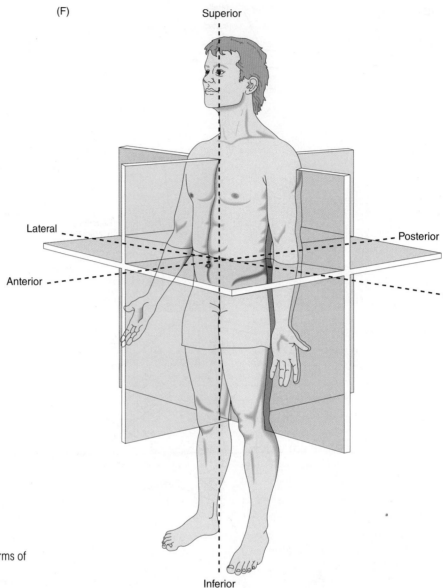

(F)

Superior

Lateral

Anterior

Posterior

Inferior

Figure 1-1 continued. (F) Terms of spatial orientation.
© Cengage Learning®.

prone: body in horizontal position with face down

supine: body in horizontal position with face up

lateral: toward the side

from the ground) and **inferior** (below, closer to the ground) are used in situations in which gravity is important. Superior can also indicate relative location: Structures that are near the head are referred to as superior or cranial, while those near the feet are referred to as inferior or caudal (the term "caudal" is more often used in this context when referring to an embryo). The terms **prone** (on the belly) and **supine** (on the back) are also commonly used in describing the present actual position.

Often we must describe the orientation of a structure relative to another structure and subsequently disregard the anatomical position. Some terms that will assist you are **lateral** (related to the side, as in football's "lateral pass") and **medial** (toward the median plane). If a point is closer to the median plane (the one that divides the body into left and right halves), it will be medial to a point that is farther from that plane, which will be lateral. So you would say that, for instance, the tongue is medial to the molars in the mandible since it is closer to the midline or median plane.

Terms of Movement

There are specialized terms associated with movement. **Flexion** refers to bending at a joint, usually toward the ventral surface. That is, flexion usually results in two ventral surfaces coming closer together. Thus, sit-ups would be an act of flexion, because you are bending at the waist. **Extension** is the opposite of flexion, being the act of pulling two ends farther apart. Again, having completed a sit-up, you return to the extended condition. **Hyperextension**, as in arching your back at the end of your sit-up, is sometimes referred to as **dorsiflexion**.

Use of flexion and extension with reference to feet and toes is a little more complex. **Plantar** refers to the sole of the foot, the flexor surface. If you rise on your toes, you are extending your foot, but the gesture is reasonably referred to as **plantar flexion**. A **plantar grasp reflex** would be one in which stimulation of the sole of the foot causes the toes of the feet to "grasp." The term "dorsiflexion" may be used to denote elevation of the dorsum (upper surface) of the foot. You may turn the sole of your foot inward, termed **inversion**. A foot turned out is in **eversion**.

The term **palmar** refers to the palm of the hand, that is, the ventral (flexor) surface. The side opposite the palmar side is the dorsal side. If the hand is rotated so that the palmar surface is directed inferiorly, it is **pronated** (remembering that in the prone position one is lying on his or her stomach or ventral surface). **Supination** refers to rotating the hand so that the palmar surface is directed superiorly. A **palmar grasp reflex** is elicited by lightly stimulating the palm of the hand. The response is to flex the fingers to grasp.

These and other useful terms and their definitions may be found in Appendixes A and B at the end of the book, as well as in the Glossary. A good medical dictionary will be another invaluable aid in the process of sorting out anatomical terminology.

The names of muscles, bones, and other organs were mostly set down at a time in history when medical people spoke Latin and Greek as universal languages. The intention was to name parts unambiguously rather than to make things mysterious. Many of the morphemes left over from Latin and Greek are worth learning separately. When you come across a new term, you will often be able to determine its meaning from these components. For instance, when a text mentions an "**ipsilateral**" course for a nerve tract, you can see "**ipsi**" (same) and "**lateral**" (side) and conclude that the nerve tract is on the same side as something else. Your study of the anatomy and physiology of the human body will be greatly enhanced if it includes memorization of some of the basic word forms found in the appendixes.

flexion: L., flexio, bending

extension: Gr., ex, out + L., tendere, to stretch

hyperextension: extreme extension

dorsiflexion: flexion that brings dorsal surfaces into closer proximity (syn., hyperextension)

plantar: pertaining to the sole of the foot

plantar flexion: flexion of toes of the foot

inversion: L., in, in + versio, to turn

eversion: L., ex, from; out + versio, to turn

palmar: pertaining to the palm of the hand

pronate: to place an organism in the prone position

supinate: to place an organism in the supine position

ipsi: same

While you are studying the nomenclature of the field, do not let the plurals get you down. Fortunately, Latin is a well-organized language with a few general rules that will assist you in sorting through terminology. If a singular word ends in *a*, the plural will most likely be *ae* (*pleura*; *pleurae*). If a word ends in *us* (such as *locus*), the plural will be *i*. When the singular form ends in *um* (as in *datum* or *stratum*), the plural will have *a* ("data" or "strata").

Often you can feel comfortable using the Anglicized version ("hiatuses," but never "datas"), but do not assume everyone will. Many combined forms involve a possessive form, denoting ownership (the genitive case, in linguistic jargon): "corpus"—body; "corporum"—of the body.

The English pronunciation of these forms is unfortunately less predictable; the dictionary often does not agree with the pronunciations common among medical personnel.

Parts of the Body

The human body can be defined in terms of specific regions. The **thorax** is the chest region; the **abdomen** is the region represented externally as the belly, or anterior abdominal wall. Together, these two components make up the **trunk** or **torso**. The **dorsal trunk** is the region we commonly refer to as the *back*. The area of the hip bones is known as the **pelvis**. Resting atop the trunk is the head or **caput**.

The skull consists of two components: the **cranial portion**, the part of the skull that houses the brain and its components, and the **facial part**, the part of the skull that houses the mouth, pharynx, nasal cavity, and structures related to the upper airway and mastication (chewing).

The upper and lower extremities are attached to the trunk. The **upper extremity** consists of the arm (from the shoulder to the elbow), the forearm, wrist, and hand. The **lower extremity** is made up of the thigh, leg, ankle, and foot.

Within these components of the body are five enclosed spaces, or cavities, within which organs reside. Specific neuroanatomical cavities include the cranial cavity, in which the brain resides, and the vertebral canal, within which is found the spinal cord. Within the trunk are found the thoracic cavity (housing lungs and related structures), the pericardial cavity (housing the heart), and the abdominal cavity, within which are found the structures of the digestive system. While these spaces are particularly important because of the structures they house, they may also become infected as a result of trauma or other condition.

✔ *To summarize:*

- The **axial skeleton** consists of the trunk and head, whereas the **appendicular skeleton** comprises the upper and lower extremities.
- The **trunk** consists of the abdominal and thoracic regions.
- Anatomical terminology is the specialized set of terms used to define the position and orientation of structures.
- The **frontal plane** divides the body into front and back halves, whereas the **median** or **sagittal plane** divides the body into right and left halves. Sections that are parallel to these planes are referred to as **frontal sections** or **sagittal sections**, respectively.

---

thorax: the part of the body between the diaphragm and the seventh cervical vertebra

abdomen: L., belly

dorsal trunk: the region commonly referred to as the back of the body

pelvis: the area formed by the sacrum, coccyx, and innominate bones of the body

cranial portion: the part of the skull that houses the brain and its components

facial part: the part of the skull that houses the mouth, pharynx, nasal cavity, and structures related to the upper airway and mastication

lower extremity: portion of the body made up of the thigh, leg, ankle, and foot

- A **transverse section** divides the body into upper and lower portions.
- **Anterior** and **posterior** refer to the front and back surfaces of a body, respectively, as do **ventral** and **dorsal** for the erect human.
- **Superficial** refers to the surface of a body, while **peripheral** and **deep**, respectively, refer to directions toward and away from the surface.
- **Distal** and proximal refer to being away from and toward the midline of a free extremity, respectively.
- **Medial** refers to something closer to the median plane, while **lateral** refers to something farther from that plane.
- **Superior** refers to an elevated position, whereas **inferior** is closer to the ground.
- **Prone** and **supine** refer to being on the belly and back, respectively.
- **Lateral** refers to the side, **proximal** refers to a point near the point of attachment of a free extremity, and **distal** refers to a point away from the root of the extremity.
- **Flexion** and **extension** refer to bending at a joint. Flexion refers to bringing ventral surfaces closer together and extension is moving them farther apart.
- **Plantar** refers to the sole of the foot, while **palmar** refers to the palm of the hand. Both are ventral surfaces.

In the sections that follow, we will present the building blocks of the physical system you are preparing to study. These blocks include the basic tissues, organs, and structures made up of these tissues and the systems made up of the organs. Let us turn our attention to the basic elements of which all bodies are composed.

BUILDING BLOCKS OF ANATOMY: ORGANS, TISSUES, AND SYSTEMS

Organs

The body is composed of cells, living tissue that contains a nucleus and a variety of cellular material specialized to the particular function of the individual cell. Cells differ based on the type of **tissue** they comprise. Our study of anatomy will focus on muscle cells, nerve cells, and cells, as these cells combine to form the structures involved in speech and hearing. Four basic tissues constitute the human body, and variants of these combine to make up the structures of the body. These are epithelial, connective, muscular, and nervous tissue. These tissues have numerous subclasses, as shown in Table 1-1. Let us look at each tissue in turn.

tissue: L., texere, to weave

Tissues

Epithelial Tissue

Epithelial tissue refers to the superficial (outer) layer of mucous membranes and the cells constituting the skin, as well as the linings of major body cavities and all of the "tubes" that pass into, out of,

epithelial tissue: the superficial (outer) layer of mucous membranes and the cells constituting the skin, as well as the linings of major body cavities and all of the "tubes" that pass into, out of, and through the body

Table 1-1 **Tissue types**

I. Epithelial

A. Simple epithelium: Single layer of cells

Squamous (pavement) epithelium: Single layer of flat cells; linings of blood vessels, heart, alveoli, lymphatic vessels.

Cuboidal (cubical) epithelium: Cube-shaped; secretory function in some glands, such as thyroid.

Columnar epithelium: Single layer, cylindrical cells; inner lining for stomach, intestines, gall bladder, bile ducts.

Ciliated epithelium: Cylindrical cells with cilia; lining of nasal cavity, larynx, trachea, bronchi.

B. Compound epithelium: Different layers of cells

Stratified epithelium: Flattened cells on bed of columnar cells; epidermis of skin, lining of mouth, pharynx, esophagus; conjunctiva.

Transitional epithelium: Pear-shaped cells; lining of bladder, etc.

C. Basement membrane (baseplate)

Made predominantly of collagen; underlies epithelial tissue; serves stabilizing and other functions, including joining epithelial and connective tissues.

II. Connective

A. Areolar: Elastic; supports organs, between muscles.

B. Adipose: Cells with fat globules; between muscles and organs.

C. White fibrous: Strong, closely packed; ligaments binding bones; periosteum covering bone; covering of organs; fascia over muscle.

D. Yellow elastic: Elastic; in areas requiring recoil, such as trachea, cartilage, bronchi, lungs.

E. Lymphoid: Lymphocytes; make up lymphoid tissue of tonsils, adenoids, lymphatic nodes.

F. Cartilage: Firm and flexible.

1. Hyaline cartilage: Bluish white and smooth; found on articulating surfaces of bones, costal cartilage of ribs, larynx, trachea, and bronchial passageway.
2. Fibrocartilage: Dense, white, flexible fibers; intervertebral disks, between surfaces of knee joints.
3. Yellow (elastic) cartilage: Firm elastic; pinna, epiglottis.

G. Blood: Corpuscles (cells: red, white), platelets, blood plasma.

H. Bone: Hardest connective tissue.

1. Compact bone: Has haversian canal, lamellar structure.
2. Cancellous (spongy) bone: Spongy appearance, larger haversian canal, red bone marrow producing red and white blood cells and plasma.

III. Muscular

A. Striated: Skeletal, voluntary.

B. Smooth: Muscle of internal organs, involuntary.

C. Cardiac: Combination of striated and smooth, involuntary.

IV. Nervous

A. Neurons: Transfer information; communicating tissue.

B. Glial cells: Nutrient transfer; blood–brain barrier.

Compiled from Taxonomy from Foundations of Anatomy and Physiology by J. S. Ross & K. J. W. Wilson, 1966, pp. 1–32. Baltimore, MD: Williams & Wilkins.

and through the body. The hallmark of epithelial tissue is its shortage of intercellular material. This is in contrast to bone, cartilage, and blood, all of which have significant quantities of intercellular matter. The absence of intercellular material lets the epithelial cells form a tightly packed sheet, which has a protective quality. This is the common quality of all epithelia: They serve as a barrier to prevent or permit substances to pass to the structures being contained by them. This comes strongly into play with the epithelial lining of the vocal folds, which keeps the tissues from becoming dehydrated (a very important function, as any singer will attest). There may be many layers of epithelium. We are most familiar with the surface covering of the human body, but epithelial tissue lines nearly all of the cavities of the body as well as the tubes that connect them. Some forms of epithelium are secretory (glandular epithelium), some allow for absorption (the linings of our intestines), and others have **cilia** or hairlike protrusions that actively beat to remove contaminants from the epithelial surface (beating ciliated epithelia) of the respiratory passageway. Generally, epithelial tissue can regenerate if damaged.

Cilia can be found throughout the body on surfaces and are unique in that they are motile, which means that their function involves movement. Cilia are found in the cavities of the respiratory passageway, within the ventricles of the brain, in the lining of the central canal in the spinal cord, as part of the olfactory receptor (sense of smell), and even in portions of the rods and cones of the retina. Ciliated tissues share a common characteristic, which is the beating behavior of their hairlike protrusions: The cilia move rapidly in one direction, and more slowly in the opposite or return direction. In this manner, they are able to move materials from one location to another during the slow stroke but return to their original position using a rapid stroke. This extraordinary function removes pollutant-laden mucus from the respiratory passageway and moves molecules of materials onto (and off of) the surface of an olfactory sensor. While this may seem at first glance to be an esoteric discussion, realize that the same motile elements that drive cilia to move "gunk" from the lungs also provide the most exciting discovery in the last decade in hearing science, which is the active movement of the outer hair cells of the cochlea in response to sound stimulation.

A **baseplate** or **basement membrane** made predominantly of collagen underlies epithelial tissue, serving a number of functions, depending on the location of the epithelium. Basement membrane may act as a filter (for instance, in the kidneys) or stabilize the epithelial tissue (as in the juncture of connective tissue with epithelium). The basement membrane is important in the process of directing growth patterns for epithelial cells.

The role of epithelial tissue is to provide a barrier to some material. For instance, the surface epithelium we know as "skin" is an amazing barrier to hostile agents in the environment (although it is not impermeable, particularly to modern solvents, many of which can pass quickly through the epithelial barrier). Epithelia can protect

baseplate or **basement membrane:** the tissue that underlies the epithelium, which is made predominantly of collagen

skin from dehydration and leakage of fluid. Specialized versions of epithelia can also have a secretory function (such as secreting epithelia that make up glands), or serve as sensory elements, such as the sensory epithelia of the olfactory system (sense of smell).

Connective Tissue

Connective tissue is perhaps the most complex of the tissue categories, being specialized for the purposes of support and protection. Unlike epithelium, connective tissue is composed predominantly of intercellular material, known as the **matrix**, within which the cells of connective tissue are bound. Connective tissue may be solid, liquid, or gel-like. The matrix is the defining property of a specific connective tissue.

Areolar tissue, also referred to as *loose connective tissue*, is supportive in nature. This elastic material is found between muscles and as a thin, membranous sheet between organs. It fills the **interstitial** space between organs, and its fibers form a mat or weave of flexible collagen. **Adipose** tissue is areolar tissue that is highly impregnated with fat cells. **Lymphoid tissue** is specialized connective tissue found in tonsils and adenoids. A **mucous** membrane lines many cavities, and it arises from an embryonic mucosal tissue. This membrane includes an epithelial lining (that may have mucosal glands that secrete mucus), loose connective tissue (referred to as the lamina propria), and a thin layer of muscle, which may help move material within the cavity. **Mucus** is a secretion by specialized cells that derive from epithelium.

Fibrous tissue binds structures together and may contain combinations of fiber types. **White fibrous tissue** is strong, dense, and highly organized. It is found in ligaments that bind bones together, as well as in the fascia that encases muscle, as will be described shortly. **Yellow elastic** tissue is found where connective tissue must return to its original shape after being distended, such as in the cartilage of the trachea or bronchial passageway. **Collagenous** and **reticular fibers** provide a flexible structure to fibrous connective tissue, while **elastic fibers** provide recoil to this tissue where needed.

Cartilage is a particularly important tissue because it has unique properties of strength and elasticity. The **tensile strength** of cartilage keeps the fibers from being easily separated when pulled, while the **compressive strength** lets it retain its form by being resistant to crushing, compressing forces. **Hyaline cartilage** is smooth and has a glassy, blue cast. It provides a smooth mating surface for the articulating surfaces of bones, as in the cartilaginous portion of the rib cage, constituting the larynx, trachea, and bronchial passageway. **Fibrocartilage** contains collagenous fibers, providing the cushion between the vertebrae of the spinal column, as well as the mating surface for the temporomandibular joint between the lower jaw and the skull. Fibrocartilage acts as a shock absorber and provides a relatively smooth surface for gliding. **Yellow (elastic) cartilage**

---

matrix: a material that holds or constrains another material. Intercellular material

tissue: L., texere, to weave

interstitial: L., interstitium, space or gap in tissue

fibrous tissue: tissue that binds structures together and that may contain combinations of fiber types

White fibrous tissue: connective tissue that is strong and dense, providing the means for binding structures of the body

collagenous fibers: connective fibers containing collagen

reticular fibers: extremely fine connective fibers

elastic fibers: connective fiber that returns to its original shape after being deformed

fibrocartilage: connective tissue fibers that contain collagen, providing a cushioning for structures

Yellow (elastic) cartilage: cartilaginous connective tissue that has reduced collagen and increased numbers of elastic fibers. See yellow cartilage

has less collagen, endowed rather with elastic fibers. It is found in the structure of the outer ear (pinna), nose, and the epiglottis, a cartilage of the larynx.

You might be surprised to know that **blood** is connective tissue. The fluid component of blood is called plasma, and blood cells (including red and white corpuscles) are suspended in this matrix. The blood cells arise from within the marrow of another type of connective tissue, bone.

Bone is the hardest of the connective tissues. The characteristic hardness of bone is a direct function of the inorganic salts that make up a large portion of bone. Bone is generally classified as being compact or spongy. **Compact bone** is characterized microscopically by its lamellar or sheet-like structure, whereas **spongy bone** looks porous. Spongy bone contains the marrow that produces red and white blood cells as well as the blood plasma matrix.

The protective function of connective tissue is played out by several different classes of cells. **Fibroblasts** are responsible for production of the extracellular matrix, so are able to synthesize and secrete protein. Another important function of fibroblasts is wound repair: Fibroblasts infiltrate a wound site and lay down a matrix, which becomes infiltrated with vascular supply to become granulations. In this manner, the wound area is closed and sealed, and blood supply is restored to the wound region. The matrix will ultimately contract as a result of contractile properties of the fibroblast, at least partially closing the wound area.

Macrophages are another very important class of "healing" connective tissue. They are responsible for the collection of waste or necrotic (dead) tissue. Macrophages engulf bacteria and dead tissue, and digest them by secreting soluble proteins. The process of digestion and removal of dead tissue is a critical stage preceding regeneration of tissue. We will return to this topic when we discuss tissue regeneration within the nervous system.

Two other important protective cells types include lymphocytes and mast cells. B-lymphocytes arise from bone marrow and are stimulated to proliferate within lymph tissue by the presence of foreign matter. They ultimately generate and secrete antibodies to defend against the viral attack. T-lymphocytes also arise from bone marrow but end up in the thymus. Their proliferation is stimulated by viruses, and their job is to seek and destroy viral agents. Mast cells are found in loose connective tissues and some organs. They provide the "first response" to irritation, namely inflammation. Apparently the inflammation of connective tissues promotes migration of other cells to the damaged site for protective purposes. This protective function can go awry, as seen in anaphylactic shock, which is a runaway hypersensitive inflammatory reaction.

Muscle Tissue

Muscle is specialized contractile tissue, unlike any other tissue of the body. Although the connective tissues discussed previously have important supportive roles, muscle fibers are capable of being stimulated to contract.

blood: connective tissue comprised of plasma and blood cells suspended in this plasma matrix

bone: the hardest of the connective tissues

compact bone: bone characterized microscopically by its lamellar or sheet-like structure

spongy bone: bone that appears porous, and contains marrow that produces red and white blood cells

fibroblast: L., fibra, fibrous + Gr., blastos, germ; tissue element able to synthesize and secrete protein

Muscle function is described in Chapter 12.

striated: L., stria, striped; streaked

smooth muscle: muscle that is found in the viscera, including digestive tract and blood vessels

cardiac muscle: muscle of the heart, composed of cells that interconnect in a net-like fashion

autonomic: Gr., autos, self + nomos, law; self-regulating

Muscle is generally classified as being striated, smooth, or cardiac (see Figure 1-2). **Striated** muscle is so called because of its striped appearance on microscopic examination. Striated muscle is known as **skeletal muscle** as well, because it is the muscle used to move skeletal structures. Likewise, it is known as **voluntary** or **somatic muscle**, because it can be moved in response to conscious, voluntary processes. This is in contrast to **smooth muscle**, which includes the muscular tissue of the digestive tract and blood vessels. Smooth muscle is generally sheet-like, with spindle-shaped cells. **Cardiac muscle** is composed of cells that interconnect in a net-like fashion. Smooth and cardiac muscle are generally outside of voluntary control, relegated to the **autonomic** or involuntary nervous system, which will be discussed in Chapter 12.

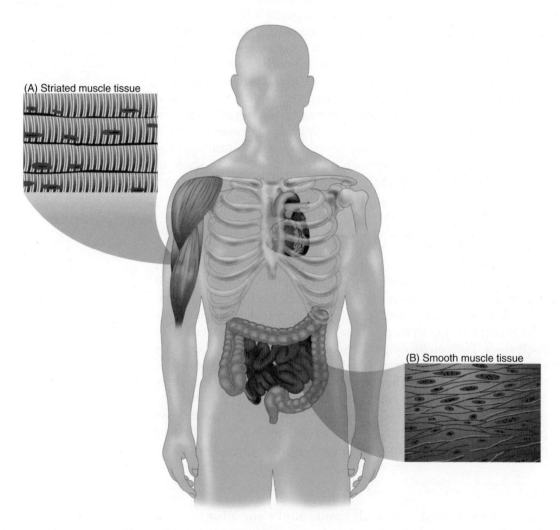

(A) Striated muscle tissue

(B) Smooth muscle tissue

Figure 1-2. Striated (A) and smooth muscle (B).
© Cengage Learning®.

Nervous Tissue

Nervous tissue is a highly specialized communicative tissue. Nervous tissue consists of **neurons** or nerve cells that take on a variety of forms. The function of nervous tissue is to transmit information from one neuron to another, from neurons to muscles, or from sensory receptors to other neural structures.

✔ *To summarize:*

- Four **basic tissues** constitute the human body: epithelial, connective, muscular, and nervous.
- **Epithelial tissue** includes the surface covering of the body and linings of cavities and passageways. **Mucous membranes** arise from epithelial tissue, and are specialized structures that line cavities, and sometimes secrete mucus.
- **Connective tissue** varies as a function of the intercellular material (matrix) surrounding it.
- **Areolar connective tissue** is loose and thin. **Adipose tissue** is areolar tissue with significant fat deposits.
- White **fibrous connective** and **yellow elastic tissues** are found in ligaments, tendons, and cartilage.
- **Cartilage** has both tensile and compressive strength and is elastic (fibers of cartilage resist being torn apart or crushed, and cartilage tends to return to its original shape upon being deformed).
- **Hyaline cartilage** is smooth, while fibrocartilage provides a collagenous cushion between structures.
- **Yellow cartilage** is highly elastic.
- **Blood** is a fluid connective tissue, whereas **bone** is a highly dense connective tissue.
- **Muscle** is the third type of tissue, consisting of **voluntary** (striated), **involuntary** (smooth), and **cardiac** muscle.
- **Nervous tissue** is specialized for communication.

Tissue Aggregates

The basic body tissues (epithelial, connective, muscular, and nervous) are used to form larger structures. For instance, **organs** are aggregates of tissues with **functional unity**, by which we mean that the tissues of the organ all serve the same general purpose (for example, the heart or the lungs or the tongue). In the same sense, we speak of **muscles** (such as the diaphragm) as being structures made up of muscular tissue, and the muscles must be attached to bone or cartilage in some fashion. Let us examine some of the larger organizational units.

Fascia. As mentioned in the previous section, **fascia** surrounds organs, being a sheet-like membrane that may be either dense or nearly transparent, thin or thick. Striated muscle is surrounded by **perimysium**, fascia sufficiently thick that the muscle cannot be seen clearly through it. It is usually sheet-like and interwoven in structure,

Nervous tissue structure is described in Chapter 11.

nervous tissue: highly specialized communicative tissue consisting of neurons or nerve cells

neurons: nerve cell tissue whose function is to transmit information from one neuron to another, from neurons to muscles, or from sensory receptors to other neural structures

organs: tissue of the body with functional utility

muscle: contractile tissue

fascia: L., band

and does not have the highly organized and compact form that tendons take on. It is the "packing material" around organs, peripheral nerves, and blood vessels, providing some physical isolation and stability.

Ligaments. The term **ligament** refers specifically to "binding" structures of the body together. Visceral ligaments bind organs together or hold structures in place. **Ligaments** must withstand great pressure, as they typically bind bone to bone. To achieve this, the connective tissue fibers course in the same direction, giving ligaments great tensile strength. Most ligaments have little stretch, although some (such as the posterior spinal cord ligaments) are endowed with elastic fibers to permit limited stretching. Ligaments that stretch appear yellow, while inelastic ligaments have a white cast.

Tendons. **Tendons** provide a means of attaching muscle to bone or cartilage (see Figure 1-3). The fibers of tendons are arrayed longitudinally (as opposed to interwoven or matted), giving them a great tensile strength but reduced compressive strength. Because tendon is actually part of the muscle, it always binds muscle to another structure (typically bone), attaching to the connective tissue of that skeletal structure. Tendons tend to have the **morphology** (or form) of the muscles they serve. Compact, tubular muscles tend to have long, thin tendons. Flat muscles, such as the diaphragm, will have flat tendons. The microscopic structure of a tendon makes it quite resistant to damage. Because the collagenous fibers intertwine, the forces placed on the tendon are distributed throughout the entire bundle of fibers. Tendons may stretch up to 10 percent of their length without being injured. They are flexible, so can course around bone as needed. They have a blood supply and a sensory nerve supply.

When a tendon is sheet-like, it is called an **aponeurosis**. Aponeuroses greatly resemble fascia, but are much denser. In addition, an aponeurosis will retain the longitudinal orientation of the connective tissue fibers, whereas a fascia is made up of matted fibers.

viscera: L., body organs

ligaments: connective tissue that binds bone to bone

morphology: Gr., morphe, form + mys, muscle

aponeurosis: Gr., apo, from + neuron, nerve; sheet-like tendon

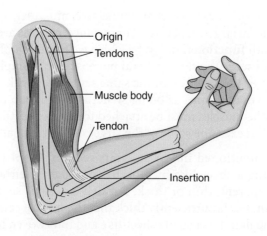

Figure 1-3. Tendon attaching muscle to bone.
© Cengage Learning®.

Osteoporosis

Osteoporosis is a condition wherein bone becomes increasingly porous due to loss of calcium. The reduction in calcium may be the result of aging or may arise from vitamin D deficiency, as in osteomalacia. Loss of calcium may also arise from disuse, as found in individuals confined to bed during illness. Individuals with osteoporosis are particularly susceptible to bone fractures arising from what would be considered normal application of force. The elderly individual who has fallen and broken a hip may actually have broken the hip prior to the fall. An individual with osteoporosis may break ribs while coughing.

Osteoporosis may be localized, as seen in the bones of the skull in Paget's disease (osteitis deformans).

The dense packing of longitudinal fibers makes tendons quite strong. A tendon can withstand pulling of more than 8,000 times the stretching force that a muscle the same diameter can. In fact, the tendon for a given muscle will be able to withstand at least twice the pulling force of the muscle itself. That is to say, a sudden pull on a muscle will damage the muscle itself or the musculo-tendinous junction well before the tendon itself is actually damaged.

Bones. Bones and cartilage have an interesting relationship. Developing bone typically has a portion that is cartilage, and all bone begins as a cartilaginous mass. Many points of **articulation** or joining between bones are comprised of cartilage, because cartilaginous surfaces are smoother and glide across each other more freely than surfaces of bone. Likewise, cartilage will replace bone where elasticity is beneficial. We will see this in the cartilaginous portion of the rib cage (Chapter 2), in the cartilage of the larynx (Chapter 4), and in the nasal cartilages (Chapter 6). As cartilage becomes impregnated with inorganic salts, it begins to harden, ultimately becoming bone.

Bones provide rigid skeletal support and protect organs and soft tissues. Thirty percent of a bone is collagen, providing great tensile strength. The rigidity and compressive strength of bone tissue comes from the even greater proportion of calcium deposited within it. Indeed, bones of the aged become more susceptible to compression as a result of loss of calcium through aging.

Bones are broadly characterized by length (long or short) or shape (flat), or generally as having irregular morphology. The periosteum (fibrous membrane covering of a bone) extends along its entire surface, with the exception of regions endowed with cartilage. This outer periosteum layer is most tightly bound to the bone at the tendinous junctures. Although the outer periosteum layer is tough and fibrous, the inner layer of periosteum contains cells that facilitate bone repair, fibroblasts.

Blood cell production occurs within the cavities of the spongy bone trabeculae (trabeculae are supporting "beams" of a structure).

Cartilage becomes quite important as we discuss the respiratory system (Chapter 2), the phonatory system (Chapter 4), and the articulatory/resonatory system (Chapter 6).

articulation: the point of union between two structures

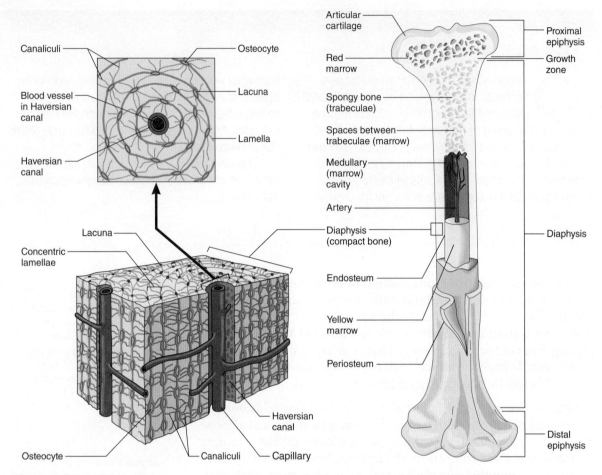

Figure 1-4. Microscopic structure of bone, revealing periosteum, haversian canals, and spongy bone trabeculae.
© Cengage Learning®.

As you can see from Figure 1-4, the cavities within the spongy bone are well protected by the compact bone. Notice the periosteum bound to the compact bone, and the blood supply to the entire bony structure.

Bone growth and development stand as a classic example of "use it or lose it." The density of a bone and its conformation are directly related to the amount of force placed on the bone. Use of muscles actually causes bone to strengthen and become denser in regions stressed by that activity. Males tend to have greater muscle mass than females, and the bones of males often have more readily identifiable landmarks.

Joints. The union of bones with other bones, or cartilage with other cartilage, is achieved by means of **joints** (see Figure 1-5). Joints take a variety of forms. Generally, joints are classified based on the degree of movement they permit: high mobility (**diarthrodial** joints), limited mobility (**amphiarthrodial**), or no mobility (**synarthrodial**) (see Table 1-2). The joints are classified in parallel form based on the primary component involved in the union

diarthrodial: the class of joints of the skeletal system that permits maximum mobility

amphiarthrodial: the class of joints of the skeletal system that permit limited movement

synarthrodial: the class of joints of the skeletal system that permit no movement

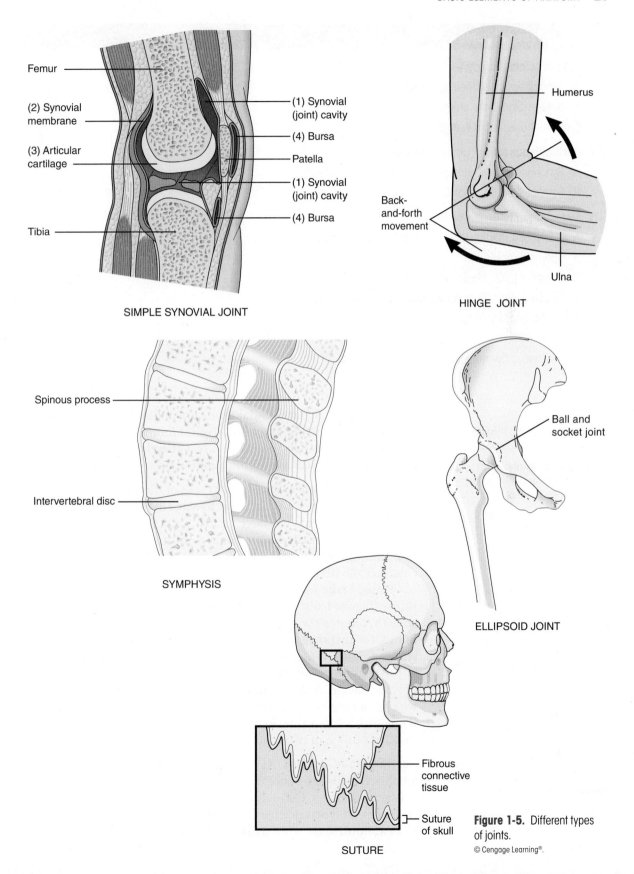

Figure 1-5. Different types of joints.
© Cengage Learning®.

Table 1-2 **Types of joints**

I. **Fibrous joints** (Immobile)

   A. Syndesmosis: Banded by ligament.

   B. Suture: Skull bone union.

   C. Gomphosis: Tooth in alveolus.

II. **Cartilaginous joints** (Limited movement)

   A. Synchondrosis: Cartilage that ossifies through aging.

   B. Symphysis: Bone connected by fibrocartilage.

III. **Synovial joints** (Highly mobile)

   A. Plane joint (gliding joint; arthrodia): Shallow or flat surfaces.

   B. Spheroid (cotyloid).

   C. Condylar joint: Shallow ball-and-socket joints.

   D. Ellipsoid joint: "Football" shaped ball-and-socket joint.

   E. Trochoid joint (pivot).

   F. Sellar joint.

   G. Ginglymus (hinge) joint.

fibrous joints: joints that are connected by fibrous tissue

cartilaginous joints: joints in which cartilage serves to connect two bones

synovial joints: a type of diarthrodial joint that has encapsulated fluid as a cushion

syndesmosis: Gr., syndesmos, ligament + osis, condition

sutures: L., sutura, seam; immobile joints between plates of bone

gomphosis: Gr., bolting together

synchondrosis: Gr., syn, together + chondros, cartilage + osis, condition

between bones. Synarthrodial joints are anatomically classified as **fibrous joints**; while amphiarthrodial joints are **cartilaginous joints**; and diarthrodial joints are **synovial joints**, or joints containing synovial fluid within a joint space.

Fibrous Joints. There are two major types of fibrous or synarthrodial joints: syndesmoses and sutures. **Syndesmosis** joints are bound by fibrous ligaments but have little movement. **Sutures** are joints between bones of the skull that are not intended to move at all. The mating surfaces of the bones form a rough and jagged line that enhances the strength of the joint.

    Sutures take several forms (see Figure 1-6). A serrate or dentate suture (Figure 1-6B) gains its strength from the jagged (i.e., serrated) edge that mates the two bones together. This is the type of suture found, for instance, between the two parietal bones. A squamous suture (Figure 1-6C) is one in which the two mating bones actually overlap in a "keying" formation, much like current-day joining of wood sheets. A third suture type is a **gomphosis** (Figure 1-6A), which is a hole-and-peg arrangement. A socket (alveolus) and tooth is one such joint. A final joint, the plane joint (Figure 1-6D), is simply the direct union of two edges of bone.

Cartilaginous Joints. As the name implies, cartilaginous or amphiarthrodial joints are those in which cartilage provides the union between two bones. Considering that bone arises from cartilage during development, it makes sense that in some cases cartilage would persist. In **synchondrosis**, the cartilaginous union is maintained, as in the

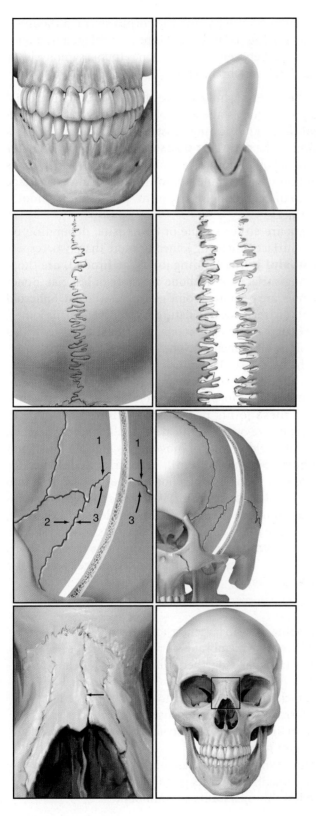

(A) Gomphosis or peg suture

(B) Dentate (serrated) suture

(C) Squamous suture (arrows)

(D) Plane suture (arrow)

Figure 1-6. Sutures are immobile joints between plates of bone. (A) Gomphosis or peg suture, in which a structure such as a tooth is embedded in an alveolus or hole; (B) Dentate (serrated) suture, so called because of the jagged edge; (C) Squamous suture, in which the two plates of bone are "keyed" by means of interlocked, overlapping phalanges; and (D) Plane sutures, which involve simple edge-to-edge union between two bones.

© Cengage Learning®.

junction of the manubrium sterni and the corpus sterni, although it ossifies as the individual ages. The second type of cartilaginous joint is a **symphysis**, as found between the pubic bones (pubic symphysis) or between the disks of the vertebral column.

symphysis: Gr., growing together

Synovial Joints. The distinguishing feature of synovial or diarthrodial joints is that they all include some form of joint cavity within which is found **synovial fluid**, a lubricating substance, and around which is an articular capsule. The **articular capsule** is made up of an outer fibrous membrane of collagenous tissue and ligament to which binds the bone and an inner synovial membrane lining. Hyaline cartilage covers the surface of each bone of the joint, providing a smooth, strong mating surface.

articular capsule: the fibrous connective tissue covering of a synovial joint

Synovial joints are either simple or composite, depending on whether two bone surfaces are being joined or more than two, respectively. **Plane synovial joints** (gliding joints; arthrodial) are those in which the mating surfaces of the bone are more or less flat. Bones joined in this manner are permitted some gliding movement. **Spheroid** (or **cotyloid**) joints are **reciprocal** in nature (as are all but plane joints), in that one member of the union has a convex portion that mates with a concave portion of the other member. The spheroid joint is a ball-and-socket joint, in which a convex ball or head fits into a cup or **cotylica**. This joint permits a wide range of movement, including rotation.

plane synovial joints: joints with mating surfaces that are predominantly flat

cotyloid: Gr., kotyloeides, cup-shaped

Condylar joints are more shallow versions of the ball-and-socket joint, and these joints permit more limited movement. **Ellipsoid joints** capitalize on an elliptical (football-shaped) member. These joints permit a wide range of movements, but obviously not rotation. A **trochoid joint** (**pivot joint**), in contrast, is designed for rotation, and little else. It consists of a bony process protruding into a space. A **saddle joint** (or **sellar joint**) is perhaps the most descriptive of the joint names. One member of the saddle joint is convex, like a saddle, while the other concave member "sits" on the saddle. A **hinge joint** (**ginglymus**) acts like the hinge of a cabinet door: One member rotates on that joint with a limited range, permitting only flexion and extension.

condylar joint: a shallow ball-and-socket joint with limited mobility

trochoid joint (pivot joint): a joint consisting of a process and fossa, permitting only rotation

sellar: L., sella, Turkish saddle

saddle or sellar joint: a ball-and-socket joint in which the concave member rests on an elongated convex member (syn., sellar joint)

hinge joint: a joint that acts like a hinge, permitting only flexion and extension

✔ *To summarize:*

- Tissues combine to form larger structures.
- **Fascia** is a sheet-like membrane surrounding organs.
- **Ligaments** bind organs together or hold bones to bones or cartilage.
- **Tendons** attach muscle to bone or to cartilage; if a tendon is flat, it is referred to as an **aponeurosis**.
- Bones and cartilage provide the structure for the body, articulating by means of joints.
- **Diarthrodial** (synovial) **joints** are highly mobile, **amphiarthrodial** (cartilaginous) **joints** permit limited mobility, and **synarthrodial** (fibrous) **joints** are immobile.

Craniosynostosis

As the infant develops, the sutures of the skull become ossified, a process called **synostosis**. Complete synostosis normally occurs well into childhood, but in some instances synostosis may occur prenatally. Continued normal growth of the brain, especially during the first postnatal year, places pressure on the skull. The effects of premature synostosis or **craniosynostosis** on skull development are quite profound. With **premature sagittal synostosis**, the child's head becomes peaked along the suture and elongated in back. In Apert syndrome, a genetic condition, the affected child's stereotypic "peaked head" is the result of premature closure of the coronal suture, resulting in pronounced bulging along that articulation.

- **Fibrous joints** bind immobile bodies together, **cartilaginous joints** are those in which cartilage serves the primary joining function, and **synovial joints** are those in which lubricating synovial fluid is contained within an articular capsule.
- Among synovial joints are **plane** (gliding) joints, **spheroid**, **condylar**, **trochoid**, **sellar**, and **ellipsoid** joints (all variants of ball-and-socket joints), as well as **hinge** joints.

synostosis: ossification of sutures

craniosynostosis: premature closure of cranial sutures

premature sagittal synostosis: premature closure of sagittal suture

Muscles. The combination of muscle fibers into a cohesive unit is both functionally and anatomically defined. Anatomically, muscles are bound groups of muscle fibers with functional unity. A fascia of connective tissue termed the **epimysium** surrounds the muscles, and the muscles are endowed with a tendon to permit attachment to skeletal structure. Muscles have a nerve supply to provide stimulation of the contracting bundle of tissue; muscles also have a vascular supply to meet their nutrient needs. Muscle morphology or form varies widely, depending on function. Fibers of wide, flat muscles tend to radiate from a broad point of origination to a more focused insertion. More cylindrical muscles will have unitary points of attachment on either end. In all cases, the orientation of the muscle fibers defines the region on which force will be applied, because muscle fiber can only actively shorten.

epimysium: Gr., epi, upon; over + mys, muscle

A muscle can contract to approximately one-third its original length, and thus long muscles can contract greater distances than short muscles. The diameter of a muscle is directly related to its strength, because that represents the number of muscle fibers allocated to perform the task.

The work performed by the body is widely varied between extremes of muscular effort (very little to great amounts) and extremes of muscle rate of contraction (very rapid to slow and sustained). Although muscle morphology accounts for much of the variation in function, the physical relationship between muscle and bone provides a great deal of flexibility in muscle use.

See Chapter 12 for a discussion of neuromuscular function.

Muscles can exert force only by shortening the distance between two points and can contract only in a straight line (with the exception of sphincteric muscles). By convention, the point of attachment of the least mobile element is termed the **origin**, and the point of attachment that moves as a result of muscle contraction is termed the **insertion**. When referring to limbs, the insertion point is more distant from the body. Muscles that move a structure are referred to as **agonists** or **prime movers**, whereas those that oppose a given movement are called **antagonists**. Thus, an agonist for one movement may become an antagonist for the opposite movement. Muscles that stabilize structures are termed **synergists** or **fixators**. For example, in the middle ear, when the stapedius muscle contracts it pulls the stapes posteriorly, so that it inhibits movement of the footplate in the oval window. When the tensor tympani of the middle ear contracts it pulls the malleus anteromedially, reducing the movement of the malleus and, subsequently, the movement of the tympanic membrane in response to sound. In this sense, these two muscles are antagonistic to each other (the stapedius works to oppose the action of the tensor tympani). In another sense, these two muscles work together, since co-contraction causes the ossicular chain to stiffen or become relatively less mobile, reducing sound conduction to the inner ear. Thus, acting together these muscles work synergistically to stabilize the ossicular chain, reducing the impact of loud noise.

Another, more direct example of the fixative function is the interaction of the genioglossus and intrinsic muscles of the tongue. The genioglossus is a large muscle of the tongue that moves the tongue into its gross position, but the intrinsic muscles of the tongue do the job of making fine movements. In this sense, the genioglossus is responsible for stabilizing the tongue so that the fine gestures associated with articulation can be accomplished.

Muscle action that does not result in movement of a structure is termed **isometric**. Agonists and antagonists often co-contract, providing a **fixator** function that stabilizes a structure. This is a critically important component of motor control. We need to make another very important point here, specifically related to speech and hearing. As we mentioned earlier, humans have done a marvelous job of getting double duty from systems. For instance, the larynx is responsible for protecting the airway from foreign matter, but we use it for voice production. When we discuss origins and insertions of muscles, we define those as the *functional* origins and insertions. We will differ from with classical anatomical texts in some cases, because *our* speech-based piggybacked function differs from the *stated* classic or primary functions for a few of the muscles. For instance, contraction of the pectoralis major adducts the humerus and with it the shoulder, so for its primary (classical) function the origin is at the sternum, and the insertion is the greater tubercle of the humerus. The pectoralis major is also a muscle of respiration, in which case its job is to expand the rib cage. When we use pectoralis to help us expand the chest cavity and inhale, the origin is the humerus, while the insertion is

agonist: muscle contracted for purpose of a specific motor act (as contrasted to the antagonist)

prime mover: agonist. this is the muscle responsible for the primary or desired movement

antagonist: a muscle that opposes the contraction of another muscle (the agonist)

fixators: muscles that stabilize structures through contraction

isometric: muscle action that does not result in movement

fixator: muscle responsible for stabilizing a structure

Neuromuscular Diseases

A host of neuromuscular conditions prey on the muscular system and the nerve components that supply it. Amyotrophic lateral sclerosis is a condition in which the motor neuron is destroyed, resulting in loss of muscle function. Myelin destruction occurs in multiple sclerosis, with manifestation of the disease varying by site of lesion. Myasthenia gravis is a condition in which the nerve–muscle junction is compromised as a result of an immune system response. The result is weakness and loss of muscle range due to inability of the nerve and muscle to communicate.

the sternum (the humerus is holding still and the sternum is moving). We will remind you of this again later, but recognize that we are using the functional definition of origin and insertion as related to speech function. As you can see in Figure 1-7, the points of muscle attachment have a great deal to do with how much force can be exerted by muscle contraction to achieve work. A muscle attached closer to a joint will move the bone farther and faster than the one attached farther from the joint. In contrast, the muscle farther from the joint will be able to exert more force through its range, because of the leverage advantage. Thus, the more distally placed muscle will have an advantage for lifting, while the muscle closer to the joint will provide greater range to the bone to which it is attached.

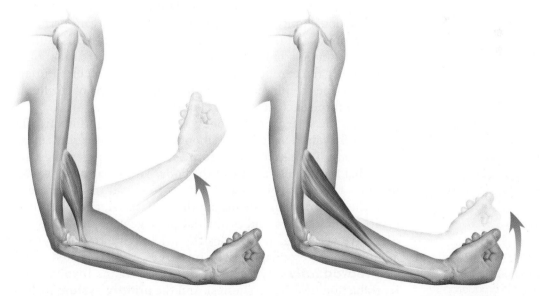

Figure 1-7. Mechanical advantage derived from point of insertion. On the left, the muscle inserts closer to the point of rotation and the movable point will undergo a greater excursion on contraction of the muscle. On the right, the muscle is attached a greater distance from the point of rotation so that the bone will move a smaller distance, but the muscle is capable of exerting greater force in the direction of movement.

© Cengage Learning®.

innervation: stimulation of a muscle, gland or structure by means of a nerve

afferent: L., ad, to + ferre, carry

efferent: L., ex, from + ferre, carry

Muscles are **innervated** or supplied by a single nerve. **Innervation** refers to the process of stimulating a muscle or gland, or receiving output from a body sensor. Innervation can be sensory (generally termed **afferent**) or excitatory (**efferent**) in nature. A **motor unit** consists of one efferent nerve fiber and the muscle fibers to which it attaches. Every muscle fiber will be innervated. In addition, muscles have sensory components providing information to the central nervous system concerning the state of the muscle.

✔ *To summarize:*

- **Muscle** is contractile tissue, with muscle bundles capable of shortening to about half their length.
- The point of attachment with the least movement is termed the **origin**, while the **insertion** is the point of attachment of relative mobility.
- Muscles that move a structure are **agonists** and those that oppose movement are called **antagonists**.
- Muscles that stabilize structures are termed **synergists** or **fixators**.
- Muscles are innervated by a single nerve.
- A **motor unit** is the efferent nerve fiber and muscle fibers it innervates.

BODY SYSTEMS

system: a functionally defined group of organs

muscular system: the anatomical system that includes smooth, striated, and cardiac muscle

skeletal system: the anatomical system that includes the bones and cartilages that make up the body

respiratory system: the physical system involved in respiration, including the lungs, bronchial passageway, trachea, larynx, pharynx, oral cavity, and nasal cavity

reproductive system: the system of the body involved in reproduction

urinary system: they body system including kidneys, ureters, bladder and urethra

endocrine system: the system involved in production and dissemination of hormones

nervous system: the system of nervous tissue, comprising the central and peripheral nervous systems

In the same way that tissues combine to form organs, organs combine to form functional systems. **Systems** of the body are groups of organs with functional unity. That is, the combination of organs performs a basic function, and failure or deficiency of an organ will result in a change in function of the system. Because systems are functionally defined, organs can belong to more than one system. Similarly, we can define the physical communication systems of the human organism through combinations of organs.

The basic systems of the body are fairly straightforward. The **muscular system** includes the smooth, striated, and cardiac muscle of the body. The **skeletal system** includes the bones and cartilages that form the structure of the body. The **respiratory system** includes the passageways and tissues involved in gas exchange with the environment, including the oral, nasal, and pharyngeal cavities; the trachea and bronchial passageway; and lungs. The **digestive system** also includes the oral cavity and pharynx, in addition to the esophagus, liver, intestines, and associated glands. The **reproductive system** includes the organs involved with reproduction (ovaries and testes), and the **urinary system** includes the kidneys, ureters, bladder, and urethra. The **endocrine system** involves production and dissemination of hormones, so it includes glands, such as the thyroid gland, testes, and ovaries. The **nervous system** includes the nerve tissue and structures of the central and peripheral nervous systems that are responsible for muscle control and sensory function.

Systems of Speech

Speech is an extraordinarily complex process that capitalizes on these systems. The functionally defined systems of speech combine organs and structures in a unique fashion.

Our definition of systems of speech is truly a convenience. None of the systems operates in isolation. Speech requires the integrated action of all of the systems, and the level of coordination involved in this task is complicated (see Figure 1-8).

A classical categorization of the systems of speech includes respiratory, phonatory, articulatory, resonatory, and nervous systems. The respiratory system is a precise match with the anatomical respiratory system, including the respiratory passageway, lungs, trachea, and so forth. The **phonatory system** is involved in the production of voiced sound and utilizes a significant protective component of the respiratory system (the larynx). The **articulatory system** is the combination of structures that are used to alter the characteristics of the sounds of speech, including parts of the anatomically defined digestive and respiratory systems (the tongue, lips, teeth, soft palate, etc.). The **resonatory system** includes the nasal cavity and soft palate and portions of the anatomically defined respiratory and digestive systems. Although some speech scientists view the resonatory system as separate from the articulatory system, we take an alternate view in this text, combining them into the articulatory/resonatory

The logic of combining the articulatory and resonatory systems will become clear in Chapter 6.

phonatory system: the system including the laryngeal structures through which phonation is achieved

articulatory system: in speech science, the system of structures involved in shaping the oral cavity for production of the sounds of speech

resonatory system: the portion of the vocal tract through which the acoustical product of vocal fold vibration resonates (usually the oral, pharyngeal, and nasal cavities combined; sometimes referring only to the nasal cavities and nasopharynx)

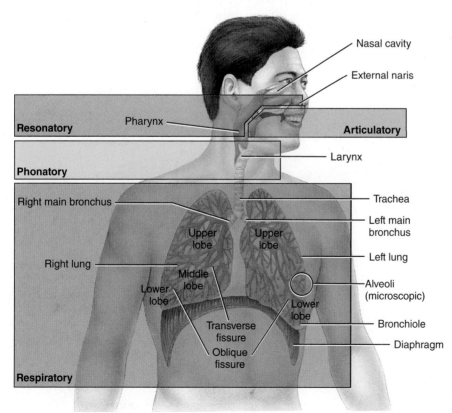

Figure 1-8. Relationship of anatomical systems and overlaid speech systems.
© Cengage Learning®.

system of speech production. The nervous system used for sensation and control of the body is the same one used for the control of speech structures, but with some special twists. Speech, language, and hearing related to speech and language have developed as very special systems in humans, as you will see in the chapters on neuroantomy and neurophysiology. Because the nervous system is a thread woven throughout all of our discussions of anatomy and physiology, we want to spend a little more time on the nervous system before we dive into anatomy for speech and hearing.

The Nervous System

The nervous system is the most complex of the systems of the body. The nervous system is broken into two major components: the **central nervous system** (CNS) and **peripheral nervous system** (PNS) (see Figure 1-9). The CNS is comprised of some large and major structures, including the cerebral cortex, the cerebellum, thalamus, basal ganglia, brain stem, and spinal cord. You'll notice that all of these are encased in bone. The PNS, in contrast, serves the peripheral body: Nerves leave the brain stem or spinal cord to activate muscles of the head or body, and sensations from these "peripheral" regions are translated to the CNS by means of these peripheral nerves as well. We will return to these shortly, because there are some peripheral nerves that will come up in the next chapter.

Together the CNS and PNS provide the means by which we can receive and process information, perceive and make sense of that information, and then act on that information. Let's talk in broad terms about how these systems operate so that you will have some context for muscle and sensory function.

central nervous system: portion of the nervous system comprised of the cerebral cortex, the cerebellum, thalamus, basal ganglia, brain stem, and spinal cord

peripheral nervous system: portion of the nervous system serving the peripheral body

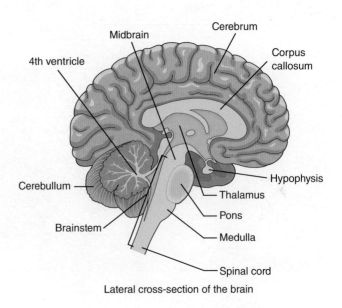

Figure 1-9. Schematic showing basic elements of the central and peripheral nervous system.
© Cengage Learning®.

Lateral cross-section of the brain

Building Blocks of the Nervous System

Both the PNS and CNS are composed of neurons or nerve cells. Neurons are specialized tissues that are responsible for communicating information between the environment and the brain, for communicating among the components of the nervous system, and for activating glands and muscles. The processes of receiving or sensing information are termed sensory or afferent processes, and the processes of activating muscles and glands are called motor or efferent processes. We refer to sensory pathways as afferent pathways, and motor pathways as efferent pathways. Both of these broad neurophysiological processes are the product of interactions among neurons, so let us look at some of the basic parts so they make sense in the following chapters.

A neuron is made up of three basic components: the dendrite, soma, and axon (Figure 1-10). The dendrite or dendritic tree is the input side of a neuron. Information, such as touch sensation, is received by the dendrite. The soma is the cell body of the neuron, and it houses many organelles

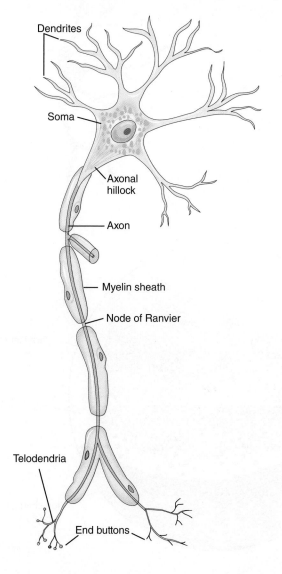

Figure 1-10. Schematic of basic elements of a neuron.
© Cengage Learning®.

or components that are essential for the function and maintenance of the neuron. The axon is the point at which information leaves the neuron.

If the information at the dendrite is sufficiently robust or "loud" enough to cause the neuron to be excited, an impulse will travel from the dendrite, through the soma, and to the axon. At the axon, an action potential is generated that will cause a wave of depolarization down the axon to its end, the end *bouton*. Depolarization is the process whereby the membranous surface of the axon opens up to allow passage of ions that, in turn communicate information toward the end of the axon, an area known as the *end bouton* (or "end button"). End boutons have small sacs or vesicles filled with neurotransmitter (Figure 1-11), and the

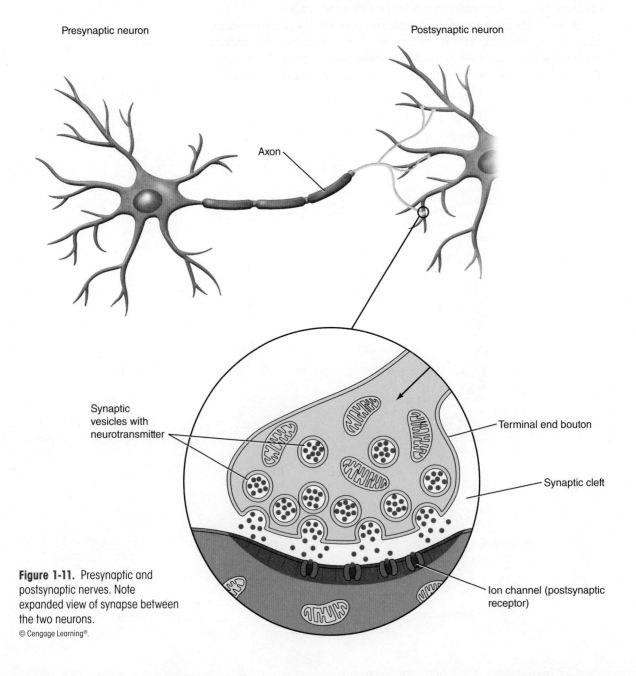

Presynaptic neuron

Postsynaptic neuron

Axon

Synaptic vesicles with neurotransmitter

Terminal end bouton

Synaptic cleft

Ion channel (postsynaptic receptor)

Figure 1-11. Presynaptic and postsynaptic nerves. Note expanded view of synapse between the two neurons.
© Cengage Learning®.

wave of depolarization passing through the axon causes these vesicles to migrate into the space between the axon of the first neuron and the next neuron, known as the synaptic cleft or synapse. Axons are frequently covered in myelin, a fatty sheathe that insulates the axon and speeds up transmission through the axon.

In this way, information is passed from neuron to neuron, or from neuron to muscle. In the case of muscle activation, an impulse arising, for instance, from the cerebral cortex will pass through a chain of neurons and synapses to a terminal point in the spinal cord (Figure 1-12). If my goal is to move a muscle in my body such as to flex my toe, a specific peripheral nerve will be activated. In this case, a *spinal nerve* will be activated, because nerves arising from the spinal cord activate the muscles of my toes. For us in speech and hearing the peripheral nerves that arise from the brain stem are critically important: These are called the **cranial nerves**, because they arise from the cranium or skull. Let us spend a few minutes talking about cranial nerves,

cranial nerves: peripheral nervous system components arising from the brain stem that innervate primarily the structures associated with speech and hearing

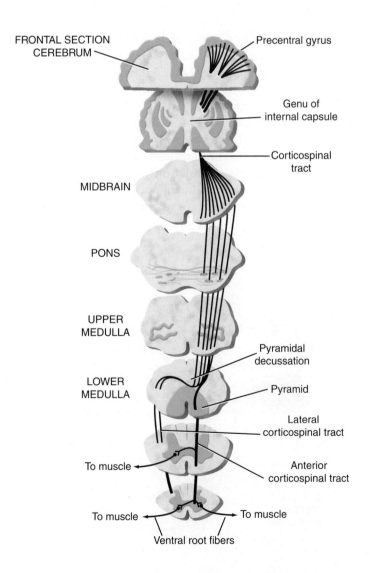

Figure 1-12. Corticospinal pathway, carrying impulses from cerebral cortex to spinal cord for motor activation via spinal nerves.

© Cengage Learning®.

because they are going to come up again and again in our discussion of anatomy and physiology.

Cranial nerves. Cranial nerves are those peripheral nerve components of the PNS that arise from the brainstem. They have the same basic properties of spinal nerves, in that the motor (efferent) nerves receive their orders from the **cerebral cortex** or other higher brain structures (such as the basal ganglia). Likewise, sensory cranial nerves will convey their information from the periphery (for instance, the sensation of a fly walking on your forehead) to the central nervous system so that the CNS can decide what to do about it (such as shooing the fly away). So, in that way cranial nerves and spinal nerves share a great deal of responsibility, with cranial nerves serving the area of the head and neck, and spinal nerves serving the rest of the body. Another shared feature between these two is the presence of simple and complex reflexes. Reflexes are the "rapid response team" of the nervous system. If you touch a hot pan, you will reflexively pull your hand away well before your cerebral cortex even knew anything had happened. Reflexes are protective circuits that we have evolved, often designed to get us out of harm's way. The basic reflex circuit is embodied in the spinal reflex arc. If you take a look at Figure 1-13, you will see that the tap of a hammer on the patellar tendon region causes a tendon to stretch, sending a signal to the spinal cord, which in turn causes a muscle to shorten in response. This type of circuit does not rely on the cerebral cortex to operate, and in fact can function in the case of spinal cord injury that separates the cortex from the area below the injury.

Cranial nerves may also have reflexes. In this case, the reflexes govern head- and neck-related functions, such as stretching of the muscles of the jaw, chewing, swallowing, heart rate deceleration, and breathing. Notice that these reflexes we just mentioned seem pretty

cerebral cortex: the highest integrating system of the nervous system, responsible for conscious thought and voluntary action

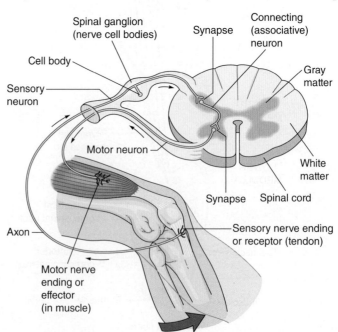

Figure 1-13. Spinal arc reflex.
© Cengage Learning®.

important, since we all need to keep breathing. The reflexes mediated by cranial nerves tend to be more complex than spinal reflexes, so the stakes are much higher when we have damage to the **brain stem** area from which cranial nerves arise. This damage usually comes in the form of a stroke (cerebrovascular accident), and those of you choosing to be speech-language pathologist will be very much involved in rehabilitation of a person with this kind of a problem.

What follows is a brief discussion of cranial nerves so that you are familiar with them as you delve into anatomy and physiology. Please realize that some cranial nerves have multiple functions: Some will be only sensory, some will be only motor, and some will be mixed sensory and motor. Some will serve not only skeletal muscle but also smooth muscle, and some of the sensations mediated by cranial nerves would not even reach consciousness. We'll cover the cranial nerves in more depth in the chapters on neuroanatomy and neurophysiology. We use the convention here of giving number and name of the cranial nerve, and we always use the Roman numerals (see Figure 1-14). We have found that if we always refer to the cranial nerve by name and number we will always have those two mentally linked. Pay particular attention to cranial nerves I olfactory, V trigeminal, VII facial, VIII vestibulocochlear, IX glossopharyngeal, X vagus, XI accessory, and XII hypoglossal. These are all important to speech and hearing function.

> **brain stem:** the subcortical region including the medulla, pons, and midbrain

   I. Olfactory nerve: This afferent cranial nerve mediates the sense of smell through sensors within the mucous membrane of the nasal cavity. It is only sensory in nature. This is an important cranial nerve related to eating and swallowing, as damage to it can affect our taste perception.
  II. Ophthalmic nerve: This afferent cranial nerves mediates the special sense of vision.
 III. Occulomotor nerve: This efferent cranial nerve mediates most of the movement of the eyeball. It also is responsible for accommodation to light.
  IV. Trochlear nerve: This efferent cranial nerve is responsible for moving the eyeball down.
   V. Trigeminal nerve: This is an important mixed cranial nerve that mediates the sense of touch for the face (sensory) and controls many of the muscles of chewing (mastication). It is divided into three branches: the V trigeminal ophthalmic branch, V trigeminal maxillary branch, and V trigeminal mandibular branch. The ophthalmic branch mediates the sense of touch for the upper face, including forehead, front of scalp, upper eyelid, and iris. The maxillary branch sends information about sensation from the lower eyelid, nose, palate, upper teeth and upper jaw (maxilla) region. The maxillary branch has a double function: The sensory component mediates sensory information for the lower teeth and jaw (mandible), cheeks, and touch sense for the anterior 2/3 of tongue; the motor component controls contraction of the muscles of mastication, one muscle of the soft palate, and one of the tiny muscles in the middle ear.

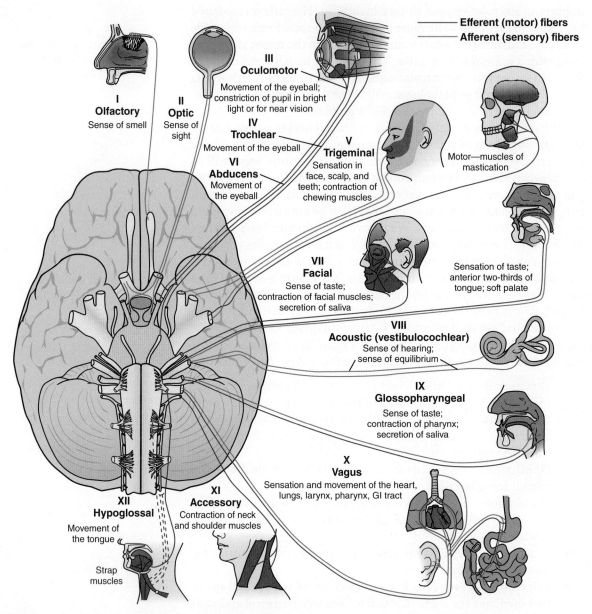

Efferent (motor) fibers
Afferent (sensory) fibers

I
Olfactory
Sense of smell

II
Optic
Sense of sight

III
Oculomotor
Movement of the eyeball; constriction of pupil in bright light or for near vision

IV
Trochlear
Movement of the eyeball

VI
Abducens
Movement of the eyeball

V
Trigeminal
Sensation in face, scalp, and teeth; contraction of chewing muscles

Motor—muscles of mastication

VII
Facial
Sense of taste; contraction of facial muscles; secretion of saliva

Sensation of taste; anterior two-thirds of tongue; soft palate

VIII
Acoustic (vestibulocochlear)
Sense of hearing; sense of equilibrium

IX
Glossopharyngeal
Sense of taste; contraction of pharynx; secretion of saliva

X
Vagus
Sensation and movement of the heart, lungs, larynx, pharynx, GI tract

XII
Hypoglossal
Movement of the tongue

Strap muscles

XI
Accessory
Contraction of neck and shoulder muscles

Figure 1-14. Brainstem and cranial nerves serving the head and neck.
© Cengage Learning®.

VI. Abducens: This motor nerve is responsible for abduction of the eyeball.

VII. Facial nerve: This mixed nerve provides motor activation of the muscles of the face and the lacrimal (tearing), sublingual and submandibular (salivary) glands. The sensory component includes body sense of the ear canal and skin of the outer ear, as well as taste for the anterior 2/3 of the tongue.

VIII. Vestibulocochlear nerve: This sensory nerve is often called the auditory nerve because it mediates the sense of sound from the cochlea to the brain stem. It also transmits information from the vestibular mechanism of the inner ear, which is critical for balance and movement.

IX. Glossopharyngeal nerve: This is a mixed motor/sensory nerve, responsible for many important functions. The sensory component mediates sense of taste and body sense for the posterior 1/3 of the tongue and upper airway region (upper pharynx), as well as body sense for the ear (in conjunction with the VII facial). It also mediates the sensation associated with initiating the swallow, gag, and vomit reflexes. The motor component is responsible for helping to constrict the upper airway (pharynx) for swallowing, as well as for elevation of the pharynx.

X. Vagus nerve: This mixed nerve has various functions, but we will just mention a few here. There are two main branches of concern for us right now. The X vagus recurrent laryngeal nerve (RLN) controls almost all of the musculature of the larynx, so it is responsible for protection of the airway. The X vagus superior laryngeal nerve controls the muscles associated with pitch changing in voice. The sensory components of the X vagus provide body sensation for the pharynx, larynx, trachea, esophagus, thorax, and abdomen. There are even taste sensors in the entry to the larynx that are innervated by the X vagus.

XI. Accessory nerve: This efferent nerve joins with the X vagus to serve the intrinsic muscles of the larynx, as well as innervating two muscles associated with respiration.

XII. Hypoglossal nerve: This efferent nerve is responsible for controlling all of the muscles of the tongue. As you can probably guess, it's highly important for articulation.

Cerebral Cortex and Subcortical Structures

The cerebral cortex is by far the most complex structure of the nervous system. It is responsible for all conscious thought and voluntary action. It is the seat of cognitive function and is responsible for making sense of the world we live in. It is composed of two hemispheres (left and right), with five lobes in each hemisphere (Figure 1-15). Because of the construction of the pathways to and from the cortex, the left hemisphere governs motor activity on the right side of the body, while the right hemisphere governs the left. Likewise, sensations from the right body are sent to the left hemisphere (fortunately, there is a structure—the corpus callosum—that guarantees the right side knows what the left side knows).

Frontal lobe. This lobe is responsible for cognition, which is how we make sense of the world. It is also responsible for initiation of all voluntary motor activity, through activation of the motor strip (precentral gyrus). Immediately anterior to the motor strip is the premotor region, responsible for motor planning. A very important cortical structure within the dominant hemisphere for speech and language is the area known as **Broca's area**, which is responsible for the expression of language (i.e., spoken language).

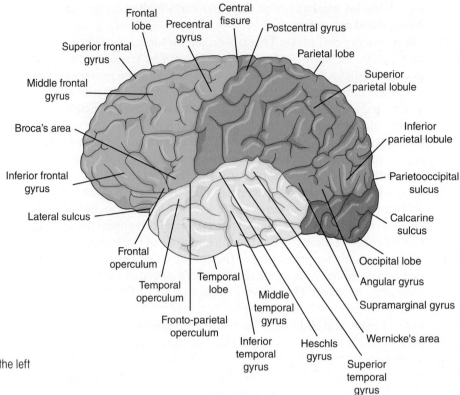

Figure 1-15. Landmarks of the left cerebral hemisphere.
© Cengage Learning®.

Parietal lobe. This lobe is responsible for processing body (somatic) sense. Body sense includes the sense of touch, vibration, pressure, pain, and temperature sense, but not the special senses of hearing, smell, vision, and speech. Information arriving in the parietal lobe is used by the frontal lobe to plan the motor act as well as to identify the environment in which cognition functions (i.e., if you have a significant pain, you'll direct your cognitive functions to figuring out how to stop it). The parietal lobe is also an area of integration with other areas, particularly with vision. Damage to the parietal lobe can result in dressing apraxia, a problem in which a person cannot organize their motor plan to put clothes on his or her body.

Occipital lobe. This lobe has the responsibility for receiving and processing visual information. It projects its output to many different areas, including the parietal and temporal lobes.

Temporal lobe. This is a very important lobe for those of us in speech and hearing. This lobe receives the auditory input that arose from the cochlea. The left temporal lobe also houses the very important language zone, Wernicke's area. Wernicke's area is responsible for auditory comprehension, particularly of language, and damage to this area can result in a severe form of receptive language deficit, receptive (Wernicke's) aphasia. The temporal lobe also houses the hippocampus, which is responsible for mediating short-term memory.

Insular lobe. This lobe is hidden from view, residing beneath Broca's area of the frontal lobe. The left insular lobe is critically important for planning and organization of speech output: Damage to the left insular lobe will result in apraxia of speech, which is a difficulty planning the speech act. The insular cortex has many other functions as well, including mediating the sense of taste (gustation) and a sense of self.

Cerebellum

The cerebellum is the second largest structure of the nervous system. It is situated beneath the cerebral cortex and behind the brain stem. It is responsible for integrating all body sense with the motor plan so that what we do (motor act) is planned appropriately for the context of our body condition. That is to say, picking up a glass from the floor while standing is a completely different task from picking up the same glass while lying on the floor, so the motor plan needs to take all body conditions into consideration. The cerebellum is the great coordinator for motor activity.

Brain Stem

The brain stem is divided into three regions: the medulla oblongata (medulla), pons, and midbrain. The medulla houses many cranial nerve nuclei and other nuclei that are critical for life function. The pons is a major communication bridge (*pons* is Latin for "bridge") among the spinal cord, vestibular mechanism, brain stem, cerebral cortex, and cerebellum. The midbrain has cranial nerve nuclei and is also the recipient of the motor pathway as the fibers exit the cortex to enter the brain stem.

Subcortical structures. Beneath the cortex are a group of nuclei that are very important for sensory and motor function. The basal ganglia are responsible for repetitive movement, muscle tone control, and control of background movement (such as arm swing when walking). The thalamus is the last way station for sensory information that will go to the cortex. The subthalamus works with the basal ganglia for motor control.

Neural processes. As you can guess, this is a very complex system: The cerebral cortex alone contains between 20 and 25 billion neurons, and each neuron has at least 1,000 connections with other neurons. It is the interaction of the neurons with each other that translates into functional subsystems that are responsible for processing the continually varying information sent to the brain and making sense of that information.

✔ *To summarize:*

- Organs combine to form **functional systems**, including the system concerned with muscles (**muscular system**), with the framework of the body (**skeletal system**), breathing (**respiratory system**), digestion (**digestive system**), reproduction (**reproductive system**), the **urinary** and **endocrine systems**, and **nervous system**.

- Within the discipline of speech pathology, we have functionally defined four systems.

- The **respiratory system** is concerned with respiration, the **phonatory system** is made up of the components of the respiratory and digestive systems associated with production of voiced sounds (the larynx), the **articulatory/resonatory system** (including the structures of the face, mouth, and nose), and the **nervous system** (related to central nervous system's control of speech process).

- The nervous system is broken into the peripheral nervous system (PNS) and central nervous system (CNS). The basic unit of the nervous system is the neuron, which is responsible for communication within the nervous system. Glial cells support neuron function and are responsible for development of myelin, which greatly reduced conduction time in the nervous system.

- The PNS is made up of cranial and spinal nerves, with cranial nerves being the most critical part of the PNS for speech and hearing.

- Cranial nerves include the I olfactory that is responsible for the sense of smell, II ophthalmic, which mediates vision. The III oculomotor, IV trochlear, and VI abducens serve eye movement. The V trigeminal innervates muscles of mastication, some muscles of the soft palate, and a muscle of the middle ear. The VII facial nerve innervates muscles of facial expression, as well as the sense of taste for a portion of the tongue. The VIII vestibulocochlear nerve is responsible for hearing and balance, and the IX glossopharyngeal is involved in both sensory and motor function related to swallowing. The X vagus innervates a number of motor systems, including laryngeal musculature. The XI accessory functions largely as a support system for IX and X. The XII hypoglossal nerve innervates the tongue muscles.

- The CNS is made up of larger neural structures, including the cerebral cortex, brain stem, cerebellum, spinal cord, and other subcortical structures.

- The cerebral cortex is responsible for conscious and voluntary function, while the cerebellum coordinates sensory and motor plans. The brain stem mediates many life functions, as well as serving as the origination for cranial nerves. The thalamus is the last way-station for sensation from the body, while the basal ganglia control muscle tone and some stereotyped movements.

CHAPTER SUMMARY

Anatomy and physiology are the study of structure and function of an organism, respectively. Subspecializations of anatomy interact to provide the detail required for understanding the anatomy and physiology of speech. Descriptive anatomy relates the individual parts of the body to functional systems and pathological anatomy relates to changes in structure from disease. Disciplines such as cytology and histology study cells and tissues, respectively, and myology examines muscle form and function. Arthrology refers to the study of the joint system for bones, while osteology is the study of form and function of bones. Neurology relates to the study of diseases of the nervous system.

The axial skeleton is that supporting the trunk and head, and the appendicular skeleton is related to the extremities. Anatomical terminology relates position and orientation of the body and its parts. A frontal plane is that involving a cut that produces front and back halves of a body, a sagittal plane is produced by a cut dividing the body into left and right halves, and a transverse plane is produced by dividing the body into upper and lower halves. Anterior and posterior refer to front and back of a body, respectively, as do ventral and dorsal for the human. Peripheral refers to a direction toward the surface or superficial region, while deep refers to direction away from the surface. Distal and proximal refer to away from and toward the root of a free extremity, respectively. Superior and inferior refer to upper and lower regions, respectively. Lateral and medial refer to the side and midline, respectively. Flexion refers to bending ventral surfaces toward each other at a joint, and extension is moving those surfaces farther apart. Plantar and palmar refer to ventral surfaces of the feet and hands, respectively.

The four basic tissues of the human body are epithelial, connective, muscular, and nervous. Epithelial tissue provides the surface covering of the body and linings of cavities and passageways. Connective tissue provides the variety of tissue linking structures together, those comprising ligaments, tendons, cartilage, bone, and blood. Muscular tissue is contractile in nature, comprised of striated, smooth, and cardiac. Nervous tissue is specialized for communication.

Tissues combine to form structures and organs. Fascia surrounds organs, ligaments bind bones or cartilage, tendons attach muscle to bone or to cartilage, and bones and cartilage provide the structure for the body. Joints between skeletal components may be diarthrodial (synovial; highly mobile), amphiarthrodial (cartilaginous; slightly mobile), and synarthrodial (fibrous; immobile). Fibrous joints bind immobile bodies together, cartilaginous joints are those in which cartilage serves the primary joining function, and

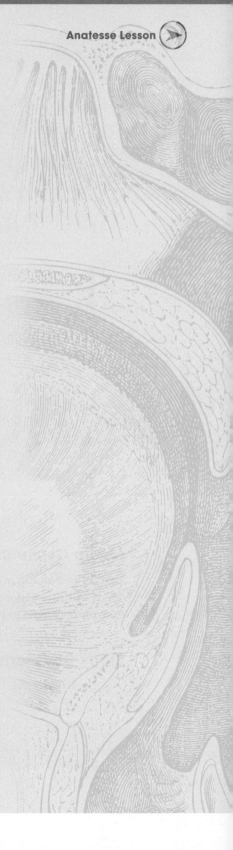

Anatesse Lesson

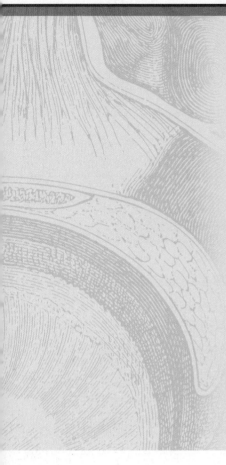

synovial joints are those in which lubricating synovial fluid is contained within an articular capsule.

Muscle bundles are capable of shortening to about half their length. The origin is the point of attachment with the least movement, and the insertion is the relatively mobile point of attachment. Agonists are muscles that move a structure, antagonists oppose movement, and synergists stabilize a structure. Muscles are innervated by a single nerve, and innervation can be afferent or efferent. A motor unit is the efferent nerve fiber and muscle fibers it innervates.

Systems of the body include the muscular, skeletal, respiratory, digestive, reproductive, urinary, endocrine, and nervous systems. Systems of speech production include the respiratory, phonatory, articulatory/resonatory, and nervous systems. The peripheral nervous system (PNS) and central nervous system (CNS) are made up of neurons, which transmit information, and glial cells, which support neuron function. The PNS is made up of cranial and spinal nerves. The CNS is made up of larger structures, including the cerebral cortex, brain stem, cerebellum, spinal cord, and others. The cerebral cortex is responsible for conscious and voluntary function, while the cerebellum coordinates sensory and motor plans. The brain stem mediates many life functions, as well as serving as the origination for cranial nerves. The thalamus is the last way station for sensation from the body, while the basal ganglia control muscle tone and some stereotyped movements.

Media Connection

Go to the accompanying online resources at CengageBrain.com and have fun learning! Study with the Anatesse software program, play games, view animations and videos, and take practice tests to help reinforce the key concepts you learned in this chapter.

Study Questions

1. _____ is the study of the structure of an organism.

2. _____ is the study of the function of a living organism and its parts.

3. _____ anatomy is anatomical study for diagnosis and treatment of disease.

4. _____ anatomy is involved in the description of individual parts of the body without reference to disease conditions, viewing the body as a composite of systems that function together.

5. _____ is the study of structure and function of cells.

6. _____ is the study of structure and function of bones.

7. _____ is the study of form and function of muscle.

8. _____ is the study of diseases of the nervous system.

9. _____ Skin and mucous membrane are made up of this type of tissue.

10. _____ is a particularly important connective tissue because it is both strong and elastic.

11. _____ is a contractile tissue.

12. _____ bind organs together or hold bones to bone or cartilage.

13. _____ is a sheet-like membrane surrounding organs.

14. _____ attach muscle to bone or to cartilage.

15. The relatively immobile point of attachment of a muscle is termed the

   _____.

16. The relatively mobile point of attachment of a muscle is termed the

   _____.

17. Identify the systems defined below:

   a. _____ This system includes smooth, striated, and cardiac muscle of the body.

   b. _____ This system includes the bones and cartilages that form the structure of the body.

   c. _____ This system includes the passageways and tissues involved in gas exchange with the environment, including the oral, nasal, and pharyngeal cavities, the trachea and bronchial passageway, and lungs.

   d. _____ This system includes the esophagus, liver, intestines, and associated glands.

   e. _____ This system includes the nerve tissue and structures of the central and peripheral nervous system.

18. Identify the systems of speech defined below:

   a. _____ This system includes the passageways and tissues involved in gas exchange with the environment, including the oral, nasal, and pharyngeal cavities, the trachea and bronchial passageway, and lungs.

   b. _____ This system is involved in production of voiced sound and utilizes components of the respiratory system (the laryngeal structures).

c. _____ This system is the combination of structures used to alter the characteristics of the sounds of speech, including parts of the anatomically defined digestive and respiratory systems (the tongue, lips, teeth, soft palate, etc.).

d. _____ This system includes the nasal cavity and soft palate and portions of the anatomically defined respiratory and digestive systems.

19. Terms of orientation: On the following figure, identify the descriptive terms indicated.

a. _____ plane

b. _____ plane

c. _____ plane

d. _____ aspect

e. _____ aspect

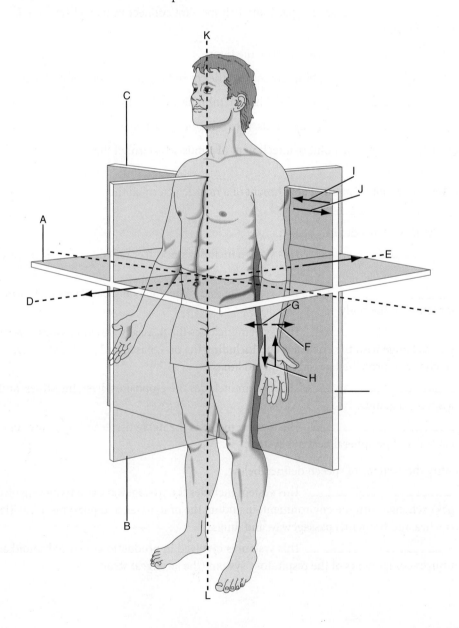

     f. _____ (movement away from midline)

     g. _____ (movement toward midline)

     h. _____ (movement away from midline)

     i. _____ (movement toward midline)

     j. _____ (related to the side)

     k. _____ (above)

     l. _____ (below)

20. The _____ system refers to that group of nervous system components that include the cerebrum, cerebellum, brain stem, and spinal cord.

21. The _____ system includes cranial and spinal nerves.

22. The _____ is responsible for coordinating the motor act by integrating motor and sensory information.

23. The _____ contains the medulla oblongata, pons, and midbrain.

24. The _____ (number and name) nerve mediates the sense of smell.

25. The _____ (number and name) nerve mediates the sense of taste for the anterior 2/3 of the tongue.

26. The _____ (number and name) nerve is responsible for activation of muscles of the face.

27. The _____ (number and name) nerve is responsible for movement of the muscles of mastication.

28. The _____ (number and name) nerve mediates the sense of taste for the posterior 1/3 of the tongue.

29. The _____ (number and name) nerve innervates all of the tongue muscles.

30. As our field has developed, the professionals working with speech and language became known as "speech-language pathologists." Reflecting on the terminology you have just reviewed, to what does the term "pathologist" refer?

Study Question Answers

1. **ANATOMY** is the study of the structure of an organism.

2. **PHYSIOLOGY** is the study of the function of a living organism and its parts.

3. **CLINICAL OR APPLIED** anatomy is anatomical study for diagnosis and treatment of disease.

4. **SYSTEMIC ANATOMY** is involved in the description of individual parts of the body without reference to disease conditions, viewing the body as a composite of systems that function together.

5. **CYTOLOGY** is the study of structure and function of cells.

6. **OSTEOLOGY** is the study of structure and function of bones.

7. **MYOLOGY** is the study of form and function of muscle.

8. **NEUROLOGY** is the study of the nervous system.

9. Skin and mucous membrane are made up of **EPITHELIAL** tissue.

10. **CARTILAGE** is a particularly important connective tissue because it is both strong and elastic.

11. **MUSCLE** is a contractile tissue.

12. **LIGAMENTS** bind organs together or hold bones to bone or cartilage.

13. **FASCIA** is a sheet-like membrane surrounding organs.

14. **TENDONS** attach muscle to bone or to cartilage.

15. The relatively immobile point of attachment of a muscle is termed the **ORIGIN**.

16. The relatively mobile point of attachment of a muscle is termed the **INSERTION**.

17. Identify the systems defined below:
    a. **MUSCULAR SYSTEM** This system includes smooth, striated, and cardiac muscle of the body.
    b. **SKELETAL SYSTEM** This system includes the bones and cartilages that form the structure of the body.
    c. **RESPIRATORY SYSTEM** This system includes the passageways and tissues involved in gas exchange with the environment, including the oral, nasal, and pharyngeal cavities, the trachea and bronchial passageway, and lungs.
    d. **DIGESTIVE SYSTEM** This system includes the esophagus, liver, intestines, and associated glands.
    e. **NERVOUS SYSTEM** This system includes the nerve tissue and structures of the central and peripheral nervous system.

18. Identify the systems of speech defined below.
    a. **RESPIRATORY SYSTEM** This system includes the passageways and tissues involved in gas exchange with the environment, including the oral, nasal, and pharyngeal cavities, the trachea and bronchial passageway, and lungs.
    b. **PHONATORY SYSTEM** This system is involved in production of voiced sound and utilizes components of the respiratory system (the laryngeal structures).
    c. **ARTICULATORY SYSTEM** This system is the combination of structures used to alter the characteristics of the sounds of speech, including parts of the anatomically defined digestive and respiratory systems (the tongue, lips, teeth, soft palate, etc.).
    d. **RESONATORY SYSTEM** This system includes the nasal cavity and soft palate and portions of the anatomically defined respiratory and digestive systems.

19. Terms of orientation: On the figure below, identify the descriptive terms indicated.
    a. **TRANSVERSE** plane
    b. **SAGITTAL OR MEDIAN** plane
    c. **CORONAL OR FRONTAL** plane
    d. **ANTERIOR OR VENTRAL** aspect
    e. **POSTERIOR OR DORSAL** aspect

      f. **ABDUCT** (movement away from midline)

      g. **ADDUCT** (movement toward midline)

      h. **DISTAL** (located away from root of free extremity)

      i. **PROXIMAL** (located near root of free extremity)

      j. **LATERAL** (related to the side)

      k. **SUPERIOR** (above)

      l. **INFERIOR** (below)

20. The **CENTRAL NERVOUS** system refers to that group of nervous system components that include the cerebrum, cerebellum, brain stem, and spinal cord.

21. The **PERIPHERAL NERVOUS** system includes cranial and spinal nerves.

22. The **CEREBELLUM** is responsible for coordinating the motor act by integrating motor and sensory information.

23. The **BRAIN STEM** contains the medulla oblongata, midbrain, and pons.

24. The **I OLFACTORY** (number and name) nerve mediates the sense of smell.

25. The **VII FACIAL** (number and name) nerve mediates the sense of taste for the anterior 2/3 of the tongue.

26. The **VII FACIAL** (number and name) nerve is responsible for activation of muscles of the face.

27. The **V TRIGEMINAL** (number and name) nerve is responsible for movement of the muscles of mastication.

28. The **IX GLOSSOPHARYNGEAL** (number and name) nerve mediates the sense of taste for the posterior 1/3 of the tongue.

29. The **XII HYPOGLOSSAL** (number and name) nerve innervates all of the tongue muscles.

30. Pathology is the study of diseased tissue. By extension, a speech-language pathologist is one who studies the "pathology" of our field, communication disorders.

Bibliography

Agur, A. & Dalley, A. (2012). *Grant's atlas of anatomy* (13th ed.). New York: Lippincott Williams and Wilkins.

Barnett, H. L. (1972). *Pediatrics*. New York: Appleton-Century-Crofts.

Bateman, H. E., & Mason, R. M. (1984). *Applied anatomy and physiology of the speech and hearing mechanism*. Springfield, IL: Charles C. Thomas.

Duffy, J. R. (2012). *Motor speech disorders,* (3rd ed.). St. Louis, MO: Mosby.

Fink, B. R., & Demarest, R. J. (1978). *Laryngeal biomechanics*. Cambridge, MA: Harvard University Press.

Gilroy, A. M., MacPherson, B. R., & Ross, L. M. (2012). *Atlas of anatomy* (2nd ed.). New York: Thieme.

Gosling, J. A., Harris, P. F., & Humpherson, J. R. (2009). *Human Anatomy: Color atlas and text book,* (5th ed.). St. Louis, MO: Mosby.

Grant, J. C. B., Basmajian, J. V., & Sloneker, C. E. (1989). *Grant's method of anatomy: A clinical problem-solving*. Baltimore, MD: Williams & Wilkins.

Kaplan, H. (1960). *Anatomy and physiology of speech*. New York: McGraw-Hill.

Kuehn, D. P., Lemme, M. L., & Baumgartner, J. M. (1991). *Neural bases of speech, hearing, and language.* Boston: Little, Brown.

Moore, K. L., Persaud, T. V. N., & Torchia, M. G. (2013). *The developing human: Clincally oriented embryology* (9th ed.). Philadelphia: W. B. Saunders.

Rohen, J. W., Lutjen-Drecoll, E., & Yokochi, C. (2010). *Color atlas of anatomy: A photographic study of the human body.* New York: Lippincott Williams & Wilkins.

Ross, J. S., & Wilson, K. J. W. (1966). *Foundations of anatomy and physiology.* Baltimore, MD: Williams & Wilkins.

Standring, S. (2008). *Gray's anatomy* (40th ed.). London: Churchill Livingstone Elsevier.

Zemlin, W. R. (1998). *Speech and hearing science: Anatomy and physiology* (4th ed.). Needham Heights, MA: Allyn & Bacon.

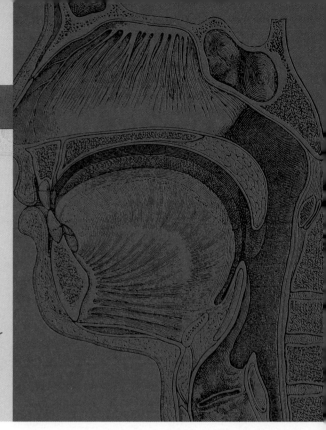

Chapter 2

ANATOMY OF RESPIRATION

"Breathe! You are alive!"

— *Thich Nhat Hanh, Zen Master*

We *must* breathe with great regularity to maintain body systems that are dependent on efficient oxygen exchange. Respiration is simultaneously a very robust and a very delicate system. Our respiratory rate and depth of breathing are governed by a number of involuntary sensory systems, and we take these involuntary processes for granted as they meet our everyday needs. On the other hand, changes in respiratory tissues arising from environmental or disease-related issues can quickly destabilize this system, leaving the individual in peril for his or her life. Indeed, we will see that most of the degenerative neurological diseases with which we work in speech-language pathology will end with respiratory failure. In parallel with these automatic life processes, we, as humans, have hijacked the respiratory system to provide the energy source for oral communication. As you will see in our discussion of respiratory physiology, we exercise a great deal of external control over the respiratory mechanism while still working within the bounds of the biological requirements for life. First, let us discuss respiration as it is needed to sustain life, and then we'll discuss respiration for speech.

Respiration is defined as the exchange of gas between an organism and its environment. We bring oxygen to the cells of the body to sustain life by breathing in, the process of **inspiration**, and eliminate waste products by breathing out, or **expiration**.

Gas exchange happens within the minuscule air sacs known as the **alveoli** after gas has been drawn into the system. Bringing air into the lungs is an active, muscular process. It capitalizes on the fact that all forces in nature seek balance and equilibrium. The basic mechanism for inspiration may be likened to that of a hypodermic needle. When

Anatesse Lesson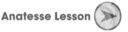

inspiration: Gr. Spiro, breath

alveoli: L., small hollows or cavities in a structure

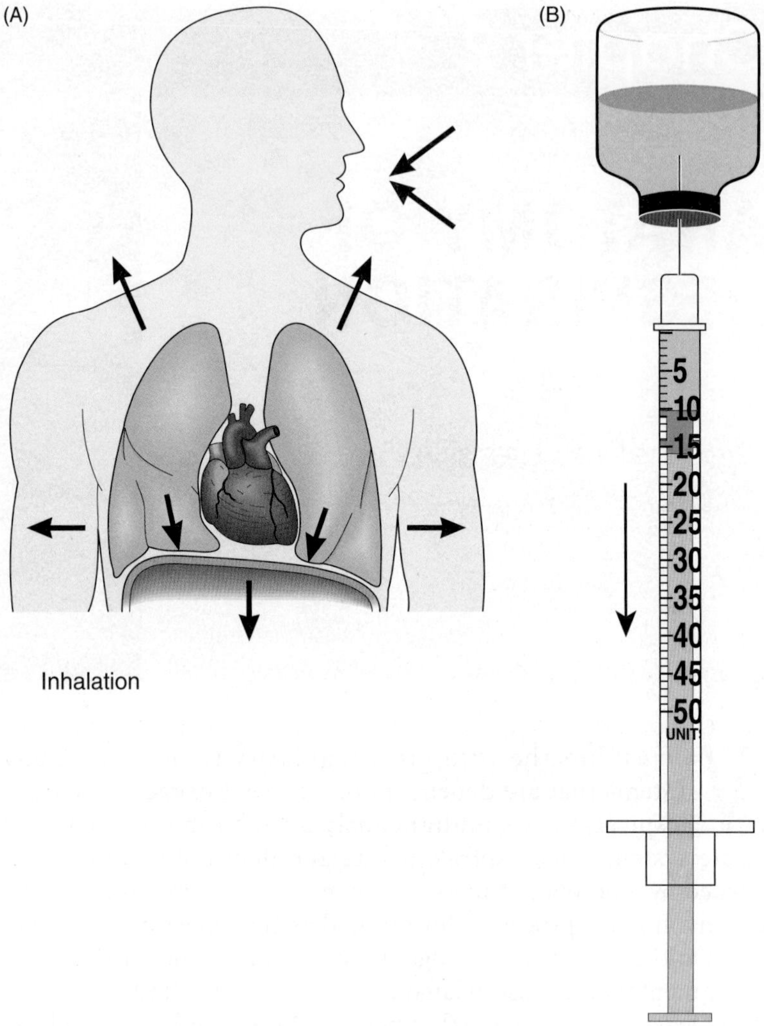

(A)   (B)

Inhalation

Figure 2-1. Comparison of the action of the diaphragm with that of a plunger on a syringe. As the diaphragm pulls down (A) air enters the lungs, just as it enters the chamber of the syringe when the plunger is pulled down (B).
© Cengage Learning®.

air pressure: the force exerted on a surface by air molecules

the plunger on the hypodermic needle in Figure 2-1 is pulled down, whatever is near the opening will enter the tube and be drawn into the awaiting chamber. If you envision the respiratory system as a syringe, with your mouth or nose as the tip, you will realize that pulling on the plunger (your diaphragm) causes air to enter the chamber (your lungs). If you were to hold your finger over the opening as you pulled back the plunger, you would feel the suction of the device on your finger. This suction is the product of *lowering* the relative air pressure within the chamber, producing an imbalance in relation to atmospheric pressure. Let us examine the physical principles involved a little more deeply.

Before we can talk about the forces driving respiration, you need an intuitive feel for what air pressure really is. **Air pressure** is the force exerted on the walls of a chamber by molecules of air. Because of the molecular charge, air molecules tend to keep their distance from other air molecules. If the chamber is opened to the atmosphere, the pressure exerted on the inner walls of the chamber will be the same as that exerted on the outer walls.

The action starts when you close the chamber and change the volume. Making the chamber smaller does not change the forces that keep molecules apart, but rather lets those forces be manifest on the walls of the chamber. Although the forces have not changed, the area on which they exert themselves has (you made it smaller, remember?), and that results in an increase in pressure. That is, **pressure** is *Force* exerted on *Area*, or P = F/A. You have just increased pressure by decreasing area.

Boyle's law states that, given a gas of constant temperature, if you increase the volume of the chamber in which the gas is contained, the pressure will decrease. If you increase the size (volume) of the chamber of a syringe, the air pressure within that chamber will decrease. The opposite is also true: If you decrease the volume of the chamber, the pressure will increase. Once again we see that forces seek stability and equilibrium. When volume increases, pressure decreases, and natural law says that air will flow to equalize that pressure. Thus, air flows into the chamber—in our case, the lungs.

Figure 2-2 shows the same effect graphically. The chamber has 11 molecules in it in both cases. On the left, the volume of the chamber has been reduced, so the 11 molecules are much closer together and the pressure has increased (known as **positive pressure**). Likewise, when you pull the plunger back so the molecules are farther apart than the forces dictate, the pressure decreases, and the pressure is now referred to as **negative pressure**. The beauty of this arrangement is that it provides all the principle we need to discuss respiratory physiology at the macro- or microscopic level. The forces that draw air into the lungs are also responsible for drawing carbon dioxide out.

positive pressure: air pressure that exceeds atmospheric pressure

negative pressure: air pressure that is less than atmospheric pressure

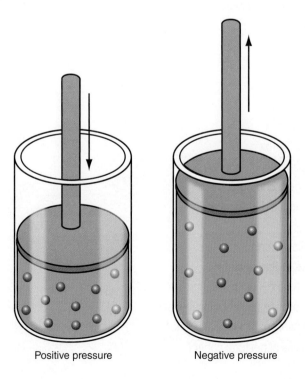

Positive pressure   Negative pressure

Figure 2-2. The piston on the left has been depressed, compressing the air in the chamber and increasing the air pressure. On the right, the piston has been retracted, increasing the space between the molecules and creating a relatively negative pressure.
© Cengage Learning®.

✔ *To summarize:*

- **Pressure** is defined as force distributed over area, P = F/A.
- **Boyle's law** tells us that as the volume of a container increases, the air pressure within the container decreases.
- This relatively **negative pressure** will cause air to enter the container until the pressure is equalized.
- If volume is decreased, pressure increases and air flows out until the pressures inside and outside are equal.
- This principle forms the basis for movement of air into and out of the lungs.

THE SUPPORT STRUCTURE OF RESPIRATION
Overview

The respiratory system consists of a gas-exchanging mechanism supported and protected by a bony cage (see Table 2-1). Gas exchange is carried out by the lungs, while the rib cage performs a protective function.

Table 2-1 **Structures of respiration**
Bony Thorax
Vertebrae and vertebral column
Ribs and their attachment to vertebral column
Pectoral girdle
Scapula and clavicle
Sternum
Pelvic girdle
Ischium
Pubic bone
Sacrum
Ilium
Visceral Thorax
Respiratory passageway
Mouth and nose
Trachea and bronchi
Lungs
Mediastinum
Muscles of Respiration
Diaphragm
Accessory muscles of inspiration
Accessory muscles of expiration
Muscles of postural control

Let us take a guided tour of the respiratory system. To begin, pay attention to your own breathing. Try the following. Sit up straight and close your eyes while taking 10 quiet breaths through your nose. First, concentrate attention on your nose, feeling the air entering and leaving your nostrils. Then feel your abdominal region stretch out a little with each inspiration, and then become aware that your thorax (rib cage) is expanding a little with each inhalation. Now take a good, deep breath (still through your nose) and feel your whole chest rise and your shoulders straighten out a little.

Besides relaxing you, attending to your breathing has given you a sense of the parts of your body that are activated for inspiration and expiration. At first you directed your attention to your nostrils, the part of the respiratory passageway that warms and moistens the air going into the lungs. Then you noticed your abdomen protruding, which is a natural process associated with inspiration, because the diaphragm is pushing against the abdomen when it contracts to bring air in. Then you noticed that your thorax was expanding a little as you breathed in quietly, and then you noted that your thorax expanded markedly as you breathed in deeply. If you missed any of these things happening, take a minute and breathe a little more. This will set the stage for understanding what is going on with the bones and muscles of respiration.

Developing an understanding of respiratory function requires knowledge of the skeletal system. The lungs are housed within the thorax, an area bounded in the superior aspect by the first rib and clavicle, and in the inferior by the 12th rib (see Figure 2-3). The lateral and anterior aspects are composed of the ribs and **sternum**. The entire thorax is suspended from the **vertebral column** (spinal column), a structure that doubles as the conduit for the **spinal cord**, the nervous system supply for the body and extremities.

sternum: L., sternum, breastplate

vertebral column: the bony structure made of vertebrae

spinal cord: the nerve tracks and cell bodies within the spinal column

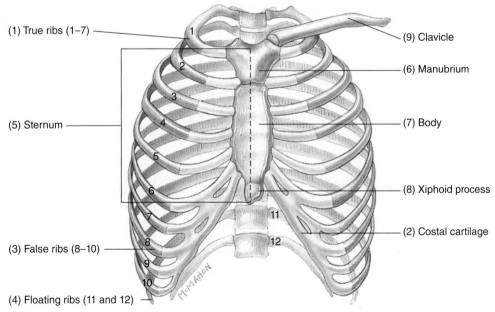

(1) True ribs (1–7)

(9) Clavicle

(6) Manubrium

(5) Sternum

(7) Body

(8) Xiphoid process

(2) Costal cartilage

(3) False ribs (8–10)

(4) Floating ribs (11 and 12)

Figure 2-3. Anterior view of the thorax.

© Cengage Learning®.

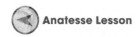

vertebra: bony segment of the vertebral (spinal) column

cervical vertebra: vertebra of the cervical spinal column

thoracic vertebra: vertebra of the thoracic spinal column

lumbar vertebra: vertebra of the lumbar spinal column

sacral vertebra: vertebral components of the sacrum

coccygeal vertebra: vestigial vertebral components of the coccyx

Vertebral Column

The functional unit of the vertebral column is the **vertebra** (plural, vertebrae) or vertebral column segment. The vertebral column has five divisions: cervical, thoracic, lumbar, sacral, and coccygeal (see Figure 2-4). The anatomical shorthand associated with the vertebral column and spinal nerves is as follows. The vertebrae are numbered sequentially from superior to inferior by section, so that the uppermost **cervical vertebra** is C1, the second is C2, and so forth to C7. Likewise, the first **thoracic vertebra** is T1, and the last is T12. **Lumbar vertebrae** include L1 through L5, **sacral vertebrae** include S1 through S5, and the **coccygeal vertebrae** are considered to be a fused unit, known as the coccyx. The vertebrae are separated by intervertebral discs, which are made of fibrocartilage. Each disc consists of a gelatinous core that equalizes forces placed on the disc (the *nucleus pulposus*) and a fibrous ring known as the *annulus fibrosus*. The role of the disc is to keep the vertebrae separated, to cushion the forces exerted on the vertebrae, and to allow free space for passage of the spinal nerves from the spinal cord to the periphery.

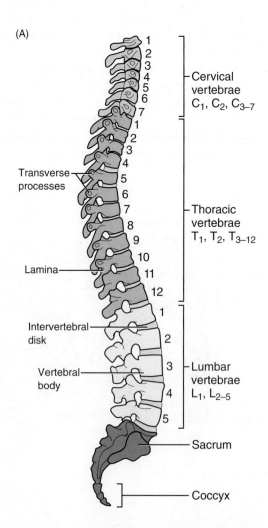

(A)

Cervical vertebrae C_1, C_2, C_{3-7}

Transverse processes

Thoracic vertebrae T_1, T_2, T_{3-12}

Lamina

Intervertebral disk

Vertebral body

Lumbar vertebrae L_1, L_{2-5}

Sacrum

Coccyx

Figure 2-4. (A) Components of the vertebral column. (continues).
© Cengage Learning®.

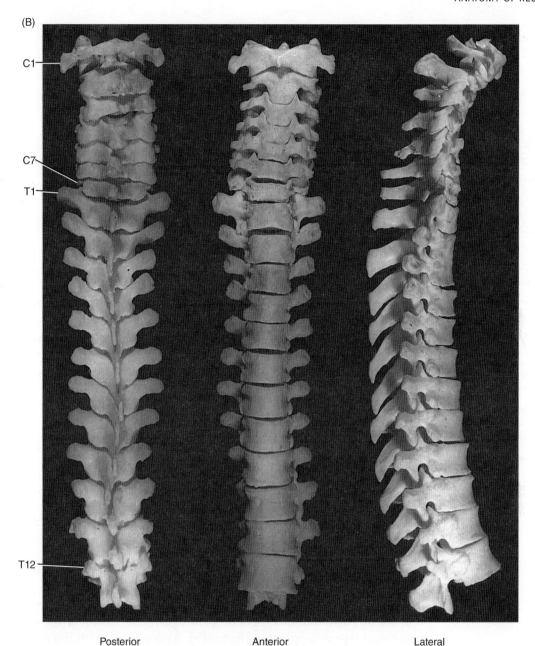

Figure 2-4 continued. (B) Articulated cervical and thoracic vertebrae.
© Cengage Learning®.

The vertebral column is composed of 33 segments of bone with a rich set of fossa and protuberances clearly designed for function. Although vertebrae have roughly the same shape, their form and landmarks vary depending on the location and the area they serve, their attachments (such as ribs), and their neural payload. The area serving the head requires more security for the vertebral artery and vein, so there are protected **foramina** (or openings) for that purpose. In lower regions, there is a great deal more bone in the **corpus** or body of the vertebra, reflecting the power of the muscles used for lifting.

foramina, foramen: L., opening

corpus: L., body

Palpation

Palpation, or the process of examining structures with the hands, can be a very useful tool to understanding anatomy. When you perform an oral peripheral examination as a clinician, you will need to be comfortable with the process of palpating because it is a means of gathering information about your client's physical condition that may help you in your diagnosis and in the remediation of speech problems. For instance, palpation of the temporomandibular joint, the joint forming the articulation of the mandible and the temporal bone, while your client moves his or her jaw will provide you with insight into the integrity of the joint as well as the degree of muscular control your client is able to exert.

Throughout these chapters we will provide you with palpation activities that you can perform on yourself. Identifying these landmarks will help you understand the structures with which we deal in speech-language pathology.

Cervical Vertebrae

spinous process: posterior-most process of vertebra

transverse process: lateral process of vertebra

vertebral foramen: foramen of vertebral segment through which spinal cord passes

intervertebral foramen: foramen through which spinal nerve exits and/or enters the spinal cord

Major landmarks of the vertebrae include a prominent **spinous process** (the collection of which can be felt by rubbing the spine of your friend's back) and **transverse processes** on both sides (see Figure 2-5). The corpus of the vertebra makes up the anterior portion, with a prominent hole or **vertebral foramen** just posterior to that. It is through this foramen that the tracts of the spinal cord pass. The spinal nerves must somehow exit and enter the spinal cord; the **intervertebral foramina** on either side of the vertebra permits this. Vertebral segments ride one atop another to form the vertebral column. This articulation is completed by means of the superior and inferior articular facets. These facets provide the mating surfaces for two adjacent vertebrae, limiting movement in the anterior–posterior dimension, thus protecting the spinal cord and allowing limited rotatory and rocking motion. We must be able to move freely, but not *too* freely, considering the importance of the spinal cord within that column.

tubercle: L., tuberculum, little swelling

facet: Fr., facette, small face

dens: L., tooth

The uppermost cervical vertebra, C1, is the **atlas**, so named for its singular role in supporting the skull for rotation (after the mythical figure supporting the earth). Articulating with the inferior surface of the atlas is C2, the **axis**, on which the skull pivots (see Figure 2-6). C1 and C2 differ markedly from C3 through C7. The posterior of C1 has a reduced prominence, here called the posterior **tubercle**. The superior articular **facet** is larger than those of C3 through C7, providing increased surface area for vertebra-skull articulation. Similarly, the vertebral foramen is larger than those in the lower cervical vertebrae, reflecting the transition from spinal cord to brain stem that begins at that level. The **dens** process of the axis (also known as the odontoid process) protrudes through it. The relationship between the odontoid process and vertebral foramen is protective, because unchecked movement could result in damage to the spinal cord at this level, which would be life threatening.

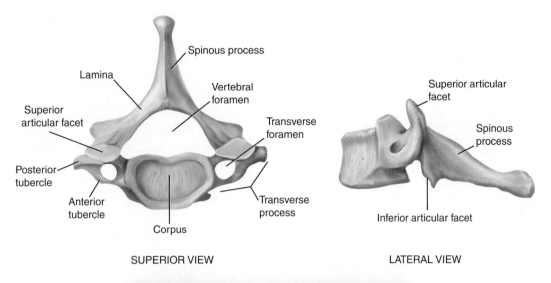

SUPERIOR VIEW   LATERAL VIEW

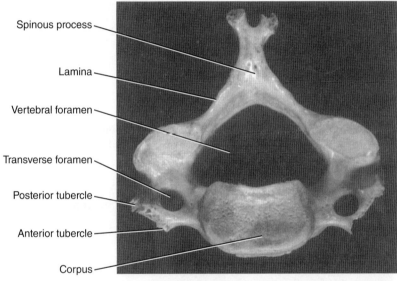

Figure 2-5. Superior and lateral views of cervical vertebra.
© Cengage Learning®.

You might notice that the axis (C2) has a rudimentary spinous process, although the atlas does not. The articulation of C1 and C2 is shown in Figure 2-6.

As you can see in Figure 2-5, a typical cervical vertebra has a number of landmarks. The corpus and spinous process provide a clue to orientation, because the corpus is in the anterior aspect and the posterior spinous process will slant downward.

Examination of Figure 2-5 also reveals lateral wings known as the transverse processes, which are directed in a posterolateral (*postero* = back; *lateral* = side) direction. The superior surface is marked by a superior articular facet, which rests atop the **pedicle**. The inferior surface contains an inferior articular facet. In the articulated vertebral column, these facets mate. The paired transverse foramina shown in Figure 2-5 are found only in the cervical vertebrae and may even be absent in C7. Figure 2-7 shows that the vertebral artery and vein pass

pedicle: L., pedalis, foot

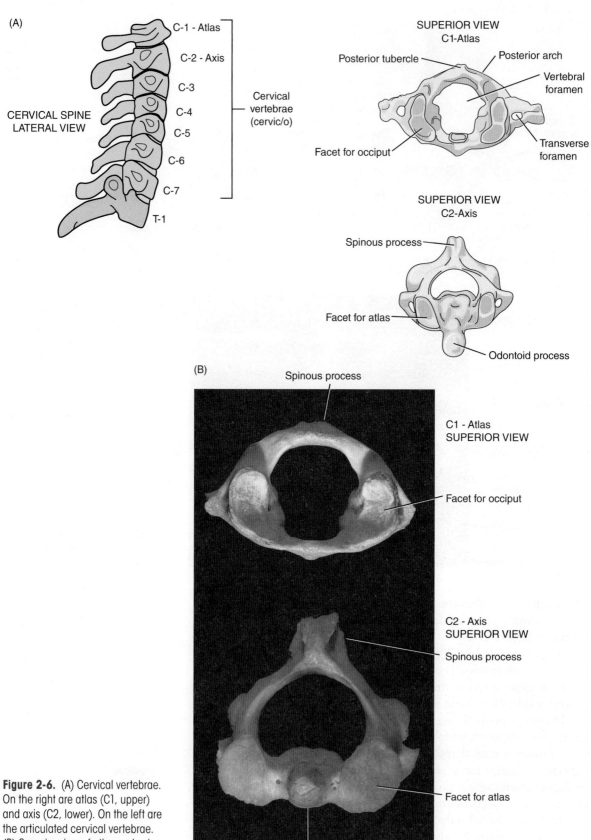

(A)

C-1 - Atlas
C-2 - Axis
C-3
C-4
C-5
C-6
C-7

Cervical
vertebrae
(cervic/o)

CERVICAL SPINE
LATERAL VIEW

T-1

SUPERIOR VIEW
C1-Atlas

Posterior tubercle
Posterior arch
Vertebral
foramen
Facet for occiput
Transverse
foramen

SUPERIOR VIEW
C2-Axis

Spinous process
Facet for atlas
Odontoid process

(B)

Spinous process

C1 - Atlas
SUPERIOR VIEW

Facet for occiput

C2 - Axis
SUPERIOR VIEW

Spinous process

Facet for atlas

Odontoid process

Figure 2-6. (A) Cervical vertebrae.
On the right are atlas (C1, upper)
and axis (C2, lower). On the left are
the articulated cervical vertebrae.
(B) Superior view of atlas and axis.
© Cengage Learning®.

Odontoid Malformations

Odontoid malformations are those in which the odontoid process of C2 fails to develop. In cases such as these the atlas (C1) is free to rotate on the axis (C2), providing the potential for significant spinal cord and medulla oblongata injury during hyperrotation or hyperextension. Because the medulla oblongata is a vital component of the brainstem, these malformations can be life threatening. The individual with undiagnosed odontoid malformation may complain of joint pain or stiffness in the neck, but otherwise may be asymptomatic. It is not until a radiograph of the neck region is performed for other purposes that the absent process is identified. Often the individual will undergo a minor trauma, such as a fall, that has a result that is greater than expected. In the literature on odontoid malformations are cases of wrestlers who suffer repeated syncope (significant reduction in blood pressure that results in light-headedness), transient limb weakness, and even seizure disorder. A more serious malformation is the *os odontoideum* malformation, in which the anterior tip of the vertebra is separated. In this condition, the tip typically continues to receive vascular supply and often grows into the foramen magnum. The result is that the tip places pressure on the spinal cord and lower brainstem, resulting in muscular weakness, pain, and reduction in motor coordination (ataxia), depending upon the location of the injury. If the tip compresses an artery, there can be further complications due to reduction in vascular supply.

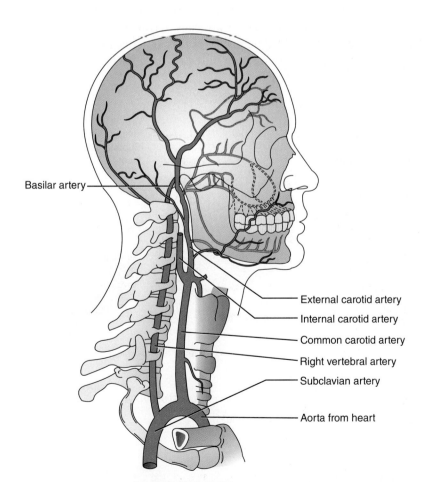

Basilar artery

External carotid artery

Internal carotid artery

Common carotid artery

Right vertebral artery

Subclavian artery

Aorta from heart

Figure 2-7. Course of vertebral artery through the transverse foramina of cervical vertebrae.
© Cengage Learning®.

through this foramen. You can palpate the seventh cervical vertebra by bending your head forward so that your chin touches your chest. The first prominent spinous process you feel on your neck is C7. You can also palpate the large transverse processes of the atlas, inferior to the mastoid process of the temporal bone.

Thoracic Vertebrae

The 12 thoracic vertebrae (T1 to T12) provide the basis for the respiratory framework, because they form the posterior point of attachment for the ribs of the bony thorax. As seen in Figure 2-8, the thoracic vertebrae have larger spinous and transverse processes. Between vertebrae is the intervertebral foramen, the product of the inferior and superior vertebral notches of articulating vertebrae, through which spinal nerves communicate with the spinal cord. You should pay particular attention to the superior and inferior costal facets, because these are the points of attachment for the ribs, as seen in Figure 2-9.

The articulation of rib and thoracic vertebrae is complicated. Although it would have been simpler for us had the second rib been attached to the second vertebra, had the third rib been attached to the third vertebra, and so forth, only the first rib and the last three ribs (1, 10, 11, 12) have this nice one-to-one arrangement. Each of the remaining ribs (2 through 9) attaches to the transverse process and corpus of the same-numbered vertebra and also attaches to the body of the vertebra above it (e.g., rib 2 attaches to transverse process of T2 and body of T1 and T2). The utility of this articulation will become apparent as we discuss movement of the rib cage for respiration.

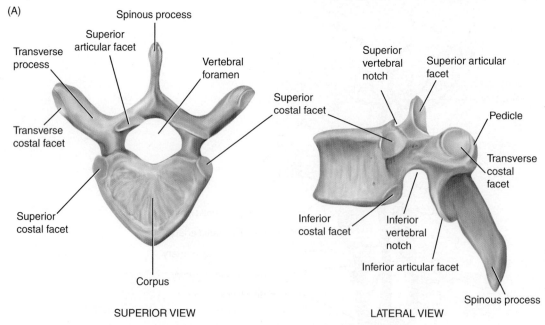

Figure 2-8. (A) Superior and lateral views of thoracic vertebrae. (continues).
© Cengage Learning®.

(B)

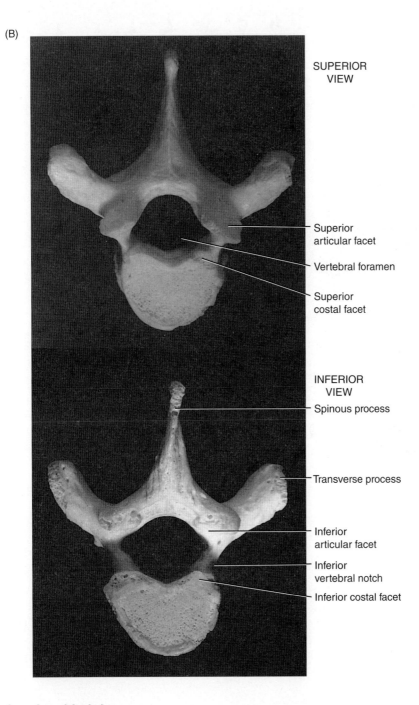

SUPERIOR
VIEW

Superior
articular facet

Vertebral foramen

Superior
costal facet

INFERIOR
VIEW

Spinous process

Transverse process

Inferior
articular facet

Inferior
vertebral notch

Inferior costal facet

Figure 2-8 continued. (B) Superior (upper) and inferior (lower) view of thoracic vertebra.
© Cengage Learning®.

Lumbar Vertebrae

The five lumbar vertebrae are quite large in comparison to those of the thoracic or cervical region, reflecting the stress placed on them during lifting and **ambulation** (walking). They provide direct or indirect attachment for a host of back and abdominal muscles, as well as for the posterior fibers of the diaphragm. The transverse and spinous processes are relatively smaller, and the corpus is much larger than in the thoracic and cervical vertebrae.

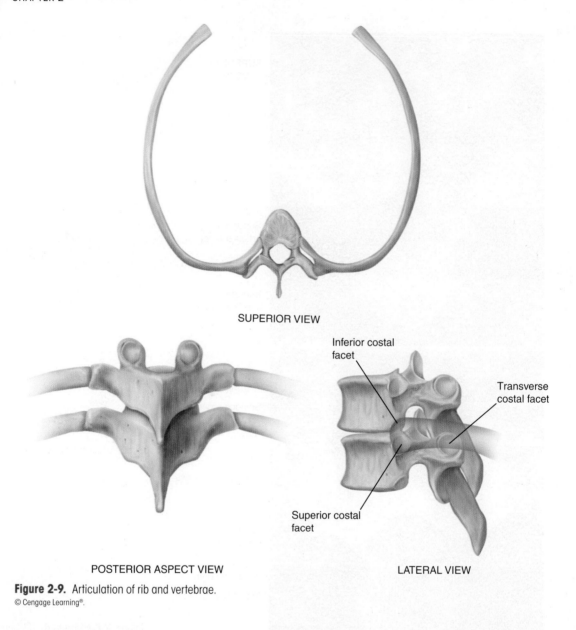

SUPERIOR VIEW

Inferior costal facet

Transverse costal facet

Superior costal facet

POSTERIOR ASPECT VIEW

LATERAL VIEW

Figure 2-9. Articulation of rib and vertebrae.
© Cengage Learning®.

Sacrum and Coccyx

The five sacral vertebrae are actually a fused mass known as the **sacrum**. The sacrum and its ossified intervertebral discs retain vestiges of the vertebrae from which they are formed, with remnants of spinous and transverse processes. The sacral foramina perform the function of the intervertebral foramina, providing a passage for the sacral nerves (see Figure 2-10).

The **coccyx** is composed of the fused coccygeal vertebrae. It is so named because of its beaklike appearance, and it articulates with the inferior sacrum by means of a small disc.

sacrum: L., sacralis, sacred

coccyx: Gr., kokkus, cuckoo
(shaped like a cuckoo's beak)

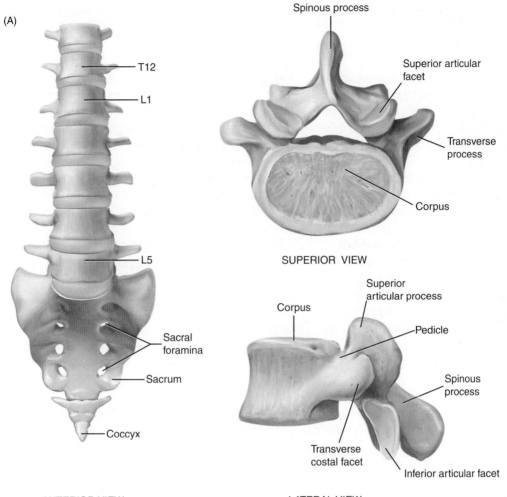

(A)

T12

L1

L5

Sacral
foramina

Sacrum

Coccyx

ANTERIOR VIEW

Spinous process

Superior articular
facet

Transverse
process

Corpus

SUPERIOR VIEW

Corpus

Superior
articular process

Pedicle

Spinous
process

Transverse
costal facet

Inferior articular facet

LATERAL VIEW

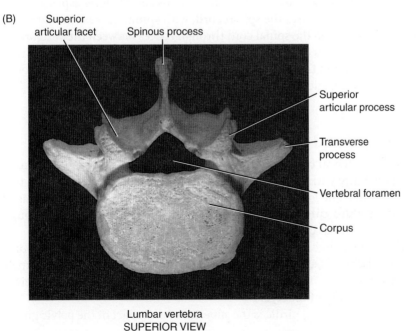

(B)

Superior
articular facet

Spinous process

Superior
articular process

Transverse
process

Vertebral foramen

Corpus

Lumbar vertebra
SUPERIOR VIEW

Figure 2-10. (A) Lumbar vertebrae articulated with sacrum and coccyx (left). Upper right shows the superior view of lumbar vertebra, and lower right shows the lateral view. (B) Superior view of lumbar vertebra.

© Cengage Learning®.

Herniation of Intervertebral Discs

The vertebral column is made up of individual vertebrae that are separated by intervertebral discs. These discs are an elegant solution to the problem of how to allow the vertebral column to move while still protecting the integrity of the column and its precious cargo, the spinal cord. Each intervertebral disc is made up of a ring of fibrocartilage surrounding a gelatinous core. The spinal cord takes a tremendous beating in day-to-day life. Every time you lift something or push on an object, or throw a baseball you are putting compressive force on the vertebral column as muscles attached to the thorax and or vertebral column contract forcefully. Discs are exquisite in design, as the fibrocartilage rings flex with each movement. The gelatinous core distributes forces placed on the ring evenly throughout the disc. (As an example, blow up a balloon and push your finger into it. The compression of your finger causes the entire balloon to change shape and expand because the forces are distributed evenly throughout the balloon.)

The problem with this design is age. Nothing lasts forever, and the intervertebral disc is no exception. The fibrocartilage weakens and bulges under the pressure. Sometimes the disc ruptures and allows the core (the nucleus pulposus) to leak out. When the disc collapses it allows the vertebrae to come closer, and the disc will tend to bulge in the process. Both of these processes can compress the spinal nerve roots that emerge through the intervertebral foramina. This can result in pain and muscular weakness of the areas and muscles served by the nerve.

✔ *To summarize:*

- The **vertebral column** is composed of vertebral segments that combine to form a strong but flexible column.
- **Vertebrae** are identified based on their level: C1 to C7 (**cervical**), T1 to T12 (**thoracic**), L1 to L5 (**lumbar**), S1 to S5 (**sacral**).
- The fused **coccygeal** vertebrae are referred to as the *coccyx*.
- This spinal column provides the points of attachment for numerous muscles by means of the **spinous** and **transverse processes**.
- It also houses the **spinal cord**, with **spinal nerves** emerging and entering the spinal cord through spaces between the vertebrae.
- The ribs of the rib cage articulate with the spinal column in a fashion that permits the rib cage some limited movement for respiration.

Pelvic and Pectoral Girdles

The vertebral column is central to the body, and if we are to interact physically with our environment, we must attach appendages to this column. The lower extremities are attached to this axis by means of the **pelvic girdle**, and the upper extremities are attached through the **pectoral girdle**.

The pelvic girdle is comprised of the ilium, sacrum, pubic bone, and ischium (see Figure 2-11). The combination provides an extremely strong structure capable of bearing a great deal of translated weight from the use of the legs.

The pectoral girdle is the superior counterpart of the pelvic girdle.

pelvic girdle: the area comprised of the ilium, sacrum, pubic bone, and ischium

pectoral, pectoralis: L., pertaining to the chest

Spinal Cord Injury

The spinal cord is well protected by the osseous vertebral column, in that the vertebrae fit together in a partial lock-and-key fashion to inhibit motion. The vertebral column is richly bound together by ligaments and surrounded by muscles of the back.

Despite this degree of redundant protection, the spinal cord is frequently traumatized. The most frequent cause of spinal cord injury is vehicle accidents, especially those in which the occupant is not properly restrained. When a person is ejected from a vehicle, the vertebral column can undergo rotatory stresses that can tear the spinal cord, and the impact can compress the vertebral column, resulting in distention of the spinal cord. Both ejection and whiplash injuries can result in hyperextension of the cervical vertebrae, which can cause damage to the odontoid process, compress and distend the disc, and stretch or tear the spinal cord. Typically the compression occurs in the corpus. Significant transverse forces can cause a shearing of the spinal cord as well.

The result of spinal cord injury is frequently the loss of motor and sensory function to the area below the spinal cord injury, with subsequent paraplegia (legs paralyzed) or quadriplegia (both arms and legs paralyzed). For an exhaustive review of spinal cord injury, see Mackay, Chapman, and Morgan (1997).

(A)

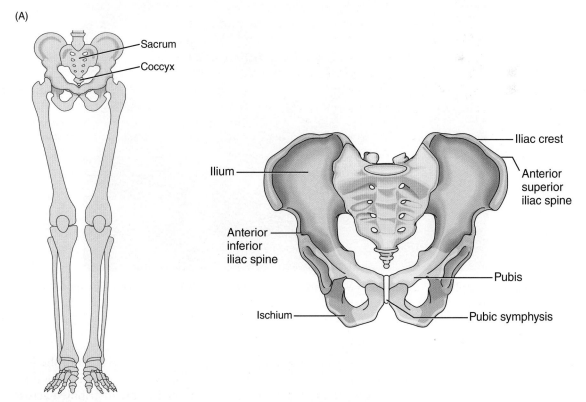

Figure 2-11. (A) Pelvic girdle, consisting of the ilium, pubis, and ischium. (continues).

© Cengage Learning®.

(B)

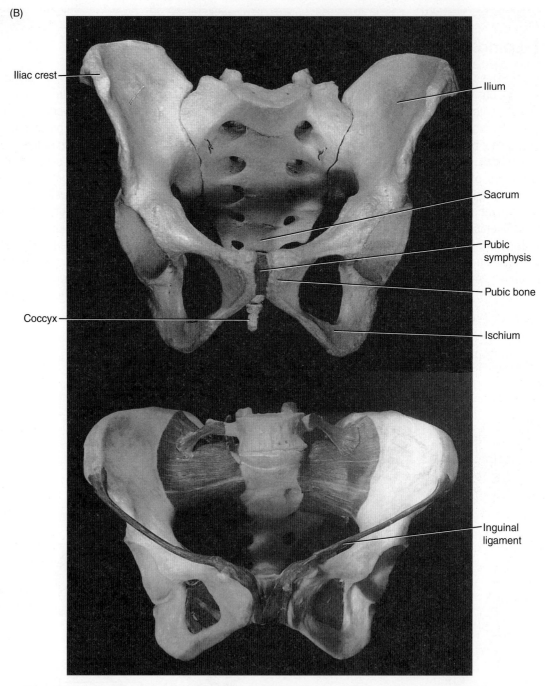

Iliac crest

Ilium

Sacrum

Pubic symphysis

Pubic bone

Coccyx

Ischium

Inguinal ligament

Figure 2-11 continued. (B) Anterior view of pelvis. Lower view shows location of the inguinal ligament.
© Cengage Learning®.

Pelvic Girdle

The pelvic girdle provides a strong structure for attaching the legs to the vertebral column (see Figure 2-11). By means of this structure, forces generated through movement of the legs are distributed across a mass of bone, which, in turn, is attached to the vertebral column.

The pelvic girdle is made up of the ilium, sacrum, pubic bone, and ischium. The **ilium** is a large, wing-like bone (similar in this way to the **scapula** or shoulder blade of the upper body) that provides the bulk of the support for the abdominal musculature and the prominent hip bone on which many parents carry their children. The iliac crest of the superior-lateral surface is an important landmark: The anterior-superior iliac spine (ASIS) marks the termination of the crest as well as the superior point of attachment for the inguinal ligament. The inguinal ligament runs from ASIS of the iliac crest to the **pubic symphysis**, which is the point of union between the two pubic bones. Deep to the ilium is the massive medial structure, the sacrum. As may be seen in Figure 2-11, the sacrum articulates with the fifth lumbar vertebra. The iliac bones articulate with the sacrum laterally, forming the sacroiliac joints. The coccyx is the inferior-most segment of the spinal column, consisting of four fused vertebrae articulating at the inferior aspect of the sacrum. The structure comprised of the iliac, ischium, and pubis bones is referred to as the *innominate* or *hip bone*: *innominate* means, literally, *unnamed*.

ilium: one of the bones of the pelvic girdle

scapula: the major structure of the pectoral girdle

pubic symphysis: joint between the paired pubic bones

Pectoral Girdle

The pectoral or **shoulder girdle** includes the scapula and **clavicle**, bones that support the upper extremities. The clavicle, also known as the collarbone, is attached to the superior sternum, running laterally to join with the winglike scapula. The clavicle provides the anterior support for the shoulder (see Figure 2-12). The scapula has its only skeletal attachment via the clavicle, which in turn has its only skeletal attachment at the sternum. From the scapula are slung several muscles that hold it in a dynamic tension that facilitates flexible upper body movement without compromising strength. The downside of this precarious arrangement is the vulnerability of the junction of the scapula and clavicle. Disarticulation of these two bones will cause a collapse of the structure so that the shoulder rotates forward and inward.

shoulder girdle: another term for pectoral girdle

clavicle: L., clavicula, little key

The physical arrangement of the pectoral girdle provides an "A-frame" of support to distribute force through relatively solid articulation at the scapula and through muscular attachment in the form of the massive muscles of the thorax and back.

When taken together, one can view the human skeleton as a tube with two A-frames attached at the ends. The tube provides flexible yet strong support for the trunk, even as the A-frames give that trunk the opportunity to explore its environment by means of the arms and legs. The A-frame design provides maximum strength for these extremities with a minimum of bone mass.

✔ *To summarize:*

- The bony support structure of the respiratory system is composed of the **rib cage** and **vertebral column**.
- At the base of the vertebral column is the **pelvic girdle**, composed of the **ilium**, **sacrum**, **pubic bone**, and **ischium**.

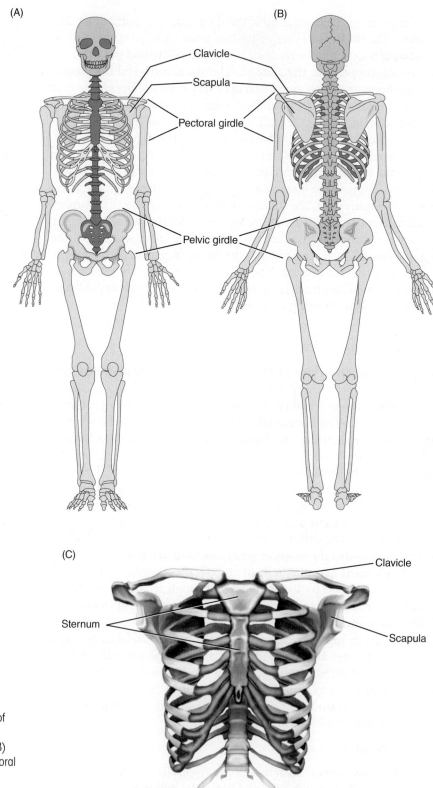

Figure 2-12. (A) Anterior view of skeleton, showing components of pelvic and pectoral girdles. (B) Posterior view. (C) Isolated pectoral girdle. (continues).

© Cengage Learning®.

(D)

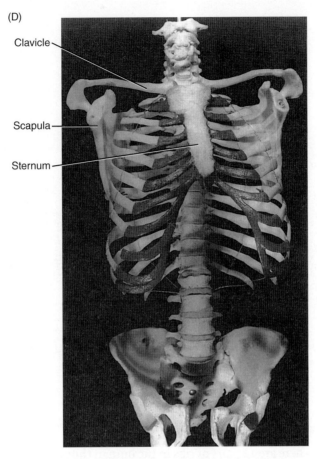

Clavicle

Scapula

Sternum

PELVIC AND PECTORAL GIRDLES

Figure 2-12 continued.
(D) Photograph of articulated thorax with pelvic and pectoral girdles.
© Cengage Learning®.

- The **pectoral girdle** is comprised of the **scapula** and **clavicle**, which attach to the **sternum**.
- These structures provide the points of attachment for the lower and upper extremities.

Ribs and Rib Cage

Anatesse Lesson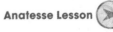

Ribs are capable of a degree of movement so that the rib cage can rock up in front and flare out via lateral rotation, being hinged on the vertebral articulation with the rib cage. The rib cage is made up of 12 ribs, with all but the lowest two attached by means of cartilage to the sternum in the front aspect. Figure 2-13 shows that the sternum provides a focal point for the rib cage, and the sternum turns out to be a significant structure in respiration.

Another thing you might notice in Figure 2-13 is that the rib cage tends to slant down in front. With the mobility of the rib cage granted by the articulation of the vertebrae and ribs, the rib cage is quite capable of elevating during inspiration to increase the size of the thorax.

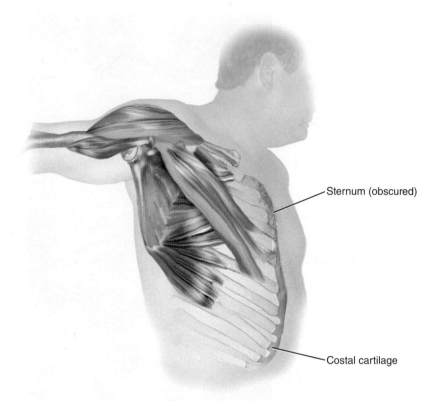

Sternum (obscured)

Costal cartilage

Figure 2-13. Lateral view of rib cage showing relationship between ribs and sternum. Note that the rib cage slants down in the front.
© Cengage Learning®.

shaft of rib: the long, relatively straight component of a rib, between the neck and the angle of the rib

angle of rib: the portion of the rib between the head and shaft, at which the direction of the rib takes an acute turn

true rib: a.k.a. vertebrosternal ribs, consisting of those ribs making direct attachment with the sternum (ribs 1 through 7)

false rib: a.k.a. vertebrochondral ribs, consisting of those ribs making indirect attachment with the sternum (ribs 8, 9 and 10)

floating rib: those ribs that do not articulate with the sternum (ribs 11 and 12)

chondral: Gr., chondros, cartilaginous

Ribs

There are 12 pairs of ribs in the human **thorax**, with each rib generally consisting of four components; the **head**, **neck**, **shaft**, and **angle** (see Figure 2-14). The head provides the articulating surfaces with the spinal column, and the angle represents the point at which the rib begins the significant curve in its course forward. The barrel shape of the thorax is created by the relatively small superior and inferior ribs as compared to the longer middle ribs. The rib cage provides attachment for numerous muscles that provide strength, rigidity, continuity, and mobility to the rib cage.

Ribs are of three general classes: **true ribs**, **false ribs**, and **floating ribs**. The true (or vertebrosternal) ribs consist of the upper ribs (1 through 7), all of which form a more or less direct attachment with the sternum. Their actual attachment is by means of a cartilaginous union through the **chondral** (i.e., cartilaginous) portion of the rib (see Figure 2-15). The false, or vertebrochondral, ribs (ribs 8, 9, and 10) are also attached to the sternum by means of cartilage, although this chondral portion must run superiorly to attach to the sternum. The floating or vertebral ribs (ribs 11 and 12) articulate only with the vertebral column.

While we like to think of the rib cage as being constant and consistent across humans, it is not really. Most of us have 12 pairs of ribs, but fully 8 percent of adults will reveal a 13th rib. That 8 percent is in good company, as both chimpanzees and gorillas sport the full complement of 13 ribs. Similarly, 1 percent of the human population may have neck ribs attached to the cervical vertebrae. This rare

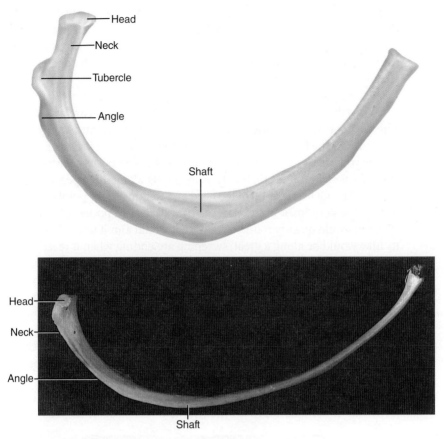

Figure 2-14. Schematic of second rib with landmarks.
© Cengage Learning®.

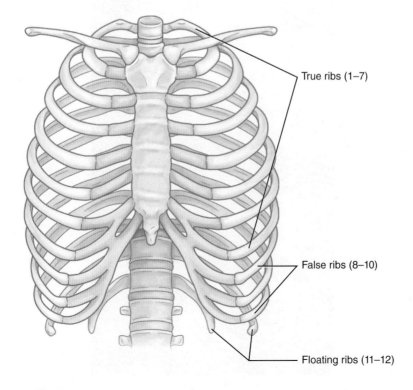

Figure 2-15. Schematic of relationships among true, false, and floating ribs.
© Cengage Learning®.

phenomenon can cause problems with the vascular supply. Similarly, the coccyx is thought to be the vestigial remnant of a mammalian tail.

The elastic properties of cartilage permit the ribs to be twisted on the long axis (torqued) without breaking. Thus, the rib cage is quite strong (being made up predominantly of bone), but capable of movement (being well endowed with resilient cartilage).

The rib cage gives significant protection to the heart and lungs. The rib cage also provides the basis for respiration, and the general structure of the barrel deserves some attention at this juncture.

As you can see in Figure 2-16, the ribs make their posterior attachment along the vertebral column. If a fly were to walk along the superior surface of a rib, starting from the tip of the head and walking to the point of attachment at the sternum, it would start out by walking in a posterolateral direction, but would quickly round a curve that would aim it toward the front. Its hike would be along a great, sweeping arc ending when it reached the cartilaginous portion of the sternal attachment. In short, the rib's course—running posterolateral and then arching around to the anterior aspect of the body—provides the bony structure for most of the posterior, lateral, and anterior aspects of the thorax. In addition, the fly would have hiked downhill, because the ribs slope downward when the rib cage is inactive and at equilibrium. The beauty of the rib cage, the vertebral attachments, and the chondral (cartilaginous) portion of the sternal attachment is that the rib cage can elevate, providing an increase in lung capacity for respiration.

The posterior attachment of the rib is made through a gliding (arthrodial) articulation with the thoracic vertebrae, thus permitting

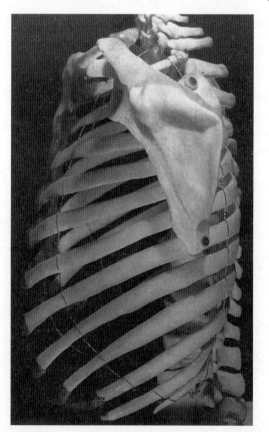

Figure 2-16. Lateral view of the rib cage. The downward tilt of the rib cage in front provides one of the mechanisms for increasing the volume of the thorax during respiration.
© Cengage Learning®.

the rib to rock up in both lateral and anterior aspects during inspiration. As mentioned, most of the ribs actually attach to two vertebrae.

Sternum

The sternum has three components: the **manubrium sterni**, the **corpus** (body), and the **xiphoid** or **ensiform** process (see Figure 2-17). The sternum has articular cavities for costal attachment, with the manubrium sterni providing the attachment for the clavicle and first rib, and the second rib articulating at the juncture of the manubrium and corpus, known as the **manubrosternal angle**. The corpus provides articulation for five more ribs by means of relatively direct costal cartilage, and the remaining (false) ribs 8, 9, and 10 are attached by means of more indirect costal cartilage.

manubrium sterni: L., handle of sternum

xiphoid: Gr., sword

ensiform: L., swordlike

manubrosternal angle: the point of articulation of manubrium sterni and corpus sterni

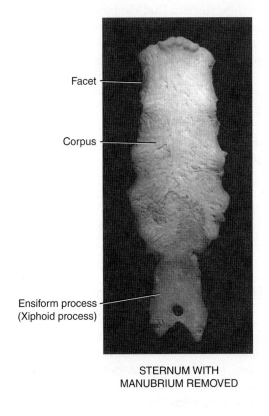

Facet

Corpus

Ensiform process
(Xiphoid process)

STERNUM WITH
MANUBRIUM REMOVED

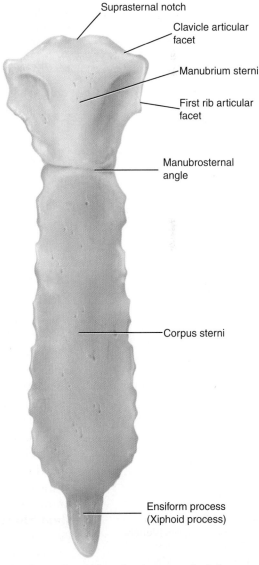

Suprasternal notch

Clavicle articular facet

Manubrium sterni

First rib articular facet

Manubrosternal angle

Corpus sterni

Ensiform process
(Xiphoid process)

Figure 2-17. Schematic and photo of sternum. Note that the manubrium has been removed from the sternum on the left.

The sternum provides an excellent opportunity to investigate anatomy with your own hands. As you look at Figure 2-17 of the sternum, you can palpate your own sternal structures. First, find your "Adam's apple" (actually, the thyroid cartilage of the larynx) and then bring your finger downward until you reach the significant plateau at about the level of your shoulders. This is the superior surface of the manubrium sterni, and is known as the **suprasternal or sternal notch**. Ignoring the tendon that you can feel on either side, palpate the bone that is directed laterally. This is the clavicle. If you can feel the place where the clavicle articulates with the manubrium, you can probably find the articulation of the first rib immediately inferior to it. If you once again find the sternal notch and draw your finger downward about two inches, you may feel a very prominent bump, which is the manubrosternal angle or junction. Now if you draw your finger downward another four or five inches, you can find the point at which the sternum and xiphoid process articulate, an important landmark for individuals performing cardiopulmonary resuscitation (CPR). You have also found the anterior-most attachment of your diaphragm.

✔ *To summarize:*

- The **rib cage** is composed of 12 ribs (7 true ribs, 3 false ribs, and 2 floating ribs).
- The **cartilaginous attachment** of the ribs to the sternum permits the ribs to rotate slightly during respiration, allowing the rib cage to elevate.
- The construction of the rib provides the characteristic curved barrel shape of the rib cage.
- At rest the ribs slope downward, but they elevate during inspiration.

Soft Tissue of the Thorax and Respiratory Passageway

Deep to the rib cage lies the core of respiration. Gas exchange for life occurs within the lungs—spongy, elastic tissue that is richly perfused with vascular supply and air sacs. Healthy, young lungs are pink, whereas older lungs that have undergone the stresses of modern, polluted life are distinctly gray. Communication between the lungs and the external environment is by means of the respiratory passageway, which includes the oral and nasal cavities, larynx, trachea, and bronchial tubes.

The **trachea** is a flexible tube, approximately 11 cm in length and composed of a series of 16 to 20 hyaline cartilage rings that are open in the posterior aspect. This tube runs from the inferior border of the larynx for about 11 cm, where it bifurcates (divides) at a point known as the **carina trachea** to become the left and right **main stem bronchi** (or **bronchial tubes**), which serve the left and right lungs, respectively (see Figure 2-18).

The tracheal rings are 2 to 2.5 cm in diameter, and 0.4 to 0.5 cm wide. They are connected by a continuous mucous membrane lining, which provides both continuity and flexibility. The ring is discontinuous in the

---

suprasternal notch: a.k.a. sternal notch. the notch on the superior aspect of the manubrium sterni

Anatesse Lesson

trachea: Gr., tracheia, rough

carina: L., keel of boat

bronchi: Gr., bronchos, windpipe

bronchial tubes: another name for mainstem bronchi, the cartilaginous tubes connecting the trachea to the lungs

Congenital Thorax Deformities

A number of congenital (present at birth) problems may occur within the thoracic wall. *Pectus excavatum* is a condition in which the sternum and costal cartilages are depressed relative to the rib cage. This depression may be bilateral or asymmetrical, providing the individual with costal flaring, a broad-but-thin chest and hook-shoulder deformity. The deformity can be repaired surgically but may reoccur, especially during the period of rapid growth in puberty. The opposite deformity, *pectus carinatum*, involves protrusion of the sternum anteriorly. Surgical repair is typically successful.

Poland's syndrome is a congenital condition in which both the pectoralis major and minor muscles are absent, and the child has fusion of the fingers or toes (syndactyly). The muscles may be partially or completely absent, and the breast is typically involved. In significantly affected individuals, the anterior portions of ribs 2 through 5 and their cartilaginous portions may be absent as well. Although the muscle cannot be restored, surgery can correct the defect of the rib cage to establish thoracic symmetry.

Cleft sternum is a rare congenital deformity that can have devastating consequences. In the simple and more benign case, the sternum has a simple cleft as a result of failure of the sternal bars during gestation. The cleft is covered with skin, and the heart and diaphragm are normal. *Ectopia cordis* is a life-threatening form of cleft sternum, in which the infant is born with the heart exposed extrathoracically. Repair of this condition is extremely difficult.

You may wish to examine the thorough discussion of these disorders in Schamberger (2000).

---

posterior aspect, allowing for increase and decrease of the diameter of the ring, an action largely controlled by the trachealis muscle. The gap between the rings is spanned by smooth muscle that is in a steady state of contraction until oxygen needs of an individual increase, at which time the muscle relaxes. That is, the tube is in a state of slight constriction until oxygen needs are sufficiently great that the muscle action is inhibited, at which time the diameter of the trachea increases to improve air delivery to the lungs. The inner mucosal lining of the trachea is infused with submucosal glands that assist in cleaning the trachea.

The cartilaginous rings of the trachea are particularly well suited for the task of air transport. Because the process involves drawing air into the lungs and expelling it, pressures (negative and positive) must be generated to get that gas moving, but pressure tends to collapse or expand tissue that is not reinforced for strength. However, a strictly rigid tube will not permit the degree of flexibility dictated by an active life (i.e., differential head and thorax movement). Thus, the trachea must be both rigid and flexible. In response to this need, the trachea is built of hyaline cartilage rings connected by fibroelastic membrane. The cartilage provides support, while the membrane permits freedom of movement.

Posterior to the trachea is the **esophagus**. The esophagus is a long, collapsed tube running parallel to and behind the trachea, providing a conduit to the digestive system. It retains its collapsed condition except when occupied with a **bolus** of food being propelled by gravity and peristaltic contractions to the waiting stomach.

The trachea bifurcates to form the right and left main stem (or main) bronchi. The right side forms a 20–30° angle relative to the trachea, and the left forms a 45–55° angle. (This explains why the

esophagus: the tube connecting the laryngopharynx with the stomach, through which food passes during swallowing

bolus: L., lump

(A)

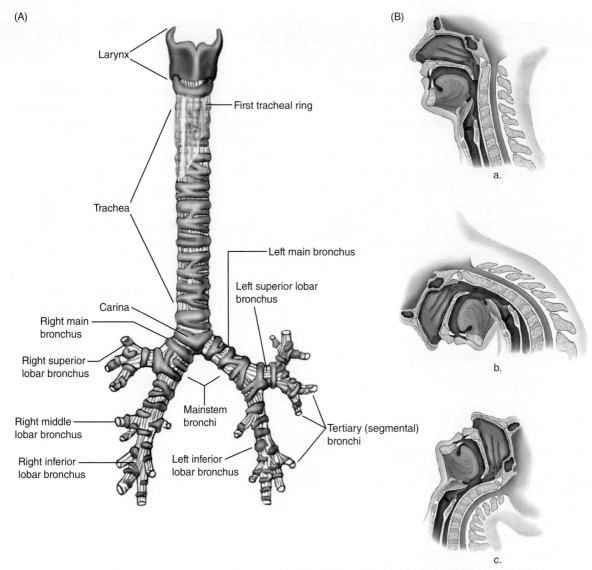

(B)

a.

b.

c.

Figure 2-18. (A) Bronchial passageway, including trachea, mainstem bronchi, secondary (lobar) bronchi, and tertiary (segmental) bronchi. (B) Effect of head posture on airway patency. (continues).
© Cengage Learning®.

right lung is most often the landing site for the errant peanut that makes it past the protective laryngeal structure.)

The lungs are a composite of blood, arterial and venous network, connective tissue, the respiratory pathway, and tissue specialized for gas exchange.

The **bronchial tree** is characterized by increasingly smaller tubes as one progresses into the depths of the lungs, but the total surface area at any given level of the tree is greater than that of the level before it. There are 14 generations of the bronchial tree in the left lung, and 28 generations in the right lung, beginning with the single trachea. The left and right main stem bronchi bifurcate off the trachea to serve the left and right lungs, respectively, while **lobar** (intermediate, secondary) bronchi supply the lobes of the lungs (see Figure 2-18).

lobar bronchi: bronchial passageways connecting the mainstem bronchi with individual lobes of the lungs

(C)

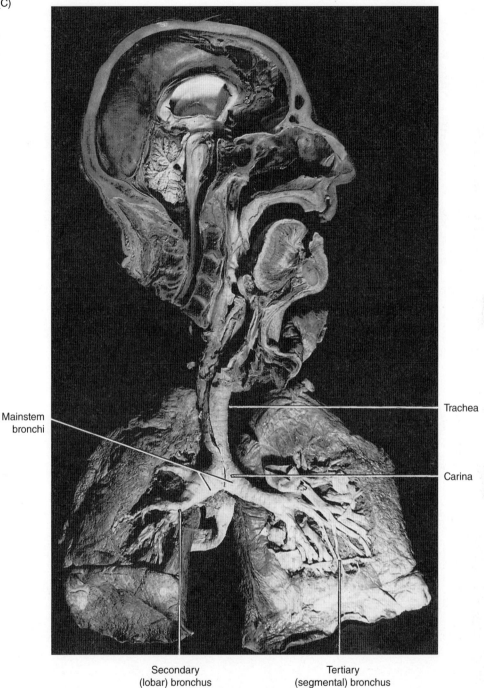

Mainstem bronchi

Trachea

Carina

Secondary (lobar) bronchus

Tertiary (segmental) bronchus

Figure 2-18 continued. (C) Respiratory passageway from oral cavity to segmental bronchi. Note that lungs have been dissected to reveal the bronchi within.

© Cengage Learning®.

Further branching occurs, down to the final **terminal respiratory bronchioles**. This division process is shown in Table 2-2 and Figure 2-19. Within the cartilaginous passageway, there are 1 trachea, 2 main stem bronchi, 5 lobar bronchi, 19 segmental bronchi, and so forth.

terminal respiratory bronchioles: the last bronchioles in the respiratory tree, connecting the respiratory tree to the alveoli

Table 2-2 Divisions of the bronchial tree

	Generation From			Number	Diameter	Cross-Section
	Trachea	Segmental Bronchus	Terminal Bronchiole			
Trachea	0			1	2.5 cm	5.0 cm^2
Main bronchi	1			2	11–19 mm	3.2 cm^2
Lobar bronchi	2–3			5	4.5–13.5	2.7 cm^2
Segmental	3–6	0		19	4.5–6.5 mm	3.2 cm^2
Subsegmental bronchi	4–7	1		38	3–6 mm	6.6 cm^2
Bronchi		2–6		Variable	Variable	Variable
Terminal bronchi		3–7		1,000	1.0 mm	7.9 cm^2
Bronchioles		5–14		Variable	Variable	Variable
Terminal bronchioles		6–15	0	35,000	0.65 mm	116 cm^2
Respiratory bronchioles			1–8	Variable	Variable	Variable
Terminal respiratory bronchioles			2–9	630,000	0.45 mm	1,000 cm^2
Alveolar ducts and sacs			4–12	14×10^6	0.40 mm	1.71 m^2
Alveoli				300×10^6	0.24–0.3 mm	70 m^2

From *Respiratory Emergencies* by K. M. Moser & R. G. Spragg. 1982. p. 15. St. Louis, MO: C. V. Mosby. Copyright 1982 C. V. Mosby Co. Reprinted with permission.

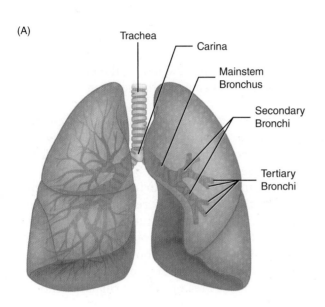

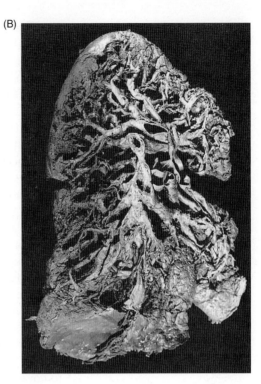

Figure 2-19. (A) Bronchial tree. (B) Lung dissected to reveal bronchial passageway.
© Cengage Learning®.

Nanotechnology and the Body

As technology advances, our susceptibility to design errors increases. Nanotechnology is the field involved in the production of nanoscale devices that include micromotors, molecule-sized robots, and chemical delivery systems. The nanoscale devices are proliferating as production abilities develop, but there remain questions about the body's response to them. The fact that the lungs are not capable of eliminating pollutants that are very small has prompted research into the impact of airborne nanoscale particles on respiration.

Recent evidence indicates that the effects of nanoscale particles may extend to the vascular supply as well. We know that particulate pollution from automobiles in the 2.5 micrometer (called PM2.5 particles, or 2.5 parts per million) range is related to increases in heart disease. Recent evidence reveals that particles 1/10 the size (PM0.25) cause increases in the buildup of atherosclerotic plaque.

These particles enter the lungs as pollution and, because of their minute size, are able to enter the blood stream. There they act like "cement," closing off the arteries of the vascular system. While the causal link has only been proven in mice (Araujo et al., 2008) there remains the distinct probability that what you cannot see will hurt you. That having been said, dust-level products have existed for some time (e.g., erionite and quartz dust), and much research is needed into the nature of their toxicology as well (Donaldson & Seaton, 2012).

On the flip side of the "nano-coin" is use of the technology as filters. Nanoscale materials are being developed that absorb specific toxins within the body and are being designed to greatly enhance our ability to image cancer and even to treat diseases (Sargent, 2011). Nanoscale technology has the potential for being an exceptionally powerful societal force in the coming years.

The lobar or secondary divisions serve the lobes of the lungs. The right lung is composed of three lobes, separated by fissures. The left lung has only two lobes (see Figure 2-19). Space on the left is taken up by the heart and **mediastinal** or "middle space" structures. The right main stem bronchus divides to supply the superior, middle, and inferior lobes of the right lung. The left main stem bronchus bifurcates to serve the superior and inferior lobes of the left lung, although there is a vestigial middle lobe (called the *lingula*). The space of the missing lobe is taken up by the heart on the left side (see Figure 2-20).

The third level of branching serves the segments of each lobe. At this third level of division, the bronchi divide repeatedly into smaller and smaller cartilaginous tubes, with the final tube being the **terminal** (end) **bronchiole** (see Figure 2-21).

This repeated branching has an important effect on respiratory function. Examination of Table 2-2 reveals that there are 28 generations of subdivisions in the respiratory tree, providing a truly amazing amount of surface area for respiration. Although the cross-sectional area of the trachea is about 5 cm^2 (about the size of a quarter), the cross-sectional area of the 300,000,000 alveoli would equal 70 m^2, or the area of a throw rug large enough to cover a 10 × 24 room.

The first nine divisions of the bronchial tree are strictly conductive and cartilaginous, being designed only to transport gas between the environment and the lungs. Successive divisions of the noncartilaginous airway reach a minimal diameter of 1 mm. This conducting zone, which includes the conducting regions of both the upper and lower respiratory tracts and terminates with the terminal bronchioles, makes up approximately 150 mL in the adult, a volume known as *dead air* because air that does not descend below the space cannot undergo gas exchange with the blood.

The final seven divisions are actual respiratory zones comprised of the respiratory bronchioles, alveolar ducts, and alveoli. The respiratory bronchioles ("little bronchi") are the terminal bronchioles, serving the alveoli.

The terminal bronchiole is small (about 1 mm in diameter) and at its end becomes the alveolar duct, which in turn communicates with the alveolus. The alveoli are extremely small (approximately 1/4 mm in diameter) but extremely plentiful, with approximately 300 million in the mature lungs.

You might think of the final respiratory exchange region as a series of apartment houses. As you can see in Figure 2-21, the respiratory bronchioles are the entryways for each apartment building, and the alveolar duct is the passageway to the individual "apartment," the alveolus. Each of these alveoli is between 200 and 300 microns in diameter, which is quite small because a micron is one thousandth of a millimeter. Put another way, you could place five alveoli in the space between the millimeter marks on your ruler and 8 within the "o" in alveoli.

(A)

Right lung		Left lung	
Superior lobe		Superior lobe	
Apical	1	Upper division	
Posterior	2	Apical/Posterior	1 & 2
Anterior	3	Anterior	3
Middle lobe		Lower division (lingular)	
Lateral	4	Superior lingula	4
Medial	5	Inferior lingula	5
Inferior lobe		Inferior lobe	
Superior	6	Superior	6
Medial basal	7	Anterior medial basal	7 & 8
Anterior basal	8	Lateral basal	9
Lateral basal	9	Posterior basal	10
Posterior basal	10		

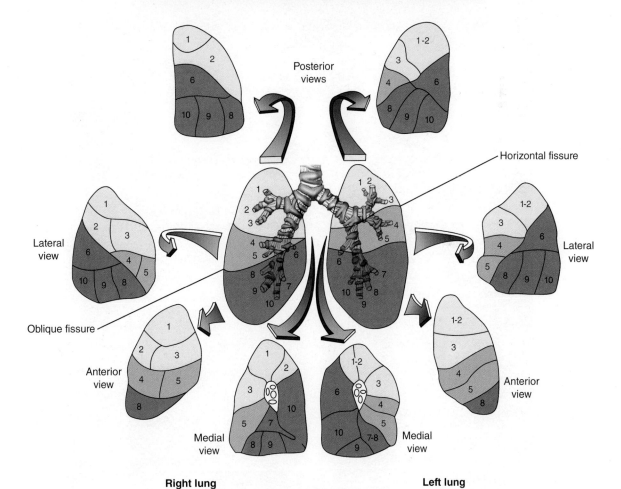

Figure 2-20. (A) Schematic representation of lungs, showing lobes and segments. (continues).
© Cengage Learning®.

(B)

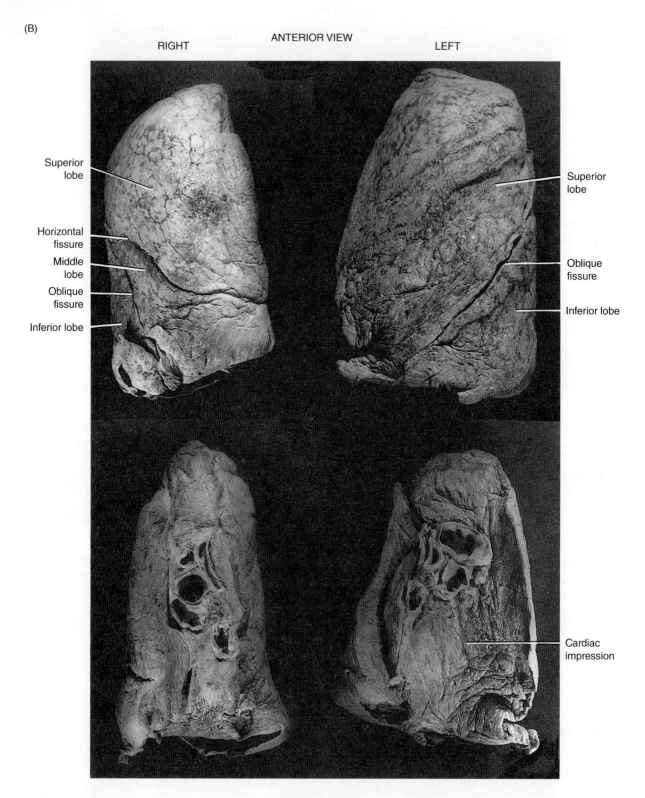

ANTERIOR VIEW

RIGHT   LEFT

Superior
lobe

Superior
lobe

Horizontal
fissure

Middle
lobe

Oblique
fissure

Oblique
fissure

Inferior lobe

Inferior lobe

Cardiac
impression

MEDIAL VIEW

Figure 2-20 continued. (B) Anterior and medial view of lungs. (continues).

(C)

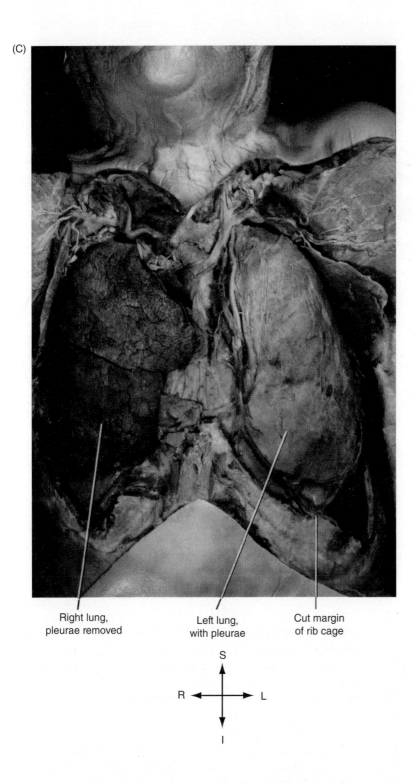

Right lung,
pleurae removed

Left lung,
with pleurae

Cut margin
of rib cage

S

R ← → L

I

Figure 2-20 continued.
(C) Anterior view of lungs in situ.
Note that the pleural lining has
been removed from the right lung,
while it remains on the left lung.
© Cengage Learning®.

This "apartment house" analogy will serve you as you read about
the devastating effects of emphysema on respiration. Among other
things, emphysema removes the "walls" within individual "apart-
ments," greatly reducing the surface area available for participation
in gas exchange.

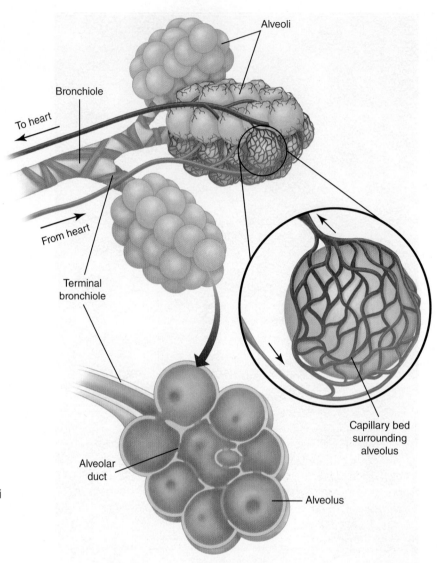

Figure 2-21. Schematic representation of cluster of alveoli with capillary bed. Lower portion shows a cross-section through alveoli and terminal bronchiole.
© Cengage Learning®.

The alveoli at this terminal point do the real work of respiration by virtue of their architecture and relationship with the vascular supply (see Figure 2-21). The alveolar lining is made up of two types of cells, Type I and Type II pneumocytes. Type I pneumocytes (membranous pneumocytes) are flat cells that are directly involved in gas exchange. Type II cells (cuboidal cells) are the source of the surfactant, a substance that reduces surface tension, which is released into the alveolus to alter the surface tension to keep the alveoli from collapsing during respiration. When Type I cells are damaged, Type II cells will proliferate, becoming Type I cells in a regenerative process. The rich investment with alveoli makes the lungs spongy, because the surfactant at that level promotes inflation of the alveoli.

Each alveolus is richly supplied with blood for gas exchange from more than 2,000 capillaries. A little multiplication will reveal that there are more than 600,000,000,000 (600 billion) capillaries involved

Keeping the Airway Open in Respiratory Emergency

In times of respiratory emergency, it sometimes becomes necessary to ensure that the respiratory pathway remains patent (open). In a conscious patient, the normal head and neck orientation places the mouth at a 90° angle with the airway above the larynx (pharynx). If an unconscious individual's head drops forward (see Figure 2-18B), the airway may become occluded and limit respiration.

In some cases, there may be concern that the vocal folds or airway above the larynx will not remain open, so an emergency tracheostomy will be performed (*trachea*, trachea; *stoma*, mouth). This medical procedure involves opening an artificial passageway into the trachea, typically 1–3 cm below the cricoid cartilage.

Gastroesophageal Reflux

The esophageal orifice is situated in the inferior laryngopharynx and is enveloped by the musculature of the inferior pharyngeal constrictors. The cricopharyngeus muscle, which is actually part of the inferior constrictor, controls the size of the orifice by contracting to constrict the opening.

Gastroesophageal reflux refers to the reintroduction of gastrointestinal contents into the esophagus and respiratory passageway. This condition may be found in the newborn and very young child who has a weak esophageal sphincter or hypersensitivity of the esophageal sphincter, resulting in reflux, inability to retain nourishment, and life-threatening malnutrition. It is not uncommon among children with cerebral palsy, typically resulting in frequent vomiting, loss of nutrition, and aspiration pneumonia (see clinical note on aspiration).

The size of the esophageal opening may be reduced surgically through a procedure known as

Nissen fundoplication ("sling"), thereby inhibiting regurgitation of stomach contents. Nissen fundoplication involves surgical narrowing of the esophageal opening by releasing a flap of tissue from the stomach, followed by elevation and suturing of the flap to the esophageal orifice. The individual may receive nutrition through a tube run through the nasal cavity into the esophagus (nasogastric tube; naso = nose; gastric = stomach) or through orogastric feeding (oral feeding a.k.a. "gavage") again via tube.

Surgical placement of a gastronomy tube may be required if reflux cannot be controlled adequately to guarantee nutrition. This procedure, referred to as "gastronomy," results in surgical placement of a feeding tube into the stomach wall. Similarly, "jejunostomy" is the placement of a feeding tube into the small intestine. For a more detailed discussion of these problems in cerebral palsy, see Langley and Lombardino (1991).

in gas exchange, reminding us of the amount of vascular tissue in the lungs. The lungs also have an intricate lacework of cartilage, because the bronchial tree is invested with this supportive tissue, and because most of the levels of branching of this tree contain cartilage.

The alveolar wall is extraordinarily thin, ranging from 0.35 to 2.5 microns (by comparison, a red blood cell is 7 microns in diameter), and this quality promotes rapid transfer of gas across the membrane. The capillaries in the lungs are the most dense in the body, being approximately 10 microns long and 7 microns wide. Their extremely small size and prolific presence permit 100 to 300 mL of blood to be

Aspiration

Although not directly related to respiratory anatomy or physiology, aspiration *is* an issue in maintaining respiratory function. *Aspiration* refers to entry of liquid or solid materials into the lungs. Fluids or solids may enter the lungs as a result of some failure in strength, coordination, sensation, or awareness. Patients who are intubated to support respiration during crisis are *also* at risk for aspiration because the airway is artificially kept open. Vomitus or reflux from the stomach (logically via the esophageal opening at the level of the larynx) readily enters the unprotected lungs through the larynx. To prevent aspiration of foreign matter into the lungs, the endotracheal tube is surrounded by an inflatable cuff. This cuff completely seals off the airway above the tube. When the cuff is to be removed, the area above the cuff can be suctioned to remove any material that may be lodged in the airway. Aspiration of foreign matter into the lungs is a very real danger in cases of neurological deficit, and an individual who has had a stroke, or who has cerebral palsy or another compromising condition, is particularly vulnerable. The patient may demonstrate diminished or ineffective (nonproductive) cough, as well as reduced muscular strength and control of the muscles of deglutition, and perhaps diminished ability to recognize the threat involved. In children with cerebral palsy, reduction in coordinated movement ability may also arise from the neurological deficit.

Because the client with neurological deficit may not be aware or competent to seek help, it is wise to know the signs of aspiration. If the client's voice sounds wet or gurgly, or if the client has a history of respiratory illnesses, the client is at risk for aspiration pneumonia. Likewise, the client may have a weak, breathy vocalization or cry, indicating laryngeal muscle weakness and the potential for lack of adequate protective function.

---

pulmonary: L., pulmonarius, pertaining to the lungs

spread over 70 square meters of surface. Moser and Spragg (1982) note that this is the equivalent of spreading one teaspoon of blood over a square meter of surface.

During normal quiet respiration, the blood spends only about half a second in the capillaries, with gas exchange occurring within the first quarter of its transit through the pulmonary system. The **pulmonary** artery branches to follow the bronchial tree, ultimately serving the gas exchange process at the alveolar level. There is a parallel vascular supply to oxygenate the lung tissue (the bronchial arteries). The maintenance of lung tissue via the bronchial arteries requires only about 50 mL of blood per minute, whereas the pulmonary system will process approximately 5000 mL per minute.

The bronchial tree and trachea are obvious conduits for contaminants as well as air. The nasal and oral passageways provide some protection from respiratory contamination, but nature has not caught up with the heavily polluted modern society (Shaffer & Rengasomy, 2009). The respiratory pathway has multiple filtering functions to safeguard the lungs against pollutants. The nostril hairs provide a first line of defense, catching most particulate matter greater than 10 microns (a micron is one millionth of a meter) before it enters the trachea. The moist mucous membrane of the upper respiratory system provides another receptacle for foreign matter. Goblet cells within the mucosal lining and submucosal glands secrete lubricant into the respiratory tract to trap pollutants as they enter the trachea and larynx. The respiratory passageway from the nose to the beginning of the bronchi is lined with

Protection Against Trauma

The lungs are obviously important for life function and are designed with damage control in mind. The two lungs are encased in separate pleural linings, so that if one lung is penetrated by an object (such as happens when a lung is punctured by a broken rib), the other lung will continue to function. Likewise, the segmented nature of lungs is a protective device. If a lung is punctured, the extremely rich vascular bed will cause significant and dangerous bleeding. The segmented nature of the lungs provides some protection against total lung failure: Bleeding in one segment is confined to that segment, at least until the bronchial tree is filled with blood.

Blast trauma is a different story, unfortunately. The concussive forces of explosions put an overpressure on the respiratory system, causing a condition known as blast lung (pulmonary barotrauma). Essentially, the overpressure can cause hemorrhaging of the vascular supply and rupturing of the alveoli (Cernak & Noble-Haeusslein, 2010).

tall columnar epithelium covered by **cilia** (hairlike processes) that beat more than 1,000 times per minute. In the lower pathway, the beating action drives pollutants upward and posteriorly.

The beating epithelia progressively move the material up the bronchi to the level of the vocal folds in the larynx, at which time the individual feels the stimulation of secretion at the vocal folds and clears the throat. That "ahem" creates just enough force to blow the mucus off the folds (**mucus** is the dense fluid product of mucous membrane tissue), where it can be swallowed without further ado. Unfortunately, these beating epithelia may be damaged by pollutants such as cigarette smoke, resulting in failure of this system. Particles in the 2 to 10 micron range will settle on the walls of the bronchi, where they will be eliminated by these beating epithelia. If a particle is less than 2 microns, it will generally reach the alveolus.

The lymphatic system provides a final cleaning stage for the respiratory tissue. Particles not eliminated by the beating epithelia are removed by means of the lymphatic system, which serves even the minute terminal bronchiole. Pollutants are suspended in mucus and migrate to the bronchioles through coughing, where they can be eliminated by the lymphatic system.

The respiratory passageway also protects the lungs by warming and humidifying the air as it enters. Cold air reduces the ability of the lungs to exchange gasses, and the lower humidity of cold air dries the delicate alveolar tissue, reducing mobility and making the tissues more susceptible to infection. The mucous membrane is highly vascularized, permitting rapid transfer of heat from blood to air.

✔ *To summarize:*

- A critical organ of the respiratory systems is the **lungs**, the right and left lung having three and two **lobes** respectively.
- Communication between the external and internal environments is by means of the **trachea** and **bronchial tree**.
- Repeated subdivisions of this bronchial tree end with the **alveoli**, the site of gas exchange.

Emphysema

Emphysema is generally considered to be a product of a modern society that has not solved its pollution problems. Often the disease results from tobacco smoking, but it may also arise from living in an industrial environment. Its progression is slow and may be arrested to some degree by altering the respiratory environment by, for example, eliminating smoke and other pollutants.

The overwhelming cause of emphysema in modern society is smoking cigarettes, although it is not the only source. Alpha-1 antitrypsin deficiency, an inherited disorder, can result in the absence of an enzyme that regulates lung cleansing. The result is a form of self-destruction wherein the cleansing mechanism destroys the lung tissue. You will recall that the bronchial passageway is lined with ciliated epithelia that beat continuously to remove contaminants from the respiratory tract. This continuous waste removal process is seriously hampered by pollutants that, in the early stages of emphysema, destroy the cilia. The mechanism for emphysema appears to be as follows.

The absence of cilia greatly reduces the cleaning ability of the respiratory system and hampers the removal of waste products, promoting deposition of pollutants within the alveoli. The alveoli undergo a significant morphological (form) change: The walls of the alveoli break down and alveoli recombine so that clusters of alveoli become a single sac. Although this may seem benign, it has a devastating effect in that the surface area for gas exchange is greatly reduced.

A second morphological change arises as a compensation for the first. An individual with emphysema is faced with a continuous shortage of oxygen and is forced to attempt continually deeper inspirations to compensate, and a characteristic "barrel chest" results from these excessive efforts. (The thorax must be greatly expanded to accommodate the compromised alveolar surface area.)

This second morphological change causes a third pathological response. You will recall that the lower margin of the rib cage marks the point of attachment of the diaphragm. Because the rib cage is flared out due to emphysema, contraction of the diaphragm (which pulls on the rib cage) causes the rib cage to pull down and in medially, which actually *reduces* the size of the thorax rather than increasing it.

The final change arising from this triad of tragedies is respiratory failure. The respiratory mechanism is highly compromised, leaving the individual susceptible to respiratory diseases such as pneumonia.

- These highly vascularized alveoli provide the mechanism by which oxygen enters and carbon dioxide exits the bloodstream.
- Pollutants entering the respiratory tract are removed through the cleansing action of the **beating epithelia** that line the bronchial passageway.

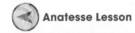

Anatesse Lesson

vertical dimension (of thoracic expansion): the superior-inferior dimension of thorax movement, generated by contraction of the diaphragm

MOVEMENT OF AIR THROUGH THE SYSTEM

The lung tissue is particularly prepared to process the gasses of life by virtue of its construction. Such great design, however, would be useless without a mechanism for taking air into and out of the lungs.

We have already discussed the mechanics of the system, so you should be familiar with the idea that the lungs expand as a result of enlargement of the structure surrounding them. We contract the diaphragm to enlarge the **vertical dimension** (superior-inferior dimension) and elevate the rib cage to enlarge the **transverse dimension** (antero-posterior and lateral dimensions). You might be curious about *how* these changes cause the lungs to expand. The key is having a closed system.

You will recall that the cavity holding the lungs is supported by muscle and bone that cover every centimeter of the thoracic wall. Likewise, the bottom of the thoracic cavity is completely sealed by the diaphragm, making the thorax almost impervious to the outside world, were it not for the respiratory passageway. The only way air can enter or leave the lungs is by means of the tubes connected to them (the bronchial tree, continuous with the upper respiratory passageway).

Now comes the tricky part. The lungs are simply placed inside this cavity, not held to the walls by ligaments or cartilage. It is as if you placed a too-small sponge in a too-large bottle, because the thoracic volume is *greater* than that of the lungs at rest.

The lungs and inner thoracic wall are each completely covered with a **pleural lining** (Figure 2-22) that provides a means of smooth contact for rough tissue, as well as a mechanism for translating the force of thorax enlargement into inspiration. The lungs are encased in linings referred to as the **visceral pleurae** and the thoracic linings are the **parietal pleurae**. The regions of the parietal pleurae are identified by location: mediastinal, pericardial, diaphragmatic, parietal, and apical pleurae. The **mediastinal pleura** covers the mediastinum and the **diaphragmatic pleura** covers the diaphragm. The **costal pleurae** cover the inner surface of the rib cage. The **apical pleurae** cover the superior-most region of the rib cage.

transverse dimension of thorax expansion: the antero-posterior and lateral dimensional expansion of the thorax generated by contraction of the accessory muscles of inspiration

pleural: Gr., pleura, a side

visceral pleurae: pleural lining encasing the lungs

parietal pleurae: pleural linings of the thoracic cavity

mediastinal pleura: parietal pleural lining covering the mediastinum

diaphragmatic pleurae: parietal pleural lining covering the diaphragm

costal: L., costae, coast

apical pleurae: parietal pleural linings covering the lung superior aspect

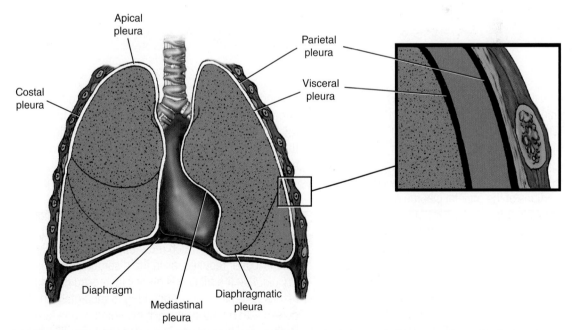

Figure 2-22. Pleural linings of the lungs and thorax. Parietal pleurae include costal, diaphragmatic, mediastinal, and apical pleurae. Visceral pleurae line the surface of the lungs.
© Cengage Learning®.

venules: L., venula, tiny veins

The pleural membranes are composed of elastic and fibrous tissue and are endowed with **venules** and lymphocytes. Although it is convenient to think of the pleural linings as being separate entities, the visceral and parietal pleurae are actually continuous with each other. These wrappings completely encase both the lungs and the inner thorax, with the reflection point being the hilum (root of lung, at about the level of T4 or T5). This continuous sheet provides the airtight seal required to permit the lungs to follow the movement of the thorax.

Understanding how these pleura help us breathe will take a little thought. You have probably experienced the difficulty involved in separating two pieces of plastic food wrap, especially if there is fluid between the two sheets. There is a degree of surface tension arising from the presence of fluid and highly conforming surfaces that helps keep the sheets together. Cuboidal cells within the pleural lining produce a mucous solution that is released in the space between the parietal and visceral pleurae. This surfactant reduces the surface tension in the lungs and provides a slippery interface between the lungs and the thoracic wall, permitting easy, low-friction gliding of the lungs within the thorax. The presence of surfactant keeps the two sheets from clinging to each other. The two surfaces conform to each other as a result of the fluid bond between them, and a negative pressure is maintained by lack of contact with the outside atmosphere. (If you puncture the membrane, the bond is broken.)

diaphragm: the primary, unpaired muscle of respiration that completely separates abdomen and thorax

We have discussed the lungs and hinted at the second most important muscle of the body (the diaphragm), but have glossed over the fact that the most important muscle of the body (the heart) is located

Pleurisy

Pleurisy is a condition in which the pleural linings of the thoracic cavity are inflamed. When the inflammation results in "dry pleurisy," the patient will experience extreme pain upon breathing as a result of the loss of lubricating quality of the intrapleural fluid. "Adhesions" may result, in which portions of the parietal pleurae adhere to the visceral pleurae. (The patient may experience "breaking up" of these adhesions for quite some time following his or her bout with pleurisy.) Pleurisy may be unilateral or bilateral and may result in excessive fluid (potentially purulent) in the pleural space.

When you contract the **diaphragm**, the pleural lining of the diaphragm maintains its contact with the visceral pleurae of the two lungs above it, causing the lungs to expand. Likewise, if you expand the thorax transversely by elevating the rib cage, you will find that the lungs will follow faithfully. In this manner, the lungs are able to follow the action of the muscles without actually being attached to them.

The pleural linings serve another function as well. Because the mating surfaces of the two linings are infused with a serous secretion, the friction of movement of the two linings is greatly reduced, making respiration much more efficient. When this fluid is lost or reduced, as in the disorder known as *dry pleurisy*, the friction is greatly increased and pain results. As a protection, each lung is separately endowed with a pleural lining. If the lining of one lung is damaged through disease or trauma, we still have the other lung in reserve.

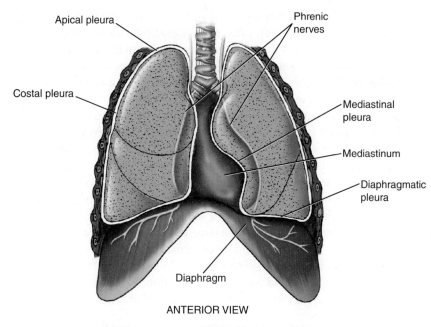

Apical pleura

Phrenic nerves

Costal pleura

Mediastinal pleura

Mediastinum

Diaphragmatic pleura

Diaphragm

ANTERIOR VIEW

Figure 2-23. Relationship among pleural linings of mediastinum, diaphragm, and lungs. Note the phrenic nerve innervation of the diaphragm.
© Cengage Learning®.

deep within the thorax, in a region known as the **mediastinum**. The heart is encased in the mediastinal pleurae, along with nerves, blood vessels, lymphatic vessels, and the esophagus (see Figure 2-23).

The mediastinum is the most protected region of the body. This space is occupied primarily by the heart, as well as by the trachea, the major blood vessels, nerves, the thymus gland, lymph nodes, and the conducting portion of the gastrointestinal tract known as the esophagus.

The mediastinum lies deep to the bony thorax and its muscular coverings and is nestled deep in the lungs. Its central location in the body betrays its importance to all regions, and its critical placement surrounded by lung tissue guarantees efficient transfer of gas to (and from) the blood pumped by the heart.

Because the heart is such an important muscle, it is located deep within several layers of thick muscle and bone. In the posterior are the vertebrae and the massive muscles of the back, and the antero-lateral aspect of the thorax is a strong wall of bone and muscle. The heart is well protected against most trauma, with the exception of romantic disappointment!

The organs and structures of the mediastinum are encased by a continuation of the parietal pleurae. This lining provides a low-friction mating surface between the lungs and the middle space. The visceral pleural lining of the lungs adjacent to the mediastinum is termed the *mediastinal pleurae*. The left and right phrenic nerves serving the diaphragm pass anterior to the root structures of the lungs, coursing along the lateral surfaces of the pericardium (the membranous sac enclosing the heart) to innervate the diaphragm. The left and right vagus nerves enter the posterior mediastinum to innervate the heart, first passing behind the root structures of the lung, coursing inferiorly to the anterior and posterior surfaces

mediastinum: L., medius, middle

hiatus: L., an opening

of the esophagus. They descend through the diaphragm adjacent to the esophagus through the esophageal **hiatus** to innervate the abdominal viscera. The vagal pulmonary branches provide a parasympathetic nerve supply for the lungs, with nerve fibers found even in the smallest bronchioles. The vagus mediates the cough reflex and control of the airway diameter.

Movement of the rib cage for inspiration requires muscular effort. Muscles of respiration may be divided into muscles of inspiration and expiration (see Table 2-3). Before delving into these muscles, we should give you a word of caution. The primary muscles of respiration are relatively easy to identify, but we will inevitably make some assumptions about function of secondary muscle groups based on muscle attachment. It is also wise to explain at the start that expiration can be either forced or passive but is much more often a passive process. Thus, the muscles of expiration are not always active and depend on some other forces to help us eliminate carbon dioxide–laden air. A second, very important note is that *identification of origin and insertion are determined by function.* Remember that our

Table 2-3 Muscles of respiration

Inspiration	Expiration
Muscles of Trunk	**Muscles of Trunk**
Primary of thorax	**Muscles of thorax, back, and upper limb anterior**
Diaphragm	Internal intercostal (interosseous portion)
Accessory of thorax Anterior	Transversus thoracis
External intercostal	**Posterior**
Interchondral portion, Internal Intercostal	Subcostal
Posterior	Serratus posterior inferior
Levatores costarum (brevis and longis)	Innermost intercostal
Serratus posterior superior	Latissimus dorsi
Muscles of Neck	**Abdominal Muscles Anterolateral**
Sternocleidomastoid (superficial neck)	Transversus abdominis
Scalenus (anterior, middle, posterior)	Internal oblique abdominis
Trapezius	External oblique abdominis
Muscles of thorax, back, and upper limb	Rectus abdominis
Pectoralis major	**Posterior**
Pectoralis minor	Quadratus lumborum
Serratus anterior	
Subclavius	
Levator scapulae	
Rhomboideus major	
Rhomboideus minor	

speech mechanisms are built on nonspeech functions: sometimes we use muscles for speech in a manner that is different from the basic function, which means that *the origin and insertion may be different from what you might find in basic anatomy texts.* This reality reflects just how ingenious we humans have been at making the basic human physiology work for speech, language, and hearing.

✔ *To summarize:*

- The lungs are covered with **pleural linings**, which, in conjunction with the thoracic wall, provide the mechanism for air movement through muscular action.
- When the diaphragm contracts, the lungs are pulled down because of the association between the pleurae and the diaphragm.
- **Diaphragmatic contraction** expands the lungs, drawing air into them through the bronchial passageway.
- Origins and insertions are based on the function of the muscle as used for speech, and this may be at odds with classical anatomy.

MUSCLES OF INSPIRATION

As with many voluntary bodily functions, inspiration is a graded activity. Depending on the needs of your body, you are capable of **quiet inspiration**, which involves primarily the diaphragm, and **forced inspiration**, which calls on many more muscles. We enlist the help of increasingly larger numbers of muscles as our respiratory needs increase. You may wish to refer to Appendix C for a summary of the muscles of respiration.

If the lungs are to expand and fill with air, the thorax must increase in size as well. As mentioned, there are only two ways this can happen. The first way to expand the thorax is to increase its vertical (superior-inferior) dimension, a process that occurs for both quiet and forced inspiration. First, picture the lungs encased in bone around the barrel-shaped midsection of the rib cage and bounded above by the clavicle and first rib. Remember that the rib cage is open at the bottom.

A thin but strong muscle placed across the bottom margin of the rib cage, configured like a drum-head, would be an economical means of expanding the size of the rib cage without having to manipulate the bony portion at all. The thorax and abdominal cavity below are separated by one of the most important muscles of the body, the diaphragm.

The diaphragm takes the form of an inverted bowl, with its attachments along the lower margin of the rib cage, sternum, and vertebral column. It forms a complete separation between the upper (thoracic) and lower (abdominal) chambers, and when it contracts, the force of contraction is directed downward toward the abdominal

Anatesse Lesson

quiet inspiration: inspiration that involves minimal muscular activity, primarily that of the diaphragm

forced inspiration: inspiration that involves both diaphragm and accessory muscles of inspiration

viscera. This contraction results in elongation of the cavity formed by the ribs, so that the lungs expand and air enters through the respiratory passageway.

Primary Inspiratory Muscle of Thorax

Diaphragm

The primary muscle of inspiration is the diaphragm. As seen in Figure 2-24, the diaphragm completely separates the abdominal and thoracic cavities (with the exception of vascular and esophageal hiatuses). The edges attach along the inferior boundary of the rib cage, to the xiphoid process, and to the vertebral column in the posterior aspect. The intermediate region is made up of a large, leafy aponeurosis called the **central tendon**. When the muscle contracts, muscle fibers shorten and the diaphragm pulls the central tendon down and forward. Let us look at this extremely important muscle in detail.

The muscle fibers of the diaphragm radiate from the central tendon, forming the sternal, costal, and vertebral attachments. The anterior-most sternal attachment is made at the xiphoid process, with fibers coursing up and back to insert into the anterior central

central tendon: large aponeurosis making up the central portion of the diaphragm

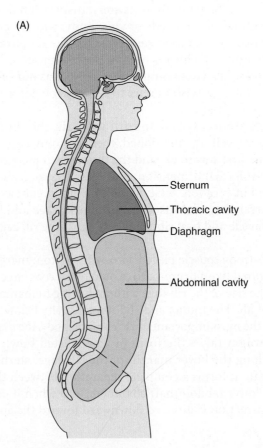

(A)

Sternum

Thoracic cavity

Diaphragm

Abdominal cavity

Figure 2-24. (A) Lateral-view schematic of the diaphragm and thorax. Notice that the diaphragm courses markedly down from the sternum to the vertebral attachment, completely separating the thorax from the abdomen. (continues).

© Cengage Learning®.

(B)

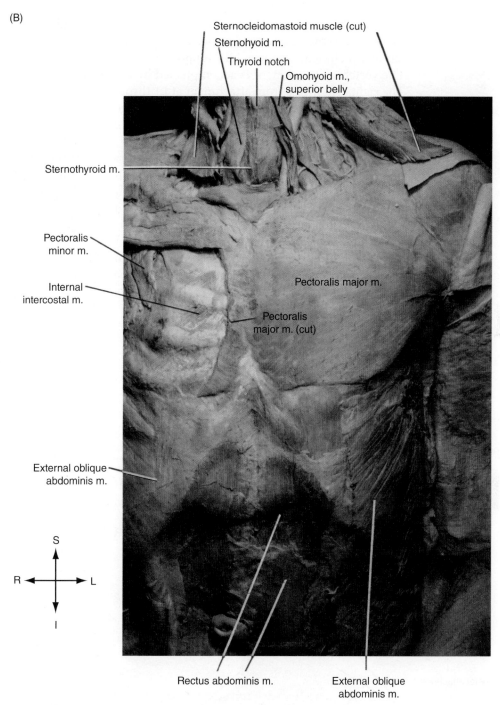

Sternocleidomastoid muscle (cut)

Sternohyoid m.

Thyroid notch

Omohyoid m.,
superior belly

Sternothyroid m.

Pectoralis
minor m.

Internal
intercostal m.

Pectoralis major m.

Pectoralis
major m. (cut)

External oblique
abdominis m.

S

R ◄────►L

I

Rectus abdominis m.

External oblique
abdominis m.

Figure 2-24 continued. (B) Anterior view of rib cage.
© Cengage Learning®.

tendon. Lateral to the xiphoid, the fibers of the diaphragm attach to
the inner border of ribs 7 through 12 and to the costal cartilages to
form the costal attachment. In the posterior aspect, the vertebral diaphragmatic attachment is made with the corpus of L1 through L4 and
transverse processes of L1.

crura: L., crosses

The fibers from these attachments course upward and inward to insert into the central tendon (see Figure 2-25). The posterior vertebral attachment also provides support for the esophageal hiatus. The vertebral attachment is accomplished by means of two **crura**. The right crus arises from attachment at L1 through L4, wherein the fibers ascend and separate to encircle the esophageal hiatus. Fibers of the left crus also arise from L1 through L4, passing to the left of the hiatus.

Although the diaphragm separates the thorax from the abdomen, the need for nutrients dictates that there be communication between the oral cavity and abdominal region. The region below the diaphragm also has vascular needs, and these require supply routes through the diaphragm.

There are three openings (diaphragmatic hiatuses) through which structures pass. As seen in Figure 2-25, the *descending abdominal aorta* passes through the aortic hiatus located adjacent and lateral

(A)

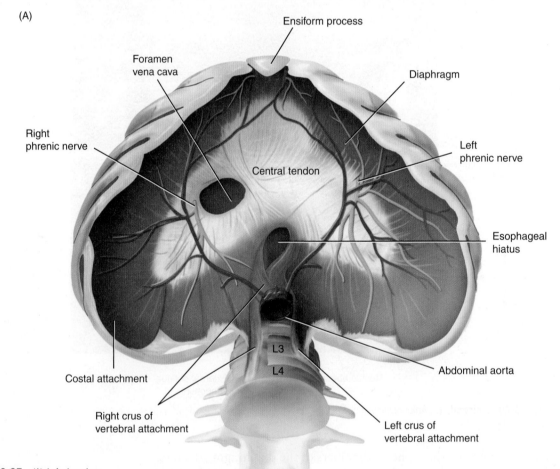

INFERIOR VIEW

Figure 2-25. (A) Inferior-view schematic of diaphragm, as seen from the abdominal cavity. (continues).
© Cengage Learning®.

(B)

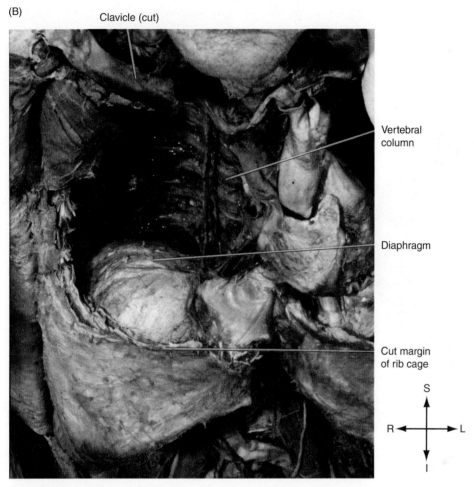

Clavicle (cut)

Vertebral column

Diaphragm

Cut margin of rib cage

S

R ◄───►L

I

Figure 2-25 continued. (B) Photograph of superior view of diaphragm.
© Cengage Learning®.

to the vertebral column. The *esophageal hiatus*, through which the esophagus passes, is found immediately anterior to the aortic hiatus, while the *inferior vena cava* traverses these two cavities by means of the foramen vena cava (which is in the right-central aspect of the diaphragm as viewed from above).

The actual muscle fibers of the diaphragm radiate from the imperfect center formed by the central tendon. Careful examination of the forces of muscular contraction will be most helpful in later discussion of muscular contraction and action. Realize, again, that muscle can perform only one task and that is to shorten. If a muscle is attached to two points, shortening will tend to bring those two points closer together, or simply tense the muscle if neither point is capable of moving. The diaphragm will stretch your understanding of this basic muscle function somewhat. Movement of the diaphragm will not make a great of sense, although the principles of muscle action and resulting shortening of the muscle still hold, until you realize where the points of attachment really are.

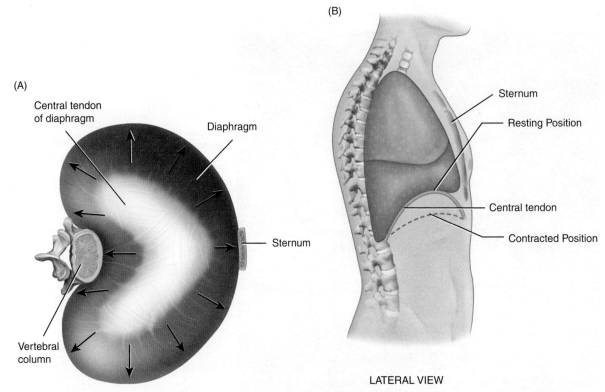

Figure 2-26. (A) Schematic of transverse view of the diaphragm with central tendon. The arrows depict the direction of force upon contraction of the diaphragm. (B) This lateral view of the diaphragm shows that contractions of the diaphragm pull the central tendon down.

© Cengage Learning®.

Figure 2-26 is a schematic drawing of the diaphragm and central tendon. First, look at the upper portion of the figure. If you choose some subset of those fibers and shorten them, the end result will be that the central tendon moves toward the point of firm attachment, the origin. But when the diaphragm contracts, all fibers contract together, which means that all fibers will pull equally on the central tendon. Now look at the second part of the figure and trace the same effect. If you contract (shorten) one fiber, the central tendon will move down toward the origin of the fiber. If you contract the entire diaphragm, the net result will be that the diaphragm is pulled down as a unit. The fibers in the front are longer than those in the back. *Contraction of the diaphragm has the result of pulling the central tendon down and forward.* It is directly analogous to placing someone in the middle of a blanket while a host of his or her friends pull on all of the corners of the blanket. When the friends pull together, the person in the middle flies up. Because the diaphragm has the shape of an inverted bowl, pulling on the edges (muscular contraction) draws the center down, but (gravity notwithstanding) the analogy holds.

The prominent central tendon is the last element of the diaphragm that we need to consider. Look again at Figure 2-26 and notice that the central tendon is a crescent-shaped aponeurosis that is white and translucent. The tendon tends to conform to the prominence of the vertebral column in the thoracic cavity, so its shape mimics the curvature of the transverse thoracic cavity. It has the flexibility of an aponeurosis, but has no contractile qualities. It depends on the radiating fibers of the diaphragm for movement. Above the central tendon is the heart, and this tendon provides a strong and secure floor for that mediastinal organ.

Innervation of the diaphragm is by means of the **phrenic nerves** (see Figure 2-23). The diaphragm can be placed under voluntary control (you can hold your breath), but it is primarily under the control of the autonomic system (you have no choice but to breathe eventually). Nature has provided bilateral innervation of the diaphragm, supporting the notion that this is an exceptionally important unpaired muscle. The phrenic nerves originate in the **cervical plexus** (a *plexus* is a group of nerves coming together for a common purpose) from spinal nerves C1, C2, C3, and C4 on both sides of the spinal cord.

The phrenic nerve descends deep to the omohyoid and sternocleidomastoid muscles and superficial to the anterior scalenus muscle, into the mediastinal space on the left and right sides of the heart. The nerve fibers descend and divide to innervate the superior surface of the diaphragm. One branch (the left and right phrenicoabdominals) descends deep to innervate the inferior surface. The left branch is longer than the right, because it has a greater distance to travel around the mediastinum. The phrenic nerves mediate both motor and sensory information. The lower intercostal nerve serves the inferior-most boundary of the diaphragm.

One final comment is warranted on the diaphragm and its action. Throughout this description we have ignored the abdominal viscera; beneath the diaphragm are numerous organs that undergo continual cycles of compression during respiration, a fact that will work to the advantage of anyone wishing to forcefully exhale (or perform the Heimlich maneuver, as we shall see).

✔ *To summarize:*

- The primary muscle of inspiration is the **diaphragm**, the dividing line between the thorax and the abdomen.
- The fibers of the diaphragm pull on the **central tendon**, resulting in the downward motion of the diaphragm during inspiration. This movement expands the lungs in the **vertical dimension**.

phrenic nerve: the nerve arising from the cervical plexus that innervates muscular activity of the diaphragm

cervical plexus: group of nerves that anastomoses from the spinal nerves c1, c2, c3, and c4

Muscle:	Diaphragm, Sternal head
Origin:	Xiphoid process of sternum
Course:	Superiorly and medially
Insertion:	Central tendon
Innervation:	Phrenic nerve arising from cervical plexus of spinal nerves C1, C2, C3, & C4
Function:	Depresses central tendon of diaphragm; enlarges vertical dimension of thorax; distends abdomen and compresses abdominal viscera

Muscle:	Diaphragm, Costal head
Origin:	Inferior margin of ribs 7–12
Course:	Superiorly and medially
Insertion:	Central tendon
Innervation:	Phrenic nerve arising from cervical plexus of spinal nerves C1, C2, C3, & C4
Function:	Depresses central tendon of diaphragm; enlarges vertical dimension of thorax; distends abdomen and compresses abdominal viscera

Muscle:	Diaphragm, Vertebral head
Origin:	Transverse processes of L1, corpus of L1–L4
Course:	Superiorly and medially
Insertion:	Central tendon
Innervation:	Phrenic nerve arising from cervical plexus of spinal nerves C1, C2, C3, & C4
Function:	Depresses central tendon of diaphragm; enlarges vertical dimension of thorax; distends abdomen and compresses abdominal viscera

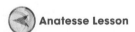 Anatesse Lesson

Accessory Muscles of Inspiration

Although the diaphragm is the major contributor to inspiration, it needs help to meet the needs of your body for forced inspiration. If you take a look at Figure 2-27, you will see the rib cage from the side. Direct your attention first to the way the ribs run: They are directed distinctly downward as they make their path to the front of the skeleton. Next, imagine raising the ribs in front, and realize that when you do that, the front of the rib cage expands. Swinging those ribs up means that they will swing out a bit in both anterior and lateral aspects, thereby increasing the volume of the rib cage.

For a demonstration of this function in everyday terms, look at Figure 2-27 showing venetian blinds from the side. When they are closed, they are similar to the rib cage at rest, and when they are tilted, so that you can see through them, they are similar to the point of elevation of the ribs. That elevation brings the ribs more nearly

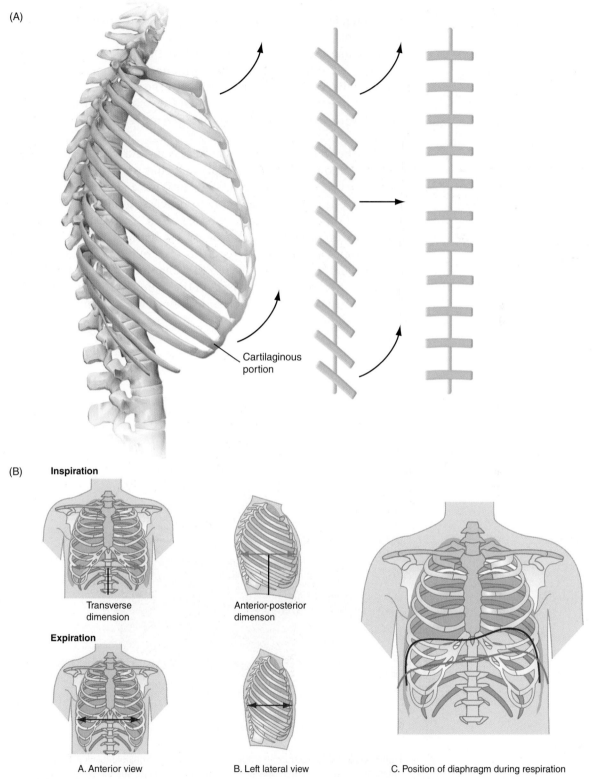

Figure 2-27. (A) Schematic of rib cage from the side. Notice that the ribs slant down as they run forward. During inspiration the rib cage will elevate, as shown by the arrows. On the right side, the "Venetian blinds" shown from the side demonstrate the change in volume achieved by elevation of the rib cage. (B) Schematic showing changes in thoracic dimensions during inspiration and at resting state.

© Cengage Learning®.

horizontal, just like the blinds, which increases the overall front–back dimension.

Because the goal is to raise all of the ribs and all parts of the ribs, we must have muscles attached to broad areas of the ribs to achieve this. The **external intercostal** muscles (see Figure 2-28) are positioned so that when they contract, the entire rib cage elevates, with most of the distance moved being in the front aspect.

By labeling these muscles as accessory muscles of inspiration we are acknowledging the simple fact that we could perform the respiratory act without them. They provide a significant increase in the amount of air we are able to process, but one is capable of surviving on diaphragmatic support alone, in the absence of the accessory muscles. You most likely are using little of the accessory muscles as you quietly read this text, but you would probably invoke them to help you discuss this chapter in front of the class. We will differentiate these based on the region of the body: anterior and posterior thoracic muscles, neck muscles, and muscles of the arm and shoulder.

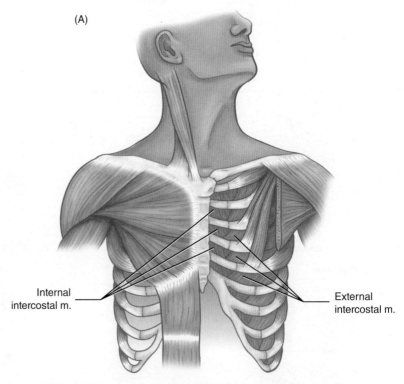

(A)

Internal intercostal m.

External intercostal m.

Figure 2-28. (A) Rib cage with external and internal intercostal muscles. External intercostals are absent near the sternum, and thus one can see the deeper internal intercostals within that region. (continues).
© Cengage Learning®.

(B)

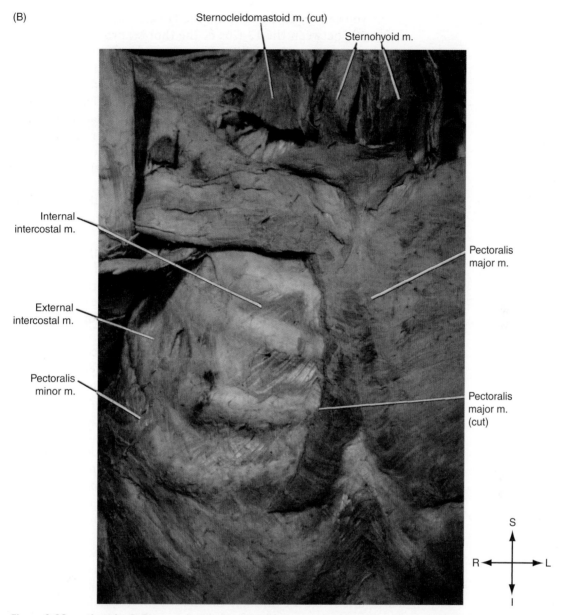

Sternocleidomastoid m. (cut)

Sternohyoid m.

Internal intercostal m.

External intercostal m.

Pectoralis minor m.

Pectoralis major m.

Pectoralis major m. (cut)

Figure 2-28 continued. (B) Photograph showing some accessory muscles of inspiration and expiration.
© Cengage Learning®.

Anterior Thoracic Muscles of Inspiration

- **External Intercostal**
- **Interchondral Portion, Internal Intercostal**

External Intercostal and Interchondral Portion, Internal Intercostal Muscles. The external intercostal muscles are among the most significant respiratory muscles for speech. They not only provide a significant proportion of the total respiratory capacity, but they also perform functions that are uniquely speech-related.

As you can see in Figure 2-28, the 11 external intercostal muscles reside between the 12 ribs of the thorax, providing the ribs with both unity and mobility. The external intercostal muscles originate in the lower surface of each rib (except rib 12) and course downward and inward to insert into the upper surface of the rib immediately below. These muscles provide a unified surface of diagonally slanting striated muscle on all costal surfaces of the rib cage with the exception of the region near the sternum, because contraction of external intercostal fibers in that region would provide little benefit (and perhaps some negative effect) to the job of increasing cavity size.

The external intercostal muscles are covered with the translucent intercostal membrane that separates them from the internal intercostal muscles.

The internal intercostal muscles (to be discussed) are predominantly muscles of expiration, with the exception of the chondral (cartilaginous) portion. The **parasternal** (near the sternum) portion of the internal intercostal muscles encompassing the chondral aspect of the ribs has been shown to be active during forced inspiration. The musculature is quite capable of segmental activation, so that one portion of this muscle can contract while contraction of the rest of the muscle is inhibited. The cross-laced effect of external and internal intercostal muscles forms a strong protective barrier for the lungs and heart and an impervious cavity for the forces of gas exchange.

Functionally, the external intercostal muscles elevate the rib cage. When the rib cage is elevated, the flexible coupling of the costo-sternal attachment permits the chondral portion of the ribs to rotate as they elevate. The net result is that the sternum remains relatively parallel to the vertebral column even as the rib cage expands, increasing the anterior dimension and thus the volume of the lungs (see Figure 2-27).

Innervation of the external intercostal muscles is achieved by the anterior divisions of the 11 pairs of thoracic spinal nerves, identified by the location of the region they innervate. The thoracic intercostal nerves arise from T1 through T6, and the thoracoabdominal intercostal nerves that pass into the abdominal wall arise from T7 through T11. These intercostal nerves supply not only the intercostal muscles but also a number of other muscles of respiration located in the anterior abdominal wall (see Figure 2-29).

Although the external intercostals account for most of the second dimensional change (the anterior-posterior dimension), there are other muscles that, by virtue of their arrangement, are assumed to be of help. Any muscle that attaches to the rib cage or sternum, and could feasibly elevate either, could assist in the process of inspiration.

Some other possible assistants in respiration are the **levatores costarum** (brevis and longis) and **serratus posterior superior**, shown in Figure 2-30. They elevate the rib cage on contraction.

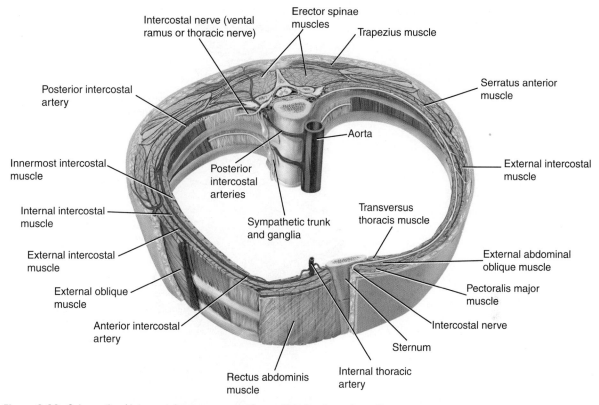

Figure 2-29. Schematic of intercostal nerves as seen from within the thoracic cavity.
© Cengage Learning®, After view and data of Netter, F. (2006). Atlas of Human Anatomy, 4e. Philadelphia, PA: Saunders.

Muscle:	External intercostal muscles
Origin:	Inferior surface of ribs 1–11
Course:	Down and obliquely in
Insertion:	Upper surface of rib immediately below
Innervation:	Intercostal nerves: thoracic intercostal nerves arising from T1 through T6 and thoracoabdominal intercostal nerves from T7 through T11
Function:	Elevate rib
Muscle:	Internal intercostal muscles, interchondral portion
Origin:	Superior margin of ribs 1–11
Course:	Down and in
Insertion:	Inferior surface of the rib above
Innervation:	Intercostal nerves: thoracic intercostal nerves arising from T1 through T6 and thoracoabdominal intercostal nerves from T7 through T11
Function:	Elevate ribs 1–11

(A)

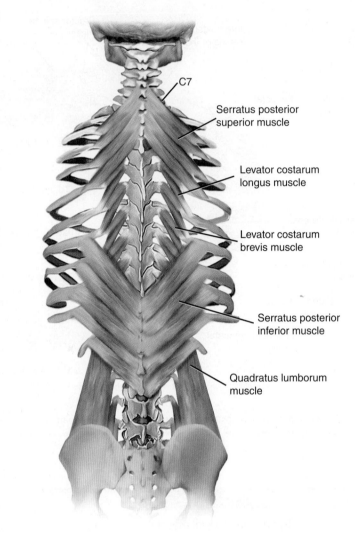

C7

Serratus posterior
superior muscle

Levator costarum
longus muscle

Levator costarum
brevis muscle

Serratus posterior
inferior muscle

Quadratus lumborum
muscle

Figure 2-30. (A) Posterior thoracic muscles of inspiration. Note that the levatores costarum are present on all ribs, but in the superior aspect they are deep to the serratus posterior muscles. (continues).
© Cengage Learning®.

Posterior Thoracic Muscles of Inspiration

- **Levatores Costarum (Brevis and Longis)**
- **Serratus Posterior Superior**

Levator Costarum (Brevis and Longis). If you examine the course of the levator costarum (levator = elevator, costarum = of the rib) shown in Figure 2-30A you will see that shortening these muscles tends to elevate the rib cage. Although these muscles may appear to be muscles of the back, they are considered to be thoracic muscles. The **brevis** (brief) portions of the levator costarum originate on the transverse processes of vertebrae C7 through T11, for a total of 12 levator costarum brevis muscles. Fibers course obliquely down and out to insert into the tubercle of the rib below.

The **longis** portions originate on the transverse processes of T7 through T11, with fibers coursing down and obliquely out. The fibers bypass the rib below the point of origin, inserting rather into the next

(B)

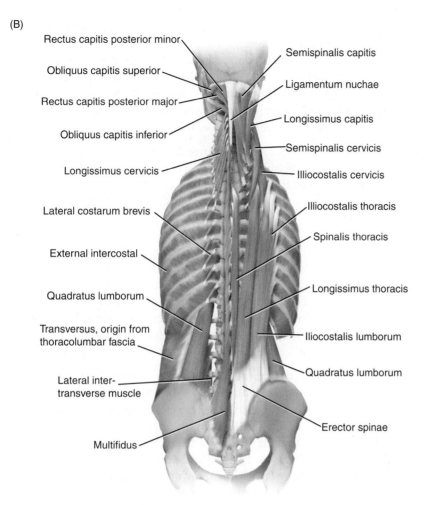

Rectus capitis posterior minor

Obliquus capitis superior

Rectus capitis posterior major

Obliquus capitis inferior

Longissimus cervicis

Lateral costarum brevis

External intercostal

Quadratus lumborum

Transversus, origin from thoracolumbar fascia

Lateral inter-transverse muscle

Multifidus

Semispinalis capitis

Ligamentum nuchae

Longissimus capitis

Semispinalis cervicis

Illiocostalis cervicis

Illiocostalis thoracis

Spinalis thoracis

Longissimus thoracis

Iliocostalis lumborum

Quadratus lumborum

Erector spinae

Figure 2-30 continued.
(B) Components of erector spinae muscle group, responsible for the movement and alignment of the vertebral column.
© Cengage Learning®.

Muscle:	Levator costarum, brevis
Origin:	Transverse processes of vertebrae C7–T11
Course:	Obliquely down and out
Insertion:	Tubercle of the rib below
Innervation:	Dorsal rami (branches) of the intercostal nerves arising from spinal nerves C7–T11
Function:	Elevate ribs cage

Muscle:	Levator costarum, longis
Origin:	Transverse processes of T7–T11
Course:	Down and obliquely out
Insertion:	Bypass the rib below the point of origin, inserting into the next rib
Innervation:	Dorsal rami (branches) of the intercostal nerves arising from spinal nerves C7–T11
Function:	Elevate rib cage

rib. You can see that the longis portion will have a greater effect on the elevation of the rib cage.

Much like the intercostal muscles, the levatores costarum take their innervation from the dorsal rami (branches) of the intercostal nerves. Upon exiting the spinal column, the dorsal rami course abruptly back, dividing into medial and lateral branches. The lateral branch of the dorsal ramus provides innervation of the levatores costarum.

Serratus Posterior Superior. In Figure 2-30A you can see that, given their course, contraction of the serratus posterior superior muscles could contribute to the elevation of the rib cage, though evidence of function in respiration is elusive (Vilensky, Baltes, Weikel, Fortin, & Fourie 2001).

The serratus posterior superior muscles take their origins on the spinous processes of C7 and T1 through T3. Fibers from these muscles course down and laterally to insert just beyond the angles of ribs 2 through 5. This more lateral insertion provides a significant enhancement of the mechanical advantage afforded this muscle, as compared with the levatores costarum brevis or longis. Innervation of the serratus posterior superior is completed by means of the ventral intercostal portion of the spinal nerves T1 through T4 or T5.

Erector Spinae (Sacrospinal Muscles). The erector spinae (or sacrospinal muscles) are not specifically involved in the process of respiration but rather serve to stabilize the vertebral column and thus the rib cage as well (Cala, Edyvean, & Engel, 1992). These muscles are divided into three major types that appear as a single mass on superficial examination. In the lumbar and thoracic regions, the muscle is covered by the thoracolumbar fascia (Figure 2-30B). The erector spinae are deep to the serratus posterior inferior and rhomboids. The erector spinae muscles arise from a tendon attached to the sacral crest, lumbar vertebrae, and 11th and 12th thoracic vertebrae. The muscles arise as a unit from this tendon and then get subdivided into three bundles: lateral (iliocostocervicalis), intermediate (longissimus), and medial (spinalis). Let us briefly look at each bundle in turn (see Figure 2-30B).

Lateral (Iliocostocervicalis) Bundle. This bundle is subdivided into three muscles: iliocostalis lumborum, iliocostalis thoracis, and

Muscle:	Serratus posterior superior
Origin:	Spinous processes of C7 and T1–T3
Course:	Down and laterally
Insertion:	Just beyond the angles of ribs 2–5
Innervation:	Ventral intercostal portion of the spinal nerves T1–T4 or T5
Function:	Elevate ribs 2–5

iliocostalis cervicis. The iliocostalis lumborum is attached to the angles of the lower seven ribs. Iliocostalis thoracis continues from those ribs (6–12) and courses to insert into ribs 1–6, as well the transverse process of the seventh cervical vertebra. Iliocostalis cervicis arises as a continuation from ribs 3 through 6 to insert into the fourth through sixth cervical vertebrae.

Intermediate (Longissimus) Bundle. This bundle consists of three muscles: longissimus thoracis, longissimus cervicis, and longissimus capitis. The longissimus thoracis arises partially from the transverse processes of the lumbar vertebrae as well as the middle aspect of the thoracolumbar fascia. It inserts into the transverse processes of all of the thoracic vertebrae and the lower 10 ribs. The longissiumus cervicis is the apparent extension of the longissimus thoracis, arising from the upper four or five thoracic vertebrae and inserting into the transverse processes of the second through sixth cervical vertebrae. The longissimus capitis arises from the transverse processes of the upper 4th and 5th cervical vertebrae, as well as from the articular processes of C3 and C4, to insert into the posterior mastoid process of the temporal bone. Together, these muscles provide great support for the vertebral column and become major players in neck extension during development.

Muscle:	Iliocostalis lumborum
Origin:	Sacral crest, L1–L5, T11–T12
Course:	Up
Insertion:	Angles of ribs 6–12
Innervation:	Dorsal rami of lower cervical nerves and thoracic and lumbar nerves
Function:	Stabilize and move vertebral column
Muscle:	Iliocostalis thoracis
Origin:	Ribs 6–12
Course:	Up
Insertion:	Ribs 1–6 and C7 vertebra
Innervation:	Dorsal rami of lower cervical nerves and thoracic and lumbar nerves
Function:	Stabilize and move vertebral column
Muscle:	Iliocostalis cervicis
Origin:	Ribs 3–6
Course:	Up
Insertion:	C4–C6 vertebrae
Innervation:	Dorsal rami of lower cervical nerves and thoracic and lumbar nerves
Function:	Stabilize and move vertebral column

Muscle:	Longissimus thoracis
Origin:	L1–L5 transverse processes and thoracolumbar fascia
Course:	Up
Insertion:	T1–T12 vertebrae, transverse processes and ribs 3–12
Innervation:	Dorsal rami of lower cervical nerves and thoracic and lumbar nerves
Function:	Stabilize and move vertebral column
Muscle:	Longissimus cervicis
Origin:	T1–T5 vertebrae
Course:	Up
Insertion:	C2–C6 vertebrae, transverse processes
Innervation:	Dorsal rami of lower cervical nerves and thoracic and lumbar nerves
Function:	Stabilize and move vertebral column
Muscle:	Longissimus capitis
Origin:	C1–C5 vertebrae
Course:	Up
Insertion:	Posterior mastoid process of temporal bone
Innervation:	Dorsal rami of lower cervical nerves and thoracic and lumbar nerves
Function:	Stabilize and move vertebral column

Medial (Spinalis) Bundle. This bundle consists of three muscles as well: spinalis thoracis, spinalis cervicis, and spinalis capitis. The spinalis thoracis is medial to the longissiumus thoracis, arising from the posterior spines of the 11th –12th thoracic vertebrae and L1–L3. It inserts into the upper fourth–eighth thoracic vertebrae (T4–T8). The muscle spinalis cervicis is often absent, but if it is present it courses from the nuchal ligament and posterior spine of C7 to insert into C2. Spinalis capitis is often indistinct from the semispinalis capitis, which arises from the posterior spine of T1–T6 and C7, as well as the articular processes of C4–C6, by means of a tendonous slip. The muscle inserts into the nuchal line of the skull and aids in neck extension and hyperextension.

Accessory Muscles of Neck

- **Sternocleidomastoid (Sternomastoid)**
- **Scalenes (Anterior, Middle, Posterior)**

Several neck muscles assist in inspiration (see Figure 2-31). The **sternocleidomastoid** (alternately sternomastoid) muscle makes a direct attachment to the sternum and elevates that structure and the rib cage with it. Other potential muscles of inspiration are the **scalenus anterior**, **medius**, and **posterior** muscles, which are muscles of the neck. When they contract, they elevate the first and second ribs.

scalenus: L., uneven

Muscle:	Spinalis thoracis
Origin:	T-11 and T-12, L1–L3 vertebrae
Course:	Up
Insertion:	T1–T8
Innervation:	Dorsal rami of lower cervical nerves and thoracic and lumbar nerves
Function:	Stabilize and move vertebral column

Muscle:	Spinalis cervicis
Origin:	Nuchal ligament and C7 vertebra
Course:	Up
Insertion:	C2 vertebra
Innervation:	Dorsal rami of lower cervical nerves and thoracic and lumbar nerves
Function:	Stabilize and move vertebral column

Muscle:	Spinalis capitis
Origin:	T1–T6, C4–C7
Course:	Up
Insertion:	Nuchal line of skull
Innervation:	Dorsal rami of lower cervical nerves and thoracic and lumbar nerves
Function:	Stabilize and move vertebral column

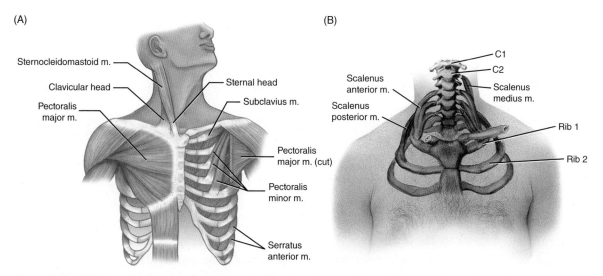

Figure 2-31. (A) Schematic of pectoralis major, pectoralis minor, sternocleidomastoid, subclavius, and serratus anterior muscles. (B) Schematic of scalenus anterior, medius, and posterior muscles.

© Cengage Learning®.

As with virtually all anatomical structures involved in speech, the muscles of the neck serve double duty. Although the muscles that will be discussed in this section are important for respiration, they are also sources of stability and control for neck flexion and extension. As an infant develops, it is the early control of neck musculature that marks the shift from the neonatal flexion position to one of balance between flexion and extension. When flexion and extension are balanced, the infant is well on the road toward whole-body stability required for speech.

Sternocleidomastoid. The sternocleidomastoid courses from its origin on the mastoid process of the temporal bone to its insertion at the sternum (sterno) and clavicle (cleido) (see Figure 2-31). This muscle is prominent and its outline is easily visible on an individual, especially when the head is turned toward one side. When contracted separately, the sternocleidomastoid will rotate the head toward the side of contraction. When both left and right sternocleidomastoid muscles are simultaneously contracted, the sternum and the anterior rib cage will elevate.

The sternocleidomastoid and trapezius muscles derive their innervation from the 11th cranial nerve, spinal branch (XI) accessory. The spinal portions of the accessory nerves originate from rootlets that arise from the side of the spinal cord in the regions of C2 through C4 or C5. These fibers join to become the spinal root, ascending within the vertebral column behind the denticulate ligament. The spinal root enters the skull via the foramen magnum, where it joins with the cranial root to exit the skull through the jugular foramen. The spinal and cranial branches separate, with the spinal branch coursing to innervate the sternocleidomastoid. This is supported in this by its interconnection with C2 spinal nerve, which also innervates the muscle. This branch continues, descending deep to the trapezius muscle and above the clavicle, finally communicating with C3 and C4 to form a pseudoplexus, subsequently innervating the trapezius. The fibers of the cranial parts of the accessory nerve join the vagi to be distributed among skeletal muscles as vagal fibers.

Scaleni Anterior, Middle, Posterior. The scaleni (or *scalenes*, as they also are called) are muscles of the neck that provide stability to the head and facilitate rotation. By virtue of their attachment to the first

Muscle:	Sternocleidomastoid (sternomastoid)
Origin:	Mastoid process of temporal bone
Course:	Down
Insertion:	Sternal head: superior manubrium sterni
Clavicular head:	Superior surface of clavicle
Innervation:	XI accessory, spinal branch arising from spinal cord in the regions of C2–C4 or C5
Function:	Elevates sternum and, by association, rib cage

Clavicular Breathing

Clavicular breathing is a form of respiration in which thorax expansion arises primarily through the elevation of the rib cage via contraction of the accessory muscles of inspiration, most notably the sternocleidomastoid. Clavicular breathing is often an adaptive response by an individual to some previous or present pathological condition, such as chronic obstructive pulmonary disease, which prohibits use of other means to expand the thorax. Because elevation of the sternum results in only a small increase in thorax size, clavicular breathing is a less-than-perfect solution to the problem of respiration.

Use of accessory muscles of inspiration to augment diminished respiratory support most typically includes the anterior, middle, and posterior scalene muscles (to elevate the first and second ribs) and the sternocleidomastoid (to elevate the sternum and increase the antero-posterior dimension of the rib cage). You may have seen patients with severe respiratory difficulties stretch out their arms and hold onto the back of a chair to breathe: when they do this, they give the pectoralis major muscles something to work against, thus allowing these muscles to increase the antero-posterior dimension. You may have also seen "shrugging" action by these patients, a sure sign that the trapezius muscle is in use to raise the rib cage.

Muscle:	Scalenus anterior
Origin:	Transverse processes of vertebrae C3–C6
Course:	Down
Insertion:	Superior surface of rib 1
Innervation:	C4–C6
Function:	Elevates rib 1
Muscle:	Scalenus medius
Origin:	Transverse processes of vertebrae C2–C7
Course:	Down
Insertion:	Superior surface of the first rib
Innervation:	Cervical plexus derived from C1, C2, C3, & C4 and spinal nerves C5–C8
Function:	Elevates rib 1
Muscle:	Scalenus posterior
Origin:	Transverse processes of C5–C7
Course:	Down
Insertion:	Second rib
Innervation:	Spinal nerves C5–C8
Function:	Elevates rib 2

and second ribs, they have the potential of increasing the vertical dimension of the thorax (see Figure 2-31).

The anterior scaleni originate on the transverse processes of vertebrae C3 through C6, with fibers coursing down to insert into the superior surface of the first rib. The middle scaleni take their origin on transverse processes of vertebrae C2 through C7, also inserting into the first rib. The posterior scaleni insert into the second rib, having coursed from the transverse processes of C5 through C7.

The scaleni anterior are innervated by spinal nerves C4 through C6. The middle scalenes are innervated primarily by the cervical plexus C1, C2, C3 & C4(although spinal nerves C5 through C8 are also involved in their innervation). Spinal nerves C5 through C8 innervate the posterior scalenes.

Muscles of Upper Arm and Shoulder

The accessory muscles of the arm may assist the external intercostal in elevation of the thorax by virtue of their attachment to the sternum and ribs. Although not all have been confirmed through physiological study, the action of each of the following muscles has been thought to have the potential to increase the anterior–posterior dimension of the thorax.

- Pectoralis Major
- Pectoralis Minor
- Serratus Anterior
- Subclavius
- Levator Scapulae
- Rhomboideus Major
- Rhomboideus Minor
- Trapezius

Pectoralis Major and Minor. The pectoralis major is a large, fan-shaped muscle that originates from two heads (see Figure 2-31). The sternal head attaches along the length of the sternum at the costal cartilages, while the clavicular head arises from the anterior surface of the clavicle. The pectoralis major runs from the sternal and clavicular origins up and out to insert into the greater tubercle of the humerus. The muscle converges at the crest of the greater tubercle of the humerus. In respiration, the pectoralis major elevates the sternum and thus increases the transverse dimension of the rib cage.

The pectoralis minor originates on the anterior surface of ribs 2 through 5, with fibers coursing up to converge on the coracoid process of the scapula. As with the pectoralis major, respiratory function involves elevation of the rib cage. The pectoralis major has been shown to be active during respiration (Cerqueira & Garbellini, 1999).

Innervation of the pectoralis major and pectoralis minor is by the pectoral nerves arising from the medial and lateral cords of the brachial plexus, a formation of C5 through C8 and T1 spinal nerves (see Figure 2-32).

Muscle: Pectoralis major

Origin: Sternal head: length of sternum at costal cartilages; Clavicular head: anterior clavicle

Course: Fan out laterally, converging at humerus

Insertion: Greater tubercle of humerus

Innervation: Superior branch of the brachial plexus (spinal nerves C5–C8 and T1)

Function: Elevates sternum, and subsequently increases transverse dimension of rib cage

Muscle: Pectoralis minor

Origin: Anterior surface of ribs 2–5 near chondral margin

Course: Up and laterally

Insertion: Coracoid process of scapula

Innervation: Superior branch of the brachial plexus (spinal nerves C5–C8 and T1)

Function: Increases transverse dimension of rib cage

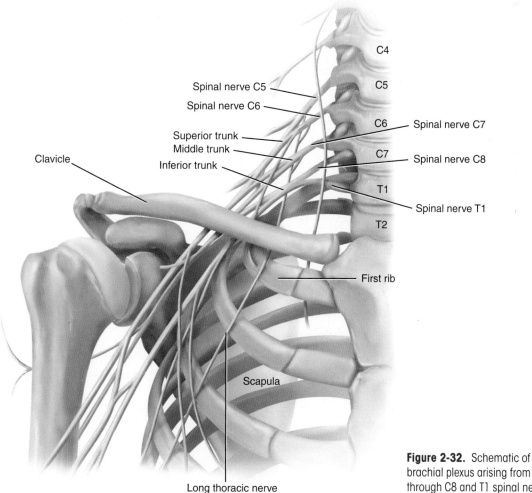

Figure 2-32. Schematic of brachial plexus arising from C5 through C8 and T1 spinal nerves.
© Cengage Learning®.

serratus: L., serratus, toothed; notched

Serratus Anterior. The sawlike fingers of this muscle give it its name (*serratus* as in *serrated knife*). Fibers of the **serratus** anterior arise from ribs 1 through 9 along the side of the thorax, coursing up to converge on the inner vertebral border of the scapula. Contraction of the muscle may elevate the ribs to which it is attached and subsequently the rib cage (see Figure 2-31).

As with the pectoralis major and minor, the serratus anterior receives innervation from the brachial plexus. The long thoracic nerve arises from C5 through C7 and passes between the middle and posterior scalene neck muscles to descend to the level of the serratus anterior.

Subclavius. As the name implies, the subclavius muscle courses under the clavicle, originating from the inferior margin of the clavicle and taking an oblique and medial course to insert into the superior surface of the first rib at the chondral margin. It is a small muscle that may elevate the first rib during inspiration (see Figure 2-31). The subclavius muscle is innervated by branches from the brachial plexus, with fibers originating in the fifth and sixth spinal nerves. The subclavius is not present in all people and is most likely a holdover from the days when our ancestors were quadrupeds.

Muscle:	Serratus anterior
Origin:	Ribs 1–9, lateral surface of thorax
Course:	Up and back
Insertion:	Inner vertebral border of scapula
Innervation:	Brachial plexus, long thoracic nerve from C5 through C7
Function:	Elevates ribs 1–9

Muscle:	Subclavius
Origin:	Inferior surface of clavicle
Course:	Oblique and medial
Insertion:	Superior surface of rib 1 at chondral margin
Innervation:	Brachial plexus, lateral branch, from spinal nerves 5 and 6
Function:	Elevates rib 1

Muscle:	Levator scapulae
Origin:	Transverse processes of C1–C4
Course:	Down
Insertion:	Medial border of scapula
Innervation:	C3–C5
Function:	Neck support: elevates scapula

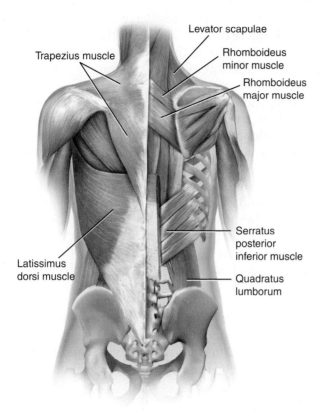

Levator scapulae

Trapezius muscle

Rhomboideus minor muscle

Rhomboideus major muscle

Serratus posterior inferior muscle

Latissimus dorsi muscle

Quadratus lumborum

POSTERIOR VIEW

Figure 2-33. Accessory muscles of respiration: trapezius, levator scapulae, rhomboideus minor, rhomboideus major, serratus posterior inferior, latissimus dorsi, and quadratus lumborum.
© Cengage Learning®.

Levator Scapulae. The levator scapulae provides neck support secondarily as a result of its function as an elevator of the scapula. This muscle originates from the transverse processes of C1 through C4, and courses down to insert into the medial border of the scapula (see Figure 2-33). As with the scaleni anterior, middle, and posterior, the levator scapulae derives its innervation from C3 through C5.

Rhomboideus Major and Minor. The rhomboids (major and minor) lie deep to the trapezius, originating on the spinous processes of T2 through T5 (**rhomboideus** major) and from C7 and T1. The muscle courses down and laterally to insert into the medial border of the scapula. The primary speech function of the rhomboids is the support they provide for the upper body, and especially for the stability of the shoulder girdle (De Freitas & Vitti, 1980).

The rhomboids receive their innervation from the dorsal scapular nerves off the upper roots of the brachial plexus (C5). The dorsal scapular nerves pass through the scaleni medius muscles in their course to the rhomboids.

Trapezius. The trapezius muscle (see Figure 2-33) is a massive muscle making up the superficial upper back and neck, originating along the spinous processes of C2 to T12 by means of fascial connection.

rhomboideus: L., rhombus, parallelogram + oid, like

(The trapezius is alternately considered a muscle of the arm.) Fibers of this muscle fan laterally to insert into the acromion of the scapula and the superior surface of the clavicle. Contraction of this muscle clearly plays a significant role in elongation of the neck and for head control.

For respiration, support is the primary function of the back muscles, although there are distinct respiratory actions, as we shall see. Back muscles provide a dense, multilayered mass of tissue that supports and protects (see Figure 2-33). Perhaps the most important function of these muscles is the maintenance of the delicate balance of upper body mobility in the face of required stability. To experience this firsthand, place both feet firmly on the ground while sitting erect, and then with one arm reach straight ahead as if you were about to grasp an object beyond your reach. You will need to overextend when you do this, but if you attend to the musculature of your head, shoulders, and back, you will feel them tighten to support your efforts. Your shoulders rotated while the rest of your trunk remained relatively stable.

In the "big picture" of trunk control, the following back muscles are key players. The trapezius and levator scapulae muscles serve clear roles in neck elongation and head stability. Support for the vertebral column is provided by the trapezius muscle and the rhomboideus

Muscle:	Rhomboideus major
Origin:	Spinous processes of T2–T5
Course:	Down and laterally in
Insertion:	Scapula
Innervation:	Spinal C5 from the dorsal scapular nerve of upper root of brachial plexus
Function:	Stabilizes shoulder girdle

Muscle:	Rhomboideus minor
Origin:	Spinous processes of C7 and T1
Course:	Down and laterally in
Insertion:	Medial border of scapula
Innervation:	Spinal C5 from the dorsal scapular nerve of upper root of brachial plexus
Function:	Stabilizes shoulder girdle

Muscle:	Trapezius
Origin:	Spinous processes of C2 to T12
Course:	Fan laterally
Insertion:	Acromion of scapula and superior surface of clavicle
Innervation:	XI accessory, spinal branch arising from spinal cord in the regions of C2–C4 or C5
Function:	Elongates neck: controls head

Trunk Stability and Upper Body Mobility

Infant motor development is a process of increasing the control of motor function: Control of speech musculature depends in large part on the development of trunk control. It is truly a "for want of a nail" situation: If the infant fails to develop neck extension, he or she will not develop the ability to balance neck extensors and flexors. Once the normal extension begins development, the back muscles begin to come under control, again becoming dynamically opposed by anterior trunk muscles. Through this interplay of antagonist and agonist trunk muscles, the infant develops the ability to rotate the trunk, stabilize the hips (and, of course, walk), and elevate the head in preparation for speech. Once controlled, the infant can rotate his or her head, differentiate mandible movement from head movement, and tongue from mandible. All the while, the infant is developing the dynamic aspects of laryngeal control that permit the larynx to descend and the tongue to become controlled.

This is a long-winded way of saying that, although the respiratory function of the back muscles is open to question, the absence of controlled use of the back muscles would most certainly result in loss of head control for speech, reduced differentiation of facial muscle control, and lack of laryngeal control due to the tonic imbalance of the torso. The indirect effects of muscle imbalance within the trunk are innumerable.

major and minor muscles, and this support serves respiration in a stabilizing manner. Finally, the erector spinae, discussed earlier, play a vital role in head, neck, and trunk stability. The clinical note on the development of motor coordination emphasizes the importance of trunk and back muscle development from an oral motor perspective.

✔ *To summarize:*

- The **diaphragm** is an exceptionally important muscle of inspiration, but there are many **accessory muscles** of inspiration and expiration that also serve respiration.
- Generally, muscles of the thorax and neck that elevate the rib cage serve some accessory function for inspiration.

In the next section we shall see that muscles that compress the abdomen or pull down on the rib cage also assist in expiration.

MUSCLES OF FORCED EXPIRATION

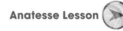

Anatesse Lesson

Active expiration requires that musculature act on the lungs indirectly to "squeeze" the air out of them. This is achieved in two ways. Because the rib cage expands in two dimensions, it makes sense that it will contract in two dimensions as well. The front-to-back dimension is expanded by elevating the rib cage, so active expiration should reduce that dimension. The rib cage can be pulled down by the internal intercostal muscles, the innermost intercostal muscles, and the transversus thoracis muscles. The second means of expanding the volume of the thorax is by increasing the vertical dimension through

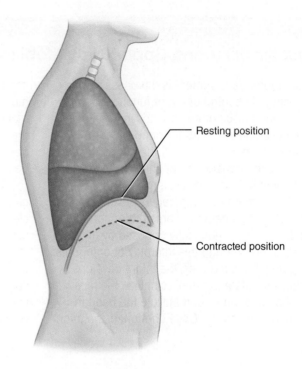

- Resting position
- Contracted position

LATERAL VIEW

Figure 2-34. Lateral-view schematic of diaphragm showing relative position during inspiration and passive expiration.
© Cengage Learning®.

contraction of the diaphragm. If you examine Figure 2-34, you will realize that relaxing the diaphragm will return it to its original position, and no farther. If you note the viscera of the abdomen below the diaphragm, you can now see the second means of active expiration. If I can somehow squeeze my abdominal viscera, I will be able to push my diaphragm higher into the thorax and remove more air from my lungs. (If you want to verify this, have one of your friends perform a gentle version of the Heimlich maneuver on you and feel what happens with your respiration. Do you inhale or exhale?)

We can forcefully expire by contracting the muscles of the abdominal region which, in turn, squeeze the abdomen and force the viscera upward, reducing the size of the thorax. This is half of the reason you get "the wind knocked out of you" when someone punches you in the abdomen. See the clinical note for the other half of that story.

If you examine the abdominal muscles of expiration (see Figure 2-35), you will see that they are very much like a cummerbund, wrapping the abdomen into a neat package in the front, side, and back. The major players in the anterior abdomen are the internal and external oblique abdominis, transversus abdominis, and the **rectus** abdominis muscles. In the posterior abdomen, the quadratus lumborum, iliacus, and psoas major and minor muscles serve this function. If you look at Figure 2-33, you will see that the latissimus dorsi muscles appear to be useful in maintaining an open, expanded thorax during respiration in professional singers and could well have

rectus: L., straight (not crooked)

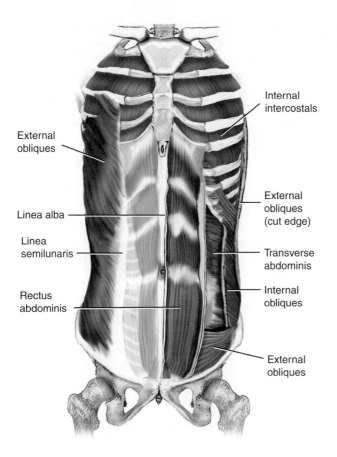

External
obliques

Internal
intercostals

Linea alba

External
obliques
(cut edge)

Linea
semilunaris

Transverse
abdominis

Rectus
abdominis

Internal
obliques

External
obliques

Figure 2-35. Accessory muscles of expiration and landmarks of the abdominal aponeurosis.
© Cengage Learning®.

that function in everyday speaking as well, particularly if the speaker is projecting his or her voice (Watson, Williams & James, 2012).

The layers of abdominal muscles provide excellent support for the rib cage during lifting and other body gestures. These gestures virtually demand fixing the thorax by inflating the lungs and closing off the vocal folds, and the abdominal muscles help to compress the viscera while simultaneously stabilizing the thorax.

Muscles of Thorax: Anterior/Lateral Thoracic Muscles

- Internal Intercostal (Interosseous Portion)
- Transversus Thoracis
- Innermost Intercostals

Internal Intercostal, Interosseous Portion

The interosseous portion of the internal intercostal muscles are significant contributors to forced expiration. As seen earlier in Figure 2-28, the internal intercostal muscles are pervasive in the thorax, originating on the superior margin of each rib (except the first) and running up and medially to insert into the inferior surface of the rib above. They are conspicuously absent in the posterior aspect of the rib cage near the vertebral column. Because the external intercostal muscles run at nearly right angles to the internals, these two sets of muscles provide significant support for the rib cage and protection for the ribs within, as well as maintenance of rib spacing.

The course of the muscle fibers is constant from the front to side to back of the rib cage. That is, while the fibers run up and medially in front, that translates to running up and laterally in the dorsal aspect.

Besides of their support function, the internal intercostal muscles also provide a mechanism for depressing the rib cage. As you can see from the schematic of Figure 2-36, when the interosseous portion of the internal intercostals contracts and shortens, the direction of movement is downward, and the expanded rib cage will become smaller.

Muscle:	Internal intercostal, interosseous portion
Origin:	Superior margin of ribs 1–11
Course:	Up and in
Insertion:	Inferior surface of the rib above
Innervation:	Intercostal nerves: thoracic intercostal nerves arising from T2 through T6 and thoracoabdominal intercostal nerves from T7 through T11
Function:	Depresses ribs 1–11

"Getting the Wind Knocked Out of You"

Why *does* a blow to the abdomen result in your losing your breath? Logic would dictate that you would lose your breath from being hit in the chest. You will want to take a look at the explanation of reflexive responses in the clinical note entitled "paradoxical respiration," because that will go a long way toward explaining this response as well.

Try to recall what happened the last time you had the wind knocked out of you. First, something hit you in the abdominal region. From what you now know, forced expiration depends in large part on the contraction of the abdominal muscles, which, in turn, causes the abdominal viscera to push the diaphragm upward and pull the thorax down. Both of these gestures remove air forcefully from the lungs.

This does not explain the agony you experience trying to regain respiratory control, however. When those muscles are passively moved (stretched), a stretch reflex is triggered, which causes the muscle to contract involuntarily. This contraction only serves to increase the effect of being hit in the abdomen, because it is essentially doing the same thing the blunt force did. To cap it all, your attempts to contract your diaphragm add a third dimension to the problem, because that will once again stretch the abdominal muscles and promote further reflexive contraction.

Use of Abdominal Muscles for Childbirth and Other Biological Functions

Nature has a way of getting the most use out of structures, and the abdominal muscles are a great example. Clearly, we use the abdominal muscles to force air out of the lungs, but they serve several other worthwhile (even vital) functions. The act of vomiting requires evacuation of the gastric or even intestinal contents and doing so necessitates forceful action from the abdominal muscles.

A less obvious function has to do with thoracic fixation. For the muscles of the upper body to gain maximum benefit, they need to pull against a relatively rigid structure. The thorax can be made rigid by inhaling and then capturing the respiratory charge by closing off the vocal folds. To demonstrate this process, take a very deep breath and hold it: To do this you must close off the vocal folds.

This thoracic fixing gives leverage for lifting (notice that you may "grunt" when you lift because some air is escaping past the vocal folds, having been compressed by your muscular effort), but it also gives leverage for expulsion in the other direction. Defecation is facilitated by compression of the abdomen and an increase in abdominal pressure, and that process also demands thoracic fixation for efficiency.

Another not immediately obvious use for abdominal muscle contraction is childbirth. Although you may not have experienced this directly, you are probably familiar with midwives, nurses, or partners whose job it is to remind the mother-to-be to "breathe." It shouldn't surprise you to realize that the mother has not forgotten this basic biological process, but rather she has an overwhelming, deep biological urge to "push." Besides providing supportive encouragement, the person who is cheerleading is doing so to synchronize breathing with contractions and to keep the mother from closing the vocal folds (you can't breathe through closed folds) because if she does, she will start pushing the baby to its new home before the time has come (Creasy, 1997).

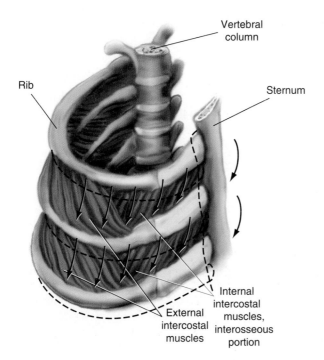

Figure 2-36. Effect of contraction of the interosseous portion of the internal intercostals is the rib cage down, thereby decreasing the volume of the lungs.
© Cengage Learning®.

Innermost Intercostal (Intercostales Intimi)

The innermost intercostal muscles are the deepest of the intercostal muscles, with fibers coursing between the inner costal surfaces of adjacent ribs. The innermost intercostals have a course parallel to those of the internal intercostal muscles, with fibers originating on the superior surface of the lower rib and coursing obliquely up to insert into the rib above. As with the external intercostals, the innermost intercostals are absent in the chondral portion of the ribs, becoming apparent first in the lateral aspect of the inner rib cage. The innermost intercostals are absent near the vertebral and sternal borders, are sparse in the upper thorax, and parallel the morphology of the internal intercostals. The innermost intercostals interdigitate with the subcostal muscles (see Figure 2-29).

Transversus Thoracis

As the name implies, the transversus thoracis muscles (transverse muscles of the thorax) are found on the inner surface of the rib cage. The muscles originate on the margin of the sternum, with fibers coursing to the inner chondral surface of ribs 2 through 6. As seen in Figure 2-37, contraction of the muscles would tend to resist elevation of the rib cage and decrease the volume of the thoracic cavity.

Considering the proximity of the transversus thoracis to the internal intercostal muscles, it should not be surprising that the transversus thoracis takes its innervation from the same source (the thoracic intercostal nerves), as well as from the thoracoabdominal intercostal nerves and subcostal nerves derived from T2 through T1 spinal nerves.

Posterior Thoracic Muscles

- **Subcostals**
- **Serratus Posterior Inferior**

Subcostals. The subcostals are widely variable but generally take a course parallel to the internal intercostals and thus have the potential

Muscle:	Innermost intercostal
Origin:	Superior margin of ribs 1–11; sparse or absent in superior thorax
Course:	Upward and forward
Insertion:	Inferior surface of the rib above
Innervation:	Intercostal nerves: thoracic intercostal nerves arising from T2 through T6 and thoracoabdominal intercostal nerves from T7 through T11
Function:	Depresses ribs 1–11

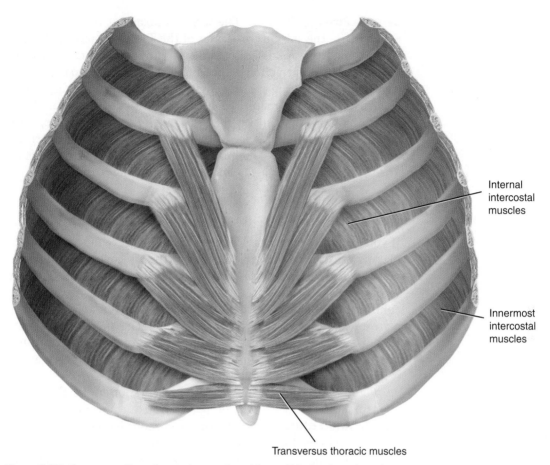

Figure 2-37. Transversus thoracis muscles, as viewed from within the thoracic cavity.
© Cengage Learning®.

Muscle:	Transversus thoracis
Origin:	Inner thoracic lateral margin of sternum
Course:	Laterally
Insertion:	Inner chondral surface of ribs 2–6
Innervation:	Thoracic intercostal nerves, thoracoabdominal intercostal nerves, and subcostal nerves derived from T2 through T12 spinal nerves
Function:	Depresses rib cage for expiration

of aiding expiration. The subcostals are found on the inner posterior wall of the thorax. Unlike the intercostal muscles, the subcostals may span more than one rib. The subcostals are innervated by the intercostal nerves of the thorax, arising from the ventral rami of the spinal nerves.

Serratus Posterior Inferior. The serratus posterior inferior muscles originate on the spinous processes of the T11, T12, and L1 through L3 and course up and laterally to insert into the lower margin of the lower five ribs. Contraction of these muscles would tend to pull the rib cage down, supporting expiratory effort, although neither anatomical (Loukas, Louis, Wartmann, Tubbs, Gupta, Apaydin, & Jordan, 2008) nor physiological (Vilensky, Baltes, Weikel, Fortin, & Fourie, 2001) studies have found evidence of this (see Figure 2-33). The serratus posterior inferiors derive their innervation from the intercostal nerves arising from T9 through T11 and the subcostal nerve from T12.

Abdominal Muscles of Expiration

If you examine, once again, the skeleton in Figure 2-3 and imagine placing muscles in the region between the rib cage and the pelvis, you will realize that there are few places from which muscles can originate. Clearly one could attach muscles to the rib cage, vertebral column, and the pelvic girdle to give some structure, but that leaves a great deal of territory to cover in the anterior aspect. To deal with this, nature has provided a tendinous structure, the **abdominal aponeurosis**. Let us examine how it is constructed and then attach some muscles to that structure.

Figure 2-38 shows a schematic representation of the abdominal aponeurosis from the front, as well as in transverse section.

The **linea alba** (white line) runs from the xiphoid process to the pubic symphysis, forming a midline structure for muscular attachment. As the linea alba progresses laterally, it differentiates into two sheets of aponeurosis, between which is placed the rectus abdominis. This aponeurotic wrapping comes back together to form another

abdominal aponeurosis: the aponeurotic complex of the anterior abdominal wall that forms points of origination for abdominal musculature

linea alba: L., white line

Muscle:	Subcostal
Origin:	Inner posterior thorax; sparse in upper thorax; from inner surface of rib near angle
Course:	Down and lateral
Insertion:	Inner surface of second or third rib below
Innervation:	Intercostal nerves of thorax, arising from the ventral rami of the spinal nerves
Function:	Depresses thorax

Muscle:	Serratus posterior inferior
Origin:	Spinous processes of T11, T12, L1–L3
Course:	Up and laterally
Insertion:	Lower margin of ribs 7–12
Innervation:	Intercostal nerves from T9 through T11 and subcostal nerve from T12
Function:	Contraction of these muscles tends to pull the rib cage down, supporting expiratory effort

band of tendon, the linea semilunaris. This tendon once again divides, but this time into three sheets of aponeurosis, which will provide us with a way to attach three more muscles to this structure.

In the posterior aspect, the fascia of the abdominal muscles join to form the lumbodorsal fascia. This structure provides for the union of three abdominal muscles (transversus abdominis, internal, and external oblique abdominis) with the vertebral column.

The external oblique aponeurosis communicates directly with the fascia covering the rectus abdominis, forming a continuous layer of connective tissue from the linea alba to the external oblique muscle.

(A)

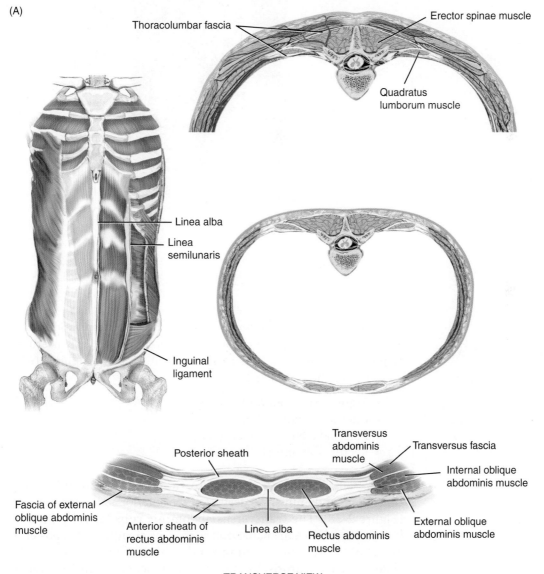

TRANSVERSE VIEW

Figure 2-38. (A) Schematic of abdominal aponeurosis as related to the abdominal muscles of expiration. (continues).

© Cengage Learning®.

(B)

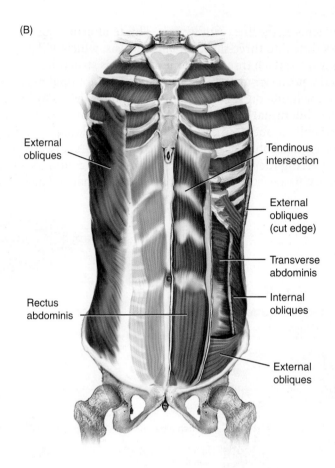

External obliques

Tendinous intersection

External obliques (cut edge)

Transverse abdominis

Internal obliques

Rectus abdominis

External obliques

Figure 2-38 continued.
(B) Transversus abdominis, rectus abdominis, external and internal oblique abdominis muscles.
© Cengage Learning®.

Anterolateral Abdominal Muscles

The abdominal muscles of expiration function by compression of the abdominal viscera. This compression function is not only useful in respiration but also aids in defecation, vomiting, and childbirth (with vocal folds tightly adducted).

- Transversus Abdominis
- Internal Oblique Abdominis
- External Oblique Abdominis
- Rectus Abdominis

Transversus Abdominis. Lateral to the rectus abdominis is the transversus abdominis, the deepest of the anterior abdominal muscles (Figure 2-38). The transversus abdominis runs laterally (that is, horizontally; hence the name *transversus*), originating in the posterior aspect of the vertebral column via the thoracolumbar fascia of the abdominal aponeurosis. Its anterior attachment is to the transversus abdominis aponeurosis, as well as to the inner surface of ribs 6 through 12, interdigitating at that point with the fibers of the diaphragm. Its inferior-most attachment is at the pubis. Contraction of the transversus will significantly reduce the volume of the abdomen.

Palpation of the Rib Cage

Although you cannot palpate your diaphragm, you can identify its margins easily enough. First, find your xiphoid process. This point marks part of the origin of the rectus abdominis, but the diaphragm attaches on the inner surface. Place your fingers on the xiphoid process and the muscle below, and breathe deeply in and out once. You can feel the rectus abdominis being stretched during inspiration. Now place the fingers of both hands at the bottom of the rib cage on either side of the sternum so that your fingers press into your abdominal muscles. Breathe out as deeply as you can and hold that posture while you bend slightly forward. Your fingers are marking the margin of the diaphragm, although you are palpating abdominal muscles.

Bring your fingers up to feel your ribs. Place your fingers between the ribs, with your little finger of each hand on the abdominal muscles below the rib cage. Breathe in a couple of times and feel the abdominal muscles first draw in and then tighten up as you reach maximum inspiration. Feel your rib cage elevate as you do this.

Muscle:	Transversus abdominis
Origin:	Posterior abdominal wall at the vertebral column via the thoracolumbar fascia of the abdominal aponeurosis
Course:	Lateral
Insertion:	Transversus abdominis aponeurosis and inner surface of ribs 6–12, interdigitating at that point with the fibers of the diaphragm; inferior-most attachment is at the pubis
Innervation:	Thoracic and lumbar nerves from the lower spinal intercostal nerves (derived from T7 through T12) and first lumbar nerve, iliohypogastric and ilioinguinal branches
Function:	Compresses abdomen

Innervation of the transversus abdominis is via the thoracic and lumbar nerves, specifically from the lower thoracoabdominal nerves (derived from T7 to T12) and first lumbar nerve, iliohypogastric and ilioinguinal branches.

Internal Oblique Abdominis. The internal oblique abdominis is located between the external oblique abdominis and the transversus abdominis. As seen in Figure 2-38, this muscle fans out from its origin on the inguinal ligament and iliac crest to the cartilaginous portion of the lower ribs and the portion of the abdominal aponeurosis lateral to the rectus abdominis, and thus, by association, inserts into the linea alba. Contraction of the internal oblique abdominis assists in the rotation of the trunk, if unilaterally contracted, or flexion of the trunk, when bilaterally contracted. The internal oblique abdominis is innervated by the first eight intercostal nerves, as well as the ilioinguinal and iliohypogastric nerves.

Muscle:	Internal oblique abdominis
Origin:	Inguinal ligament and iliac crest
Course:	Fans medially
Insertion:	Cartilaginous portion of lower ribs and the portion of the abdominal aponeurosis lateral to the rectus abdominis
Innervation:	Thoracic and lumbar nerves from the lower spinal intercostal nerves (derived from T7 through T12) and first lumbar nerve, iliohypogastric and ilioinguinal branches
Function:	Rotates trunk; flexes trunk; compresses abdomen
Muscle:	External oblique abdominis
Origin:	Osseous portion of the lower seven ribs
Course:	Fan downward
Insertion:	Iliac crest, inguinal ligament, and abdominal aponeurosis lateral to rectus abdominis
Innervation:	Thoracoabdominal nerve arising from T7 through T11 and subcostal nerve from T12
Function:	Bilateral contraction flexes vertebral column and compresses abdomen; unilateral contraction results in trunk rotation

External Oblique Abdominis. The external oblique abdominis are the most superficial of the abdominal muscles, as well as the largest of this group. These muscles originate along the osseous portion of the lower seven ribs, and fan downward to insert into the iliac crest, inguinal ligament, and abdominal aponeurosis (lateral to rectus abdominis). Bilateral contraction of these muscles will flex the vertebral column, while unilateral contraction will result in trunk rotation. This muscle receives innervation from the thoracoabdominal nerve arising from T7 through T11 and the subcostal nerve from T12.

Rectus Abdominis. The rectus abdominis muscles are the prominent midline muscles of the abdominal region, which originate at the pubis inferiorly (see Figure 2-35). The superior attachment is at the xiphoid process of sternum and the cartilage of the last true rib (rib 7) and the false ribs.

These "rectangular" (i.e., rectus) muscles are manifest in a series of four or five segments connected (and separated) by tendinous slips known as *tendinous intersections*. Use of this muscle is a "must" if you are to succeed at your sit-ups, because contraction will draw the chest closer to the knees, and the only way to do this is to bend. Contraction of the rectus abdominis also compresses the abdominal contents.

Innervation is by T5 through T11 intercostal (thoracoabdominal) nerves and the subcostal nerve from T12. This segmented muscle is segmentally innervated as well: T7 supplies the uppermost segment, T8 supplies the next section, and the remaining portions are supplied by T9–T12.

Posterior Abdominal Muscles

- **Quadratus Lumborum**

Quadratus Lumborum. As seen in Figures 2-30 and 2-33, the quadratus lumborum is located in the dorsal aspect of the abdominal wall. These muscles originate along the iliac crest and fan up and inward to insert into the transverse processes of the lumbar vertebrae and inferior border of the 12th rib. Unilateral contraction of the quadratus lumborum would assist in lateral movement of the trunk, whereas bilateral contraction would fix the abdominal wall in support of abdominal compression. This muscle is innervated by the lowest thoracic nerve T12 and the first four lumbar nerves.

There are other abdominal muscles supporting abdominal wall fixation. The psoas major and minor muscles and the iliacus may provide abdominal support for forced expiration.

Muscles of the Upper Limb

- **Latissimus Dorsi**

Latissimus Dorsi. The **latissimus** dorsi muscle (see Figure 2-33) originates from the lumbar, sacral, and lower thoracic vertebrae, with fibers rising fanlike to insert into the humerus. Its primary role is in assisting the movement of the upper extremity, but it clearly plays a role in chest stability, and perhaps expiration. With the arm immobilized, contraction of the latissimus dorsi would stabilize the posterior abdominal wall, performing a function similar to that of the quadratus lumborum.

latissimus: L., widest

Muscle:	Rectus abdominis
Origin:	Originates as four or five segments at the pubis inferiorly
Course:	Up to segment border
Insertion:	Xiphoid process of sternum and the cartilage of ribs 5–7, lower ribs
Innervation:	T5–T11 intercostal (thoracoabdominal) nerves, subcostal nerve from T12 (T7 supplies upper segment, T8 supplies the second, T9–T12 supplies remainder)
Function:	Flexion of vertebral column

Muscle:	Quadratus lumborum
Origin:	Iliac crest
Course:	Fan up and inward
Insertion:	Transverse processes of the lumbar vertebrae and inferior border of rib 12
Innervation:	Thoracic nerve T12 and L1–L4 lumbar nerves
Function:	Bilateral contraction fixes abdominal wall in support of abdominal compression

Innervation for this muscle arises from the posterior branch of the brachial plexus. Fibers from the regions C6 through C8 of this plexus form the long subscapular nerve to supply the latissimus dorsi.

✔ *To summarize:*

- To inflate the lungs, you need to expand the cavity that holds them so air can rush in.
- To do this, you can either increase the long dimension fairly easily by contracting the **diaphragm**, or you can elevate the rib cage with just a little bit more effort.
- **Forced expiration** reverses this process by pulling the thorax down and in and by forcing the diaphragm higher into the thorax.
- The next chapter will provide insight into these processes.

Muscle:	Latissimus dorsi
Origin:	Lumbar, sacral, and lower thoracic vertebrae
Course:	Up fanlike
Insertion:	Humerus
Innervation:	Brachial plexus, posterior branch; fibers from the regions C6–C8 form the long subscapular nerve
Function:	For respiration, stabilizes posterior abdominal wall for expiration

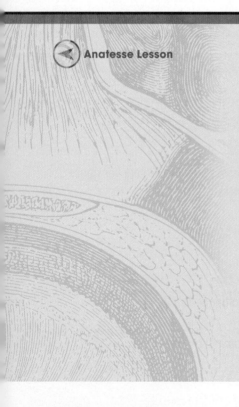

Anatesse Lesson

CHAPTER SUMMARY

Respiration is the process of gas exchange between an organism and its environment. The rib cage, made up of the spinal column and ribs, houses the lungs, which are the primary machinery of respiration. By means of the cartilaginous trachea and bronchial tree, air is brought into the lungs for gas exchange within the minute alveolar sacs. Oxygen enters the blood and carbon dioxide is removed by expiration.

Air is drawn into the lungs through muscular effort. The diaphragm, placed between the thorax and abdomen, contracts during inspiration. The lungs expand when the diaphragm contracts, drawn by pleurae linked through surface tension and negative pressure. When lungs expand, the air pressure within the lungs becomes negative with respect to the outside atmosphere, and Boyle's law dictates that air will flow from the region of higher pressure to fill the lungs. Accessory muscles also provide for added expansion of the rib cage for further inspiration.

Expiration may occur passively, through the forces of torque, elasticity, and gravity acting on the ribs and rib cage. It may also be forced, utilizing muscles of the abdomen and those that depress the rib cage to evacuate the lungs.

Media Connection

Go to the accompanying online resources at CengageBrain.com and have fun learning! Study with the Anatesse software program, play games, view animations and videos, and take practice tests to help reinforce the key concepts you learned in this chapter.

Study Questions

1. _____ is defined as force distributed over area.

2. _____ pressure causes air to enter a chamber that has expanded until the pressure is equalized.

3. How many of each of the following vertebrae are there?

   _____ cervical vertebrae
   _____ thoracic vertebrae
   _____ lumbar vertebrae
   _____ sacral vertebrae (fused)

4. On the figure below, identify the landmarks indicated.

   a. _____ process
   b. _____ process
   c. _____
   d. _____ facet
   e. _____ facet
   f. _____ facet
   g. _____ foramen

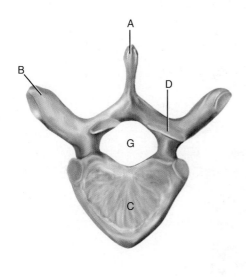

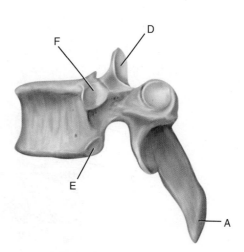

5. The _____ passes through the vertebral foramen.

6. On the following figures identify the landmarks indicated.

a. _____ (bone)

b. _____ (bone)

c. _____ (bone)

d. _____

e. _____

f. _____

g. _____ (bone)

h. _____ (bone)

i. _____ (bone)

j. _____

k. _____

l. _____

m. _____

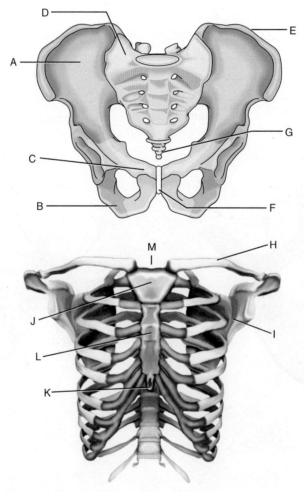

7. On the figure that follows identify the landmarks indicated.

a. _____

b. _____

c. _____

d. _____

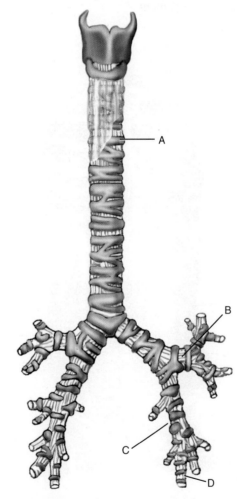

© Cengage Learning®.

8. On the following figure identify the muscles and structures indicated.

a. _____

b. _____

c. _____

d. _____

e. _____

f. _____ ligament

g. _____

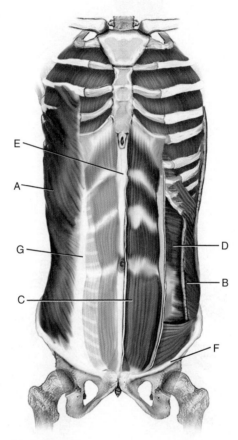

© Cengage Learning®.

9. On the following figure identify the muscles indicated.

    a. _____

    b. _____

    c. _____

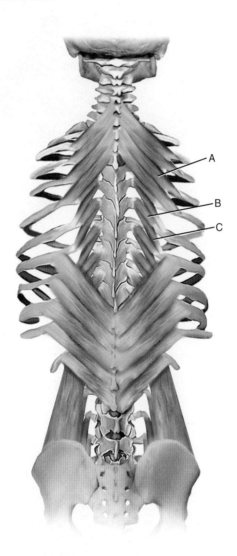

© Cengage Learning®.

10. Identify the muscles indicated on the following figure.

a. _____

b. _____

c. _____

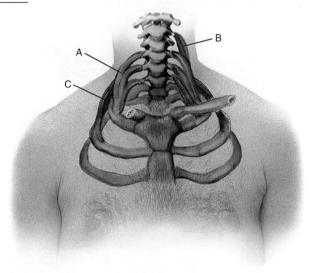

© Cengage Learning®.

11. Identify the muscles and portions of muscles indicated below.

a. _____

b. _____ head

c. _____ head

d. _____

e. _____

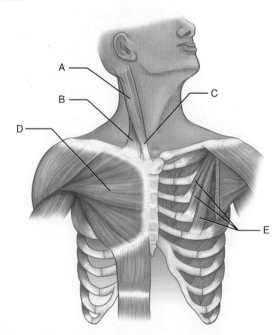

© Cengage Learning®.

12. Contraction of the diaphragm increases the _____ dimension of the thorax.

13. Contraction of the accessory muscles of inspiration increases the _____ dimension of the thorax.

14. Contraction of the muscles of expiration _____ the volume of the thorax.

15. Emphysema results in a breakdown of the alveolar wall, resulting in enlargement of alveolar clusters and consequent enlargement of the thorax known as "barrel chest." The result of this is that the diaphragm is pulled down at rest. Discuss the implications of the muscular action of inspiration and expiration on this altered system.

Study Question Answers

1. PRESSURE is defined as force distributed over area.

2. NEGATIVE pressure causes air to enter a chamber that has expanded until the pressure is equalized.

3. How many of each of the following vertebrae are there?
7 cervical vertebrae
12 thoracic vertebrae
5 lumbar vertebrae
5 sacral vertebrae (fused)

4. On the figure below, identify the landmarks indicated.
a. **SPINOUS** process
b. **TRANSVERSE** process
c. **CORPUS**
d. **SUPERIOR ARTICULAR** facet
e. **INFERIOR COSTAL** facet
f. **SUPERIOR COSTAL** facet
g. **VERTEBRAL** foramen

5. The **SPINAL CORD** passes through the vertebral foramen.

6. On the figure below, identify the landmarks indicated.
a. **ILIUM**
b. **ISCHIUM**
c. **PUBIC BONE**
d. **SACRUM**
e. **ILIAC CREST**
f. **PUBIC SYMPHYSIS**
g. **COCCYX**
h. **CLAVICLE**
i. **SCAPULA**
j. **MANUBRIUM STERNI**
k. **XIPHOID** or **ENSIFORM PROCESS**
l. **CORPUS STERNI**
m. **STERNAL NOTCH**

7. On the figure below, identify the landmarks indicated.

   a. **TRACHEA**
   b. **MAIN STEM BRONCHUS**
   c. **SECONDARY BRONCHUS**
   d. **TERTIARY BRONCHUS**

8. On the figure below, identify the muscles and structures indicated.

   a. **EXTERNAL OBLIQUE ABDOMINIS**
   b. **INTERNAL OBLIQUE ABDOMINIS**
   c. **RECTUS ABDOMINIS**
   d. **TRANSVERSUS ABDOMINIS**
   e. **LINEA ALBA**
   f. **INGUINAL LIGAMENT**
   g. **LINEA SEMILUNARIS**

9. On the figure below, identify the muscles indicated.

   a. **SERRATUS POSTERIOR SUPERIOR**
   b. **LEVATOR COSTARUM BREVIS**
   c. **LEVATOR COSTARUM LONGIS**

10. Identify the muscles indicated below.

   a. **SCALENUS ANTERIOR**
   b. **SCALENUS MEDIUS**
   c. **SCALENUS POSTERIOR**

11. Identify the muscles and portions of muscles indicated below.

   a. **STERNOCLEIDOMASTOID**
   b. **CLAVICULAR** head
   c. **STERNAL** head
   d. **PECTORALIS MAJOR**
   e. **PECTORALIS MINOR**

12. Contraction of the diaphragm increases the **VERTICAL** dimension of the thorax.

13. Contraction of the accessory muscles of inspiration increases the **TRANSVERSE** dimension of the thorax.

14. Contraction of the muscles of expiration **DECREASES** the volume of the thorax.

15. In advanced emphysema, the diaphragm is pulled down and stretched relatively flat by the flaring of the rib cage. In normal inspiration, contraction of the diaphragm causes the central tendon to pull down, causing air to enter the lungs (Boyle's law dictates that a drop in alveolar pressure will cause air to flow in). When the diaphragm of an individual with advanced emphysema contracts, it pulls the ribs closer together because they were distended by the "barrel chest." As a result, the alveoli are compressed, causing an increase in alveolar pressure and causing air to leave the lungs. Thus, the inspiratory movement of the diaphragm causes expiration. The single inspiratory avenue left to the individual is to elevate the sternum and clavicle using clavicular breathing.

Bibliography

Arnott, W. M. (1973). *Disorders of the respiratory system*. Oxford, England: Blackwell Scientific.

Araujo, J. A., Barajas, B., Kleinman, M., Wang, X., Bennett, B. J., Gong, K. W., et al. (2008). Ambient particulate pollutants in the ultrafine range promote early atherosclerosis and systemic oxidative stress. *Circulation Research*. Published online before print, January 17, 2008, doi: 0.1161/CIRCRESAHA.107.164970.

Baken, R., & Cavallo, S. (1981). Prephonatory chest wall posturing. *Folia Phoniatrica, 33,* 193–202.

Baken, R. J., & Orlikoff, R. F. (1999). *Clinical measurement of speech and voice* (2nd ed.). San Diego, CA: Singular Publishing Group.

Grant, J. C. B., Basmajian, J. V., & Sloneker, C. E. (1989). *Grant's method of anatomy: A clinical problem-solving*. Baltimore: Williams & Wilkins.

Bateman, H. E., & Mason, R. M. (1984). *Applied anatomy and physiology of the speech and hearing mechanism*. Springfield, IL: Charles C. Thomas.

Beck, E. W. (1982). *Mosby's atlas of functional human anatomy*. St. Louis, MO: C. V. Mosby Company.

Bergman, R., Thompson, S., & Afifi, A. (1984). *A catalog of human variation*. Baltimore: Urban & Schwarzenberg.

Bly, L. (1994). *Motor skills acquisition in the first year*. Tucson, AZ: Therapy Skill Builders.

Burrows, B., Knudson, R. J., & Kettel, L. J. (1975). *Respiratory insufficiency*. Chicago: Year Book Medical Publishers.

Cala, S. J., Edyvean, J., & Engel, L. A. (1992). Chest wall and trunk muscle activity during inspiratory loading. *Journal of Applied Physiology, 73*(6), 2373–2381.

Cernak, I., & Noble-Haeusslein, L. J. (2010). Traumatic brain injury: An overview of pathobiology with emphasis on military populations. *Journal of Cerebral Blood Flow Metabolism, 30*(2), 255–266.

Cerqueira, E. P., & Garbellini, D.(1999). Electromyographic study of the pectoralis major, serratus anterior, and external oblique muscles during respiratory activity in humans. *Electromyography Clinical Neurophysiology, 39*(3), 131–137.

Campbell, E., Agostoni, E., & Davis, J. (1970). *The respiratory muscles, mechanics, and neural control*. Philadelphia: W. B. Saunders.

Chusid, J. G. (1985). *Correlative neuroanatomy and functional neurology* (17th ed.). Los Altos, CA: Lange Medical Publications.

Creasy, R. K. (1997). *Management of labor and delivery*. Malden, MA: Blackwell Science.

De Freitas, V. & Vitti, M. (1980). Electromyographic study of the trapezius (pars media) and rhomboideus major during respiration. *Electromyography Clinical Neurophysiology, 20*(6), 503–507.

Des Jardins, T., & Burton, G. G. (2001). *Clinical manifestation and assessment of respiratory disease*. Chicago: Mosby.

Donaldson, K., & Seaton, A. (2012). A short history of toxicology of inhaled products. *Particle and Fiber Toxicology, 9*(13), 2–12.

Fenn, W. O., & Rahn, H. O. (Eds.). (1964). *Handbook of physiology, respiration* (Vol. 1, 3, pp. 387–409). Washington, DC: American Physiological Society; Baltimore: Williams & Wilkins.

Ganong, W. F. (2003). *Review of medical physiology* (21st ed.). New York: McGraw-Hill/Appleton & Lange.

Gilroy, A. M., MacPherson, B. R., & Ross, L. M. (2012). *Atlas of anatomy*. New York: Thieme.

Gordon, M. S. (1972). *Animal physiology: Principles and adaptations*. New York: Macmillan.

Gray, H., Bannister, L. H., Berry, M. M., & Williams, P. L. (Eds.). (1995). *Gray's anatomy*. London: Churchill Livingstone.

Grobler, N. J. (1977). *Textbook of clinical anatomy* (Vol. 1). Amsterdam: Elsevier Scientific.

Hlastala, M. P., & Berger, A. J. (1996). *Physiology of respiration*. New York: Oxford University Press.

Kahane, J. (1982). Anatomy and physiology of the organs of the peripheral speech mechanism. In N. Lass, L. McReynolds, J. Northern, & D. Yoder (Eds.), *Speech, language, and hearing. Vol. 1: Normal processes* (pp. 109–155). Philadelphia: W. B. Saunders.

Kahane, J. C., & Folkins, J. F. (1984). *Atlas of speech and hearing anatomy*. Columbus, OH: Charles E. Merrill.

Kao, F. F. (1972). *An introduction to respiratory physiology*. Amsterdam: Exerpta Medica.

Kaplan, H. (1960). *Anatomy and physiology of speech*. New York: McGraw-Hill.

Kent, R. D. (1997). *The speech sciences*. San Diego, CA: Singular Publishing Group.

Kuehn, D. P., Lemme, M. L., & Baumgartner, J. M. (1989). *Neural bases of speech, hearing, and language*. Boston: Little, Brown.

Langley, M. B., & Lombardino, L. J. (1991). *Neurodevelopmental strategies for managing communication disorders in children with severe motor dysfunction.* Austin, TX: Pro-Ed.

Lee, D. H. K. (1972). *Environmental factors in respiratory disease.* New York: Academic Press.

Logemann, J. (1998). *Evaluation and treatment of swallowing disorders* (2nd ed.). Austin, TX: Pro-Ed.

Loukas, M., Louis, R. G. Jr., Wartmann, C. T., Tubbs, R. S., Gupta, A. A., Apaydin, N., & Jordan, R. (2008). An anatomic investigation of the serratus posterior superior and serratus posterior inferior muscles. *Surgical & Radiological Anatomy, 30*(2), 119–123.

MacKay, L. E., Chapman, P. E., & Morgan, A. S. (1997). *Maximizing brain injury recovery.* Gaithersburg, MD: Aspen Publishers.

McMinn, R. M. H., Hutchings, R. T., & Logan, B. M. (1994). *Color atlas of head and neck anatomy.* London: Mosby-Wolfe.

Miller, A. D., Bianchi, A. L., & Bishop, B. P. (1997). *Neural control of the respiratory muscles.* Boca Raton, FL: CRC Press.

Mohr, J. P. (1989). *Manual of clinical problems in neurology.* Boston: Little, Brown.

Moser, K. M., & Spragg, R. G. (1982). *Respiratory emergencies.* St. Louis, MO: C. V. Mosby.

Murray, J. F. (1976). *The normal lung: The basis for diagnosis and treatment of pulmonary disease.* Philadelphia: W. B. Saunders.

Netter, F. H. (1983a). *The CIBA collection of medical illustrations. Vol. 1. Nervous system: Part I. Anatomy and physiology.* West Caldwell, NJ: CIBA Pharmaceutical Company.

Netter, F. H. (1983b). *The CIBA collection of medical illustrations. Vol. 1. Nervous system: Part II. Neurologic and neuromuscular disorders.* West Caldwell, NJ: CIBA Pharmaceutical Company.

Netter, F. H. (1997). *Atlas of human anatomy.* Los Angeles: Icon Learning Systems.

Pace, W. R. (1970). *Pulmonary physiology.* Philadelphia: F. A. Davis.

Peters, R. M. (1969). *The mechanical basis of respiration.* Boston: Little, Brown.

Rohen, J. W., Yokochi, C., Lutjen-Drecoll, E., & Romrell, L. J. (2002). *Color atlas of anatomy* (5th ed.). Philadelphia: Williams & Wilkins.

Rosse, C., Gaddum-Rosse, P., & Rosse, G. (1997). *Hollinshead's textbook of anatomy. Philadelphia:* Lippincott-Raven.

Sargent, J. R. (2011). Nanotechnology and environmental, health, and safety: Issues for consideration. *Congressional Research Service,* 7-5700, RL34614.

Schamberger, R. C. (2000). Chest wall deformities. In T. W. Shields, J. LoCicero, III, & R. B. Ponn (Eds.). *General thoracic surgery* (5th ed., pp. 535–569). Philadelphia: Lippincott/Williams & Wilkins.

Scott, J. R., Disaia, P. J., Hammond, C. B., & Spellacy, W. N. (1994). *Danforth's obstetrics and gynecology* (7th ed.). Philadelphia: J. B. Lippincott.

Shaffer, R. E. & Rengasamy, S. (2009). Respiratory protection against airborne nanoparticles: A review. *Journal of Nanoparticle Research, 11*(7), 1661–1672.

Snell, R. S. (1978). *Gross anatomy dissector.* Boston: Little, Brown.

Spector, W. S. (1961). *Handbook of biological data.* Philadelphia: W. B. Saunders Company.

Taylor, A. (1960). The contribution of the intercostal muscles to the effort of respiration in man. *Journal of Physiology, 151,* 390.

Tokizane, T., Kawamata, K., & Tokizane, H. (1952). Electromyographic studies on the human respiratory muscles. *Japan Journal of Physiology, 2,* 232.

Twietmeyer, A., & McCracken, T. D., (1992). *Coloring guide to regional human anatomy* (2nd ed.). Philadelphia: Lea & Febiger.

Vilensky, J. A., Baltes, M., Weikel. L., Fortin, J. D., & Fourie, L. J. (2001). Serratus posterior muscles: Anatomy, clinical relevance, and function. *Clinical Anatomy, 14*(4), 237–241.

Watson, A. H., Williams, C. & James, B. V. (2012). Activity patterns in latissimus dorsi and sternocleidomastoid in classical singers. *Journal of voice, 26*(3), e-95–e-105.

Whitmore, I., Willan, P. L. T., Gosling, J. A., & Harris, P. F. (2002). *Human Anatomy: Color atlas and text* (4th ed.). St. Louis, MO: Mosby.

Williams, P., & Warrick, R. (1980). *Gray's anatomy* (36th British ed.). Philadelphia: W. B. Saunders.

Zemlin, W. R. (1988). *Speech and hearing science. Anatomy and physiology.* Englewood Cliffs, NJ: Prentice-Hall.

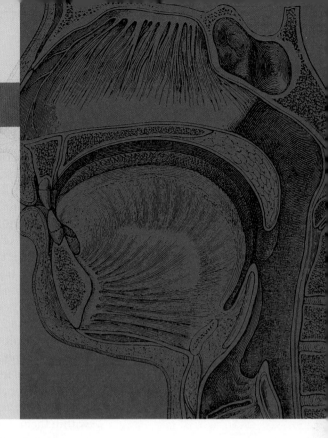

Chapter 3

PHYSIOLOGY OF RESPIRATION

Respiration requires muscular effort, and the degree to which an individual can successfully control the musculature determines, in large part, the efficiency of respiration itself. Respiratory function (physiology) changes as we exercise, age, or suffer setbacks in health. Considering its importance in speech, it is no wonder that as the respiratory system goes, so goes communication.

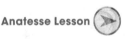

Anatesse Lesson

We are capable of both **quiet** and **forced inspiration**. There is a parallel to this in expiration, because we are capable of **passive** and **active expiration**. In passive expiration, we let the forces inherent to the tissues restore the system to a resting position after inspiration. In active expiration, we use muscular effort to push just a little farther. Let us examine these forces.

The process of expiration is one of eliminating the waste products of respiration. Attend to your own respiratory cycle to learn an important aspect of quiet expiration. Close your eyes while you breathe in and out 10 times, quietly and in a relaxed manner. Pay particular attention to the area of your body around your diaphragm, including your rib cage and your abdomen.

What you experienced is the active contraction of the diaphragm, followed by a simple relaxing of the musculature. You actively contract to breathe in, and then simply let nature take its course for expiration. You may liken this to blowing up a balloon. The balloon will expand when you blow and deflate as soon as you let go of the grip. The forces on the balloon that cause it to lose its air are among those that cause your lungs to deflate. The forces we need to talk about are elasticity and gravity.

You will recall that the lungs are highly elastic, porous tissue. They are spongelike and when they are compressed, they will tend to expand as soon as the compression is released. Likewise, if you were to grab a sponge by its edges and stretch it, the sponge would tend to return to its original shape and size when you release it.

You can think of the lungs as small sponges in a large bottle. The lungs truly will not fill up that "bottle" of the chest cavity when they are left to their own devices (i.e., permitted to deflate to their natural resting condition). In the adult body, the lungs are actually stretched beyond their resting position, but this is not so with the infant.

During early development, the lungs completely fill the thorax, so that they are not stretched to fit the relaxed rib cage. As the child develops, the rib cage grows faster than the lungs, and the pleural linings and increased negative intrapleural pressure provide a means for the lungs to be stretched out to fill that space.

The result of this stretching is greatly increased capacity and reserve in adults, but not in infants. Because the thorax and lungs are of the same size in infants, they must breathe two to three times as often as an adult for adequate respiration. The adult's lungs are stretched out and never are completely compressed, so there is always a reserve of air within them that is not at the moment undergoing gas exchange.

Upon increasing the thorax size, the lungs expand just as if you had grabbed them and stretched them out. When the muscles that are expanding the rib cage relax, the lungs tend to return to their original shape and size. In addition, when you inhale and your abdomen protrudes, you are stretching the abdominal muscles. Relaxing the inspiratory process will let those muscles return to their original length. That is, the abdominal muscles will tend to push your abdominal viscera back in and force the diaphragm up.

A second force acting in support of passive expiration is gravity. When standing or sitting erect, gravity acts on the ribs to pull them back after they have been expanded through the effort of the accessory muscles of inspiration. Gravity also works in favor of maximizing your overall capacity, because it pulls the abdominal viscera down, leaving more room for the lungs. We will talk about this more because body position becomes a significant issue in the efficiency of respiration.

There is one final "force" that bears attention. For years, speech scientists acknowledged the triad of "torque, elasticity, and gravity" as the forces driving passive expiration. It was believed that expansion of the rib cage during inspiration twisted the cartilaginous portion of the rib cage, thereby storing a restoring force that would cause the rib cage to return to rest upon relaxation. The reality, as identified by Hixon in his 2006 paper, is that the rib cage is under a negative torque at relaxation (i.e., it is pulled toward the lungs) and that inspiration, which increases the thoracic volume, only serves to move the rib cage to a neutral condition during normal respiration. Only after one has achieved upwards of 60 percent of vital capacity (i.e., taken a significantly deep inspiration) would the rib cage assist in expiration. It is worth noting that inhalation above 60 percent does occur, particularly when shouting, so torque could continue to have a role in respiration.

✔ *To summarize:*

- We are capable of quiet respiration as well as forced inspiration and expiration.
- Expiration may be passive, driven by the forces of **elasticity** and **gravity**.
- We may also use muscles that reduce the size of the thorax by compressing the **abdomen** or pulling the rib cage down, and this will force air out of the lungs beyond that which is expired in passive expiration.

THE MEASUREMENT OF RESPIRATION

The quantity of air processed through respiration is dictated primarily by bodily needs, and speech physiology operates within these limits. We will discuss respiration in terms of rate of flow in respiration, volume and lung capacities, and pressure.

Instruments in Respiration

Respiratory flow, volumes, and capacities are measured using a **spirometer** (see Figure 3-1). The classical wet spirometer consists of a tube connected to a container opened at the bottom. This container is placed inside another container that is full of water.

spirometer: device used to measure respiratory volume

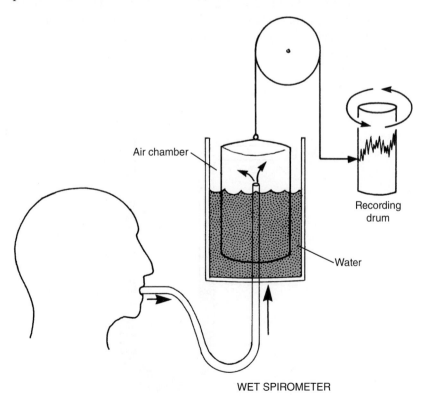

Air chamber

Recording drum

Water

WET SPIROMETER

Figure 3-1. Wet spirometer used to measure lung volumes. When the individual exhales into the tube, gas entering the air chamber displaces the water, causing the chamber to rise. These changes are charted on the recording drum.
© Cengage Learning®.

To measure lung volume, an individual breathes into the tube, causing a volume of water to be displaced. The amount of water displaced gives an accurate estimate of the air that was required to displace it. (We are ignoring the *pressure* required to raise the container and the effort involved in this process.)

In reality, spirometers take many forms. A whole-body plethymsograph is a chamber in which a subject sits. As the person's chest wall moves during respiration, the volume of the chamber changes, so volumes and capacities can be estimated more accurately than using a wet spirometer. (Biologists use a version of the whole-body plethysmograph, a microspirometer, to measure respiration in animals and insects, by placing the organism in an enclosure and reading the volume changes.) A portable spirometer outfitted with a "windmill" blade makes measurement of forced capacity readily available in any clinical site.

A pneumotachograph is a spirometer that can measure the rate of airflow, and these come in a variety of designs. One of the most reliable types uses a small turbine held within the mouthpiece: The harder an individual blows, the faster the turbine turns. The turning relates directly to how much flow has occurred, so volume over time can easily be calculated. Pneumotachographs are particularly useful for characterizing ongoing respiratory function and have the added benefit over the old wet spirometers of having fresh air for the subject to breathe. The wet spirometer was a closed system, in that you really only had one respiratory cycle before you were "recycling" your own breath.

The classic U-tube **manometer** is one means of measuring pressure, as shown in Figure 3-2. A subject is asked to place the tube in his or her mouth and to blow. The force of the subject's expiration is exerted on a column of water that rises as a result. The more force the

manometer: device for measuring air pressure differences

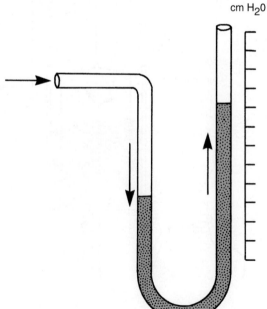

cm H$_2$O

Figure 3-2. U-tube manometer for measurement of respiratory pressure.
© Cengage Learning®.

person uses, the higher the column rises. We can measure the effects of that force in inches or in centimeters of water (barometric pressure is often reported in millimeters of mercury, which refers to how many millimeters of mercury were elevated by the pressure). Because water is considerably less dense than mercury, the same amount of pressure will elevate a column of water much higher than a similar column of mercury. For this reason, we measure the rather small pressures of respiration with the water standard.

As with spirometers, there exist an array of pressure-sensing devices that can be used for the measurement of human respiration. Portable manometers allow reliable clinical and field measurement of respiratory function, and manometers with alarms are used by respiratory therapists to monitor ventilation of patients. Similarly, inflation manometers are used to determine pressure for endotracheal cuff inflation, but these tend to be mechanical rather than electronic. We're going to see that the relationship between pressure and volume come into play as we look at issues such as the lung's ability to be distended, also known as compliance.

Breathing requires that gas be exchanged on an ongoing basis. The body has specific needs that must be met continually, so we will need to discuss respiration in terms of the **rate of flow** of air in and out of the lungs (measured as cubic centimeters per second or minute). We also need to speak of the quantities or **volumes** that are involved in this gas exchange (measured in liters [L], milliliters [mL], cubic centimeters [cc], or on occasion, cubic inches).

RESPIRATION FOR LIFE

What is obvious is that respiration is vital. If you are a swimmer, you probably remember staying under water a little too long, discovering the limits of your respiratory system and the panic you felt when you reached those limits. Let us examine why those limits are reached and how we work within those limits for speech.

When you breathe in, you are engaged in a simple gesture with very complex results. The goal of respiration, of course, is oxygenation of blood and elimination of carbon dioxide.

The basic process of gas exchange has four stages: ventilation, distribution, perfusion, and diffusion. **Ventilation** refers to the actual movement of air in the conducting respiratory pathway. This air is distributed to the 300 million alveoli where the oxygen-poor vascular supply from the right pulmonary artery is perfused to the 6 billion capillaries that supply those alveoli. **Perfusion** refers to the migration of gas or liquid through a barrier. The actual gas exchange across the alveolar-capillary membrane is referred to as **diffusion**.

The ventilation process is a direct function of the action of the diaphragm and muscles of respiration. As discussed earlier, contraction of muscles of inspiration causes expansion of the alveoli that results in a negative alveolar pressure and air being drawn into the lungs. Understanding the pressure changes in this process is critical.

ventilation: air inhaled per unit time

perfusion: migration of fluid or gas through a barrier

diffusion: migration or mixing of one material (e.g., liquid) through another

Effects of Turbulence on Respiration

When lungs expand, pressure throughout the system drops as a result of expansion of the alveoli. Air courses through the large-diameter conducting bronchi, which, being comprised of cartilage, resist the negative pressure to collapse. In healthy lungs, this results in relatively low resistance and laminar flow of air. Some slight turbulence occurs at bifurcations such as where the trachea splits to become the right and left main stem bronchi, but generally the flow is unimpeded. This is not a trivial notion, because even a small irregularity in the airway (such as mucus) greatly increases the resistance to airflow and also the difficulty in respiration.

The expiratory act is performed by decreasing the thoracic volume, thus eliminating carbon dioxide. Gas that was previously captive in the blood has migrated across the alveolar-capillary membrane and is expelled into the atmosphere.

Respiratory Cycle

During quiet respiration, adults will complete between 12 and 18 cycles of respiration per minute (see Figure 3-3). A cycle of respiration is defined as one inspiration and one expiration. This quiet breathing pattern, known as **quiet tidal respiration** (because it can be visualized as a tidal flow of air into and out of the lungs), involves about 500 mL (1/2 liter) of air with each cycle. (You can visualize this by imagining a 2-liter bottle of soda being one quarter full.) A quick calculation will reveal that we process something on the order of 6,000–8,000 mL (6–8 liters) of air every minute. (The volume of air involved in 1 minute of respiration is referred to as the **minute volume**.)

Because these values are based on quiet, sedentary breathing, it will not surprise you to learn that they increase during strenuous work. An adult male will increase his oxygen requirements by a factor of 20 on increasing work output. As you can see in Table 3-1, as work increases the ventilation requirements are met by increased respiratory flow.

minute volume: the volume of air exchanged by an organism in 1 minute

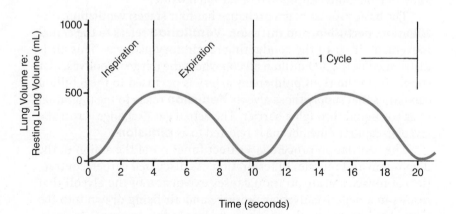

Figure 3-3. Volume display of two cycles of quiet respiration.
© Cengage Learning®.

Turbulence and Respiration

The respiratory passageway offers relatively low resistance to airflow, a fact that works in favor of efficient respiration with little effort. As resistance to airflow increases, the effort required to draw air into the lungs increases as well, which causes rapid fatigue. You may remember the exhaustion you felt the last time you had a respiratory infection that caused excessive secretions in your respiratory passageway. Part of the fatigue you felt was the product of the turbulence produced by the mucus within the passageway. The extra drag caused by these elements has to be overcome to keep the body oxygenated, and the muscles of respiration have to work overtime to do the task.

Table 3-1 **Respiratory volume as a function of work intensity**		
	Work Intensity (kg m/min)	**Ventilation (mL)**
Female	600	3470
	900	5060
Male	900	4190
	1200	5520
	1500	7090

Source: Data from *Handbook of Biological Data* by W. S. Spector, 1956, p. 352. Philadelphia: W. B. Saunders.

Developmental Processes in Respiration

There are developmental effects on respiration as well. The lungs undergo a great deal of prenatal development, as seen in Figure 3-4. By the time the infant is born, the cartilaginous conducting airway is complete, although the number of alveoli will increase from about 25 million at birth to more than 300 million by 8 years of age. We retain that number throughout life.

The conducting airways will grow steadily in diameter and length until thorax growth is complete, although the thorax will expand to a greater degree than the lungs. As the thorax expands, the lungs are stretched to fill the cavity, a fact that helps to explain two differences between adults and children. As we mentioned earlier, adults breathe between 12 and 18 times per minute while at rest, but the newborn will breathe an average of 40–70 cycles per minute. By 5 years, the child is down to about 25 breaths per minute (bpm), and this number drops to about 20 bpm at 15 years of age (see Table 3-2). The adult has a considerable volume of air that is never expelled, but the infant does

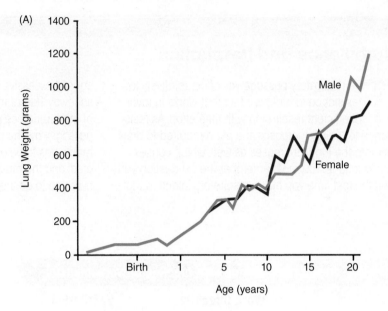

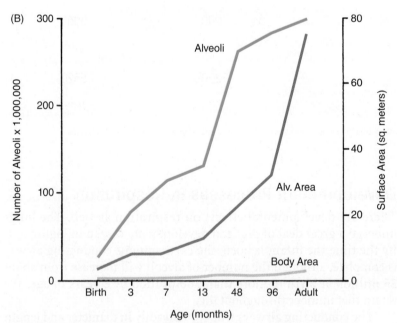

Figure 3-4. (A) Changes in lung weight as a function of age. Notice that males and females are essentially equivalent in lung weight until puberty, at which time the increased thoracic cavity size of the male is reflected in larger lung weight. (B) Changes in lung tissue with age. The number of alveoli increases radically through the fourth year of life, and the total alveolar area stabilizes around puberty when the thorax approximates its adult volume.

© Cengage Learning®. (Data from Handbook of Biological Data by W. S. Spector, 1956, pp. 162, 176–180, 353. Philadelphia: W. B. Saunders.)

Table 3-2 **Respiration rate in breaths per minute as a function of age**	
Age	**Respiration Rate (bpm)**
Newborn	60
1 year	30
2 years	25
3 years	24
5 years	20
10 years	18
15 years	18
20 years	17

Source: Data from Physical Growth and Development by J. Valadian & D. Porter, 1977, p. 311. Boston: Little, Brown, & Co.

not have this reserve. In essence, the thorax expands during growth and development and stretches the lungs beyond their natural volume.

As a result of this expansion, there is a volume of air in the adult lung that cannot be expelled (residual volume), and this volume helps to account for the reserve capacity of adults relative to infants. Infant lungs have yet to undergo the proliferation of the alveoli seen during childhood, and thus infants must breathe more frequently to meet their metabolic needs.

VOLUMES AND CAPACITIES

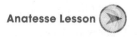

Anatesse Lesson

Respiration is the product of a number of forces and structures, and for us to make sense of them, we need to define some volumes and capacities of the lungs. When we refer to volumes, we are partitioning off the respiratory system so that we may get an accurate estimate of the amount of air each compartment can hold. (For instance, we could conceivably talk about the volume of a single alveolus, which is about 250 microns in diameter, or about 250 millionths of a meter, although this might not produce a very useful number.) We also might speak of **capacities**, which are more functional units. *Capacities* refer to combinations of volumes that express physiological limits. Volumes are discrete, whereas capacities represent functional combinations of volumes.

Both volumes and capacities are measured in milliliters (mL, which are thousandths of a liter) or cubic centimeters (cc, which is another name for the same thing). To get an idea of what these volumes and capacities really amount to, look at a 2-liter soda bottle for a reference. One liter is 1000 mL, which is also 1000 cc.

There are five volumes that we should consider. Refer to Tables 3-3 and 3-4, as well as Figure 3-5 as we discuss these.

Table 3-3 Respiratory volumes and capacities

Volumes

Tidal Volume (TV): The volume of air exchanged in one cycle of respiration.

Inspiratory Reserve Volume (IRV): The volume of air that can be inhaled after a tidal inspiration.

Expiratory Reserve Volume (ERV): The volume of air that can be expired following passive, tidal expiration. Also known as **resting lung volume**.

Residual Volume (RV): The volume of air remaining in the lungs after a maximum exhalation.

Dead Air: The volume of air within the conducting passageways that cannot be involved in gas exchange (included as a component of residual volume).

Capacities

Vital Capacity (VC): The volume of air that can be inhaled following a maximal exhalation; includes inspiratory reserve volume, tidal volume, and expiratory reserve volume (VC = IRV + TV + ERV).

Functional Residual Capacity (FRC): The volume of air in the body at the end of passive exhalation; includes expiratory reserve and residual volumes (FRC = ERV + RV).

Inspiratory Capacity (IC): The maximum inspiratory volume possible after tidal expiration (IC = TV + IRV).

Total Lung Capacity (TLC): The sum of inspiratory reserve volume, tidal volume, expiratory reserve volume, and residual volume (TLC = IC + FRC).

© Cengage Learning®.

Table 3-4 Typical respiratory volumes and capacities in adults

Volume/capacity	Males (in cc)	Females (in cc)	Average (in cc)
Resting tidal volume	600	450	525
Inspiratory reserve volume	3000	1950	2475
Expiratory reserve volume	1200	800	1000
Residual volume	1200	1000	1100
Vital capacity	4800	3200	4000
Functional residual capacity	2400	1800	2200
Inspiratory capacity	3600	2400	3000
Total lung capacity	6000	4200	5100

Note: Volumes and capacities vary as a function of body size, gender, age, and body height. These volumes represent approximate values for healthy adults between 20 and 30 years of age. Vital capacity is estimated by accounting for age (in years) and height (in cm):

Males:

VC in mL = (27.63 – [0.112 @ age in yrs]) @ height in cm

Females:

VC in mL = (21.78 – [0.101 @ age in yrs]) @ height in cm

Source: Data from Baldwin, Cournand, and Richards (1948) as cited in An Introduction to Respiratory Physiology by F. F. Kao, 1972, p. 39. Amsterdam: Excerpta Medica; and The Mechanical Basis of Respiration by R. M. Peters, 1969, p. 49. Boston: Little, Brown & Co.

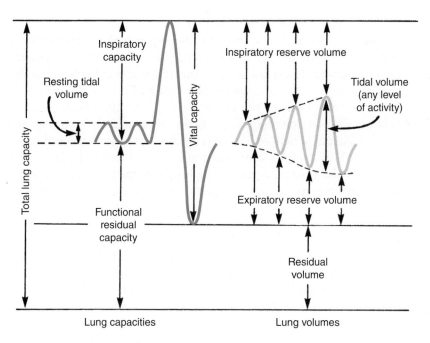

Figure 3-5. Lung volumes and capacities as displayed on a spirogram.
© Cengage Learning®. (Modified from Pappenheimer et al., 1950.)

Volumes

Tidal Volume (TV)

The volume of air that we breathe in during a respiratory cycle is referred to as tidal volume. The definition of TV makes precise measurement difficult, because it varies as a function of physical exertion, body size, and age. **Quiet tidal volume** (TV at rest) has an average for adult males of around 600 cc and for adult females of approximately 450 cc. This works out to an average of 525 cc for adults, or approximately one-quarter of the volume of a 2-liter soda bottle every 5 seconds. You will fill up three of these bottles every minute. As shown in Table 3-1, TV increases markedly as effort increases.

quiet tidal volume: the volume of air exchanged during one cycle of quiet respiration

Inspiratory Reserve Volume (IRV)

The second volume of interest is **inspiratory reserve volume** (IRV). IRV is the volume that can be inhaled after a tidal inspiration. It is the volume of air that is in reserve for use *beyond* the volume you would breathe in tidally.

To help remember the IRV, do the following exercise. Sit quietly and breathe in and out tidally until you become aware of your breath, and tag each breath mentally with the words *in* and *out*. After a few outs and ins, stop breathing at the end of one of your inspirations. This is the peak of the tidal inspiration. Instead of breathing out (which is what you want to do), breathe in as deeply as you can. The amount you inspired after you stopped is the IRV, and if you are an average adult, the volume is about 2475 cc (2.475 liters).

inspiratory reserve volume: the volume of air that can be inhaled after a tidal inspiration

Expiratory Reserve Volume (ERV)

expiratory reserve volume: the volume of air that can be expired after a tidal expiration

The parallel volume for expiration is the **expiratory reserve volume** (ERV). ERV is the amount of air that can be expired following passive, tidal expiration. To experience this, breathe as you did before, but this time stop before you breathe in following expiration. (This point is easier to reach, because you can just *relax* your muscles and air will flow out without muscular effort.) Expire as completely as you can and you will have experienced ERV: It is the amount of air you could expire after that tidal expiration, amounting to about 1000 cc (1.0 liter). This volume is also referred to as **resting lung volume** (RLV), because it is the volume present in the resting lungs after a passive exhalation.

Residual Volume (RV)

residual volume: in respiration, the volume of air remaining after a maximum exhalation

A fourth volume of interest is **residual volume** (RV), the volume remaining in the lungs after a maximum exhalation. No matter how forcefully or completely you exhale, there is a volume of air (about 1.1 liters) that cannot be eliminated. This volume exists because the lungs are stretched as a result of the relatively expanded thorax, so it should come as no shock to know that it is not present in the newborn. You might think of it as an acquired space. By the way, this does not mean we do not use that air, but rather simply that it is a *volume* that is not eliminated during expiration.

Dead Space Air

dead space air: the air within the conducting passageways that cannot be involved in gas exchange

We have accommodated the major volumes, but we must deal with the volume that cannot be involved in gas exchange. The air in the conducting passageways cannot be involved in gas exchange because there are no alveoli. You will recall that the conducting passageways of the lungs are constructed largely of cartilage, and the upper respiratory passageway (consisting of the mouth, pharynx, and nose) certainly does not have alveoli. The volume that cannot undergo gas exchange in the lungs is referred to as **dead space air** and in the adult has a volume of about 150 cc. This varies also with age and weight, but is approximately equal (in cc) to your weight in pounds. The volume associated with dead air is included in RV, because both are volumes associated with air that cannot be expelled.

The concept of dead air (and its importance) may become more vivid if you consider a swimmer using a tube or snorkel to breathe from underwater. This person has additional dead air associated with the tube: The longer the tube is, the greater the volume he or she will have to inhale to pull air from the surface into the lungs. In pathological conditions, the term *dead space* takes on new meaning. In the healthy individual, **anatomical dead space** (that described previously) and **physiological dead space** (wasted ventilation) are the same. As you found in the clinical notes of Chapter 2, there are conditions that contribute to increased physiological dead space; that is, pathological conditions of the respiratory system often result in wastage of respiratory effort and air.

Capacities

The volumes may be combined in a number of ways to characterize physiological needs. The following four capacities are useful combinations of volumes.

Vital Capacity (VC)

Of the capacities, **vital capacity** (VC) is the most often cited in speech and hearing literature, because it represents the capacity available for speech (see Figure 3-6). Vital capacity is the combination of IRV, ERV, and TV. That is, VC represents the total volume of air that can be inspired after a maximal expiration. Because VC = IRV + ERV + TV, you can quickly see that it is approximately 4000 cc in the average adult. Expiratory reserve volume (resting lung volume) is 38 percent of vital capacity, while tidal volume is only about 15 percent of VC. Inspiratory reserve volume makes up the other 47 percent of the lung capacity. Doing a quick calculation will tell you that 53 percent of your vital capacity is in your lungs at the peak of tidal inspiration.

vital capacity: the total volume of air that can be inspired after a maximal expiration

Functional Residual Capacity (FRC)

Functional residual capacity is the volume of air remaining in the body after a passive exhalation (FRC = ERV + RV). In the average adult, this comes to approximately 2200 mL.

functional residual capacity: the volume of air remaining in the body after a passive exhalation

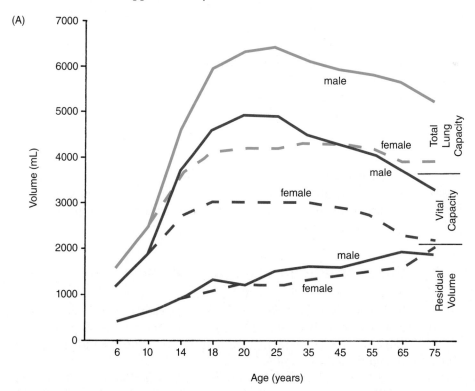

Figure 3-6. (A) Vital capacity, total lung volume, and residual volume as a function of age. (continues).

Source: Data from *Handbook of Biological Data* by W. S. Spector, 1956, p. 267. Philadelphia: W. B. Saunders.

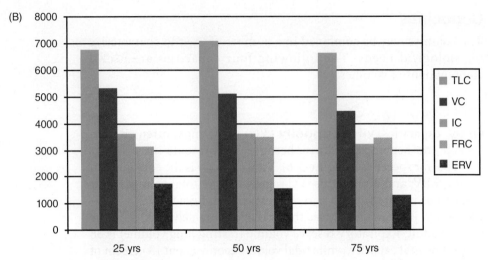

Figure 3-6 continued. (B) Effect of age on selected volumes and capacities in healthy males. Note that the total lung capacity (TLC) remains the same across the adult life-span, but vital capacity (VC), inspiratory capacity (IC), and expiratory reserve volume (ERV) diminish. Functional residual capacity (FRC) increases as one ages because it reflects the loss of inspiratory capacity of aging.

Source: From data of Hoit, J. D. & Hixon, T. J. (1987). Age and speech breathing. Journal of Speech and Hearing Research, 30, p. 357.

Total Lung Capacity (TLC)

total lung capacity: sum of tidal volume, inspiratory reserve volume, expiratory reserve volume, and residual volume

Total lung capacity is the sum of all the volumes (TLC = TV + IRV + ERV + RV), totaling approximately 5100 cc. Note that this is different from VC, which represents the volume of air that is involved in a maximal respiratory cycle, whereas TLC includes RV. RV serves as a buffer in respiration because it is not immediately involved in interaction with the environment. Oxygen-rich air is diluted by mixing with the air of the RV, so that during brief periods of fluctuating air quality relatively constant oxygenation will occur.

Inspiratory Capacity (IC)

inspiratory capacity: the maximum inspiratory volume possible after tidal expiration

Inspiratory capacity is the maximum inspiratory volume possible after tidal expiration (IC = TV + IRV). This refers to the capacity of the lungs for inspiration and represents a volume of approximately 3000 cc in the adult.

Effect of Age on Volumes and Capacities

As we age, tissue changes. What may surprise us is how rapidly our body reaches its peak function and how steady the decline is. VC is a function of body weight, age, and height, the relationship for which can be expressed mathematically, as seen in Table 3-4 and graphically in Figures 3-5 through 3-7.

What you can see from these figures is that as age increases, VC decreases by about 100 mL per year in adulthood. Figure 3-7 also shows that VC increases steadily with body growth up to about 20 years of age, holds constant through about age 25, and then begins a steady decline. Females have smaller VC throughout the life-span, as

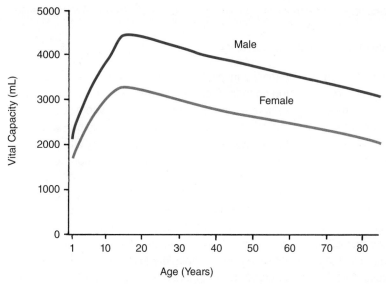

Figure 3-7. Mathematically predicted changes in vital capacity based on age and gender.
© Cengage Learning®.

reflected in the height element (males tend to be taller). As you can see in Figure 3-6B, age also has an effect on the other capacities. Hoit and Hixon (1987) showed that TLC remained essentially unaltered across the life-span for healthy Caucasian males. What can be seen, however, is a reflection of the mathematically produced curve of Figure 3-7: VC shows a clear decline with age. In addition, IC and ERV decrease. Take a look at Figure 3-6a and notice that residual capacity increases with age. We maintain the same lung capacity (TLC) throughout life, but we have a marked reduction in function as we age. As individuals age, compliance of the lungs decreases, which results in reduced ability to inflate the lungs. The lung volume is constant, but you see a *steady growth in the volume that is unavailable for direct gas exchange*, residual volume. Lung compliance is a measure of lung "distensibility," or the ability of a lung to be distended. Lung tissue is elastic, but as tissue is damaged through some disease states such as emphysema, the lungs become more distended and so the lungs become more compliant. In contrast, diseases that increase airway resistance result in less distension, and thus have less compliance.

Compliance is expressed as the change in volume (liters) divided by the change in pressure (cm H20). Essentially, an efficient lung is one in which there is maximal volume inhaled or exhaled for a given pressure change. If you have to increase the pressure to move a given volume, lung compliance drops. Normal lung compliance for an adult is about 100 cc per cm of H20 pressure. Reduced compliance, such as that found with pulmonary edema, will require greater pressure for a given volume of air. In contrast, increased compliance is seen in diseases in which the alveoli have collapsed, such as emphysema. In this case, the increased compliance in the lungs reflects reduced useable volume. Too much compliance and there will be too little volume displaced for a given pressure, while too great a compliance requires a great deal of pressure to make a volume change.

Muscle Weakness and Respiratory Function

Many disease processes reduce respiratory function, which can have a remarkable effect on other systems as well. Diseases that produce spasticity can result in paradoxical contraction of the muscles of expiration during inspiration, greatly reducing the VC. Likewise, individuals may have flaccid or hypotonic (low muscle tone) conditions that reduce the degree and strength of muscular contraction. When you think about it, it makes perfect sense that diseases that cause muscular weakness could reduce **respiratory capacity**.

We have a warning about quickly blaming the muscles of respiration for apparent deficits in vital capacity, inspiratory reserve, and so on. When testing an individual with a compromised motor system, remember that you are testing the whole system. An individual being evaluated in our clinic had weak labial muscles that caused her to have difficulty getting an adequate seal around the mouthpiece of the spirometer. Readings from this instrument thus implied respiratory deficit when, in reality, the problem was with the articulatory system. Likewise, insufficiency of the soft palate, whether due to muscular weakness or inadequate tissue, can result in nasal leakage during respiratory tasks. Again, this can masquerade as an apparent respiratory deficit.

respiratory capacities:
combinations of volumes that express physiological limits

✔ *To summarize:*

- There are several volumes and capacities of importance to your study of respiration.
- The volumes, which indicate arbitrary partitioning of the respiratory system, include **tidal volume** (the volume inspired and expired in a cycle of respiration), **inspiratory reserve volume** (air inspired beyond tidal inspiration), **expiratory reserve volume** (air expired beyond tidal expiration), **residual volume** (air that remains in the lungs after maximal expiration), and **dead air** (air that does not undergo gas exchange).
- **Vital capacity** is the volume of air that can be inspired after a maximal expiration.
- **Functional residual capacity** is the air that remains in the body after passive exhalation. **Total lung capacity** represents the sum of all lung volumes.
- **Inspiratory capacity** is the volume that can be inspired from resting lung volume.

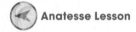
Anatesse Lesson

PRESSURES OF THE RESPIRATORY SYSTEM

There are five specific pressures for nonspeech and speech functions: alveolar pressure, intrapleural pressure, subglottal pressure, intraoral pressure, and atmospheric pressure (see Figure 3-8).

The atmosphere surrounding the earth and within which we live exerts a sizable pressure on the surface of the earth (760 mmHg; i.e., sufficient pressure to elevate a column of mercury 760 mm against gravity). Atmospheric pressure (P_{atm}) is actually our reference in discussions of the respiratory system, and so we will treat it as a constant zero against which to compare respiratory pressures. **Intraoral**, or **mouth pressure** (P_m) is the pressure that could be measured within the mouth, while

intraoral (mouth) pressure:
air pressure measured within the mouth

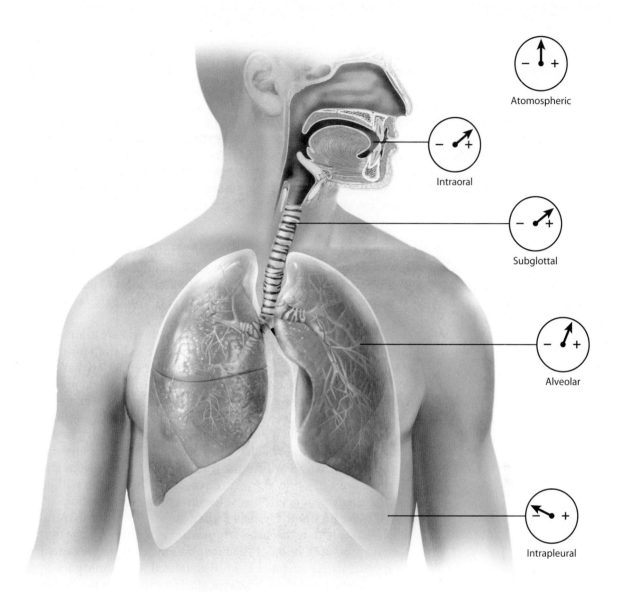

Figure 3-8. Pressures of respiration.
© Cengage Learning®.

subglottal pressure (P_s) is the pressure below the vocal folds. During normal respiration with open vocal folds, we may assume that subglottal and intraoral pressures are equal to alveolar pressure. As we progress more deeply into the lungs, we can estimate **alveolar** or **pulmonic pressure** (P_{al}), the pressure that is present within the individual alveolus. If we were to measure the pressure in the space between parietal and visceral pleurae, we would refer to it as

alveolar (pulmonic) pressure: air pressure measured at the level of the alveolus in the lung

Pneumothorax

Pneumothorax (*pneumo* = air) is aggregation of air in the pleural space between the lungs and the chest wall, with subsequent loss of the negative intrapleural pressure. It can arise through one of several means, but the product is always a "collapsed" lung. In "open" pneumothorax, air is introduced into the space through a breach of the thoracic wall, typically by means of a puncture wound (knife wound, automobile accident, etc.). When air is introduced into the intrapleural space, the result is a loss of the constant negative intrapleural pressure. Recall that this pressure maintains the close bond between the visceral pleural lining of the lungs and that of the inner thorax. When that bond is broken by the open wound, the lungs will collapse. This collapse arises from the fact that the lungs are in a state of constant outward distension, arising from the difference between adult thorax size and adult lung size (see detail on lung development).

pleural (intrapleural) pressure: pressure in the space between parietal and visceral pleurae

pleural or **intrapleural pressure** (P_{pl}). Intrapleural pressure will be negative throughout respiration. Recall that the lungs, inner thorax, and diaphragm are wrapped in a continuous sheet of pleural lining. When one attempts to separate the visceral from parietal pleurae, a negative pressure ensues.

These pressure measurements are all made relative to atmospheric pressure. When we refer to alveolar pressure as being, for instance, +3 cm H_2O, it means that, through muscular effort, we have generated +3 cm H_2O pressure *above and beyond* atmospheric pressure (if atmospheric pressure is 1033 cm H_2O, then alveolar pressure would be 1036 cm H_2O). Alveolar pressure may be indirectly estimated by having an individual swallow a balloon and breathe. Because the trachea and esophagus are adjacent structures sharing a common wall, the pressure changes within the trachea produce analogous changes in the esophagus, and a pressure sensor in the balloon will permit estimation of air pressure below the level of the vocal folds.

When the diaphragm is pulled down for tidal inspiration, Boyle's law predicts that alveolar pressure will drop (relative to atmospheric pressure). In quiet tidal inspiration, alveolar pressure drops to approximately −2 cm H_2O until equalized with atmospheric pressure by inspiratory flow. Likewise, during expiration the pressure at the alveolar level becomes positive with reference to the atmosphere, increasing to +2 cm H_2O during quiet tidal breathing.

The work of expanding the lungs is one of overcoming resistance within the lungs. Surface active solution (surfactant) is released into the alveoli, and the result is greatly reduced surface tension. This decrease in surface tension reduces the pressure of the alveoli, keeps the alveolar walls from collapsing, and keeps fluid from the capillaries from being drawn into the lungs. Pressure in any network of tubes is greatest at the source of the pressure, which in this case is at the alveolus.

The surfactant protects the alveolus, promotes airflow, and facilitates effort-free respiration. During respiration, oxygen is perfused into the bloodstream across the alveolar–capillary membrane barrier, while carbon dioxide is perfused into the alveolus.

When the thorax is expanded by means of muscular contraction, the lungs will follow faithfully, with the result being expansion of the

300 million alveoli within the lungs. Secreting cells within the visceral pleurae release a lubricating fluid into the potential space between visceral and parietal pleurae, and the presence of this fluid lets the lungs and thorax make a slippery, extremely low-friction contact. At the alveolus, oxygen and carbon dioxide diffuse across the alveolus–capillary boundary.

Figure 3-9 is a schematic of the alveolar pressures, intrapleural pressures, and change in lung volume during quiet tidal breathing.

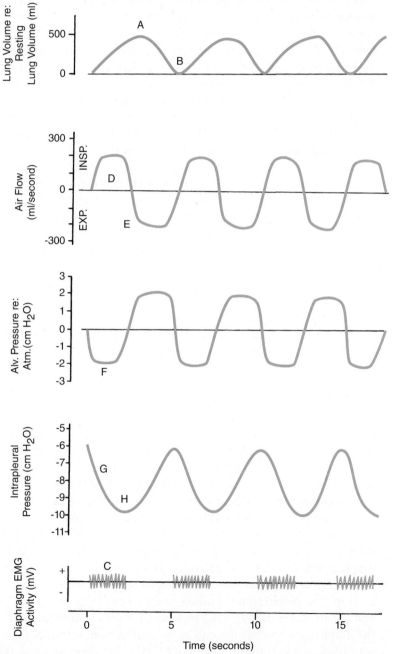

Figure 3-9. Relationships of pressures, flows, and volumes to diaphragm activity. Contraction of the diaphragm causes a drop in intrapleural pressure, which results in an increase in airflow and lung volume. The letters on the figure are explained in the text.

© Cengage Learning®. (Data from Physiology of Respiration by J. H. Comroe, 1965. Chicago: Year Book Medical Publishers.)

This figure shows the alveolar pressure associated with a cycle of respiration and illustrates what we have been talking about. We have placed markers on it so that we can discuss how this whole system of pressures and flows works together.

Look at the "volume" portion of the graph and notice the periodic function representing tidal respiration. Point "A" represents the peak of that inspiration, and the lungs have about 500 cc of air in them. Point "B" represents the end of the expiratory cycle, where our subject has relaxed the forces of inspiration and the lungs have passively evacuated down to resting lung volume. The point marked "C" represents the electromyographic activity recorded from the diaphragm as it contracts. Putting these two traces together, you can see that as the diaphragm contracts the volume increases to a maximum, ending at the point where the diaphragmatic contraction is complete.

Let us examine the "flow" component. As the diaphragm contracts, there is a fairly steady flow of air into the lungs (measured in mL/second), indicated by point "D." When the inspiratory effort is completed (represented by termination of the diaphragm activity and the volume peak at "A"), the flow of air into the lungs ends. That is, when the diaphragm stops contracting, air stops flowing. As air leaves the lungs, the airflow becomes negative at point "E" (which simply means that the air is flowing in a different direction). Alveolar pressure goes positive (+2 cm H_2O) during expiration, a change you would predict from what you know about the lungs. To summarize, when the diaphragm contracts, airflow begins and is fairly steady throughout the inspiratory cycle; when the diaphragm stops contracting, the air begins to flow out of the lungs.

This is a good point to examine the pressures driving this process. Recall that contraction of the diaphragm causes the alveolar pressure to drop, and the point marked "F" will make sense: When the diaphragm is active ("C"), pressure deep within the lungs drops. Alveolar pressure reaches its maximum negativity during this tidal respiration (−2 cm H_2O relative to atmospheric pressure), because the negative pressure is responsible for airflow into the lungs. Looking at "G" will explain why that pressure drops. You will recall that intrapleural pressure is constantly negative relative to atmospheric pressure, arising from the fact that the lungs are in a state of continued expansion within the thoracic cavity. This is reflected in the fact that the highest pressure on the intrapleural plot is negative.

When the diaphragm contracts, the intrapleural pressure becomes even more negative as the diaphragm attempts to pull the diaphragmatic pleurae away from the visceral pleurae. During the entire period of contraction of the diaphragm, the pressure continues to drop: The diaphragm is pulling farther away from its resting point and the pressure between the pleurae increases proportionately. As the diaphragm reaches the end of its contraction, intrapleural pressure reaches a maximum negativity ("H") that reverses upon relaxation of the diaphragm. When the diaphragm contracts, the volume (space) between the two pleural linings increases; Boyle's law dictates that pressure will drop, and it does. Depression of the diaphragm for quiet tidal inspiration results in an intrapleural pressure of approximately −10 cm H_2O, but relaxing the diaphragm during quiet expiration does not return the pressure to atmospheric, but rather returns it to a constant rest pressure of −6 cm H_2O. In the normal, healthy individual, intrapleural pressure remains negative at all times, becoming increasingly negative as muscles of inspiration act on the lungs.

The fact that this intrapleural pressure remains negative underscores two important notions. First, the lungs are in a state of continual expansion because the thorax is larger than the lungs that fill it. Second, the lungs are never completely deflated under normal circumstances, because of the residual volume discussed earlier.

During inspiration and expiration, two more pressures are of interest to us. Subglottal pressure is the pressure measured beneath the level of the vocal folds (*glottis* refers to the space between the vocal folds). Above the vocal folds, the respiratory pressure measured within the oral cavity is referred to as intraoral pressure. When the vocal folds are open, intraoral pressure, subglottal pressure, and alveolar pressure are the same.

The pressure beneath and above the vocal folds is directly related to what is happening in the lungs, as long as the vocal folds are open for air passage. If the lungs are drawing air in, there will be a negative pressure at both of these locations. If the lungs are in expiration, the pressure will be relatively positive. Things get more complicated when the vocal folds are closed.

When we close vocal folds for phonation (voicing), we place a significant blockage in the flow of air through the upper respiratory pathway. Closing the vocal folds causes an immediate increase in the pressure below the vocal folds (subglottal air pressure) as the lungs continue expiration. At the same time, closing the vocal folds causes the pressure above the vocal folds (intraoral pressure) to drop to near atmospheric, resulting in a large difference in pressure between the supraglottal (above vocal folds) and subglottal regions. If this increased pressure exceeds 3–5 cm H_2O, the vocal folds will be blown open and voicing will begin. This turns out to be a critical pressure in itself, because it marks the minimal requirement of respiration for speech (Netsell & Hixon, 1978). We are going to revisit this 3–5 cm H_2O pressure when we discuss checking action in another section.

The requirements for speech and nonspeech breathing are markedly different. Nonspeech respiration mandates a specific level of gas exchange to meet metabolic requirements. Respiration for speech requires, in addition, maintenance of a relatively steady flow of air at a relatively steady pressure. This is a tall order for a system that is designed for cycling air in and out of a cavity. Because we are inherently efficient creatures, we will work very hard to avoid working very hard. The most efficient range of respiration in terms of energy outlay is to maintain VC at approximately resting lung volume. Recall that as you inflate your lungs to greater and greater values above RLV, you must use increasingly more muscle activity. This is indicated by the pressure that can be generated by the contraction of the muscles at those extremes. Frankly, we do not like to spend a lot of time in these extremes, because it takes a lot of energy. Instead, we will tend to keep our VC near the RLV regions for conversational speech, ranging from 35 to 60 percent of VC. Since RLV is 38 percent of VC, you can see that we work a small bit in ERV, and considerably more in IRV, but we stay away from the extremes. Loud speech requires greater inspiration, using lung volumes upward of 80 percent of VC.

Having drawn these conclusions about volume, what can we say about maintenance of subglottal pressure? Pressure is obviously a direct function of the forces of expiration, which are generally passive above 38 percent of VC. Because we operate almost exclusively within the region above 38 percent of VC, generation of subglottal pressure is mostly a function of the forces of expiration, specifically elasticity and gravity. We must use the muscles of inspiration to check that outflow of air, so the muscular effort in speech beyond the initial inspiration is dominated by using the muscles of inspiration *again* to impede the outflow of air. By delicate manipulation of these muscles, we are able to maintain a constant subglottal pressure that can be used for the fine control of phonation by the larynx. We will discuss this in the next section, as we examine the effects of tissue characteristics on respiration, particularly as they relate to speech and this process of impeding the outflow of air, checking action.

While we readily manipulate the respiratory mechanism for speech, there is ample evidence that we take specific care to prepare for this act. Hixon, Goldman, and Mead (1979) showed that when an individual prepares for speech, he or she will expand and "set" the thorax to a greater extent than in nonspeech for a given volume of air. The authors hypothesize that this preparatory act provides the optimum thoracic positioning for production of respiratory pulses needed for speech suprasegmental aspects.

You can now view these critical pressures as a system: We are continually playing the respiratory system against the relatively stable **atmospheric pressure**. Contraction of the diaphragm and muscles of inspiration causes the intrapleural pressure to decrease markedly, which in turn causes the lungs to expand. When the lungs expand, alveolar pressure drops relative to atmospheric pressure, causing air to enter the lungs. Relaxing the muscles of inspiration permits the natural recoil of the lungs and cartilage to draw the chest back to its original position, and the relaxed diaphragm again returns to its relatively elevated position in the thorax. When this happens, intrapleural pressure increases (but still stays negative) and alveolar pressure becomes positive relative to atmospheric pressure. Air leaves the lungs.

✔ *To summarize:*

- Volumes and pressures vary as a direct function of the forces acting on the respiratory system.
- With the vocal folds open, **oral pressure**, **subglottal pressure**, and **alveolar pressure** are roughly equivalent.
- **Intrapleural pressure** will remain constantly negative, increasing in negativity during inspiration.
- These pressures are all measured relative to **atmospheric pressure**.
- During inspiration, expansion of the thorax decreases the already negative intrapleural pressure, and the increased lung volume results in a **negative alveolar pressure**.
- Air from outside the body will flow into the lungs as a result of the pressure difference between the lungs and the atmosphere.
- During expiration, this pressure differential is reversed, with air escaping the lungs to equalize the **positive alveolar pressure** with the relatively negative atmospheric pressure.

Pressures Generated by the Tissue

At this point, we should address the forces of expiration in earnest. The process of inspiration is one of exerting force to overcome gravity and the elastic forces of tissue. Inspiration is generally active, requiring muscular action to complete it.

Expiration capitalizes on elasticity and gravity to reclaim some of the energy expended during inspiration. When muscles of inspiration contract, they stretch tissue and distend the abdomen. When these muscles relax during expiration, the stretched tissues tend to return to their original dimension due to their elastic nature and gravity works to depress the rib cage. To breathe in, you have to move all of these muscles and bones, and as you relax, they return to their original positions.

These restoring forces actually generate pressures themselves. Recoil of the chest during exhalation obeys the laws applying to any elastic material: The greater you distend or distort the material, the greater is the force required to hold it in that position and the greater is the force with which it returns to rest.

You can get common-sense validation of this if you recall loading a stapler with staples. As you pull back the spring that holds the staples, you reach a point where the spring almost wins. The force required to hold the spring back is much greater as it gets farther from its point of rest. You know also the force with which your finger can get whacked if you do not get out of the way in time; the farther you have pushed the spring, the more it hurts when it is inadvertently released.

The same elastic forces govern how much effort is required to inhale. Close your eyes and breathe in as deeply as you can and hold it for a few seconds. Feel how much pressure you are fighting to hold your chest in that position. Next, take in a quiet breath and hold it: Do you feel the difference in pressure?

This relationship is described in the curve of Figure 3-10, which shows the result of pressure generated by all that force (remember that pressure is force exerted over an area). The farther the rib cage is expanded, the greater the force that is trying to return the rib cage to rest.

This curve is called the *relaxation pressure curve*, and it was generated by asking people to do what you just did with your eyes closed. The subjects were told to inhale to some percentage of their VC and then to relax their musculature while their intraoral pressure (which approximates both subglottal and alveolar pressures) was measured using a manometer. Repeated measures of this sort at various percentages of VC resulted in the upper positive portion of the curve. It is positive because the tissue is attempting to return to rest. This is a measure of the strength of those physical restoring forces. Note that you are capable of generating some reasonably large forces with this tissue recoil. Pressures on the order of 60 cm H_2O are fairly significant, considering that phonation requires only about 5 cm H_2O.

The bottom half of the curve is produced in much the same way, only this time the subjects were asked to exhale down to a percentage of their VC. The horizontal line at 38 percent is the relaxation point, the point where no pressure is generated, because all parts of the system are at equilibrium. (Breathe out and then do not breathe in again: This "relaxation" point *before you inhale a new breath* is one of three times during a respiratory cycle when atmospheric pressure equals alveolar pressure.) The relaxation point of zero pressure represents

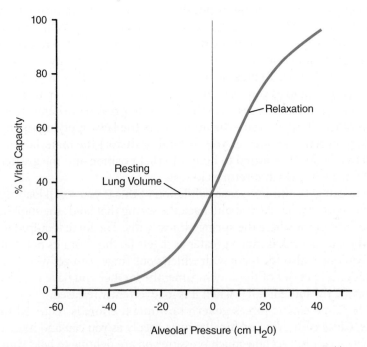

Figure 3-10. Relaxation pressure curve representing pressures generated by the passive forces of the respiratory system.
© Cengage Learning®.

about 38 percent of VC. When you relax entirely with open airway, the lungs still have 38 percent of the total directly exchangeable volume left, and this could be forcefully exhaled. Said another way, from this point you can actively inhale 62 percent of your VC.

Examine the bottom portion of the curve in Figure 3-10, and you will recognize that the pressures generated are not as great and that they are negative. These negative pressures are predominantly the result of the recoil of the chest wall attempting to return to stasis, whereas the positive pressures are governed by the contribution of lung elasticity arising from the recoil of the muscles and cartilage in bronchi, bronchioles, and blood vessels, as well as elastic tissue throughout the lung. Agostoni and Mead (1964) demonstrated that above about 55 percent of VC, the chest wall does not add anything to the pressure of the curve; below about 55 percent, the elasticity of the lungs contributes little to the curve. That is, the lungs compress the air nicely above RLV, while the chest works very hard below RLV to pull air into the system. Likewise, below 55 percent you start to use the muscles of expiration to maintain constant subglottal pressure.

The relaxation pressures reveal the recoil forces of respiration *without* considering active muscular contraction. To look at the effects of muscular activity, you can generate a similar set of responses by asking people to completely deflate their lungs and then inflate them to a specific percentage of VC, and then have them either exhale or inhale as forcefully as they can. This task measures the result of forces that can be generated by actual work associated with muscular contraction. Look at Figure 3-11 to see that the respiratory system works

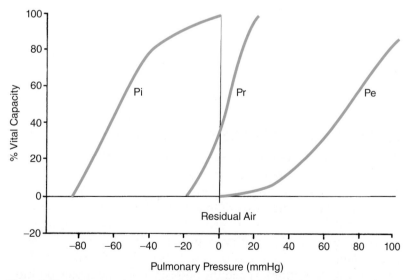

Figure 3-11. Pressure–volume relationship for muscular activity by percentage of vital capacity. P_i = Pressure from muscles of inspiration; P_e = Pressure from muscles of expiration; P_r = Pressure from relaxation of muscles of inspiration and expiration.

as you would expect. On the right side is the expiratory pressure. This is the result of trying to breathe out when you have achieved a specific lung volume. The greater your lung volume is, the more force you can generate for exhalation. On the left side, notice that your ability to draw air in is also intimately related to the amount of air in the lungs: The less air there is in your lungs, the greater is the force you can generate to bring air in. What is that curve in the middle? It is the same one we just looked at—the relaxation curve.

Hixon and Weismer (1995) view respiration as a process that involves continuing, graded contraction of musculature. Our earlier concepts of muscular action in respiration were that the muscles of inspiration ceased to function entirely during the expiratory cycle, and expiratory muscles were inactive during inspiration. We now know that all of the respiratory musculature is active throughout the respiratory cycle, with each muscle group being more or less active depending upon the needs of the moment. This permits the muscles of respiration to remain in a tonic preparatory set so that they can be called upon at any instant to contract to meet the instantaneous goal of respiration. We will see this same model arises in articulatory muscles as well, since fine adjustments require this type of preparation.

✔ *To summarize:*

- The process of contracting musculature deforms the cartilage and connective tissue, and **recoil forces** drive the respiratory system back to equilibrium after inspiration or expiration.
- **Relaxing** the musculature after inspiration results in a **positive alveolar pressure** that decreases as volume approaches RLV.
- When the pressure is measured following forced expiration, a **negative relaxation pressure** is found, increasing to equity at RLV.
- The negative pressures are a function of the chest wall recoil; the positive pressures arise from the expanded lungs and torqued cartilage.

EFFECTS OF POSTURE ON SPEECH

Body posture is a significant contributor to the efficiency of respiration, and any condition that compromises posture also compromises respiration (see Figure 3-12). As the body is shifted from an erect, sitting posture to supine, the relationship between the physical structures of respiration and gravity changes. In the sitting posture, gravity is pulling the abdominal viscera down (supporting inspiration), as well as pulling the rib cage down (supporting expiration). When the body achieves the supine position, gravity is pulling the abdominal viscera toward the spine. The result of this is spread of the viscera toward the thorax and further distension of the diaphragm into the thoracic cavity. In supine

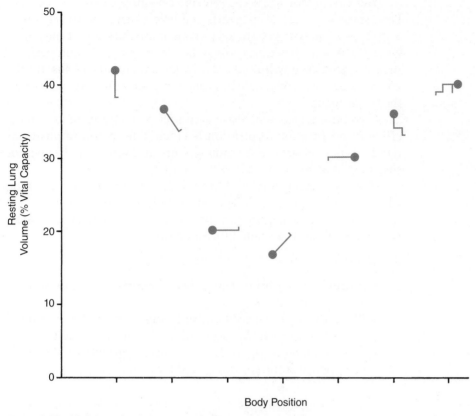

Figure 3-12. Vital capacity changes resulting from postural adjustment.

© Cengage Learning®. (Data from "Kinematics of the Chest Wall During Speech Production: Volume Displacement of the Rib Cage, Abdomen, and Lung." By T. J. Hixon, M. D. Goldman, & J. Mead, 1973. Journal of Speech & Hearing Research, 16, 78–115.)

position, gravity supports neither expiration nor inspiration: Muscles of inspiration must elevate both abdomen and rib cage against gravity. While Hixon, Goldman, and Mead (1973) found that sitting posture resulted in greater RLV than the supine posture, Roychowdhury, Pramanik, Prajapati, Pandit, and Singh (2011) found that the supine position resulted in higher VC than sitting. The practical cause of this difference is that the diaphragm is more restrained in the sitting position and is able to reach its full excursion during inspiration when the individual is in the supine position. It is entirely possible that the difference between the two studies reflected age of the subjects, since the mean age of the Hixon et al. study was 34.5 years, while that of Roychowdhury et al. used 19- to 22-year-olds.

Although VC is not affected, the ability to completely inflate the lungs is. According to the Hixon et al. data, the RLV is significantly reduced from approximately 38 percent of VC in sitting position to 20 percent in supine, arising from the shift in viscera and effects of gravity on the rib cage. The elastic forces that would normally inflate the lungs to that 38 percent point only inflate them to 20 percent, leaving muscular effort to account for the additional 18 percent.

You can demonstrate the effects of posture easily for yourself. First, stand up, take a deep breath, and hold a sustained vowel as long as you can. You will want to keep track of the duration of the vowel. Next, lie on your back (in supine), take a deep breath, and perform the same task. You will notice that you were not able to sustain the vowel for as long. Finally, lie in prone (on your stomach) and sustain the vowel again.

If you did all three of these activities, you found that the most efficient posture for respiration is erect. The reclining positions required more effort for the same gesture and were less efficient for sustained phonation.

You may have already realized the danger this poses to a person whose illness requires that he or she stay in bed for long periods of time. It should not surprise you that pneumonia is a major complication in conditions that immobilize a person.

✔ *To summarize:*

- **Posture** and **body position** play an important role in volumes for respiration.
- When the body is placed in a reclining position, the abdominal contents shift rostrally as a result of the forces of gravity.
- Aside from reducing the RLV, the force of **gravity** on the abdomen increases the effort required for inspiration.

Muscular Weakness and Respiration

Individuals with diseases that weaken the muscles of inspiration are at significant respiratory risk for a number of reasons. Although gravity is the friend of respiration in a person with normal function, we must realize that inspiration requires muscular effort and that effort is aimed very specifically at overcoming gravity.

Individuals in the later stages of neuromuscular diseases, such as amyotrophic lateral sclerosis (ALS), suffer from extreme muscular weakness as a result of the disease, but are still faced with the oxygenation demands typically met with respiratory work. If the patient is placed in the supine position (on the back), gravity will conspire against the respiratory effort, and this resting position will actually put him or her at risk for respiratory distress. Here's why: When lying in supine, gravity is pushing on the abdominal viscera, forcing them toward the patient's back. When the individual attempts to take a breath in, the abdomen should protrude, but with compromised muscular strength that will require more effort than the person is capable of. When in supine, the abdominal viscera are one more thing to overcome, and it turns out to be one thing too many.

To overcome this, patients in the later stages of ALS often remain in a semireclined position to permit rest but capitalize on gravity to assist with respiration. By the way, this might also give you a clue as to why individuals with weakened musculature are more prone to pneumonia than healthy individuals: It takes a great deal of work to clear the lungs and to keep them clear.

PRESSURES AND VOLUMES OF SPEECH

The respiratory system operates at two levels of pressure virtually simultaneously. The first level is the relatively constant supply of subglottal pressure required to drive the vocal folds, a topic with which you will become familiar in Chapter 4. To produce sustained voicing of a given intensity, this pressure is relatively constant. As we will see, the minimum driving pressure to make the vocal folds move would elevate a column of water between 3 and 5 cm (3–5 cm H_2O), with conversational speech requiring between 7 and 10 cm H_2O. Loud speech requires a concomitant increase in pressure.

The second level of pressure is one requiring microcontrol. Even as we maintain the constant pressure needed for phonation, we can rapidly change the pressure for linguistic purposes such as syllable stress. With quick bursts of pressure (and laryngeal adjustments), we can create rapid increases in vocal intensity and vocal pitch. These bursts are small and fast: We will increase subglottal pressure by about 2 cm H_2O to add stress, but we will return to the previous subglottal pressure within one-tenth of a second. We will see that these two modes of control use the same mechanical structures.

The abdominal muscles remain in a state of graded tonic contraction during expiration, which allows two things to happen. First, the abdominal muscles are poised for more rapid contraction to accommodate speech needs. Second, and more importantly, if the abdominal muscles are continually contracted to some degree, they help to restrain the abdominal viscera during pulsed contractions of the thoracic musculature. These pulses are particularly important for suprasegmental aspects of speech, particularly generation of increased vocal intensity (as we shall see in Chapter 4).

To maintain constant pressure for speech, we must first charge the system. During normal respiration, inhalation takes up approximately 40 percent of the cycle, while expiration takes up about 60 percent. When you realize that you speak only on expiration, you will also realize also that it would not take many minutes of talking like this to drive you (and your communication partner) to distraction. Imagine every 6 seconds of speaking followed by 4 seconds of silence while you inhale, and you will see why we have modified this plan for speech (see Figure 3-13). In fact, the respiratory cycle for speech is markedly different. You need a long, drawn-out expiration to produce long utterances, and you need a very short inspiration to maintain the smooth flow of communication. When you breathe in for speech, you actually spend only 10 percent of the respiratory cycle on inspiration and about 90 percent breathing out.

This does not change the amount of air we breathe in and out. We will still breathe exactly the volume we need for our metabolic processes (too much and we take in too much oxygen, or hyperventilate; too little and we take in too little oxygen and become

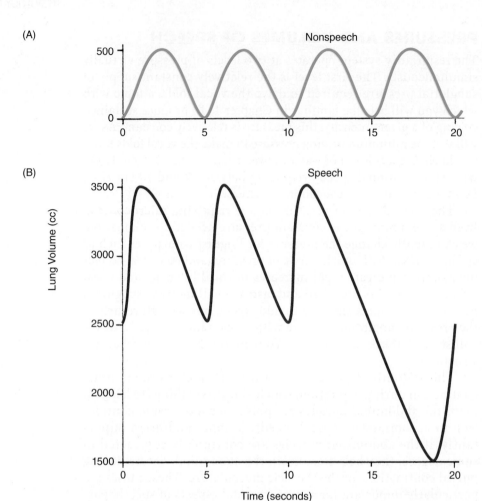

(A)

Nonspeech

(B)

Speech

Figure 3-13. Modification of respiratory cycle during speech compared with nonspeech respiratory cycle. (A) This trace represents quiet tidal respiration, with volume related to resting lung volume. (B) This trace is related to total lung capacity. The speaker rapidly inhales a markedly larger volume than during quiet tidal inspiration and then slowly exhales the air during speech. Note that inspiration occurs with the same timing in both speech and nonspeech, but that the expiratory phase is proportionately longer during speech. In the final portion of the trace, the speaker is called on to speak on expiratory reserve volume.

© Cengage Learning®.

hypoxic). All we need to do is alter how long we spend in either stage of the process. When a person initiates speaking, the adult lungs are filled to about 48 percent of vital capacity, and the person will take another breath when the lungs are just below RLV, at about 35 percent of VC (Winkworth, Davis, Adams, & Ellis, 1995). You can see that, even as we alter the cycle of respiration, we still operate in a very limited volume range. Interestingly, mildly louder speech in conversation (4–18 dB increase) does not markedly alter the volumes (Winkworth et al., 1995), but if a person produces high sound pressure levels he or she will greatly increase the inspiratory volume to capitalize on the tissue recoil to increase pressure (Hixon, Goldman, & Mead, 1973; Stathopoulos & Sapienza, 1997). Note that this increase in pressure *could* be accomplished by using muscles of expiration rather than expanding the chest wall, but that would require more effort and control. The important respiratory variable in loud speech is pressure, and increasing initial volume is the easiest way to accomplish this.

You will remember that in Chapter 2 we talked about the development of the respiratory system, with the expansion of the thorax and the stretching of the lung tissue. Children approach the task of speech differently from adults as a result of these developmental changes. Because of the limitations of their respiratory systems, young children use a greater proportion of their VC for speech than adults and inhale to a greater proportion of their vital capacity before speaking (see Figure 3-14) (Stathopoulos & Sapienza, 1997).

Earlier we said that we need to hold a reasonably constant subglottal pressure to maintain phonation, but we did not say *how* we achieve it. You already have all the pieces, so let us pose the puzzle to you. If you take in a deep breath as if you were about to speak, but just let the air flow out unimpeded, you run out of air within one or two quick words. That burst of air is not going to work for speech.

Instead of letting the air out through total relaxation, let the air out slowly. As you do this, pay attention to the fact that you are using muscles to restrain the airflow. If you remember that the lungs are attempting to empty as a result of their being stretched for inspiration, then you might realize that if you were to *hold* that inspiration position, you would impede the outflow of air. This process is called *checking action*. That is, you check (impede) the flow of air out of your inflated lungs by means of the muscles that got it there in the first place—the muscles of inspiration.

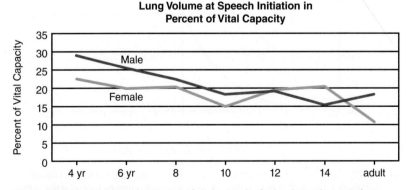

Figure 3-14. Lung volume in percent of vital capacity for low intensity speech.

Source: From data of Stathopoulos, E. T. & Sapienza, C. M. (1997). Developmental changes in laryngeal and respiratory function with variations in sound pressure level. Journal of speech, language and hearing research, 40, 595–614.

Checking action is extremely important for respiratory control of speech, because it directly addresses a person's ability to restrain the flow of air. When a person has a deficit associated with checking action (as in paralysis), the person is at a tremendous disadvantage, because he or she will be restricted to extremely short bursts of speech.

Checking action permits us to maintain the constant flow of air through the vocal tract, which in turn lets us accurately control the pressure beneath vocal folds that have been closed for phonation. We will see that this is very important when it comes to maintaining constant vocal intensity and frequency of vibration.

If you take a look at Figure 3-15, you will see the relaxation pressure curve that we talked about earlier, but with some additions. You will remember that 3–5 cm H_2O is the critical pressure required to sustain vocal fold vibration for speech. We have marked the diagram off so you can see how that pressure relates to relaxation pressures.

Recall that relaxation pressure is the pressure exerted by the tissues of the respiratory system on the lungs. As you inhale to your maximum (100 percent of vital capacity), your lung and chest recoil generate a great deal of positive pressure that is working hard to exhale

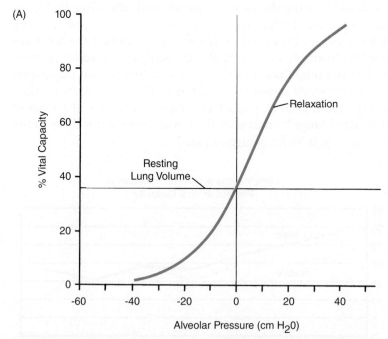

Figure 3-15. (A) Relaxation pressure curve, showing pressure generated by tissues. Note that positive pressure (upper portion of curve) is dominated by recoil forces of the lungs and muscles being distended during inspiration, while negative pressure (lower portion of curve) is governed by chest recoil. (continues).
© Cengage Learning®.

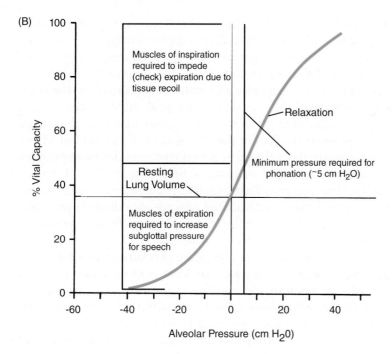

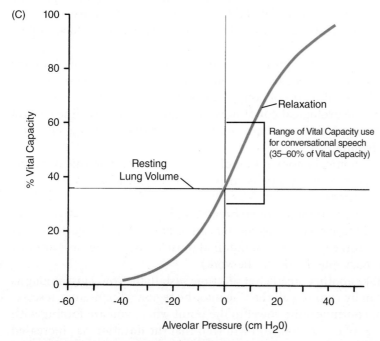

Figure 3-15 continued. (B) Relationship between relaxation pressure and minimum driving force required for phonation. The vocal folds require 5 cm H_2O pressure for onset and sustained vibration. At about 50 percent of VC the muscles of inspiration must be used to control outflow of air in order to maintain a constant 5 cm H_2O pressure (checking action). Below that point, increasing use of the muscles of expiration is required to maintain the 5 cm H_2O pressure for phonation. (C) The typical volume use range for conversational speech is 35–48 percent of vital capacity.

air. As you exhale as much air as you can (approaching 0 percent of vital capacity) your lungs are "trying" very hard to inhale. Now, look what happens when you superimpose the requirements of speech on this (the 5 cm H_2O line). In the area to the right of the figure, the forces of expiration *easily* give adequate pressure to drive the vocal folds. Not until you have exhausted down to about 50 percent of vital capacity do you need to think about using muscular force to *increase* subglottal pressure. In fact, in the region above 50 percent of VC we have to use muscular activity as a brake to impede the expiratory forces, and this is called *checking action*. You are "checking" or "impeding" the outflow of air by using the muscles of inspiration. More importantly for this discussion, you are impeding the pressure-generation so as not to exceed the 5 cm H_2O point. To do so will result in louder speech, which may not be your goal.

Notice also that once the relaxation pressure generated by the tissue is not enough to generate that 5 cm H_2O pressure, we enlist muscles of expiration to add pressure to the system. If you need to speak below the resting lung volume, you will need to enlist muscles of expiration to increase subglottal pressure. Again, you can see that speaking on expiratory reserve volume requires quite a bit of muscular activity to *increase* pressure, while speaking on inspiratory reserve requires muscular activity to *decrease* overpressure.

The take-home message here is that, as usual, we have super-imposed an added function to the respiratory system by asking it to maintain a specific pressure for speech, and once again we humans are able to do meet the challenge just fine. I think you can see, though, that diseases or conditions such as cerebrovascular accident or other neurological conditions that cause you to lose fine control of your respiratory mechanism can have a very debilitating effect on speech output.

A graphic demonstration of how well we perform this of maintaining constant pressure is fairly simple. Do the following steps and note the times:

Take a maximally deep breath, and time yourself as you hold a sustained vowel as long as you can only using your chest muscles (do not force using your abdominal muscles, but rather just let your inspiratory muscles do all the work).

Take another breath, but this time sustain the vowel just as long as you can by running all the way into the region of expiratory reserve. If you continue your vowel to the point where you are forcing with muscles of expiration, you will find that the duration has increased 40–50 percent. Of course, you do not normally speak as far down on your respiratory charge as that, but your teacher regularly gets into expiratory reserve while lecturing, we guarantee.

It is wise to say, one more time, that the speaker will always take care of business first: The body's needs will be met in a constant fashion in the face of using respiration for communication. The next time your instructor is lecturing, count the number of breaths he or she takes per minute and you will see that it is right around 15. Despite what you may have heard, teaching *is* work, so respiration may be a little faster than the 12 breaths per minute of quiet tidal respiration.

Remember, however, that this checking action and speaking on expiratory reserve do not come without a cost. We have to work to overcome the recoil forces in each case, and the deeper our inhalation or the farther we go below RLV, the greater is the force we have to overcome. If you are a cheerleader, you know exactly what we mean: Speaking loudly and with continuity requires effort. Look again at that relaxation pressure curve and realize that the effort you must exert in the upper part of the curve to keep the air from rapidly leaving the lungs is directly proportional to the pressure those forces generate. Likewise, it requires a great deal of effort to squeeze the last bit of expiratory reserve air out of the lungs.

If you look back on this discussion, you will find a common thread: Respiration is work. Generating pressure requires muscular activity, and restraining that pressure for speech requires even more effort. Respiration is truly the battery of the speech production mechanism, and it provides the energy source for our oral communication. Our next task is to see how respiration is used to produce a major component of this speech signal—voicing.

CHAPTER SUMMARY

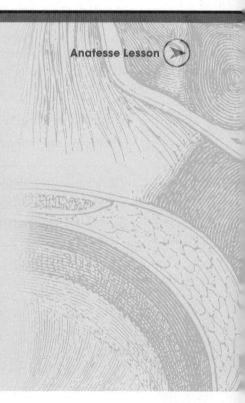

Anatesse Lesson

Respiration requires the balance of pressures. Decreased alveolar pressure is the product of expansion of the thorax. When the thorax expands, the pressure between the pleurae decreases as the thorax and diaphragm are pulled away from the lungs. The force of the distended lungs will increase the negative intrapleural pressure, and the expansion will cause a drop in alveolar pressure as well. The relatively lower alveolar pressure represents an imbalance between the pressures of the lungs and the atmosphere, and air will enter the lungs to equalize the imbalance. Expiration requires reduction in thorax size that results in a positive pressure within the alveoli, with air escaping through the oral cavity. The intrapleural **pressure** becomes less negative during expiration, but never reaches atmospheric pressure.

Several volumes and capacities may be identified within the respiratory system. Tidal volume is the volume inspired and expired in a cycle of respiration, while inspiratory reserve volume is the air inspired beyond tidal inspiration. Expiratory reserve volume is air expired beyond tidal expiration, and residual volume is air that

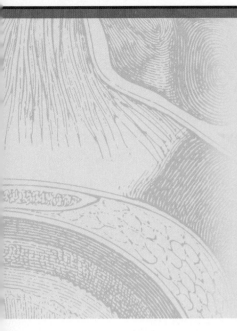

remains in the lungs after maximal expiration. Dead space air is air that cannot undergo gas exchange. Vital capacity is the volume of air that can be inspired after a maximal expiration, and functional residual capacity is the air that remains in the body after passive exhalation. Inspiratory capacity is the volume that can be inspired from resting lung volume. Total lung capacity is the sum of all lung volumes.

For speech, we must work within the confines of pressures and volumes required for life function. We alter the respiratory cycle to capitalize on expiration time and restrain that expiration through checking action. We also generate pressure through contraction of the muscles of expiration when the lung volume is less than resting lung volume. With these manipulations, we will maintain a respiratory rate to match our metabolic needs, and even use the accessory muscles of inspiration and expiration to generate small bursts of pressure for syllabic stress.

Media Connection

Go to the accompanying online resources at CengageBrain.com and have fun learning! Study with the Anatesse software program, play games, view animations and videos, and take practice tests to help reinforce the key concepts you learned in this chapter.

Study Questions

1. Passive expiration involves the forces of _____ and
_____.

2. Identify the indicated volumes and capacities described below.

   a. _____ volume: The volume of air that we breathe in during a respiratory cycle.

   b. _____ volume: The volume that can be inhaled after a tidal inspiration.

   c. _____ volume: The volume that can be exhaled after a tidal expiration.

   d. _____ volume: The volume remaining in the lungs after a maximal exhalation.

   e. _____ capacity: The combination of inspiratory reserve volume, expiratory reserve volume, and tidal volume.

    f. _____ capacity: The volume of air remaining in the body after a passive exhalation.

    g. _____ capacity: The sum of all the volumes.

3. _____ is the volume of air that cannot undergo gas exchange.

4. _____ pressure is the air pressure measured within the oral cavity.

5. _____ pressure is the air pressure measured below the vocal folds.

6. _____ pressure is the pressure within the alveolus.

7. _____ pressure is the pressure between the visceral and parietal pleural membranes.

8. When the diaphragm contracts, pressure within the alveolus _____ (increases/decreases).

9. When air pressure within the lungs is lower than that of the atmosphere, air will _____ (enter/leave) the lungs.

10. When the body is placed in a reclining position, the resting lung volume _____ (increases/decreases).

11. Use of the muscles of inspiration to impede the outward flow of air during speech is termed _____ .

12. Coordination of muscular activity is largely the responsibility of the cerebellum of the brain. An individual with neuropathology involving the cerebellum will have a deficit in coordination of motor function. What impact would this deficit have on speech function?

Study Question Answers

1. Passive expiration involves the forces of **elasticity** and **gravity**.

2. Identify the indicated volumes and capacities described below.

    a. **TIDAL VOLUME:** The volume of air that we breathe in during a respiratory cycle.

    b. **INSPIRATORY RESERVE** volume: The volume that can be inhaled after a tidal inspiration.

    c. **EXPIRATORY RESERVE** volume: The volume that can be exhaled after a tidal expiration.

    d. **RESIDUAL** volume: The volume remaining in the lungs after a maximal exhalation.

    e. **VITAL** capacity: The combination of inspiratory reserve volume, expiratory reserve volume, and tidal volume.

    f. **FUNCTIONAL RESIDUAL** capacity: The volume of air remaining in the body after a passive exhalation.

    g. **TOTAL LUNG** capacity: The sum of all the volumes.

3. DEAD SPACE AIR is the volume of air that cannot undergo gas exchange.

4. INTRAORAL pressure is the air pressure measured within the oral cavity.

5. SUBGLOTTAL pressure is the air pressure measured below the vocal folds.

6. ALVEOLAR or **PULMONIC** pressure is the pressure within the alveolus.

7. **INTRAPLEURAL** or **PLEURAL** pressure is the pressure between the visceral and parietal pleural membranes.

8. When the diaphragm contracts, pressure within the alveolus **DECREASES**.

9. When air pressure within the lungs is lower than that of the atmosphere, air will **ENTER** the lungs.

10. When the body is placed in a reclining (supine) position, the resting lung volume **DECREASES**.

11. Use of the muscles of inspiration to impede the outward flow of air during speech is termed **CHECKING ACTION**.

12. Neuromuscular conditions that affect cerebellar function can result in loss of coordination of diaphragm contraction, difficulty maintaining constant subglottal pressure due to a deficit in checking action, and difficulty coordinating the respiratory effort with phonation, among other problems.

Bibliography

Agostoni, E., & Mead, J. (1964). Statics of the respiratory system. In W. Fenn, & H. Rahn (Eds.), *Handbook of physiology, respiration* (Vol. 1, Sect. 3). Washington, DC: American Physiological Society; Baltimore: Williams & Wilkins.

Baken, R., & Cavallo, S. (1981). Prephonatory chest wall posturing. *Folia phoniatrica, 33*, 193–202.

Baken, R., Cavallo, S., & Weissman, K. (1979). Chest wall movements prior to phonation. *Journal of Speech and Hearing Research, 22*, 862–872.

Baken, R. J., & Orlikoff, R. F. (1999). *Clinical measurement of speech and voice* (2nd ed.). San Diego, CA: Singular Publishing Group.

Basmajian, J. V. (1975). *Grant's method of anatomy*. Baltimore, MD: Williams & Wilkins.

Bateman, H. E., & Mason, R. M. (1984). *Applied anatomy and physiology of the speech and hearing mechanism*. Springfield, IL: Charles C. Thomas.

Beck, E. W. (1982). *Mosby's atlas of functional human anatomy*. St. Louis, MO: C. V. Mosby.

Bergman, R., Thompson, S., & Afifi, A. (1984). *A catalog of human variation*. Baltimore: Urban & Schwarzenberg.

Burrows, B., Knudson, R. J., & Kettel, L. J. (1975). *Respiratory insufficiency*. Chicago: Year Book Medical Publishers.

Campbell, E. (1958). An electromyographic examination of the role of the intercostal muscles in breathing in man. *Journal of Physiology, 129*, 12–26.

Campbell, E., Agostoni, E., & Davis, J. (1970). *The respiratory muscles, mechanics and neural control*. Philadelphia: W. B. Saunders.

Chusid, J. G. (1985). *Correlative neuroanatomy and functional neurology* (17th ed.). Los Altos, CA: Lange Medical Publications.

Comroe, J. H. (1974). *Physiology of respiration*. Chicago: Year Book Medical Publishers.

Creasy, R. K. (1997). *Management of labor and delivery*. Malden, MA: Blackwell Science.

Des Jardins, T., & Burton, G. G. (2001). *Clinical manifestation and assessment of respiratory disease*. Chicago: Mosby.

Draper, M., Ladefoged, P., & Whitteridge, D. (1959). Respiratory muscles in speech. *Journal of Speech and Hearing Research, 2*, 16–27.

Ganong, W. F. (2003). *Review of medical physiology* (21st ed.). New York: McGraw-Hill/Appleton & Lange.

Gordon, M. S. (1972). *Animal physiology: Principles and adaptations*. New York: Macmillan.

Gosling, J. A., Harris, P. F., Humpherson, J. R., Whitmore, I., & Willan, P. L. T. (1985). *Atlas of human anatomy*. Philadelphia: J. B. Lippincott.

Gray, H., Bannister, L. H., Berry, M. M., & Williams, P. L. (Eds.). (1995). *Gray's anatomy*. London: Churchill Livingstone.

Grobler, N. J. (1977). *Textbook of clinical anatomy* (Vol. 1). Amsterdam: Elsevier Scientific.

Hixon, T. J. (1973). Respiratory function in speech. In F. D. Minifie, T. J. Hixon, & F. Williams (Eds.), *Normal aspects of speech, hearing, and language* (pp. 73–126). Englewood Cliffs, NJ: Prentice-Hall.

Hixon, T. J. (2006). Rib torque does not assist resting tidal expiration or most conversational speech expiration. *Journal of Speech, Language and Hearing Research, 49*, 213–214.

Hixon, T., & Weismer, G. (1995). Perspectives on the Edinburgh study of speech breathing. *Journal of Speech, Language and Hearing Research, 38*, 42–60.

Hixon, T. J., Goldman, M. D., & Mead, J. (1973). Kinematics of the chest wall during speech production: Volume displacement of the rib cage, abdomen, and lung. *Journal of Speech and Hearing Research, 16*, 78–115.

Hoit, J. D., & Hixon, T. J. (1987). Age and speech breathing. *Journal of Speech Language, and Hearing Research, 30*, 351–366.

Kahane, J. (1982). Anatomy and physiology of the organs of the peripheral speech mechanism. In N. Lass, L. McReynolds, J. Northern, & D. Yoder (Eds.), *Speech, language, and hearing. Vol. 1: Normal processes* (pp. 109–155). Philadelphia: W. B. Saunders.

Kao, F. F. (1972). *An introduction to respiratory physiology*. Amsterdam: Exerpta Medica.

Kaplan, H. (1960). *Anatomy and physiology of speech*. New York: McGraw-Hill.

Kent, R. D. (1997). *The speech sciences*. San Diego, CA: Singular Publishing Group.

Konno, K., & Mead, J. (1968). Measurement of the separate volume changes of rib cage and abdomen during breathing. *Journal of Applied Physiology, 22*, 407–422.

Lass, N., McReynolds, L., Northern, J., & Yoder, D. (Eds.). (1982). *Speech, language, and hearing. Vol. I: Normal processes*. Philadelphia: W. B. Saunders.

Miller, A. D., Bianchi, A. L., & Bishop, B. P. (1997). *Neural control of the respiratory muscles*. Boca Raton, FL: CRC Press.

Moser, K. M., & Spragg, R. G. (1982). *Respiratory emergencies*. St. Louis, MO: C. V. Mosby.

Murray, J. F. (1976). *The normal lung. The basis for diagnosis and treatment of pulmonary disease*. Philadelphia: W. B. Saunders.

Netsell, R., & Hixon, T. J. (1978). A noninvasive method of clinically estimating subglottal air pressure. *Journal of speech and hearing disorders, 43*, 323–330.

Netter, F. H. (1997). *Atlas of human anatomy*. Los Angeles, CA: Icon Learning Systems.

Pace, W. R. (1970). *Pulmonary physiology*. Philadelphia: F. A. Davis.

Pappenheimer, J. R., Comroe, J. H., Cournand, A., Ferguson, J. K. W., Filley, G. F., Fowler, W. S., et al. (1950). Standardization of definitions and symbols in respiratory physiology. *Federation Proceedings, Federation of the American Society for Experimental Biology* (pp. 602–605).

Peters, R. M. (1969). *The mechanical basis of respiration*. Boston, MA: Little, Brown.

Rahn, H., Otis, A., Chadwick, L. E., & Fenn, W. (1946). The pressure–volume diagram of the thorax and lung. *American Journal of Physiology, 146*, 161–178.

Rohen, J. W., Yokochi, C., Lutjen-Drecoll, E., & Romrell, L. J. (2002). *Color atlas of anatomy* (5th ed.). Philadelphia: Williams & Wilkins.

Rosse, C., Gaddum-Rosse, P., & Rosse, G. (1997). *Hollinshead's textbook of anatomy*. Philadelphia: Lippincott-Raven.

Scott, J. R., Disaia, P. J., Hammond, C. B., & Spellacy, W. N. (1994). *Danforth's obstetrics and gynecology* (7th ed.). Philadelphia: J. B. Lippincott.

Snell, R. S. (1978). *Gross anatomy dissector*. Boston: Little, Brown.

Spector, W. S. (1956). *Handbook of biological data*. Philadelphia: W. B. Saunders.

Stathopoulos, E. T. & Sapienza, C. M. (1997). Developmental changes in laryngeal and respiratory function with variations in sound pressure level. *Journal of Speech, Language and Hearing Research, 40*, 595–614.

Taylor, A. (1960). The contribution of the intercostal muscles to the effort of respiration in man. *Journal of Physiology, 151,* 390.

Tokizane, T., Kawamata, K., & Tokizane, H. (1952). Electromyographic studies on the human respiratory muscles. *Japan Journal of Physiology, 2,* 232.

Twietmeyer, A., & McCracken, T. D. (1992). *Coloring guide to regional human anatomy* (2nd ed.). Philadelphia: Lea & Febiger.

Winkworth, A. L, Davis, P. J., Adams, R. D. & Ellis, E. (1995). Breathing patterns during spontaneous speech. *Journal of speech and hearing research, 38,* 124–144.

Zemlin, W. R. (1998). *Speech and hearing science: Anatomy and physiology* (4th ed.). Needham Heights, MA: Allyn & Bacon.

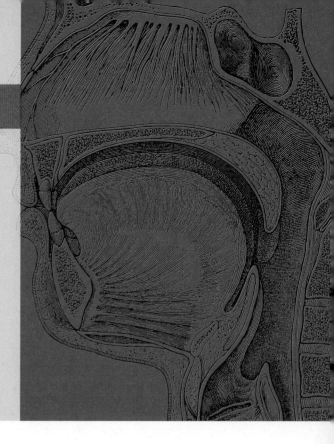

Chapter 4

ANATOMY OF PHONATION

S poken communication uses both voiceless and voiced sounds, and this chapter is concerned with that critical distinction. **Voiceless** phonemes or speech sounds are produced without the use of the vocal folds; for example, the /s/ or /f/ sounds. **Voiced** sounds are produced by the action of the vocal folds; for example, the /z/ and /v/ sounds. **Phonation**, or voicing, is the product of vibrating vocal folds, and this occurs within the larynx. Just as we referred to respiration as the source of *energy* for speech, phonation is the source of *voice* for speech. Respiration is the energy source that permits phonation to occur; without respiration there would be no voicing.

The vocal folds are actually five layers of tissue, with the deepest layer being muscle. The space between the vocal folds is called the **glottis** (or **rima glottidis**), and the area below the vocal folds is the **subglottal** region. The vocal folds are located within the course of the airstream at the superior end of the trachea. As the airstream passes between the vocal folds, they may be made to vibrate, much as a flag flaps in the wind. Try this: Place your hand on the side of your neck and hum. You will feel a tickling vibration. This is the mechanical correlate of the sound you hear. If you alternately produce /a/ and /h/, you will feel your vocal folds start vibrating and stop, because /a/ is a voiced sound and /h/ is voiceless sound.

When you felt the vibrations of the vocal folds, you might also have noted a very important aspect of phonation. You were able to turn your voice on and off to produce the alternating voiced and voiceless sounds. When you alternated those two sounds, you were actually moving the vocal folds into and out of the airstream to cause

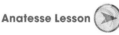

Anatesse Lesson

rima glottidis: L., "slit of the glottis"

Biological Functions of the Larynx

Although we capitalize on the larynx for phonation, it has a much more important function in nature. The larynx is an exquisite sphincter in that the vocal folds are capable of a very strong and rapid clamping of the airway in response to the threat of intrusion by foreign objects. As evidence of this function, there are three pairs of laryngeal muscles directly responsible for either approximating or tensing the vocal folds, although there is only one pair of muscles responsible for opening them. The vocal folds are wired to close immediately on stimulation by outside agents, such as food or liquids, a response that is followed quickly by the rapid and forceful exhalation of a cough. This combination of actions is designed to stop intrusion by foreign matter and to rapidly expel them from the opening of the airway.

The larynx has other important functions as well. Because the vocal folds provide an excellent seal to the respiratory system, they permit you to hold your breath, thus capturing a significant respiratory charge for such activities as swimming.

Holding your breath serves other functions. Lifting heavy objects requires you to "fix" your thorax by inspiring and clamping your laryngeal sphincter (vocal folds). This gives the muscles of the upper body a solid framework with which to work. You will also note from the margin notes in Chapter 2 that tightly clamping the vocal folds plays an important part in childbirth and defecation.

them to start and then stop vibrating. The vocal folds are bands of tissue that can be set into vibration. Now we are ready to look at the structure of the vocal mechanism (see Figure 4-1).

A TOUR OF THE PHONATORY MECHANISM

This is a good opportunity to walk you through the vocal mechanism. We will get into details soon enough, but for now let us look at the larger picture.

Framework of the Larynx

The larynx is a musculocartilaginous structure located at the superior (upper) end of the trachea. It is comprised of three unpaired and three paired cartilages bound by ligaments and lined with mucous membrane.

If you examine Figure 4-1, you can see the relation between the trachea and larynx. You might recall that the trachea is composed of a series of cartilage rings, connected and separated by a fibroelastic membrane. The larynx sits as an oddly shaped box atop the last ring of the trachea. It is adjacent to cervical vertebrae 4 through 6 in the adult, but the larynx of an infant will be higher. The average length of the larynx in adult males is 44 mm; in females it is 36 mm.

The **cricoid cartilage** is a complete ring resting atop the trachea and is the most inferior of the laryngeal cartilages. From the side, the cricoid cartilage takes on the appearance of a signet ring, with its

cricoid: Gr., krikos, ring; "ring-form"

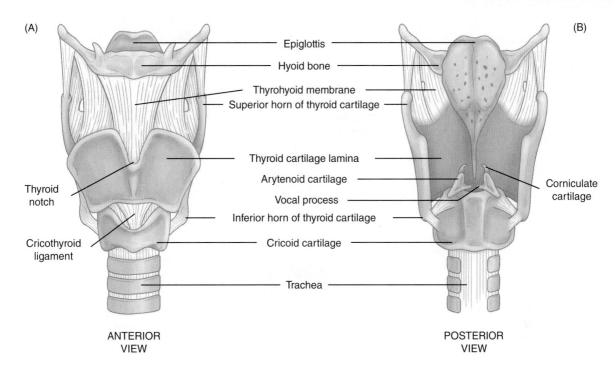

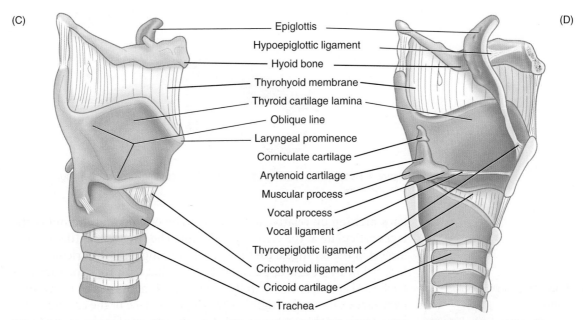

Figure 4-1. Larynx in anterior (A) and posterior (B) views (upper). (C) Lateral view of larynx. (D) View of the relationship of cricoid and arytenoids cartilages, as seen in larynx that has been cut sagittally at midline. (continues).
© Cengage Learning®.

(E)

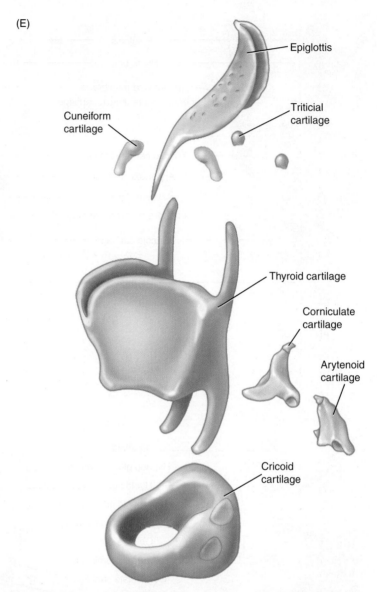

Epiglottis

Cuneiform
cartilage

Triticial
cartilage

Thyroid cartilage

Corniculate
cartilage

Arytenoid
cartilage

Cricoid
cartilage

Figure 4-1 continued. (E) Exploded view of disarticulated laryngeal cartilages.
© Cengage Learning®.

back arching up relative to the front. The cricoid and thyroid cartilages articulate at the cricothyroid joint. The **thyroid cartilage** is the
largest of the laryngeal cartilages, articulating with the cricoid cartilage below by means of paired processes that let it rock forward and
backward at that joint. With this configuration, the paired **arytenoid
cartilages** ride on the high-backed upper surface of the cricoid cartilage, forming the posterior point of attachment for the vocal folds.
The **corniculate cartilages** ride on the superior surface of each arytenoid and are prominent landmarks in the aryepiglottic folds. The
cuneiform cartilage, residing within the aryepiglotic folds, provides a
degree of rigidity to the folds. The cuneiform cartilages reside within
the aryepiglottic folds and provide stiffness to the folds.

arytenoid: Gr., arytaina, ladle;
"ladle-form"

corniculate: L., cornu, horn;
"little horn"

Laryngectomy

Patients who undergo **laryngectomy** (surgical removal of the larynx) lose the voicing source for speech. The larynx is removed and the oral cavity is sealed off from the trachea and lower respiratory passageway as a safeguard because the protective function of the larynx is also lost. **Laryngectomees** (individuals who have undergone laryngectomy) must alter their activities because they now breathe through a **tracheostoma**, an opening placed in the trachea through a surgical procedure known as a **tracheostomy**.

Loss of the ability to phonate is but one of the difficulties facing the laryngectomee. This patient will have difficulty with **expectoration** (elimination of phlegm from the respiratory passageway) and coughing, and will no longer be able to enjoy swimming or other activities that would expose the **stoma** to water or pollutants. The air entering the patient's lungs is no longer humidified or filtered by the upper respiratory passageway, and a filter must be kept over the stoma to prevent introduction of foreign objects. The patient may be restricted from having house pets that shed hair, as the hair can work its way into the unprotected airway. The flavor of foods is greatly reduced, because the patient may no longer breathe through his or her nose, and our perception of food relies heavily on the sense of smell. Depending on pre- and postoperative treatment, patients may experience extreme dryness of oral tissues (xerostomia) arising from damage to the salivary glands from radiation therapy. One result of this dryness may be a swallowing dysfunction (dysphagia). Recognize that since the trachea has been completely separated from the esophagus, the risk of aspiration is reduced after healing occurs, although the stoma will always have to be protected from intrusion of foreign bodies or liquids.

The thyroid cartilage articulates with the **hyoid bone** by means of a pair of superior processes. Medial to the hyoid bone and thyroid cartilage is the **epiglottis**, a leaflike cartilage. The epiglottis is a protective structure in that it will drop to cover the **orifice** of the larynx during swallowing. There have been questions about its protective function in protection of the airway during swallowing, but the fact that people who have had surgical removal of the epiglottis (for instance, to treat laryngeal or lingual cancer) are much more likely to have swallowing problems than those who retain the epiglottis. Indeed, reduced movement of the epiglottis after cancer surgery increases aspiration during swallowing (Halczy-Kowalik, Sulikowski, Wysocki, Posio, Kowalczy, & Rzewuska, 2012).

epiglottis: Gr., epi, over; "over glottis"

An orifice is an opening.

✔ *To summarize:*

- The **larynx** is a musculocartilaginous structure located at the upper end of the trachea. It is comprised of the **cricoid**, **thyroid**, and **epiglottis cartilages**, as well as the paired **arytenoid**, **corniculate**, and **cuneiform cartilages**.
- The thyroid and cricoid cartilages articulate by means of the **cricothyroid joint** that lets the two cartilages come closer together in front.
- The **arytenoid** and **cricoid cartilages** also articulate with a joint that permits a wide range of arytenoid motion.

- The **corniculate cartilages** rest on the upper surface of the arytenoids, while the **cuneiform cartilages** reside within the **aryepiglottic folds**.
- The epiglottis protects the airway during swallowing.

Inner Larynx

When these cartilages are combined with the trachea and the airway above the larynx, the result is a rough tubelike space with a constriction caused by the cartilages. This construction is unique, however, in that it is an *adjustable*, valve-like constriction. The vocal folds are bands of mucous membrane, connective tissue, and thyrovocalis muscle that are slung between the arytenoid cartilages and the thyroid cartilage so that they may be moved into and out of the airstream. (Alternately, some anatomists consider the vocal folds as the mucous membrane and connective tissue only, excluding the thyrovocalis muscle.) Muscles attached to the arytenoids provide both adductory and abductory functions, with which we control the degree of airflow by means of muscular contraction.

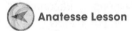
Anatesse Lesson

Laryngeal Membranes. The cavity of the larynx is a constricted tube with a smooth and reasonably aerodynamic surface (see Figure 4-1 and 4-2). This tube is created by developing a deep structure of cartilages; connecting those cartilages through sheets and cords of ligaments and membrane; and lining the entire structure with a wet, smooth mucous membrane. Let us work from the inside out to identify these connective structures. The extrinsic ligaments provide attachment between the hyoid or trachea and the cartilage of the larynx. The **thyrohyoid membrane** stretches across the space between the greater cornu of the hyoid and the lateral thyroid. Posterior to this is the **lateral thyrohyoid ligament**, which runs from the superior cornu of the thyroid to the posterior tip of the greater cornu hyoid.

Valleculae and Swallowing

The valleculae are "little valleys," formed by the membrane between the tongue and the epiglottis. During a normal swallow, the larynx elevates and the epiglottis folds down to protect the airway from food and liquid. The food and liquid pass over the back of the tongue, through the valleculae, into the pyriform sinuses, and finally into the esophagus (this will be discussed in detail in Chapter 8). When swallowing is compromised, as in the deficit arising from cerebrovascular accident (see Chapter 12), the larynx may not elevate properly (Dejaeger, Pelemans, Pouette, and Joosten 1997), or the tongue movement may be inadequate, and food can accumulate in the valleculae. From this you can see that malodorous breath in an individual who is neurologically compromised may be a significant indicator of a dangerous swallowing dysfunction, because if the epiglottis is not covering the airway, there is a good chance that the vocal folds are not doing their job in protecting the lungs and that the lungs are being exposed to food and drink.

A small **triticeal cartilage** (also known as the tritiate cartilage) may or may not be found here. In front, running from the corpus hyoid to the upper border of the anterior thyroid, is the **median thyrohyoid ligament**. Together, the median thyrohyoid ligament, thyrohyoid membrane, and lateral thyrohyoid ligament connect the larynx and the hyoid bone. There are other extrinsic ligaments. The **hyoepiglottic ligament** and **thyroepiglottic ligament** attach the epiglottis to the corpus hyoid and the inner thyroid cartilage, just below the notch, respectively. The epiglottic attachment to the tongue is made by means of the **lateral** and **median glossoepiglottic ligaments**, and the overlay of the mucous membrane on these ligaments produces the "little valleys" or **valleculae** between the tongue and the epiglottis. The trachea must attach to the larynx as well, and this is achieved through the **cricotracheal ligament**.

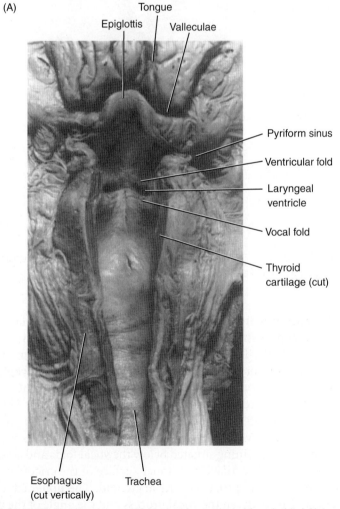

Figure 4-2. (A) Cavity of the larynx with landmarks, as viewed from behind. Note that the laryngeal space has been revealed by a sagittal incision, and the posterior laryngeal wall has been spread for access to the structure. (continues).
© Cengage Learning®.

(B)

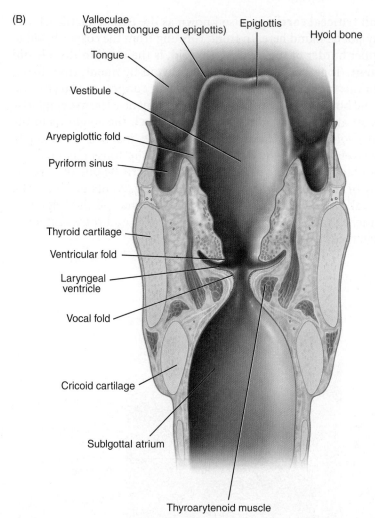

Valleculae
(between tongue and epiglottis)

Epiglottis

Hyoid bone

Tongue

Vestibule

Aryepiglottic fold

Pyriform sinus

Thyroid cartilage

Ventricular fold

Laryngeal
ventricle

Vocal fold

Cricoid cartilage

Sublgottal atrium

Thyroarytenoid muscle

Figure 4-2 continued. (B) Drawing of cavity of landmark with larynx, as viewed from behind through coronal section. (continues).
© Cengage Learning®.

quadrangular: L., quadri, four; angulus, right; "right-angled"

conus elasticus: L., elastic cone

The **intrinsic ligaments** connect the cartilages of the larynx and form the support structure for the cavity of the larynx, as well as that of the vocal folds. The **fibroelastic membrane** of the larynx is composed of the upper **quadrangular membranes** and **aryepiglottic folds**, the lower **conus elasticus**, and the **vocal ligament**, which is actually the upward free extension of the conus elasticus. The conus elasticus is also referred to as the cricovocal membrane or the crico-thyroid ligament (McHanwell, 2008). The conus elasticus is the dominant membranous lining situated below the vocal folds and attaches to the lower thyroid cartilage and upper surface of the cricoid cartilage and tip of the vocal process of the arytenoid. The upper edge of the conus elasticus between the vocal process and the angle of the thyroid cartilage forms the vocal ligament within the vocal folds (Figure 4-3). The conus elasticus has the shape and form of a vortex and is believed to reduce resistance to airflow.

(C)

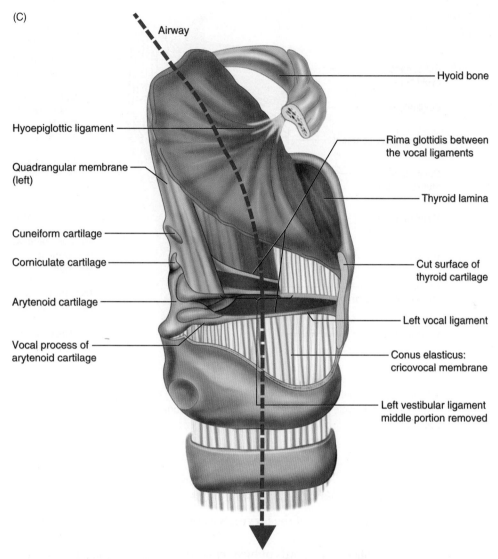

Airway

Hyoid bone

Hyoepiglottic ligament

Rima glottidis between the vocal ligaments

Quadrangular membrane (left)

Thyroid lamina

Cuneiform cartilage

Corniculate cartilage

Cut surface of thyroid cartilage

Arytenoid cartilage

Left vocal ligament

Vocal process of arytenoid cartilage

Conus elasticus: cricovocal membrane

Left vestibular ligament middle portion removed

Figure 4-2 continued. (C) Membranes and ligaments of the larynx. Note particularly the hyoepiglottic ligament, cricovocal membrane (conus elasticus), quadrangular membrane, and vocal ligament. (continues). © Cengage Learning®.

The quadrangular membranes are the undergirding layer of connective tissue running from the arytenoids to the epiglottis and thyroid cartilage and forming the false vocal folds. They originate at the inner thyroid angle and sides of the epiglottis and form an upper cone that narrows as it terminates in the free margin of the arytenoid and corniculate cartilages. The **aryepiglottic muscles** course from the side of the epiglottis to the arytenoid apex, forming the upper margin of the quadrangular membranes and laterally, the aryepiglottic folds. These folds are simply the ridges marking the highest elevation of these membranes and muscles slung from epiglottis to arytenoids. The **pyriform sinus** is the space between the aryepiglottic folds and the thyroid cartilage, marking an important point of transit for food and liquid during a swallow, as will be discussed in Chapter 8.

(D)

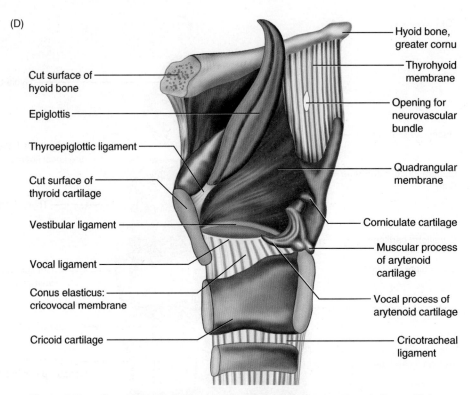

Hyoid bone, greater cornu

Thyrohyoid membrane

Opening for neurovascular bundle

Quadrangular membrane

Corniculate cartilage

Muscular process of arytenoid cartilage

Vocal process of arytenoid cartilage

Cricotracheal ligament

Cut surface of hyoid bone

Epiglottis

Thyroepiglottic ligament

Cut surface of thyroid cartilage

Vestibular ligament

Vocal ligament

Conus elasticus: cricovocal membrane

Cricoid cartilage

Figure 4-2 continued. (D) Membranes and ligaments of the larynx, viewed after sagittal cut. Note the thyrohyoid membrane, quadrangular membrane, conus elasticus, and vocal ligament.
© Cengage Learning®.

✔ *To summarize:*

- The **cavity** of the **larynx** is a constricted tube with a smooth surface.
- Sheets and cords of ligaments connect the cartilages, while a smooth **mucous membrane** covers the medial-most surface of the larynx.
- The **thyrohyoid membrane**, **lateral thyrohyoid ligament**, and **median thyrohyoid ligament** cover the space between the hyoid bone and the thyroid.
- The **hyoepiglottic** and **thyroepiglottic ligaments** attach the epiglottis to the corpus hyoid and the inner thyroid cartilage, respectively.
- The **valleculae** are found between the tongue and the epiglottis, within folds arising from the lateral and median glossoepiglottic ligaments.
- The **cricotracheal ligament** attaches the trachea to the larynx.
- The **fibroelastic membrane** is composed of the upper **quadrangular membranes** and **aryepiglottic folds**; the lower

conus elasticus and the **vocal ligament**, which is actually the upward free extension of the conus elasticus. The **pyriform sinus** is the space between the fold of the aryepiglottic membrane and the thyroid cartilage laterally.

- The **aryepiglottic folds** course from the side of the epiglottis to the arytenoid apex.
- The conus elasticus is the membranous cover beneath the level of the vocal folds. It is continuous with the vocal ligament and is thought to reduce airway resistance leading to the glottis.

Fine Structure of the Vocal Folds. The vocal folds are composed of five layers of tissue, as can be seen in Figure 4-3. The most superficial is a protective layer of squamous epithelium, approximately 0.1 mm thick, with an underlying layer of basement membrane to bind it to

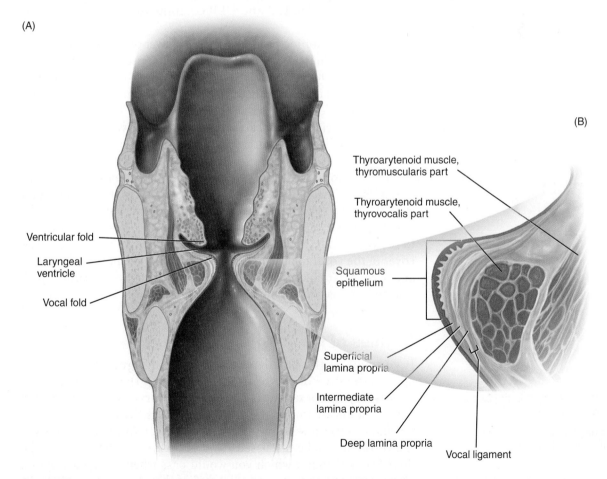

Figure 4-3. (A) Transverse section through the larynx, revealing the vocal folds. (B) Expanded view of the vocal folds, showing layers.
© Cengage Learning®.

the next layer. This epithelial layer gives the vocal folds the glistening white appearance seen during **laryngoscopic** examination (use of a **laryngoscope**, a device typically used by laryngologists or speech-language pathologists to view the larynx). This protective layer aids in keeping the delicate tissues of the vocal folds moist by assisting in fluid retention.

The next layer is the superficial lamina propria (SLP) made up of elastin fibers, so named because of their physical qualities that allow them to be extensively stretched. The fibrous and elastic elements of the SLP cushion the vocal folds. The elastin fibers of the SLP are cross-layered with the intermediate lamina propria (ILP), which is deep to it. The ILP is approximately 1–2 mm thick and is also composed of elastin fibers running in an anterior-posterior direction, making them cross-layered with the SLP. The combination of these two layers provides both elasticity and strength. The deep lamina propria (DLP) is approximately 1–2 mm thick and primarily supportive, being made up of collagen fibers that prohibit extension. The ILP and DLP combine to make up the vocal ligament.

Deep to the lamina propria is the fifth layer of the vocal folds, the thyroarytenoid muscle (thyrovocalis and thyromuscularis). This makes up the bulk of the vocal fold. Because the muscle course is anterior-posterior, the fibers are arranged in this orientation. This combination of tissues provides both active and passive elements. The thyrovocalis is the active element of the vocal folds, while the passive elements consist of the layers of lamina propria that provide strength, cushioning, and elasticity.

The **mucosal lining of the vocal folds** is actually a combination of the epithelial lining and the disorganized first lamina propria layer. The second and third layers (elastin and collagen) constitute the **vocal ligament**, a structure giving a degree of stiffness and support to the vocal folds. Some authors refer alternately to the layers as the **cover** of the vocal folds (superficial epithelium, primary and secondary layers of lamina propria) and the **body** (third layer of lamina propria and thyroarytenoid muscle) of the vocal folds.

Cavities of the Larynx

If you look at the profile of the larynx in Figure 4-4, you will appreciate some of the relationships among the structures. The **aditus laryngis** or **aditus** is the entry to the larynx from the pharynx above. (Some anatomists define the aditus as the first space of the larynx; others view it simply as the entryway to the first cavity—the vestibule—to be discussed.) You may think of the aditus as the door frame through which you would pass when entering a house. The anterior boundary of the "frame" of the aditus is the epiglottis, with the fold of membrane and muscle slung between the epiglottis and the arytenoids (the **aryepiglottic folds**) comprising the lateral

aditus laryngis: L., entrance; "laryngeal entrance"

aditus: entry to the larynx from the pharynx

aryepiglottic: ary(tenoid) epiglottis

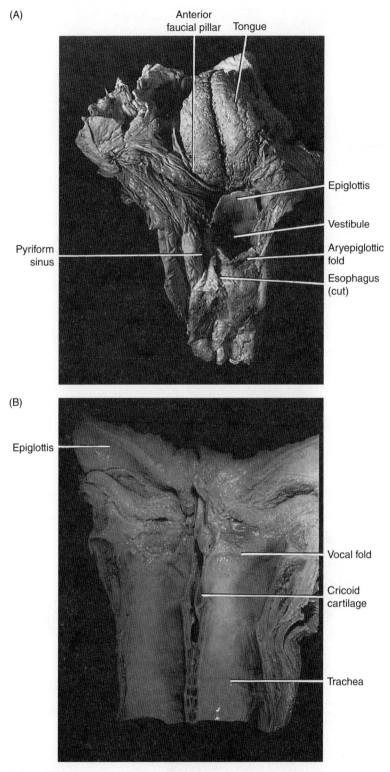

Figure 4-4. (A) Larynx, as seen from behind and above. (B) Larynx that has been cut sagittally with the sides reflected, revealing the two halves of the larynx. (continues).
© Cengage Learning®.

Figure 4-4 continued. (C) Drawing showing landmarks.
© Cengage Learning®.

Tongue

Epiglottis

Valleculae

Ventricular fold

Aryepiglottic fold

Anterior faucial pillar

Vocal fold

Pyriform sinus

Esophagus

Tongue

Anterior faucial pillar

Epiglottis

Pyriform sinus

Vestibule

Aryepiglottic fold

Esophagus (cut)

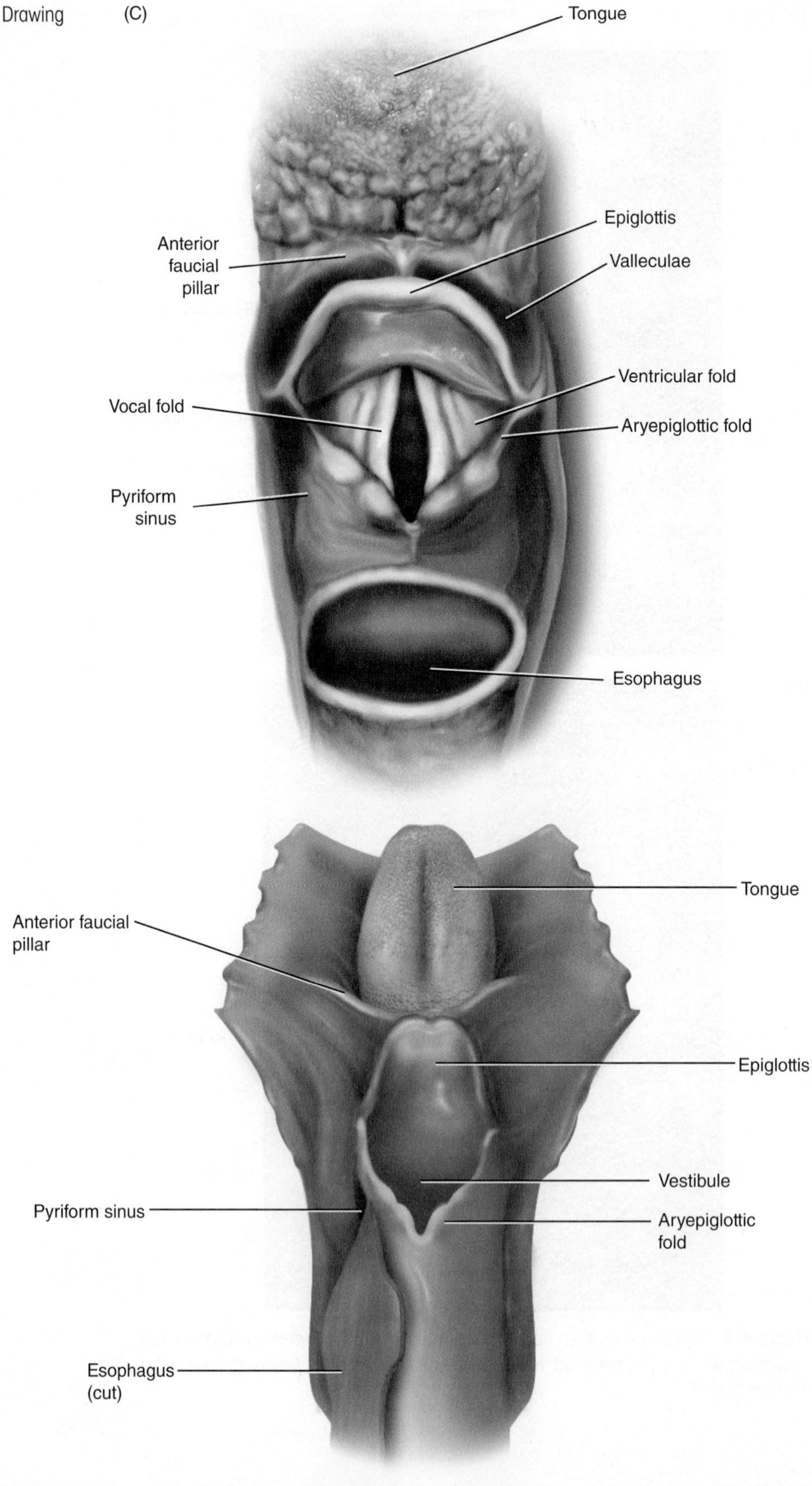

margins of the aditus. In Figure 4-5A you can see two "bumps" under the aryepiglottic folds. These are caused by the cuneiform cartilages embedded within the folds. The second set of prominences posterior to the first two are from the corniculate cartilages on the arytenoids.

The first cavity of the larynx is the **vestibule**, or entryway. The vestibule is the space between the entryway or aditus and the **ventricular** (or **vestibular**) folds. The ventricular folds are also known as the **false vocal folds**, because they are not used for phonation except in rare (and clinically significant) cases. The vestibule is wide at the aditus but narrows at the ventricular folds. The lateral walls are comprised of the aryepiglottic folds, and the posterior walls are made up of the membrane covering the arytenoid cartilages, which project superiorly to the false folds. The false vocal folds are made up of a mucous membrane and a fibrous **vestibular ligament**, but not muscular tissue. The space between the false vocal folds is termed the **rima vestibuli**.

The middle space of the larynx lies between the margins of the false vocal folds and the true vocal folds below. This space is the **laryngeal ventricle** (or **laryngeal sinus**), and the anterior extension of this space is the **laryngeal saccule** (also known as the appendix of the ventricle). The saccule (or pouch) is endowed with more than 60 mucous glands that secrete lubricating mucus into the laryngeal cavity. The thyroepiglottic muscle passes between the saccule and the

rima vestibuli: L., "slit of the vestibule"

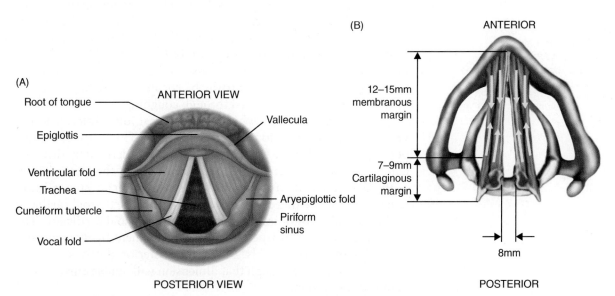

Figure 4-5. (A) Vocal folds as seen from above. Note that true vocal folds appear white upon examination as a result of the superficial layer of squamous epithelial tissue. Seen immediately superior to the true vocal folds are the ventricular or false folds. Note the corniculate and cuneiform tubercles. These prominences arise from the presence of the corniculate and cuneiform cartilages deep in the aryepiglottic folds. (B) Same view of vocal folds, but with the membranous lining and supportive muscle of larynx removed, to reveal only cartilages and the thyroarytenoid muscle (thyrovocalis and thyromuscularis). The membranous margin of the vocal folds is approximately 12–15 mm long in adults, while the cartilaginous margin is approximately 7–9 mm long. The space between the vocal folds (glottis) at rest is approximately 8 mm.
© Cengage Learning®.

Saccular Cysts and Laryngoceles

The saccule of the laryngeal ventricle is a fibrous pouch that encapsulates the mucus to be secreted into the airway for lubrication and to entrap foreign particles. The fibrous wall can break down and weaken, allowing a herniation of the saccule, and this is termed a laryngocele, and it is a rare occurrence (Gulia, Yadav, Khaowas, Basur, & Agrawal, 2012). The saccule will enlarge, expanding beyond its location in the ventricle. An internal laryngocele may expand under the aryepiglottic fold, ultimately reaching the valleculae. If it reaches the thyrohyoid membrane it may emerge superficial to the membranes, becoming an external laryngocele, which may be palpated at the neck. External laryngoceles may be quite slow in developing. Internal laryngoceles can interfere with the airway, causing hoarseness, swallowing problems (dysphagia), and laryngeal stridor (noisy inhalations and exhalations because of airway obstruction).

Saccular cysts are growths that can occur if the opening of the saccule is obstructed, for instance as a result of growth of a tumor. The saccule will enlarge and often become inflamed and infected. The expansion will take the same form as a laryngocele. Saccular cysts and laryngoceles can become health-threatening in youngsters, as they can expand to obstruct the airway, and infection of any internal tissue or organ is a significant issue.

In apes the laryngeal saccules are so well developed that they contribute to the resonance of the voice.

thyroid cartilage, and when this muscle contracts it squeezes on the saccule, causing release of mucus onto laryngeal tissue. There are, in reality, mucous glands throughout the larynx, including the surface of the epiglottis and aryepiglottic folds. These glands secrete mucus periodically to lubricate the vocal folds, since the folds themselves do not have mucous glands (McHanwell, 2008). The secretions are important for maintaining the health of the vocal folds and reducing airway resistance. The mucus also assists in eliminating errant food particles that enter the airway by encapsulating them, thereby enabling them to be eliminated through coughing.

The glottis is the space between the vocal folds, inferior to the ventricle and superior to the conus elasticus. This is the most important laryngeal space for speech, because it is defined by the *variable sphincter* that permits voicing. The length of the glottis at rest is approximately 20 mm in adults from the **anterior commissure** (anterior-most opening posterior to the angle of the thyroid cartilage) to the **posterior commissure** (between the arytenoid cartilages). The glottis area is variable, depending upon the moment-by-moment configuration of the vocal folds. At rest the posterior glottis is approximately 8 mm wide, although that dimension will double during times of forced respiration.

The lateral margins of the glottis are the vocal folds and the arytenoid cartilage. The anterior three-fifths of the vocal margin is made up of the soft tissue of the vocal folds. (You will see this referred to as the **membranous glottis**, because some anatomists define the glottis as the entire vocal mechanism. Physicians sometimes refer to this as the phonatory glottis [Merati & Rieder, 2003].) In adult males, the free margin of the vocal folds is approximately 15 mm in length, and in females it is approximately 12 mm. This free margin of the vocal folds is the vibrating element that provides voice. The posterior two-fifths of the vocal folds is comprised of the cartilage of the arytenoids. (This is often referred to as the **cartilaginous glottis**, because *glottis* is sometimes used to refer to the entire vocal mechanism. Physicians sometimes refer to it as the respiratory glottis.) This portion of the vocal folds is between 4 and 8 mm long, depending on gender and body size.

The conus elasticus begins at the margins of the true vocal folds and extends to the inferior border of the cricoid cartilage, widening from the vocal folds to the base of the cricoid.

Reinke's Edema

The larynx is lined with mucous membrane, designed to retain moisture and provide a low-resistance surface for the airway. The membrane is reasonably loose throughout, allowing movement of laryngeal structures. The exception is at the vocal ligament: at this location, the mucous membrane is fixed, and therein lies the problem. When tissue is irritated, extracellular fluid accumulates, causing swelling (edema). In the case of the larynx, that accumulation of fluid can't go anywhere because the lining is bound to the vocal ligament. The result is that the inner lining of the larynx expands, and particularly the vocal folds, become swollen. The swelling is maintained because of the poor lymphatic swelling of the space. This condition is known as Reinke's edema, because the space deep to the superficial lamina propria is called Reinke's space. The condition can arise from vocal abuse, but most often is seen in people who smoke (Móz, Domingues, Castilho, Branco, & Martins, 2013), since smoking irritates tissue.

Vocal Fold Hydration

The vocal folds are extremely sensitive to the internal and external environment. Although cigarette smoke and other pollutants are known to cause irritation to the tissues of the vocal folds, the internal environment appears to have an impact as well.

When the vocal folds are subject to abuse, several problems may arise, among them contact ulcers and vocal nodules. Hydration therapy is a frequent prescription to counteract the problems of irritated tissue. Dry tissue does not heal as well as moist tissue, so the client will be told to increase the environmental humidity, drink fluids, or even take medications to promote water retention. This type of therapy makes more than medical sense. Verdolini, Titze, and Fennell (1994) found that the *effort* of phonation increased as individuals became dehydrated, and decreased when they were hydrated beyond normal levels. Indeed, the airflow required to produce the same phonation is greatly increased by a poorly lubricated larynx. In addition, the vocal folds vibrate much more periodically (they have greatly reduced perturbation, or cycle-by-cycle variation) when lubricated (Fukida et al., 1988). When the relative periodicity of the vocal folds decreases, the voice sounds hoarse, a perception that you will agree with if you think of the last time you had laryngitis.

✔ *To summarize:*

- The **vocal folds** are made up of five layers of tissue.
- Deep to the thin **epithelial layer** is the **lamina propria**, made up of two layers of elastin and one layer of collagen fibers. The thyroarytenoid muscle is the deepest of the layers.
- The **vocal ligament** is made of elastin. The **aditus** is the entryway of the larynx, marking the entry to the **vestibule**.
- The **ventricular** and **vocal folds** are separated by the laryngeal **ventricle**.
- The glottis is the variable space between the vocal folds.

Structure of the Larynx

Cricoid Cartilage

The unpaired cricoid cartilage can be viewed as an expanded tracheal cartilage (Figure 4-6). As the most inferior cartilage of the larynx, the cricoid cartilage is the approximate diameter of the trachea. It is higher in the back than in the front.

There are several important landmarks on the cricoid. The low, anterior cricoid arch provides clearance for the vocal folds that will pass over that point, while the posterior elevation, the superior surface of the **posterior quadrate lamina**, provides the point of articulation for the arytenoid cartilages. On the lateral surfaces of the cricoid are articular facets or "faces," marking the point of articulation for the inferior horns of the thyroid cartilage. This **cricothyroid joint** is a diarthrodial, pivoting joint that permits the rotation of the two articulating structures.

One more note on the cricoid. The figures and photographs are quite misleading concerning the size of laryngeal structures. For perspective, your cricoid cartilage would fit loosely upon your little finger, which is about the diameter of your trachea. The laryngeal structures are *small*. Indeed, subglottic stenosis (narrowing of the area below the glottis) is a frequent laryngeal problem following endotracheal intubation (ventilation by means of a tube placed into the airway through the larynx) and its subsequent scarring.

Thyroid Cartilage

The unpaired thyroid cartilage is the largest of the laryngeal cartilages. As you can see in Figure 4-7, the thyroid cartilage has a prominent anterior surface made up of two plates called the thyroid laminae, joined at the midline at the **thyroid angle**. At the superior-most point of that angle you will see the **thyroid notch**, which you can palpate if you do the following. Place your finger under your chin and on your throat, and bring it downward to the point you might refer to as your Adam's apple (in adult males, the two lamina meet at about a 90 degree angle, while the angle for females is more like

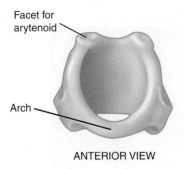

ANTERIOR VIEW

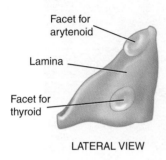

LATERAL VIEW

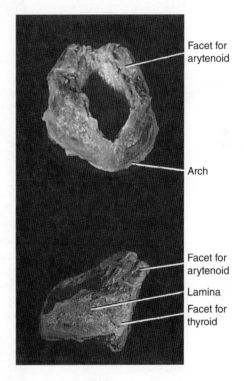

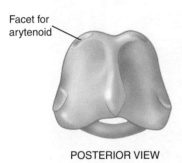

POSTERIOR VIEW

Figure 4-6. Cricoid cartilage and landmarks.
© Cengage Learning®.

120 degrees. This acute angle in males results in a more prominent "Adam's apple."). When you have found the top of that structure, you have identified the thyroid notch. Look at the drawing as you feel the indentation in your own thyroid. Now draw your finger down the midline a little until you feel the angle. If you put your index finger on the angle and your thumb and second finger on the sides, you will have digits on the angle and both laminae. Do take a moment to discover these regions on yourself, because they provide you with a reference that is near and dear to you. Incidentally, when you had your finger on the notch, you were as close as you could be to touching your vocal folds, because they attach to the thyroid cartilage just behind that point.

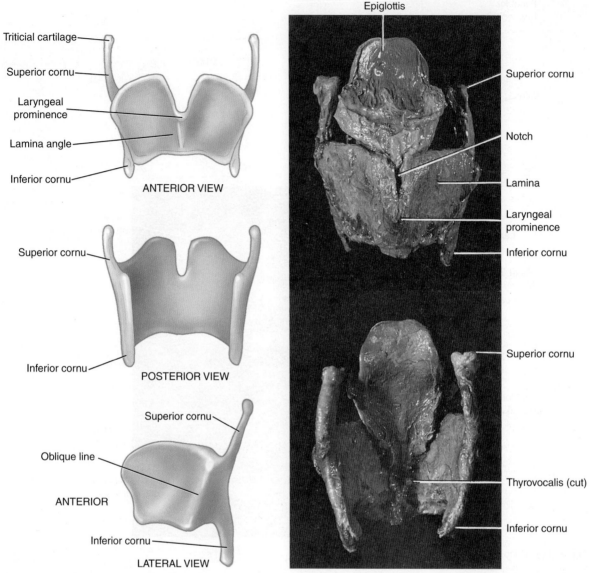

Figure 4-7. Thyroid cartilage and landmarks.
© Cengage Learning®.

cornu: L., horn (as in cornucopia, the "horn of plenty")

triticeal: L., triticeus, wheat; "wheat-like"

Drawing your attention back to Figure 4-7, on the lateral superficial aspect of the thyroid laminae you will see the **oblique line**. This marks the point of attachment for two muscles we will talk about shortly.

The posterior aspect of the thyroid is open and is characterized by two prominent sets of **cornu** or horns. The **inferior cornua** project downward to articulate with the cricoid cartilage, while the **superior cornua** project superiorly to articulate with the hyoid. In some individuals a small **triticeal** cartilage (*cartilago triticea*) may be found between the superior cornu of the thyroid cartilage and the hyoid bone.

Arytenoid and Corniculate Cartilages

The paired arytenoid cartilages are among the most important of the larynx. They reside on the superior posterolateral surface of the cricoid cartilage and provide the mechanical structure that permits onset and offset of voicing. The form of the arytenoid may be likened to a pyramid to aid in visualization (see Figure 4-8). Each cartilage has two processes and four surfaces.

The apex is the truncated superior portion of the pyramidal arytenoid cartilage, and on the superior surfaces of each arytenoid is a **corniculate cartilage**, projecting posteriorly to form the peak of the

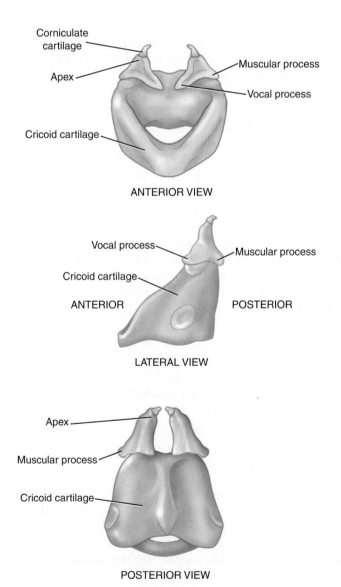

Figure 4-8. Arytenoid cartilages articulated with cricoid cartilage.
© Cengage Learning®.

distorted pyramid. The inferior surface of the cartilage is termed the **base**, and its concave surface is the point of articulation with the convex arytenoid facet of the cricoid cartilage.

The names of the two processes of the arytenoid give a hint as to their function. The **vocal processes** project anteriorly toward the thyroid notch, and it is these processes to which the posterior portion of the vocal folds themselves will attach. The **muscular process** forms the lateral outcropping of the arytenoid pyramid and, as its name implies, is the point of attachment for muscles that adduct and abduct the vocal folds.

Epiglottis

The unpaired epiglottis is a leaflike structure that arises from the inner surface of the angle of the thyroid cartilage just below the notch, being attached there by the thyroepiglottic ligament. The sides of the epiglottis are joined with the arytenoid cartilages via the aryepiglottic folds, which are the product of the membranous lining being draped over muscle and connective tissue.

The epiglottis projects upward beyond the larynx and above the hyoid bone and is attached to the root of the tongue by means of the median and lateral glossoepiglottic ligaments, with the overlying epithelium that produces the **glosso-epiglottic fold**. This juncture produces the valleculae, a landmark that will become important in your study of swallowing and swallowing deficit. During swallowing food passes over the epiglottis and, from there, laterally to the **pyriform** (also piriform) sinuses, which are small fossae or indentations between the aryepiglottic folds medially and the mucous lining of the thyroid cartilage. Together, the pyriform sinuses and valleculae are called the **pharyngeal recesses** (see Figure 4-5).

The epiglottis is attached to the hyoid bone via the **hyoepiglottic ligament**. The surface of the epiglottis is covered with a mucous membrane lining, and beneath this lining on the posterior, concave surface may be found branches of the internal laryngeal nerve of the X **vagus** that conduct sensory information from the larynx.

See Chapter 11 for a discussion of the X vagus nerve.

vagus: L., wandering

Cuneiform Cartilages

cuneiform: L., cuneus, wedge; "wedge-shaped"

The **cuneiform** cartilages are small cartilages embedded within the aryepiglottic folds. They are situated above and anterior to the corniculate cartilages and cause a small bulge on the surface of the membrane that looks white under illumination. These cartilages apparently provide support for the membranous laryngeal covering.

Hyoid Bone

Although not a bone of the larynx, the hyoid forms the union between the tongue and the laryngeal structure. This unpaired small bone articulates loosely with the superior cornu of the thyroid cartilage and has the distinction of being the only bone of the body that is not attached to another bone (see Figure 4-9).

As you can see from the view of the hyoid bone from above, this structure is U-shaped, being open in the posterior aspect. There are three major elements of the hyoid bone. The corpus or body of the hyoid is a prominent shield-like structure forming the front of the bone and is a structure you can palpate. If you place your finger on your thyroid notch and push *lightly* back toward your vertebral column, you will feel the hard structure of the corpus near your fingernail. As you are doing this, take one more look at Figure 4-1 showing the structures together to become acquainted with the relationship of these structures.

The front of the corpus is convex, and the inner surface is concave. The corpus is the point of attachment for six muscles, no small feat for such a small structure.

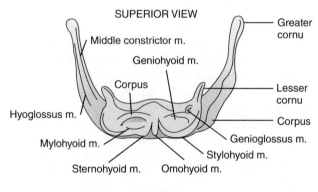

Anterior View

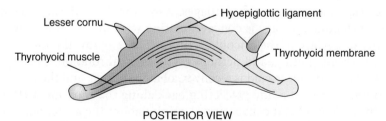

POSTERIOR VIEW

Figure 4-9. Hyoid bone as seen from above and behind. Points of attachment of muscles and membranes are indicated.
© Cengage Learning®.

Infant Larynx

Infants have different anatomy from adults, particularly as it relates to the larynx. The larynx is markedly narrow, and is higher than the adult larynx. The top of the epiglottic cartilage is visible over the back of the tongue, and all the laryngeal cartilages are softer and more pliable than those of adults. Indeed, laryngomalacia (audible breathing, or "stridor") is frequently caused by the airway being so pliant and collapsing on itself in infants, as well as the fact that the mucous membrane lining of the larynx is more loosely bound to the larynx than in adults. The thyroid cartilage is proportionately closer to the hyoid bone than in adults (the infant larynx is 1/3 the size of an adults larynx). The vocal folds are around 4.5 mm long, and the laryngeal saccule is relatively larger in infants than in adults (Standring, 2008). Because of the small size of the larynx, any conditions that cause swelling of the tissues of the airway place the infant at significant risk. By 3 years of age sex differences begin to emerge with the male larynx being larger than that of the female, but these changes come to full bloom during puberty.

The **greater cornu** arises on the lateral surface of the corpus, projecting posteriorly. At the junction of the corpus and greater cornu you can see the **lesser cornu**. Three additional muscles attach to these two structures.

Movement of the Cartilages

The cricothyroid and cricoarytenoid joints are the only functionally mobile points of the larynx, and both of these joints serve extremely important laryngeal functions.

The cricothyroid joint is the junction of the cricoid cartilage and the inferior cornu of the thyroid cartilage, as mentioned earlier. These are synovial (diarthrodial) joints that permit the cricoid and thyroid to rotate and glide relative to each other. As seen in Figure 4-10, rotation at the cricothyroid joint permits the thyroid cartilage to rock down in front, and the joint also permits the thyroid to glide forward and backward slightly, relative to the cricoid. This joint provides the major adjustment for change in vocal pitch.

The **cricoarytenoid joint** is the articulation formed between the cricoid and arytenoid cartilages. As you will recall, the base of the arytenoid cartilage is concave, mating with the smooth convex superior surface of the cricoid cartilage. These synovial joints permit rocking, gliding, and perhaps even minimal rotation. The arytenoid facet of the cricoid is a convex, oblong surface, and the axis of motion is around a line projecting back along the superior surface of the arytenoid and converging at a point above the arytenoid (see Figure 4-11). This rocking action brings the two vocal processes toward each other, permitting the vocal folds to **approximate** (make contact). The arytenoids are also capable of gliding on the long axis of the facet, facilitating changes in vocal fold length. The arytenoids also appear to rotate upon a vertical axis drawn through the apex of

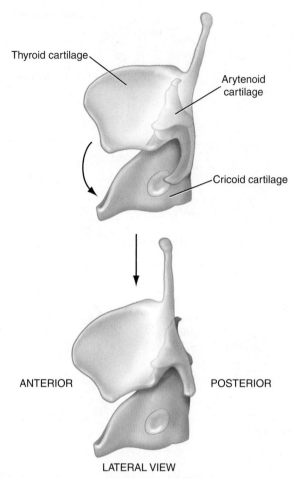

Thyroid cartilage

Arytenoid cartilage

Cricoid cartilage

ANTERIOR   POSTERIOR

LATERAL VIEW

Figure 4-10. Movement of the cricoid and thyroid cartilages about the cricothyroid joint. When the cricoid and thyroid move toward each other in front, the arytenoid cartilage moves farther away from the thyroid cartilage, tensing the vocal folds.
© Cengage Learning®.

the arytenoid, but this motion may be limited to extremes of abduction (Fink & Demarest, 1978). Recent evidence produced through the study of cadaver specimens supports the role of arytenoid rotation during phonation (Storck et al., 2012).

The combination of these movements provides the mechanism for vocal fold approximation and abduction. Your understanding of the movement of these cartilages in relation to one another will provide a valuable backdrop for understanding the laryngeal physiology presented in Chapter 5.

✔ *To summarize:*

- The laryngeal cartilages have a number of important landmarks to which muscles are attached.
- The **cricoid** cartilage is shaped like a signet ring, higher at the back.

(A)

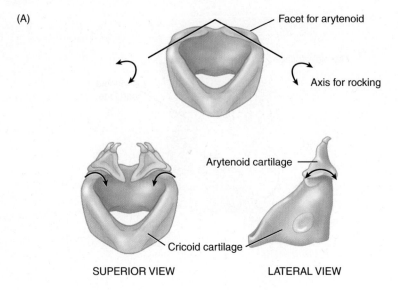

Facet for arytenoid

Axis for rocking

Arytenoid cartilage

Cricoid cartilage

SUPERIOR VIEW   LATERAL VIEW

Anatesse Lesson

(B)

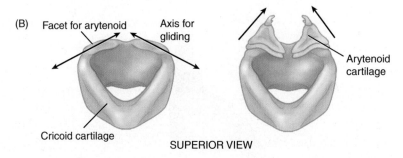

Facet for arytenoid

Axis for gliding

Arytenoid cartilage

Cricoid cartilage

SUPERIOR VIEW

Figure 4-11. The articular facet for the arytenoid cartilage permits rocking, gliding, and rotation. (A) The shape of the articular facet for the arytenoid cartilage promotes inward rocking of the arytenoid cartilage and vocal folds, as shown by the arrows. (B) The long axis of the facet permits limited anterior-posterior gliding. (C) The arytenoids may also rotate as shown, although evidence of functional movement through rotation is conflicting.

Source: (Based on data of Broad, 1973; Fink & Demarest, 1978; Netter, 1997; Zemlin, 1998.)

(C)

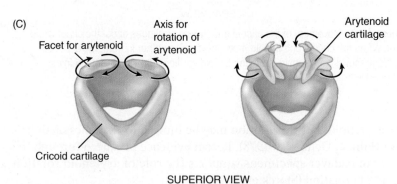

Axis for rotation of arytenoid

Arytenoid cartilage

Facet for arytenoid

Arytenoid cartilage

Cricoid cartilage

SUPERIOR VIEW

- The **arytenoid** cartilages ride on the superior surface of the cricoid, with the cricoarytenoid joint permitting rotation, rocking, and gliding.
- The **muscular** and **vocal processes** provide attachment for the **thyromuscularis** and **thyrovocalis** muscles.
- The **corniculate** cartilages attach to the upper margin of the arytenoids.

Palpation of the Larynx

To palpate the larynx, first identify the prominent thyroid notch or "Adam's apple" (see Figure 4-7). Once you have found it, place your index finger on the notch itself, with your thumb and second finger on either side. Your thumb and second finger should feel a fairly flat surface, the thyroid lamina. Now bring your index finger straight down a little bit; you will feel the prominent thyroid angle. Bring your finger back up to the top of the notch; when your finger is on top of the notch, the hard region contacting your fingernail is the corpus of the hyoid bone. In some people this is very hard to differentiate from the thyroid.

Palpate lateral to the notch on the superior surface, and you will feel the superior cornu of the thyroid. With a little discomfort, you may feel the articulation of the hyoid and thyroid. If you draw your finger down the angle again, you can find the lower margin of the thyroid and feel the cricoid beneath. After carefully placing your thumb at the junction of the cricoid and thyroid, you can hum up and down the scale and feel the thyroid and cricoid moving closer together and farther apart as you do this. You will also feel the entire larynx elevate as you reach the upper end of your range. Finally, draw your finger to find the lower margin of the cricoid, marking the beginning of the trachea. Palpate the tracheal rings.

- The **thyroid** cartilage has two prominent laminae, superior and inferior horns, and a prominent thyroid notch.
- The **hyoid bone** attaches to the superior cornu of the thyroid, while the **cricoid** cartilage attaches to the inferior horn via the cricothyroid joint.
- The **epiglottis** attaches to the tongue and thyroid cartilage, dropping down to cover the larynx during swallowing.
- The **cuneiform** cartilages are embedded within the aryepiglottic folds.

LARYNGEAL MUSCULATURE

As summarized in Table 4-1, muscles of the larynx may be conveniently divided into those that have both origin and insertion on laryngeal cartilages (**intrinsic laryngeal muscles**) and those with one attachment on a laryngeal cartilage and the other attachment on a nonlaryngeal structure (**extrinsic laryngeal muscles**). The extrinsic muscles make major adjustments to the larynx, such as elevating or depressing it, while the intrinsic musculature makes fine adjustments to the vocal mechanism itself. Extrinsic muscles tend to work in concert with the articulatory motions of the tongue, and many are important in swallowing, and some are variably active during respiration. Intrinsic muscles assume responsibility for opening, closing, tensing, and relaxing the vocal folds. We will begin with a discussion of the intrinsic muscles. The summary information of Appendix D may be helpful to your studies.

Table 4-1 **Muscles associated with laryngeal function**

Intrinsic Muscles of Larynx

  Adductors

    Lateral cricoarytenoid

    Transverse arytenoid

    Oblique arytenoid

  Abductor

    Posterior cricoarytenoid

  Tensors

    Thyrovocalis (medial thyroarytenoid)

    Cricothyroid, pars recta, and pars oblique

  Relaxers

    Thyromuscularis (lateral thyroarytenoid)

  Auxiliary Musculature

    Thyroepiglotticus[1]

    Superior thyroarytenoid

    Thyroarytenoid

    Aryepiglotticus

Extrinsic Muscles of Larynx (Suprahyoid and Infrahyoid Muscles)

  Hyoid and Laryngeal Elevators

    Stylohyoid

    Mylohyoid

    Geniohyoid

    Genioglossus

    Hyoglossus

    Inferior pharyngeal constrictor

    Digastricus anterior and posterior

  Hyoid and Laryngeal Depressors

    Sternothyroid

    Sternohyoid

    Omohyoid

    Thyrohyoid

*Note that the thyroepiglottic muscle is included here by virtue of its relevance to the swallowing function.

Intrinsic Laryngeal Muscles

Adductors

- **Lateral cricoarytenoid**
- **Transverse arytenoid**
- **Oblique arytenoid**

Lateral Cricoarytenoid Muscle. This extremely important muscle is one of the more difficult laryngeal muscles to visualize. The **lateral**

Referral in Voice Therapy

The phonatory mechanism is extremely sensitive, and vocal signs can be indicators for a broad range of problems. We must always refer an individual to a physician when we identify vocal dysfunction, even though we may be fairly certain that the problem is behavioral in nature. When a client comes to us with a hoarse voice, we may find out that the person is abusing his or her phonatory mechanism by spending too much time in loud, smoky settings that require raising the voice when speaking. What we don't know from this information is whether there is a vocal pathology, perhaps secondary to the same behavioral conditions, that is developing on the vocal folds. Although we suspect vocal nodules, the client could also be showing early signs of laryngeal cancer.

In a similar vein, a client who comes to us with a voice that is progressively weaker during the day, and for whom muscular effort of any sort is extremely difficult as the day wears on, will easily merit a referral, although it will be to a neurologist. Myasthenia gravis is a myoneural disease that results in a complex of speech disorders, including progressive weakening of phonation, progressive degeneration of articulatory function, and progressive hypernasality, all arising from the use of the speech mechanism over the course of a day or briefer time. The condition is quite treatable, but often the speech-language pathologist is the individual to first recognize the signs because the client sees it primarily as a speech problem.

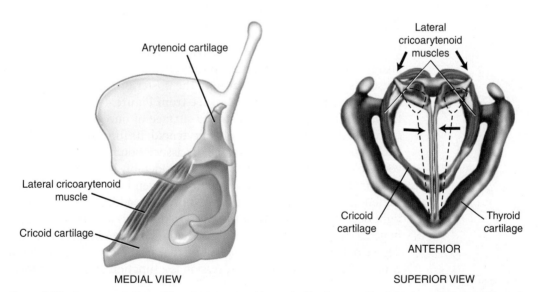

Figure 4-12. Course and effect of lateral cricoarytenoid muscle. The figure on the right shows that contraction of the lateral cricoarytenoid muscle pulls the muscular process forward, adducting the vocal folds (seen from above).
© Cengage Learning®.

cricoarytenoid muscle attaches to the cricoid and the muscular process of the arytenoid, causing the muscular process to move forward and medially (see Figure 4-12). The origin of the lateral cricoarytenoid muscle is on the superior-lateral surface of the cricoid cartilage. The muscle courses up and back to insert into the muscular process of the arytenoid cartilage. As you can see from this figure, the course of the muscle dictates that the muscular process will be drawn forward, and the motion thus induced will rock the arytenoid inward and downward. This inward-and-downward rocking is the major adjustment associated with the adduction of the vocal folds. In addition, this movement may lengthen the vocal folds (Hirano, Kiyokawa, & Kurita, 1988). Contraction of the lateral cricoarytenoid is the primary means of moving the arytenoid cartilages medially and adducting the cartilaginous portion of the vocal folds, although, as we shall see, the thyrovocalis (the medial muscle of the vocal fold) appears to be responsible for adduction of the membranous portion of the vocal folds (Chhetri, Neubauer, & Berry, 2012).

Innervation of all intrinsic muscles of the larynx is by means of the X vagus nerve. The vagus is a large, wandering nerve with multiple responsibilities for sensation and motor function in the thorax, neck, and abdomen. The vagus arises from the nucleus ambiguus of the medulla oblongata and divides into two major branches, the recurrent (inferior) laryngeal nerve (RLN) and the superior laryngeal nerve (SLN). The RLN is so named because of its course. The left RLN "re-courses" beneath the aorta, after which it ascends to innervate the larynx. The right RLN courses under the subclavian artery before ascending to the larynx. This close association to the vascular supply may cause voice problems arising from vascular disease, because **aneurysm** or enlargement of the aorta or subclavian artery may compress the left RLN and cause vocal dysfunction. See Matteucci, Rescigno, Capestro, and Torracca (2012) for a case study of Ortner's syndrome.

Transverse Arytenoid Muscle. The **transverse arytenoid muscle** may also be called the **transverse interarytenoid** muscle. This unpaired muscle is a band of fibers spanning the posterior surface of both the arytenoid cartilages. As you can see from Figure 4-13, it runs from the lateral margin of the posterior surface of one arytenoid to the corresponding surface of the other arytenoid. Its function is to pull the two arytenoids closer together and, by association, to approximate the vocal folds, but its adductory force is considerably less than the lateral cricoarytenoid (McHanwell, 2008), and even less than the oblique arytenoid muscle (to be discussed). It provides additional support for tight occlusion or closing of the vocal folds and is a component force in generating medial compression. **Medial compression** refers to the degree of force that may be applied by the vocal folds at their point of contact. Increased medial compression is a function of increased force

aneurysm: Gr., anyeurysma, widening

Muscle:	Lateral cricoarytenoid
Origin:	Superior-lateral surface of the cricoid cartilage
Course:	Up and back
Insertion:	Muscular process of the arytenoid
Innervation:	X vagus, recurrent laryngeal nerve
Function:	Adducts vocal folds; increases medial compression

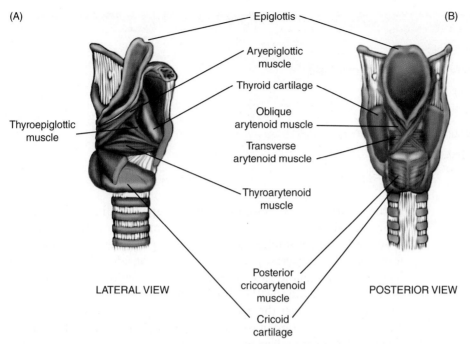

(A)

(B)

Epiglottis

Aryepiglottic muscle

Thyroid cartilage

Oblique arytenoid muscle

Transverse arytenoid muscle

Thyroepiglottic muscle

Thyroarytenoid muscle

Posterior cricoarytenoid muscle

LATERAL VIEW

POSTERIOR VIEW

Cricoid cartilage

Figure 4-13. (A) Schematic illustrating the relationship among posterior cricoarytenoid, superior thyroarytenoid, and aryepiglottic muscles. (B) Schematic of posterior cricoarytenoid muscle and transverse and oblique arytenoid muscles. Contraction of the transverse and oblique arytenoid muscles will pull the arytenoids closer together, thereby supporting adduction. Contraction of the posterior cricoarytenoid muscle pulls the muscular process back, abducting the vocal folds.
© Cengage Learning®.

Muscle:	Transverse arytenoid
Origin:	Lateral margin of posterior arytenoid
Course:	Laterally
Insertion:	Lateral margin of posterior surface, opposite arytenoid
Innervation:	X vagus, recurrent laryngeal nerve
Function:	Adducts vocal folds

of adduction, and this is a vital element in vocal intensity change, as you shall see. Motor innervation of the transverse arytenoid muscles is by means of the inferior branch of the RLN arising from the X vagus.

Oblique Arytenoid Muscles. The **oblique arytenoid muscles** are also known as the **oblique interarytenoid muscles**. The oblique arytenoid muscles are immediately superficial to the transverse arytenoid muscles and perform a similar function. The paired oblique arytenoid muscles take their origins at the posterior base of the muscular processes to course obliquely up to the apex of the opposite arytenoid. This course results in a characteristic "X" arrangement of the muscles, as well as

Muscle:	Oblique arytenoid
Origin:	Posterior base of the muscular processes
Course:	Obliquely up
Insertion:	Apex of the opposite arytenoid
Innervation:	X vagus, recurrent laryngeal nerve
Function:	Pulls the apex medially

in the ability of these muscles to pull the apex medially. This action promotes adduction, enforces medial compression, and rocks the arytenoid (and vocal folds) down and in. It generates more adductory force than the transverse arytenoid, but still considerably less than the lateral cricoarytenoid (McHanwell, 2008). Working in concert with the aryepiglottic muscle, the oblique arytenoid muscle aids in pulling the epiglottis to cover the opening to the larynx as it also serves tight adduction. Innervation of the oblique arytenoid muscles is the same as that for the transverse arytenoid muscles.

Abductor

- **Posterior cricoarytenoid muscle**

Posterior Cricoarytenoid Muscle. The **posterior cricoarytenoid muscle** is the sole abductor of the vocal folds. It is a small but prominent muscle of the posterior larynx. As you can see from Figure 4-13, the posterior cricoarytenoid muscle originates on the posterior cricoid lamina. Fibers project up and out to insert into the posterior aspect of the muscular process of the arytenoid cartilage. By virtue of their attachments to the muscular processes, the posterior cricoarytenoid muscles are direct antagonists to the lateral cricoarytenoids (see Figure 4-14), a function confirmed by Chhetri et al. (2012).

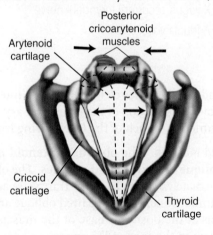

SUPERIOR VIEW

Figure 4-14. Superior view of action of the posterior cricoarytenoid muscle.
© Cengage Learning®.

Muscle:	Posterior cricoarytenoid
Origin:	Posterior cricoid lamina
Course:	Superiorly
Insertion:	Posterior aspect of the arytenoid
Innervation:	X vagus, recurrent laryngeal nerve
Function:	Rocks arytenoid cartilage laterally; abducts vocal folds

Contraction of this muscle pulls the muscular process posteriorly, rocking the arytenoid cartilage out on its axis and abducting the vocal folds. This muscle is quite active during physical exertion, broadly abducting the vocal folds to permit greater air movement into and out of the lungs. They are also active during production of voiceless consonants. The posterior cricoarytenoid is innervated by the RLN, a branch of the X vagus.

Glottal Tensors

- **Cricothyroid muscle**
- **Thyrovocalis muscle**

Cricothyroid Muscle. The primary tensor of the vocal folds achieves its function by rocking the thyroid cartilage forward relative to the cricoid cartilage. The **cricothyroid muscle** is composed of two heads, the pars recta and pars oblique, as seen in Figure 4-15.

The **pars recta** is the medial-most component of the cricothyroid muscle, originating on the anterior surface of the cricoid cartilage immediately beneath the arch. The pars recta courses up and out to insert into the lower surface of the thyroid lamina. The **pars oblique** arises from the cricoid cartilage lateral to the pars recta, coursing obliquely up to insert into the point of juncture between the thyroid laminae and inferior horns.

pars recta: L., part + straight

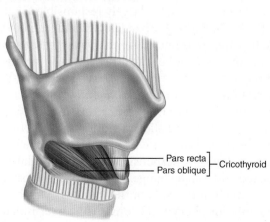

Pars recta ⎤
Pars oblique ⎦ — Cricothyroid

Figure 4-15. Cricothyroid muscle, pars recta, and pars oblique.
© Cengage Learning®.

Vocal Hyperfunction

We have emphasized the notion that the larynx is a *small* structure, but we should add that even small muscles are capable of being misused. **Vocal hyperfunction** refers to using excessive adductory force, often resulting in **laryngitis**, which is inflammation of the vocal folds. Excessively forceful contraction of the lateral cricoarytenoid and arytenoid muscles is undoubtedly the primary contributor to this problem, although it is also likely that laryngeal tension arising from the contraction of the thyroarytenoid (thyromuscularis and thyrovocalis) and cricothyroid (with support from the posterior cricoarytenoid) are contributors to this

extraordinary force. In case you did not notice, that list included virtually all of the significant intrinsic laryngeal musculature, which should emphasize the notion that vocal hyperfunction is the result of general laryngeal tension. Vocal hyperfunction can result in laryngitis, vocal nodules, contact ulcers, vocal polyps, and vocal fatigue, and is usually behavioral in etiology.

Treatment typically requires a significant behavioral change in the client, but this is not without a cost. The voice is an extremely personal entity and is very tightly woven into an individual's self-concept. Approaching a client to change his or her voice is a delicate and challenging task for a clinician.

The angle of incidence of these two segments speaks of their relative functions. Although both tense the vocal folds, individually these muscles have differing effects on the motion of the thyroid. Let us look at both of them.

By virtue of its more directly superior course, contraction of the pars recta rocks the thyroid cartilage downward, which rotates upon the cricothyroid joint. Due to the flexibility of the loosely joined tracheal cartilages below, the cricoid will also rise to meet the thyroid. This is a good time to remind you that the points of attachment of the vocal folds are the inner margin of the thyroid cartilage and the arytenoid cartilages and that the arytenoid cartilages are attached to the posterior cricoid cartilage. The effect of rocking the thyroid cartilage forward is that the vocal folds, slung between the posterior cricoid and anterior thyroid, are stretched. That is, rocking the thyroid and cricoid closer together in front makes the posterior cricoid more distant from the thyroid. The cricothyroid is largely responsible for stiffening the vocal folds (Chhetri, Berke, Lotfizadeh & Goodyer, 2009). It is worth special note that the cricothyroid is innervated by the superior laryngeal nerve, in contrast to all of the other intrinsic laryngeal muscles, which are innervated by the recurrent laryngeal nerve. We'll see that this has a direct impact on diagnosis of neurogenic voice disorders.

The cricothyroid joint also permits the thyroid to slide forward and backward. The forward sliding motion is a function of the pars oblique, and the result is to tense the vocal folds as well. Together, the pars recta and oblique are responsible for the major laryngeal adjustment associated with pitch change. The cricothyroid is innervated by the external branch of the SLN of the X vagus. This branch courses lateral to the inferior pharyngeal constrictor to terminate on the cricothyroid muscle.

Muscle:	Cricothyroid
Origin:	Pars recta: anterior surface of the cricoid cartilage beneath the arch
	Pars oblique: cricoid cartilage lateral to the pars recta
Course:	Pars recta: up and out; Pars oblique: obliquely up
Insertion:	Pars recta: lower surface of the thyroid lamina
	Pars oblique: thyroid cartilage between laminae and inferior horns
Innervation:	X vagus, external branch of superior laryngeal nerve
Function:	Depresses thyroid relative to cricoid; tenses vocal folds

Thyrovocalis Muscle. The **thyrovocalis muscle** is actually the medial muscle of the vocal folds. Many anatomists define a singular muscle coursing from the posterior surface of the thyroid cartilage to the arytenoid cartilages, labeling it as the thyroarytenoid. There is ample *functional* evidence to support the differentiation of the thyroarytenoid into two separate muscles, the thyromuscularis and the thyrovocalis, although its anatomical support is questionable. Although the thyromuscularis is discussed as a glottal relaxer, contraction of the thyrovocalis distinctly tenses the vocal folds, especially when contracted in concert with the cricothyroid muscle. It is specifically responsible for adduction of the membranous portion of the vocal folds (Chhetri et al., 2012).

The thyrovocalis (often abbreviated as vocalis) originates from the inner surface of the thyroid cartilage near the thyroid notch. The muscle courses back to insert into the lateral surface of the arytenoid vocal process. Contraction of this muscle draws the thyroid and cricoid cartilages farther apart in front, making this muscle a functional antagonist of the cricothyroid muscle (which draws the anterior cricoid and anterior thyroid closer together). This antagonistic function has earned the thyrovocalis the classification as a glottal tensor, because contraction of the thyrovocalis (in conjunction with contraction of the cricothyroid muscle) tenses the vocal folds. The thyrovocalis is innervated by the RLN, a branch of the X vagus.

Muscle:	Thyrovocalis (medial thyroarytenoid)
Origin:	Inner surface, thyroid cartilage near notch
Course:	Back
Insertion:	Lateral surface of the arytenoid vocal process
Innervation:	X vagus, recurrent laryngeal nerve
Function:	Tenses vocal folds

Relaxers

- **Thyromuscularis**

Thyromuscularis Muscle. The paired **thyromuscularis muscles** (or simply, muscularis) are considered to be the muscle masses immediately lateral to each thyrovocalis, and which, with the thyrovocalis, make up the thyroarytenoid muscle. The **thyromuscularis** or **external (lateral) thyroarytenoid** originates on the inner surface of the thyroid cartilage, near the notch and lateral to the origin of the thyrovocalis. It runs back to insert into the arytenoid cartilage at the muscular process and base.

Although there are questions about whether this muscle is truly differentiated from the vocalis, functional differences are clearly seen. As you can see from Figure 4-16, the forces exerted on the arytenoid from pulling differentially on the vocal or muscular process would produce markedly different effects. Contraction of the thyromuscularis has essentially the same effect on the vocal folds as that of the lateral cricoarytenoid. The vocal folds adduct and lengthen (Hirano, Kiyokawa, & Kurita, 1988; Zhang, 2011).

Muscle:	Thyromuscularis (lateral thyroarytenoid)
Origin:	Inner surface of thyroid cartilage near the notch
Course:	Back
Insertion:	Base and muscular process of arytenoid cartilage
Innervation:	X vagus, recurrent laryngeal nerve
Function:	Relaxes vocal folds

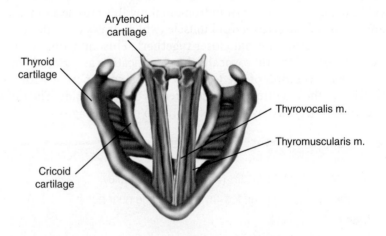

SUPERIOR VIEW

Figure 4-16. The thyromuscularis muscle is the lateral muscular component of the vocal folds; the thyrovocalis is the medial-most muscle of the vocal folds. Together they are often referred to as the thyroarytenoid muscle.
© Cengage Learning®.

Contraction of the medial fibers of the thyromuscularis may relax the vocal folds as well. By virtue of their attachment on the anterior surface of the arytenoid, these fibers pull the arytenoids toward the thyroid cartilage without influencing medial rocking. Thus, the thyromuscularis muscle is classically considered to be a laryngeal relaxer. The thyromuscularis is innervated by the RLN.

Auxiliary Musculature

- **Thyroepiglottic (thyroepiglotticus) muscle**
- **Superior thyroarytenoid muscle**
- **Aryepiglottic muscle**

Thyroarytenoid, Thyroepiglotticus, and Aryepiglotticus. As discussed previously, the thyroarytenoid muscle (see Figure 4-16), which consists of the thyrovocalis and thyromuscularis muscles, arises from the lower thyroid angle. The thyroarytenoid courses back to insert into the anterolateral surface of the arytenoid cartilages. The medial fibers of the thyroarytenoid constitute the thyrovocalis muscle, while the superior fibers are continuous with the thyroepiglotticus superiorly. The superior thyroarytenoid is inconsistently present, arising from the inner angle of the thyroid cartilage and coursing to the muscular process of the arytenoid: that is to say, it is an extension of the thyroarytenoid (thyromuscularis). The aryepiglottic muscle (see Figure 4-17) arises from the superior aspect of the oblique arytenoid muscle (i.e., the arytenoid apex) and continues as the muscular component of the aryepiglottic fold as it courses to insert into the lateral epiglottis. The thyroepiglotticus dilates the laryngeal opening, while the aryepiglotticus assists in protecting the airway during swallowing by deflecting the epiglottic cartilage over the laryngeal aditus (Gray et al., 1995). It is assumed that the superior thyroarytenoid serves as a relaxer of the vocal folds, like the thyromuscularis, although this has not been demonstrated.

Summary of Intrinsic Muscle Activity

Figure 4-17 will help us proceed with this discussion. Intrinsic muscles of the larynx include the thyrovocalis, thyromuscularis, cricothyroid, lateral and posterior cricoarytenoid, transverse arytenoid and oblique arytenoid, superior thyroarytenoid muscles, thyroepiglotticus, and aryepiglotticus. The thyrovocalis and thyromuscularis muscles make up the muscular portion of the vocal folds. The cricothyroid pulls the anterior cricoid and anterior thyroid closer together, thereby stretching the vocal folds. The lateral cricoarytenoid adducts the vocal folds by rocking the arytenoids medially, while the posterior cricoarytenoid muscle is the only abductor of the vocal folds. The oblique and transverse arytenoid muscles pull the arytenoids closer together, assisting the adductory effort of the lateral cricarytenoid. The superior thyroarytenoid muscle is variously present, serving to relax the vocal folds. The thyroepiglotticus has no apparent function in speech but is important for maintaining a well-lubricated vocal mechanism and is active during the pharyngeal stage of the swallow, as discussed in Chapter 8.

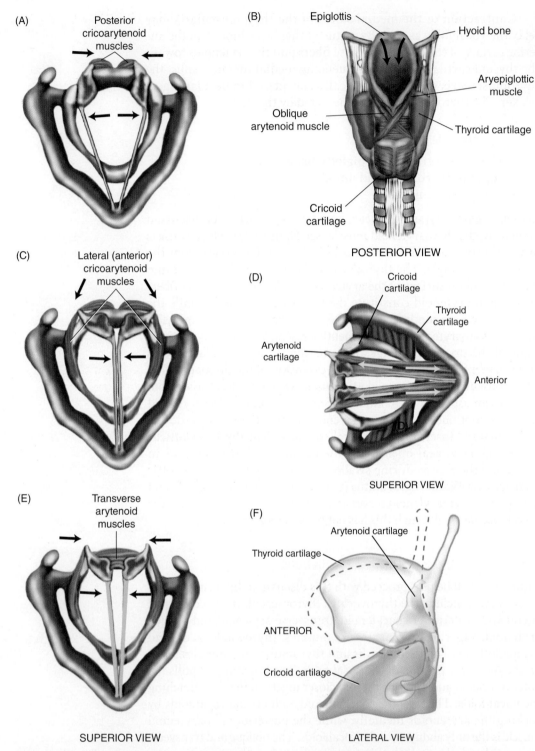

Figure 4-17. (A). Action of posterior cricoarytenoid muscles in abducting the vocal folds. (B). View of posterior intrinsic muscles of the larynx. (C) Action of lateral cricoarytenoid muscles in adducting the vocal folds. (D) Contraction of the thyromuscularis relaxes the vocal folds. (E) Contraction of the transverse arytenoid muscles moves the vocal folds toward midline, as does contraction of the lateral cricoarytenoid muscles. (F) Contraction of the cricothyroid muscle rocks the thyroid down in the anterior aspect, tensing the vocal folds.
© Cengage Learning®.

Muscle:	Superior thyroarytenoid
Origin:	Inner angle of thyroid cartilage
Course:	Back
Insertion:	Muscular process of arytenoid
Innervation:	Recurrent laryngeal nerve, X vagus
Function:	Perhaps relaxes vocal fold

Muscle:	Thyroepiglottic muscle
Origin:	Inner surface of thyroid at angle
Course:	Back and up
Insertion:	Lateral epiglottis
Innervation:	Recurrent laryngeal nerve, X vagus
Function:	Dilates airway, compresses laryngeal saccule for mucus secretion

Muscle:	Aryepiglottic muscle
Origin:	Continuation of oblique arytenoid muscle from arytenoid apex
Course:	Back and up as muscular component of aryepiglottic fold
Insertion:	Lateral epiglottis
Innervation:	Recurrent laryngeal nerve, X vagus
Function:	Constricts laryngeal opening

"Ain't Misbehavin'"

The range of phonatory misbehavior is broad and deep. The larynx is an exquisite structure made up of delicate tissues designed for use as a protective mechanism. When we use it as a phonatory source, we capitalize on its flexibility. When we overuse the mechanism, we can get into trouble. Here are a few of the problems that can occur from laryngeal misuse.

Vocal nodules arise from excessively loud phonation or excessively forceful adduction. The addition of toxins into your laryngeal environment can cause trouble as well. Alcohol consumption can irritate the vocal folds, as can cigarette and cigar smoke (primary or secondary smoke). Likewise, excessive dry air can irritate the vocal folds, leading to laryngitis. A diet that causes esophageal reflux can cause laryngeal irritation. Gastroesophageal reflux is strongly related to the development of ulcers on the posterior aspect of the vocal folds (Hanson & Jiang, 2000), and has been linked to laryngeal cancer and development of sinusitis. Surprisingly, chronic gastroesophageal reflux is related to *reduced* risk of chronic otitis media (Weaver, 2003)!

Movement of the vocal folds into and out of approximation (adduction and abduction, respectively) is achieved by the coordinated effort of many of the intrinsic muscles of the larynx. The lateral cricoarytenoid muscle is responsible for rocking the arytenoid cartilage on its axis, causing the vocal folds to tip in and slightly down. This action is directly opposed by the contraction of the posterior cricoarytenoid muscle, which rocks the arytenoid (and vocal folds) out on that same axis. Contraction of the transverse arytenoid muscle draws the posterior surfaces of the two arytenoids closer together, but the transverse arytenoid is most effective as an adductor if the lateral cricoarytenoid muscle is contracted as well. Contraction of the oblique arytenoid helps the vocal folds dip downward as they are adducted.

The thyroepiglotticus and aryepiglotticus are antagonists in that the thyroepiglotticus increases the size of the laryngeal opening while the aryepiglotticus narrows it. These two functions are probably not components of communication but rather assist in deep respiratory effort (thyroepiglotticus) and the protection of the airway (aryepiglotticus).

The fact that the vocal folds rock in and down is not trivial. The force vector associated with this movement improves the ability of the vocal folds to impede outward flow of air, because more force is directed in an inferior direction, this way, than if the arytenoid rotated on a vertical axis.

The muscles of abduction and adduction work in concert to complete their task in one more way. Although you know that the vocal folds must be adducted and abducted, you should start becoming aware that a full range of laryngeal adjustments is possible, from completely abducted to tightly adducted. We use this full range during phonation, and the bulk of the voice complaints on the caseload of a public school clinician will arise from inadequate control of this musculature (vocal nodules secondary to laryngeal hyperfunction).

Recalling the physical parameters that can be altered to change pitch will help you realize that either mass or tension is a likely candidate. Increasing the tension on the vocal folds will stretch them and thereby reduce the mass per unit length. Stretching the vocal folds does not decrease the mass of the muscle, but does decrease it relative to overall length. Both increased tension and reduced mass per unit length will increase the frequency of vibration of the vocal folds, while relaxing the vocal folds will cause the frequency to drop.

Note that when the cricothyroid is contracted, the thyrovocalis will be stretched. If you also contract the thyrovocalis, the vocal folds will become tenser and the pitch will increase.

Laryngeal Elevators and Depressors

The **extrinsic musculature** consists of muscles with one attachment to a laryngeal cartilage. These muscles include the sternothyroid, thyrohyoid, and thyropharyngeus muscles. A number of muscles attached to the hyoid also move the larynx, and these are described as **infrahyoid muscles**, which run from the hyoid to a structure below, and **suprahyoid muscles**, which attach to a structure above the hyoid.

Infrahyoid muscles consist of the sternohyoid and omohyoid muscles, while the suprahyoid muscles consist of the digastricus, stylohyoid, mylohyoid, geniohyoid, genioglossus, and hyoglossus muscles. They are often called the *strap muscles*.

A more useful categorization is based on function relative to the larynx. Muscles that elevate the hyoid and larynx are termed **laryngeal elevators** (digastricus, stylohyoid, mylohyoid, geniohyoid, genioglossus, hyoglossus, and thyropharyngeus muscles) and those that depress the larynx and hyoid are termed **laryngeal depressors** (sternohyoid, omohyoid, thyrohyoid, and sternothyroid muscles).

Hyoid and Laryngeal Elevators

- **Digastricus anterior and posterior**
- **Stylohyoid muscle**
- **Mylohyoid muscle**
- **Geniohyoid muscle**
- **Genioglossus muscle**
- **Hyoglossus muscle**
- **Thyropharyngeus muscle**

Digastricus. As seen in Figure 4-18, the **digastricus muscle** is actually composed of two separate bellies. The anterior and posterior bellies of the digastricus muscle converge at the hyoid bone, and their paired

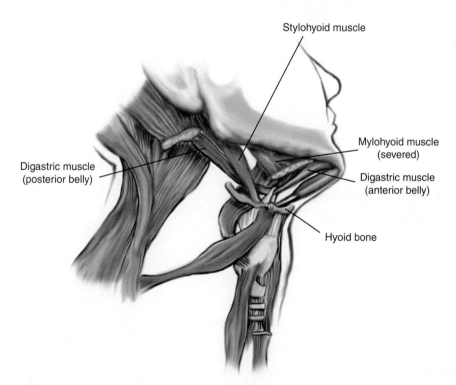

Stylohyoid muscle

Mylohyoid muscle (severed)

Digastric muscle (anterior belly)

Digastric muscle (posterior belly)

Hyoid bone

Figure 4-18. Schematic of digastricus, stylohyoid, and mylohyoid muscles.
© Cengage Learning®.

contraction elevates the hyoid. The **digastricus anterior** originates on the inner surface of the mandible at the digastricus fossa, near the point of fusion of the two halves of the mandible, the symphysis. The muscle courses medially and down to the level of the hyoid, where it joins with the posterior digastricus by means of an **intermediate tendon**. The **posterior digastricus** originates on the mastoid process of the temporal bone, behind and beneath the ear. The intermediate tendon passes through and separates the fibers of another muscle, the stylohyoid, as it inserts into the hyoid at the juncture of the hyoid corpus and greater cornu.

The structure and attachment of the digastricus bellies define their function. Contraction of the anterior component results in the hyoid being drawn up and forward, whereas contraction of the posterior belly causes the hyoid to be drawn up and back. Simultaneous contraction results in hyoid elevation without anterior or posterior migration. You will see a great deal of activity in the digastricus during swallowing.

At this point, it is wise to mention that the muscles attached to the mandible, such as the digastricus, may also be depressors of the mandible. That is, the digastricus anterior could help to pull the mandible down if the musculature *below* the hyoid were to fix it in place. You will want to retain this notion for our discussion of the role of hyoid musculature in oral motor development and control. The anterior belly is innervated by the mandibular branch of the V **trigeminal**

trigeminal: L., tres, three; gemina, twin

Muscle:	Digastricus, anterior and posterior
Origin:	Anterior: inner surface of the mandible, near symphysis; Posterior: mastoid process of temporal bone
Course:	Medial and down
Insertion:	Hyoid, by means of intermediate tendon
Innervation:	Anterior: V trigeminal nerve, mandibular branch, via the mylohyoid branch of the inferior alveolar nerve
	Posterior: VII facial nerve, digastric branch
Function:	Anterior belly: draws hyoid up and forward
	Posterior belly: draws hyoid up and back
	Together: elevate hyoid
Muscle:	Stylohyoid muscle
Origin:	Styloid process of temporal bone
Course:	Down and anteriorly
Insertion:	Corpus of hyoid
Innervation:	VII Facial
Function:	Move hyoid posteriorly

nerve via the mylohyoid branch of the inferior alveolar nerve. This branch courses along the inner surface of the mandible in the mylohyoid groove and exits to innervate the mylohyoid (to be discussed) and the anterior digastricus. The posterior belly is supplied by the digastric branch of the VII facial nerve.

Stylohyoid Muscle. The **stylohyoid muscle** originates on the prominent styloid process of the temporal bone, a point medial to the mastoid process (see Figure 4-18). The course of this muscle is medially down, such that it crosses the path of the posterior digastricus (which actually passes through the stylohyoid) and inserts into the corpus of hyoid.

Contraction of the stylohyoid elevates and retracts the hyoid bone. The stylohyoid and posterior digastricus are closely allied in development, function, and innervation. Both the stylohyoid and posterior belly of the digastricus are innervated by the motor branch of the VII facial nerve.

Mylohyoid Muscle. As with the digastricus anterior, the **mylohyoid muscle** originates on the underside of the mandible and courses to the corpus hyoid. Unlike the digastricus, the mylohyoid is fanlike, originating along the lateral aspects of the inner mandible on a prominence known as the mylohyoid line. The anterior fibers converge at the median fibrous raphe (ridge), a structure that runs from the **symphysis menti** (the juncture of the fused paired bones of the mandible) to the hyoid. The posterior fibers course directly to the hyoid. Taken together, the fibers of the mylohyoid form the floor of the oral cavity. The relationship between the digastricus and the mylohyoid muscles may be seen in Figure 4-19. As may be derived from the examination of its fiber course, the mylohyoid elevates the hyoid and projects it forward, or alternately depresses the mandible, in much the manner of the digastricus anterior. Unlike the digastricus, the mylohyoid muscle is responsible for the elevation of the floor of the mouth during the first stage of deglutition.

The mylohyoid is allied with the anterior belly of the digastricus, through proximity, development, and innervation. As with the anterior digastricus, the mylohyoid is innervated by the alveolar nerve, arising from the V trigeminal nerve, mandibular branch. As stated for the digastricus anterior, this nerve courses within the mylohyoid groove of the inner surface of the mandible, branches, and innervates the mylohyoid.

Geniohyoid Muscle. The **geniohyoid muscle** is superior to the mylohyoid, originating at the **mental spines** of the inner mandible, projecting in a course parallel to the anterior belly of the digastricus from the inner mandibular surface (see Figure 4-19). Fibers of this narrow muscle course back and down to insert into the hyoid bone at the corpus. When contracted, the geniohyoid elevates the hyoid and draws it forward. It may also depress the mandible if the hyoid is fixed. The geniohyoid is innervated by the XII **hypoglossal** nerve

mental spines: Spinous processes on the inner surface of the anterior mandible; these prominences provide a means for muscles to attach to bones

hypoglossal: L., glossa, tongue; under + tongue

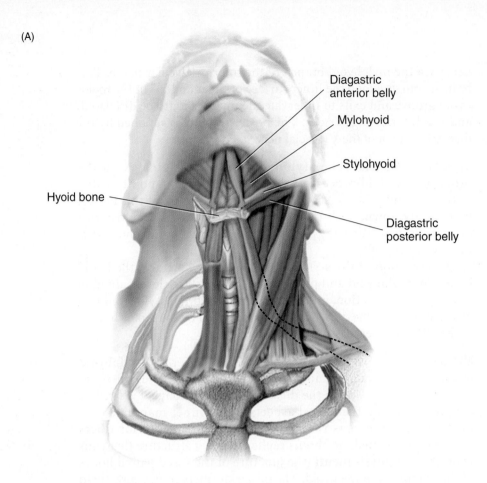

(A)

Diagastric
anterior belly

Mylohyoid

Stylohyoid

Hyoid bone

Diagastric
posterior belly

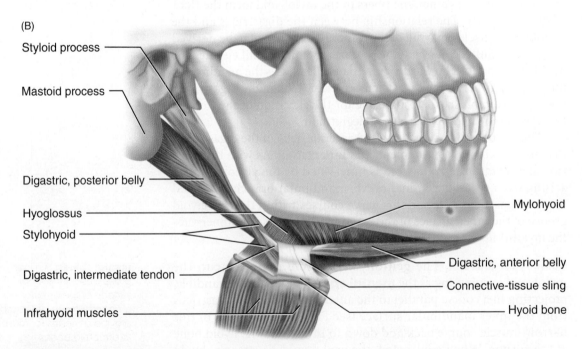

(B)

Styloid process

Mastoid process

Digastric, posterior belly

Hyoglossus

Stylohyoid

Digastric, intermediate tendon

Infrahyoid muscles

Mylohyoid

Digastric, anterior belly

Connective-tissue sling

Hyoid bone

Figure 4-19. (A) Schematic of the relationship among geniohyoid, mylohyoid, digastricus, and stylohyoid muscles. (B) Relationship among digastricus anterior, digastricus posterior, hyoglossus, mylohyoid, and stylohyoid. (continues).

© Cengage Learning®.

(C)

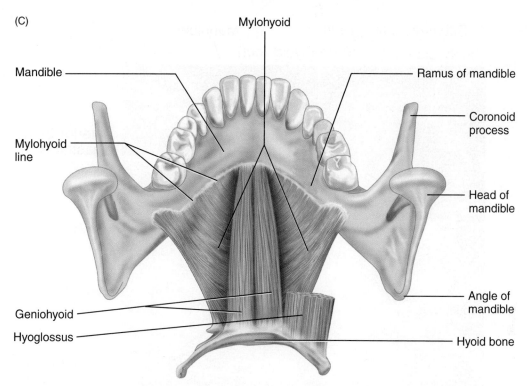

Figure 4-19 continued. (C) View of the floor of the mouth from above. Note particularly the relationship between geniohyoid and mylohyoid. (continues).
© Cengage Learning®.

and C1 spinal curve. Although most of the hypoglossal originates in the hypoglossal nucleus of the medulla oblongata of the brainstem, those fibers innervating the geniohyoid arise from the first cervical spinal nerve.

Hyoglossus Muscle. The **hyoglossus** and genioglossus provide another example of the interrelatedness of musculature. These muscles are also lingual (tongue) depressors (see Figure 6-38), because they have attachments on both of these structures. Speech-language pathologists concerned with oral motor control are painfully aware of these relationships, and studying them will benefit you as well. The hyoglossus is a laterally placed muscle. It arises from the entire superior surface of the greater cornu and corpus of the hyoid and courses up to insert into the side of the tongue. The point of insertion in the tongue is near that of the styloglossus, a muscle we will discuss in Chapter 6. The muscle has a quadrilateral appearance and is a lingual depressor or hyoid elevator. The hyoglossus muscle is innervated by the motor branch of the XII hypoglossal.

Genioglossus Muscle. Although the **genioglossus muscle** is appropriately considered a muscle of the tongue (see Figure 6-38), it definitely is a hyoid elevator as well. The genioglossus originates on the inner surface of the mandible at the symphysis and courses up, back, and down to insert into the tongue and anterior surface of the

hyoglossus: L., hyo, hyoid + glossus, tongue

See the Clinical Note in Chapter 2 for a discussion of trunk stability and upper body mobility.

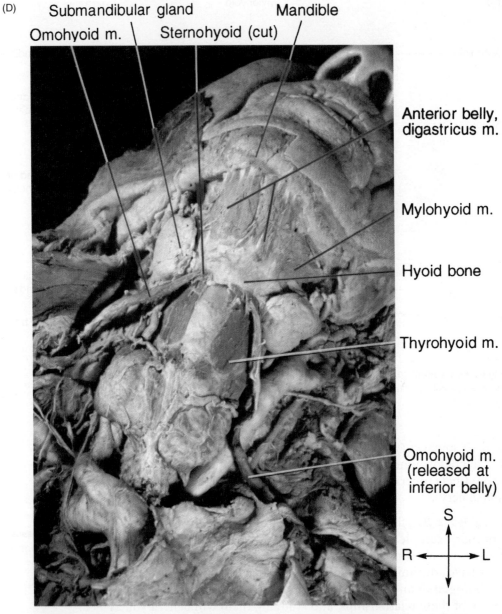

(D)
Omohyoid m.   Submandibular gland   Mandible
                    Sternohyoid (cut)

Anterior belly,
digastricus m.

Mylohyoid m.

Hyoid bone

Thyrohyoid m.

Omohyoid m.
(released at
inferior belly)

S

R ←→ L

I

Figure 4-19 continued. (d) Photograph showing the relationship among omohyoid, sternohyoid, digastricus anterior and thyrohyoid muscles.
© Cengage Learning®.

Muscle:	Mylohyoid
Origin:	Mylohyoid line, inner surface of mandible
Course:	Fanlike to median fibrous raphe and hyoid
Insertion:	Corpus of hyoid
Innervation:	V trigeminal, mandibular branch, alveolar nerve
Function:	Elevates hyoid or depresses mandible

Muscle:	Geniohyoid
Origin:	Mental spines, inner surface of mandible
Course:	Back and down
Insertion:	Corpus hyoid bone
Innervation:	XII hypoglossal nerve and C1 spinal nerve
Function:	Elevates hyoid bone; depresses mandible

Muscle:	Hyoglossus
Origin:	Hyoid bone, greater cornu, and corpus
Course:	Down
Insertion:	Sides of tongue
Innervation:	Motor branch of the XII hypoglossal
Function:	Elevates hyoid; depresses tongue

hyoid corpus. We will discuss the lingual function of this muscle in Chapter 6, but the attachment at the hyoid guarantees that this muscle will elevate the hyoid. The genioglossus muscle is innervated by the motor branch of the XII hypoglossal.

Thyropharyngeus Muscle of the Inferior Constrictor. The **thyropharyngeus** and **cricopharyngeus muscles** constitute the **inferior pharyngeal constrictor**, to be discussed in detail later. The cricopharyngeus is the sphincter muscle at the orifice of the esophagus. (Note that Mu and Sanders [2008] offer evidence that the sphincter function in humans may arise from a newly discovered muscle, the cricothyropharyngeus.) The thyropharyngeus is involved in propelling food through the pharynx. Its attachment to the thyroid provides an opportunity for laryngeal elevation (see Figure 6-43).

The thyropharyngeus arises from the thyroid lamina and inferior cornu, coursing up medially to insert into the posterior pharyngeal raphe. Contraction of this muscle promotes elevation of the larynx while constricting the pharynx. The inferior constrictors are innervated by branches from the X vagi, including the RLN and SLN.

Hyoid and Laryngeal Depressors

- **Sternohyoid muscle**
- **Omohyoid muscle**
- **Sternothyroid muscle**
- **Thyrohyoid muscle**

Laryngeal depressors depress and stabilize the larynx via attachment to the hyoid, but also stabilize the tongue by serving as antagonists to the laryngeal elevators. The interconnectedness of the laryngeal and tongue musculature may at first be daunting, but take

Muscle:	Genioglossus
Origin:	Inner surface of mandible at symphysis
Course:	Up, back, and down
Insertion:	Tongue and corpus hyoid
Innervation:	Motor branch of XII hypoglossal
Function:	Elevates hyoid

Muscle:	Thyropharyngeus of inferior pharyngeal constrictor
Origin:	Thyroid lamina and inferior cornu
Course:	Up, medially
Insertion:	Posterior pharyngeal raphe
Innervation:	X vagus, recurrent laryngeal nerve; X vagus, superior laryngeal nerve
Function:	Constricts pharynx and elevates larynx

heart. Mastery of the components will greatly enhance your clinical competency because oral motor control has its foundation in these interactions. We will discuss this in detail in Chapter 5.

Sternohyoid Muscle. As the name implies, the **sternohyoid** runs from sternum to the hyoid. It originates from the posterior-superior region of the manubrium sterni as well as from the medial end of the clavicle. It courses superiorly to insert into the inferior margin of the hyoid corpus.

Contraction of the sternohyoid depresses the hyoid or, if suprahyoid muscles are in contraction, fixes the hyoid and larynx. The lowering function is clearly evident following the pharyngeal stage in swallowing. The sternohyoid is innervated by the ansa cervicalis (*ansa* = loop; i.e., cervical loop), arising from C1 through C3 spinal nerves.

Omohyoid Muscle. As you can see in Figure 4-20, the **omohyoid** is a muscle with two bellies. The superior belly terminates on the side of the hyoid corpus, while the inferior belly has its origin on the upper border of the scapula. The bellies are joined at an intermediate tendon. As you can see from this figure, the omohyoid passes deep to the sternocleidomastoid, which, along with the deep cervical fascia, restrains the omohyoid muscle to give it its characteristic "dogleg" angle. When contracted, the omohyoid depresses the hyoid bone and larynx. The superior belly is innervated by the superior ramus of the ansa cervicalis arising from the C1 spinal nerve, whereas the inferior belly is innervated by the main ansa cervicalis, arising from C2 and C3 spinal nerves.

See Chapters 2 and 11 for the discussion of spinal nerves.

Sternothyroid Muscle. As shown in Figure 4-21, contraction of the **sternothyroid muscle** depresses the thyroid cartilage. This muscle

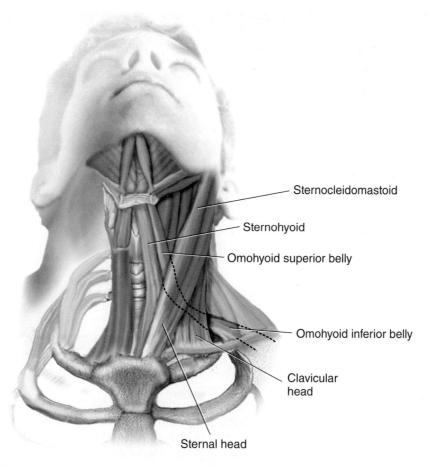

Figure 4-20. Schematic of the relationship among omohyoid, sternocleidomastoid, and sternohyoid muscles. Clavicle on left side of the image has been removed for clarity.
© Cengage Learning®.

Muscle:	Sternohyoid
Origin:	Manubrium sterni and clavicle
Course:	Up
Insertion:	Inferior margin of hyoid corpus
Innervation:	Ansa cervicalis from spinal C1 through C3
Function:	Depresses hyoid

originates at the manubrium sterni and first costal cartilage, coursing up and out to insert into the oblique line of the thyroid cartilage. It is active during swallowing, drawing the larynx downward following elevation for the pharyngeal stage of deglutition. The sternothyroid is innervated by fibers from the spinal nerves C1 and C2 that pass into the hypoglossal nerve.

Muscle:	Omohyoid, superior and inferior heads
Origin:	Superior: Intermediate tendon
	Inferior: upper border, scapula
Course:	Superior: down
	Inferior: Up and medially
Insertion:	Superior: lower border, hyoid
	Inferior: intermediate tendon
Innervation:	Superior belly: superior ramus of ansa cervicalis from C1
	Inferior belly: ansa cervicalis, spinal C2–C3
Function:	Depresses hyoid

Laryngeal Stability

Laryngeal stability is the key to laryngeal control, and this stability is gained through the development of the infra- and suprahyoid musculature. You can think of the larynx as a box connected to a flexible tube at one end (trachea) and loosely bound above. This "box" has liberal movement in the vertical dimension and has some horizontal movement as well, but there must be a great deal of control in the contraction of all of this musculature for this arrangement to work.

The larynx is intimately linked, via the hyoid bone, to the tongue so that movement of the tongue is translated to the larynx. During development an infant begins to gain control of neck musculature as early as four weeks, as seen in the ability to elevate the neck in the prone position. This ability to extend the previously flexed neck heralds the beginning of oral motor control because the ability to balance neck extension with flexion permits the child to control the gross movement of the head. During this stage, the larynx is quite elevated, so much so that you can easily see the superior tip of the epiglottis behind the tongue of a two-year-old. In the early stages, the elevated larynx facilitates the anterior tongue protrusion required in infancy for nursing.

As the child develops, the larynx descends, starting a process of muscular differentiation between the tongue and the larynx. In the "nursing" position of the tongue, laryngeal stability is not as important, but the ability to move semihard and hard food around in the oral cavity is quite important as the child begins to eat solid foods. Now the child will develop the ability to move the tongue and larynx independently, permitting a much wider set of oral movements. With this differentiation comes the control needed for accurate speech production. For information on head and neck control in children with motor dysfunction, you may wish to examine Jones-Owens (1991), and certainly you will want to read the work of Bly (1994) for insight into the development of muscle control.

Muscle:	Sternothyroid
Origin:	Manubrium sterni and first costal cartilage
Course:	Up and Out
Insertion:	Oblique line, thyroid cartilage
Innervation:	XII hypoglossal and spinal nerves C1 and C2
Function:	Depresses thyroid cartilage

(A)

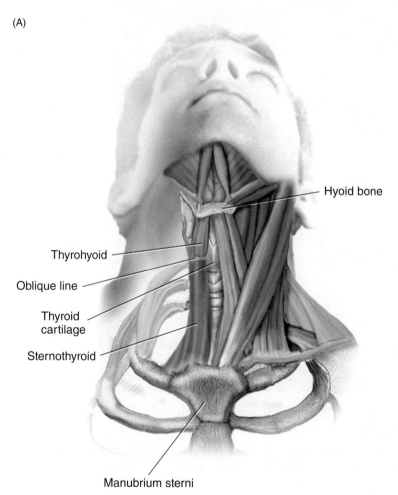

Figure 4-21. (A) The sternothyroid and thyrohyoid muscles. Clavicle on left side of the image has been removed for clarity. (continues).

© Cengage Learning®.

(B)

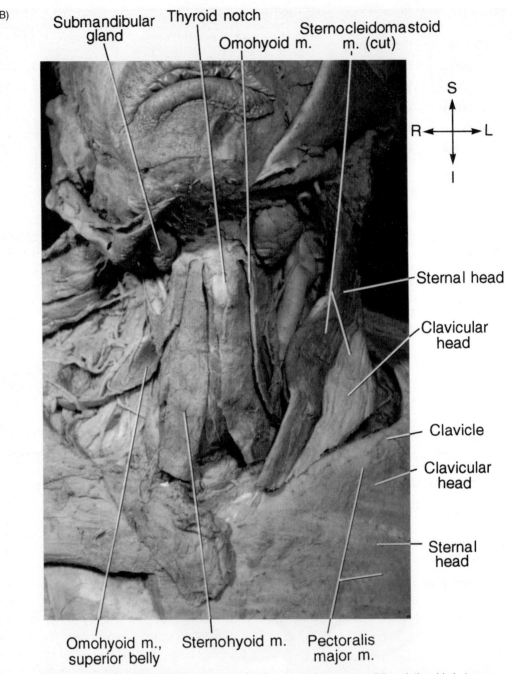

Submandibular gland

Thyroid notch

Omohyoid m.

Sternocleidomastoid m. (cut)

S

R ←→ L

I

Sternal head

Clavicular head

Clavicle

Clavicular head

Sternal head

Omohyoid m., superior belly

Sternohyoid m.

Pectoralis major m.

Figure 4-21 continued. (B) Photograph showing laryngeal placement and the relationship between sternohyoid and omohyoid muscles. Note that the omohyoid is deep to the sternocleidomastoid muscle.
© Cengage Learning®.

Thyrohyoid Muscle. This muscle is easily seen as the superior counterpart to the sternothyroid (see Figure 4-21). Coursing from the oblique line of the thyroid cartilage to the inferior margin of the greater cornu of the hyoid bone, the **thyrohyoid muscle** will either depress the hyoid or

Muscle:	Thyrohyoid
Origin:	Oblique line, thyroid cartilage
Course:	Up
Insertion:	Greater cornu, hyoid
Innervation:	XII hypoglossal nerve and fibers from spinal C1
Function:	Depresses hyoid or elevates larynx

raise the larynx. The thyrohyoid is innervated by the fibers from spinal nerve C1 that course along with the hypoglossal nerves.

✔ *To summarize:*

- The **extrinsic muscles** of the larynx include the **infrahyoid** and **suprahyoid** muscles.
- The **digastricus** anterior and posterior elevate the hyoid, whereas the **stylohyoid** retracts it.
- The **mylohyoid** and **hyoglossus** elevate the hyoid, and the **geniohyoid** elevates the hyoid and draws it forward.
- The **thyropharyngeus** and **cricopharyngeus** muscles elevate the larynx, and the **sternohyoid, sternothyroid, thyrohyoid,** and **omohyoid** muscles depress the larynx.

digastricus: L., two + belly

Interaction of Musculature

The larynx is virtually suspended from a broad sling of muscles that must work in concert to achieve the complex motions required for speech and nonspeech functions. Movement of the larynx and its cartilages requires both gross and fine adjustments. It appears that the gross movements associated with laryngeal elevation and depression provide the background for the fine adjustments of phonatory control. The supra- and infrahyoid muscles raise and lower the larynx, changing the vocal tract length, but the intrinsic laryngeal muscles are responsible for the fine adjustments associated with phonation control.

To say that the musculature works as a unit is clearly an understatement. The simple action of laryngeal elevation must be countered with the controlled antagonistic tone of the laryngeal depressors. Elevation of the tongue will tend to elevate the larynx and increase the tension of the cricothyroid, and this must be countered through intrinsic muscle adjustment to keep the articulatory system from driving the phonatory mechanism. It is time to move to Chapter 5 to see how these components work together.

Vocal Fold Paralysis

Paralysis refers to loss of voluntary motor function, whereas **paresis** refers to weakness. Either can arise from damage to the **upper motor neurons**, which are neurons that arise from the brain and end in the spinal column or brainstem; or damage to the **lower motor neurons**, which are neurons that leave the spinal column or brainstem to innervate the muscles involved.

Vocal fold paralysis may take several forms, depending on the nerve damage. If only one side of the recurrent laryngeal nerve (lower motor neuron) is damaged, the result will be unilateral vocal fold paralysis. Bilateral vocal fold paralysis would result from bilateral lower motor neuron damage.

If the result of damage is **adductor paralysis**, the muscles of adduction are paralyzed and the vocal folds remain in the abducted position. If the damage results in abductor paralysis, the individual will not be able to abduct the vocal folds, and respiration will be compromised (you may want to read the note on "laryngeal stridor" in Chapter 5 to get a notion of what happens). If the superior laryngeal nerve is involved, the individual will suffer loss of the ability to alter vocal pitch, because the cricothyroid is innervated by this branch of the vagus.

In unilateral paralysis, one vocal fold is still capable of motion. Phonation can still occur, but production will be markedly breathy. Bilateral adductor paralysis will result in virtually complete loss of phonation.

There are several causes for vocal fold paralysis, but among the leading causes are damage to the nerve during thyroid surgery and blunt trauma, such as from the steering wheel of an automobile. **Cerebrovascular accidents** (CVA: hemorrhage or other condition causing loss of blood supply to the brain) may damage the upper or lower motor neurons resulting in paralysis, and a host of neurodegenerative diseases can weaken or paralyze the vocal folds. You should also be aware that paralysis may occur as a result of aneurysm of the aortic arch. An aneurysm is a focal ballooning of a blood vessel caused by a weakness in the wall. When the aneurysm balloons out, it compresses the recurrent laryngeal nerve, causing paresis or paralysis. A **phonatory sign** (objective evidence of phonatory deficit) is not to be taken lightly.

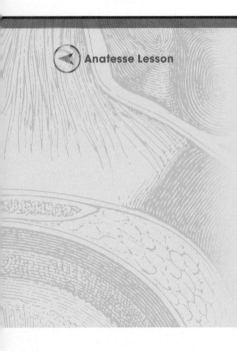

Anatesse Lesson

CHAPTER SUMMARY

The larynx consists of the cricoid, thyroid, and epiglottis cartilages, as well as the paired arytenoid, corniculate, and cuneiform cartilages. The thyroid and cricoid cartilages articulate by means of the cricothyroid joint that lets the two cartilages come closer together in front. The arytenoid and cricoid cartilages also articulate with a joint that permits a wide range of arytenoid motion. The epiglottis is attached to the thyroid cartilage and base of the tongue. The corniculate cartilages rest on the upper surface of the arytenoids, while the cuneiform cartilages reside within the aryepiglottic folds.

The cavity of the larynx is a constricted tube with a smooth surface. Sheets and cords of ligaments connect the cartilages, while a smooth mucous membrane covers the medial-most surface of the larynx. The valleculae are found between the tongue and the epiglottis, within folds arising from the lateral and median glossoepiglottic ligaments. The fibroelastic membrane is composed of the upper quadrangular membranes and aryepiglottic folds; the lower conus elasticus; and the vocal ligament, which is actually the upward free extension of the conus elasticus.

The vocal folds are made up of five layers of tissue, the deepest being the muscle of the vocal folds. The aditus is the entryway of the larynx, marking the entry to the vestibule. The ventricular and vocal folds are separated by the laryngeal ventricle. The glottis is the variable space between the vocal folds.

The intrinsic muscles of the larynx include the thyrovocalis, thyromuscularis, cricothyroid, lateral and posterior cricoarytenoid, transverse arytenoid and oblique arytenoid, superior thyroarytenoid, aryepiglotticus, and thyroepiglotticus muscles.

The thyroepiglotticus and aryepiglotticus both serve non-speech functions. The thyroepiglotticus increases the size of the laryngeal opening for forced inspiration, while the aryepiglotticus protects the airway by narrowing the aditus and vestibule.

Movement of the vocal folds into and out of approximation requires the coordinated effort of the intrinsic muscles of the larynx. The lateral cricoarytenoid muscle rocks the arytenoid cartilage on its axis, tipping the vocal folds in and slightly down. The posterior cricoarytenoid muscle rocks the arytenoid out. The transverse arytenoid muscle draws the posterior surfaces of the arytenoids closer together. The oblique arytenoid assists the vocal folds in dipping downward when they are adducted. The thyroepiglotticus has no phonatory function but is involved in the swallowing function. Vocal fundamental frequency is increased by increasing tension, a function of the thyrovocalis and cricothyroid.

Extrinsic muscles of the larynx include the infrahyoid and suprahyoid muscles. The digastricus anterior and posterior elevate the hyoid, while the stylohyoid retracts it. The mylohyoid and hyoglossus elevate the hyoid, and the geniohyoid elevates the hyoid and draws it forward. The thyropharyngeus and cricopharyngeus muscles elevate the larynx, and the sternohyoid, sternothyroid, and omohyoid muscles depress the larynx.

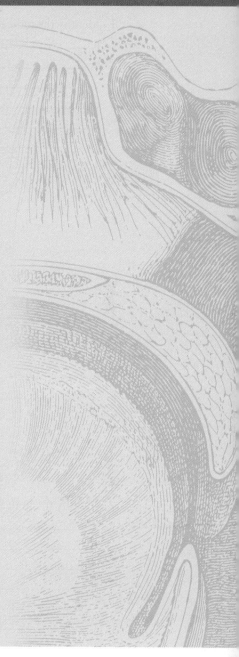

Media Connection

Go to the accompanying online resources at CengageBrain.com and have fun learning! Study with the Anatesse software program, play games, view animations and videos, and take practice tests to help reinforce the key concepts you learned in this chapter.

Study Questions

1. Identify the indicated structures in the following figure.

 a. _____ cartilage

 b. _____ cartilage

 c. _____ cartilage

 d. _____ cartilage

 e. _____ cartilage

 f. _____ bone

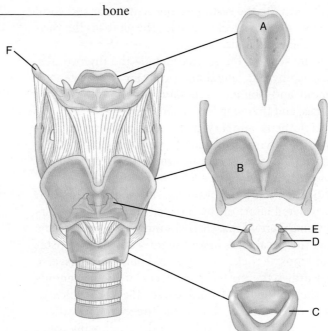

© Cengage Learning®.

2. Identify the indicated landmarks in the following figure.

 a. _____

 b. _____

 c. _____

 d. _____

 e. _____

 f. _____

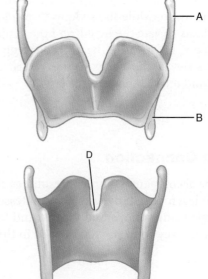

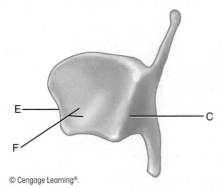

© Cengage Learning®.

3. Identify the indicated landmarks in the following figure.

   a. _____ process

   b. _____ process

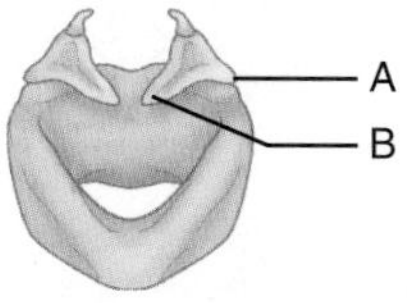

© Cengage Learning®.

4. Identify the muscles indicated.

   a. _____

   b. _____

   c. _____

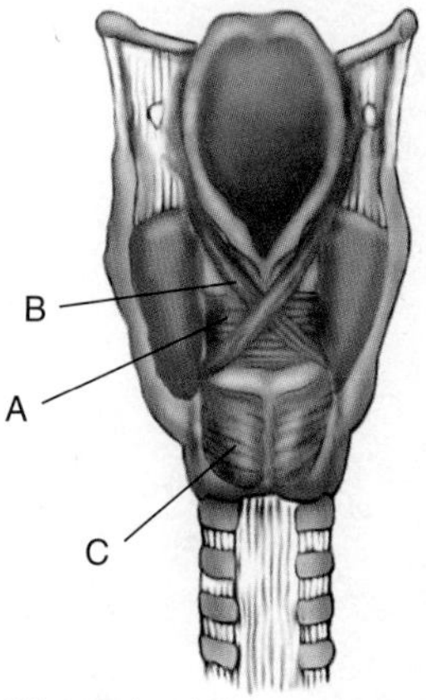

© Cengage Learning®.

5. Identify the muscles indicated in the figure.

   a. _____

   b. _____

   c. _____

   d. _____

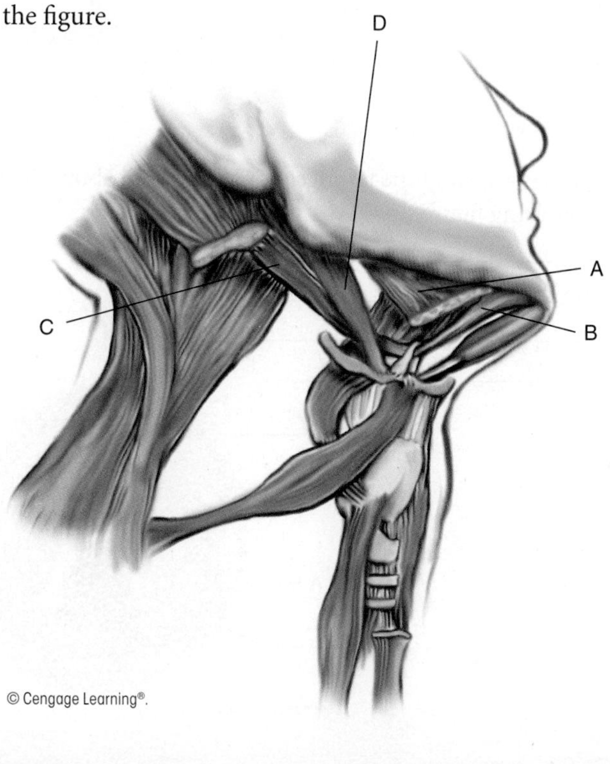

© Cengage Learning®.

6. Identify the muscles indicated in the following figure.

a. _____

b. _____

c. _____

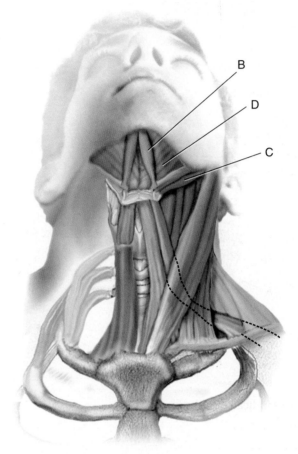

© Cengage Learning®.

7. This is a view of the laryngeal opening from above. Identify the structures indicated in the following figure.

a. _____

b. _____

c. _____

d. _____

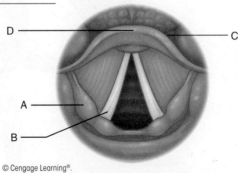

© Cengage Learning®.

8. Identify the two muscles indicated in the following figure.

a. _____

b. _____

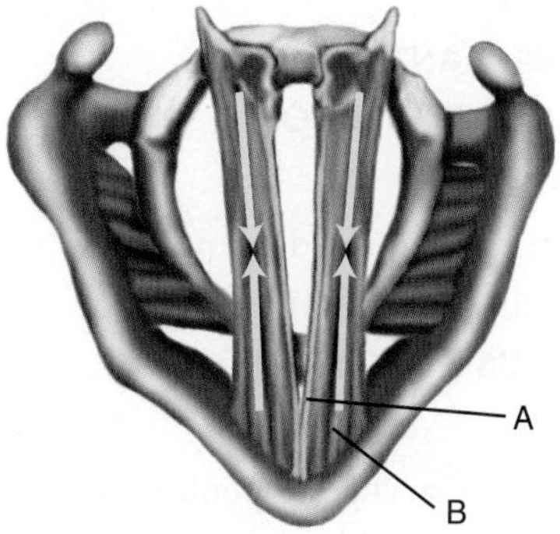

© Cengage Learning®.

9. The _____ muscle is the primary muscle responsible for the change of vocal fundamental frequency.

10. The space between the vocal folds is termed the _____.

11. Laryngeal cancer sometimes necessitates complete removal of the larynx. Because the respiratory and digestive systems share the pharynx, removal of this protective mechanism poses a problem for accounting for the needs of breathing and swallowing. What surgical changes would permit both processes?

Study Question Answers

1. Identify the indicated structures on the figure below.

a. **EPIGLOTTIS** cartilage

b. **THYROID** cartilage

c. **CRICOID** cartilage

d. **ARYTENOID** cartilage

e. **CORNICULATE** cartilage

f. **HYOID** bone

2. Identify the indicated landmarks on the figure below.

a. **SUPERIOR CORNU**

b. **INFERIOR CORNU**

c. **OBLIQUE LINE**

d. **THYROID NOTCH**

e. **ANGLE OF THYROID**

f. **LAMINA**

3. Identify the indicated landmarks on the figure below.

a. **MUSCULAR** process

b. **VOCAL** process

4. Identify the muscles indicated below.

a. **TRANSVERSE ARYTENOID**

b. **OBLIQUE ARYTENOID**

c. **POSTERIOR CRICOARYTENOID**

5. Identify the muscles indicated below.

    a. **MYLOHYOID**

    b. **DIGASTRICUS ANTERIOR**

    c. **DIGASTRICUS POSTERIOR**

    d. **STYLOHYOID**

6. Identify the muscles indicated below.

    a. **DIGASTRICUS ANTERIOR**

    b. **DIGASTRICUS POSTERIOR**

    c. **MYLOHYOID**

7. This is a view of the laryngeal opening from above. Identify the structures indicated below.

    a. **ARYEPIGLOTTIC FOLD**

    b. **TRUE VOCAL FOLDS**

    c. **VALLECULAE**

    d. **EPIGLOTTIS**

8. Identify the two muscles indicated below.

    a. **THYROVOCALIS**

    b. **THYROMUSCULARIS**

9. The **CRICOTHYROID** muscle is the primary muscle responsible for the change of vocal fundamental frequency.

10. The space between the vocal folds is termed the **GLOTTIS**.

11. Removal of the larynx would leave the airway unprotected from intrusion of foreign matter during swallowing. To avoid this danger, the airway is sealed off surgically, and a stoma is surgically opened up through the trachea to permit unhampered respiration.

Bibliography

Abrahams, P. H., McMinn, R. M. H., Hutchings, R. T., Sandy, C., & Mark, S. (2003). *McMinn's color atlas of human anatomy* (5th ed.). Philadelphia: Mosby.

Aronson, E. A. (1985). *Clinical voice disorders.* New York: Thieme.

Baer, T., Sasaki, C., & Harris, K. (1985). *Laryngeal function in phonation and respiration.* Boston: College-Hill Press.

Baken, R. J., & Orlikoff, R. F. (1999). *Clinical measurement of speech and voice* (2nd ed.). San Diego, CA: Singular Publishing Group.

Bateman, H. E. (1977). *A clinical approach to speech anatomy and physiology.* Springfield, IL: Charles C. Thomas.

Beck, E. W., Monson, H., & Groer, M. (1982). *Mosby's atlas of functional human anatomy.* St. Louis, MO: C. V. Mosby.

Berkovitz, B. K. B., & Moxham, B. J. (2002). *Head and neck anatomy: A clinical reference.* London: Martin Dunitz Ltd.

Bless, D. M., & Abbs, J. H. (1983). *Vocal fold physiology.* San Diego, CA: College-Hill Press.

Bly, L. (1994). *Motor skills acquisition in the first year.* Tucson, AZ: Therapy Skill Builders.

Boone, D. R. (1999). *The voice and voice therapy.* Englewood Cliffs, NJ: Prentice-Hall.

Broad, D. J. (1973). Phonation. In F. D. Minifie, T. J. Hixon, & F. Williams (Eds.), *Normal aspects of speech, hearing, and language.* Englewood Cliffs, NJ: Prentice-Hall.

Carrau, R. L., & Murry, T. (1999). *Comprehensive management of swallowing disorders.* San Diego, CA: Singular Publishing Group.

Childers, D. G., Hicks, D. M., Moore, G. P., Eskenazi, L., & Lalwani, A. L. (1990). Electroglottography and vocal fold physiology. *Journal of Speech and Hearing Research, 33,* 245–254.

Chhetri, D. K., Berke, G. S., Lotfizadeh, A., & Goodyer, E. (2009). Control of vocal fold cover stiffness by laryngeal muscles: A preliminary study. *Laryngoscope, 119*(1), 222–227.

Chhetri, D. K., Neubauer, J., & Berry, D. A. (2012). Neuromuscular control of fundamental frequency and glottal pressure at phonation onset. *Journal of the Acoustical Society of America, 13*(2), 1401–1412.

Chusid, J. G. (1985). *Correlative neuroanatomy and functional neurology* (17th ed.). Los Altos, CA: Lange Medical Publications.

Daniloff, R. G. (1989). *Speech science*. San Diego, CA: College-Hill Press.

Dejaeger, E., Pelemans, W., Ponette, E., & Joosten, E. (1997). Mechanisms involved in postdeglutition retention in the elderly. *Dysphagia, 12*(2), 63–67.

Doyle, P. C., Grantmyre, A., & Myers, C. (1989). Clinical modification of the tracheostoma breathing valve for voice restoration. *Journal of Speech and Hearing Disorders, 54*, 189–192.

Durrant, J. D., & Lovrinic, J. H. (1995). *Bases of hearing science*. Baltimore: Williams & Wilkins.

Eckel, F., & Boone, D. (1981). The s/z ratio as an indicator of laryngeal pathology. *Journal of Speech and Hearing Disorders, 46*, 147–149.

Fink, B. R. (1975). *The human larynx*. New York: Raven Press.

Fink, B. R., & Demarest, R. J. (1978). *Laryngeal biomechanics*. Cambridge, MA: Harvard University Press.

Frable, M. A. (1961). Computation of motion of the cricoarytenoid joint. *Archives of Otolaryngology, 73*, 551–556.

Fucci, D. J., & Lass, N. J. (1999). *Fundamentals of speech science*. Boston: Allyn & Bacon.

Fujimura, O. (1988). *Vocal fold physiology. Vol. 2. Vocal physiology*. New York: Raven Press.

Fukida, H., Kawaida, M., Tatehara, T., Ling, E., Kita, K., Ohki, K., Kawasaki, Y., & Saito, S. (1988). A new concept of lubricating mechanisms of the larynx. In O. Fujimura (Ed.), *Vocal physiology: Voice production, mechanisms and functions* (pp. 83–92). New York: Raven Press.

Ganong, W. F. (2003). *Review of medical physiology* (21st ed.). New York: McGraw-Hill/Appleton & Lange.

Gilroy, A. M., MacPherson, B. R., & Ross, L. M. (2012). *Atlas of anatomy* (2nd ed). New York: Thieme.

Gosling, J. A., Harris, P. F., Humpherson, J. R., Whitmore, I., & Willan, P. L. T. (1985). *Atlas of human anatomy*. Philadelphia: J. B. Lippincott.

Gray, H., Bannister, L. H., Berry, M. M., & Williams, P. L. (Eds.). (1995). *Gray's anatomy*. London: Churchill Livingstone.

Grobler, N. J. (1977). *Textbook of clinical anatomy* (Vol. 1). Amsterdam: Elsevier Scientific.

Gulia, J., et al. (2012) "Laryngocele: A Case Report and Review of Literature." *The Internet Journal of Otorhinolaryngology 14*(1), 1.

Halczy-Kowalik, L., Sulikowski, M., Wysocki, R., Posio, V., Kowalczy, R., & Rzewuska, A. (2012). The role of the epiglottis in the swallow process after a partial or total glossectomy due to neoplasm. *Dysphagia, 27*(1), 20–31.

Hanson, D. G., & Jiang, J. J. (2000). Diagnosis and management of chronic laryngitis associated with reflux. *American Journal of Medicine, 108*(4a), 112S–119S.

Hirano, M. (1974). Morphological structure of the vocal cord as a vibrator and its variations. *Folia Phoniatrica, 26*, 89–94.

Hirano, M., Kirchner, J. A., & Bless, D. M. (1987). *Neurolaryngology*. Boston: College-Hill Press.

Hirano, M., Kiyokawa, K., & Kurita, S. (1988). Laryngeal muscles and glottic shaping. In O. Fujimura (Ed.), *Vocal physiology: Voice production, mechanisms and functions* (pp. 49–65). New York: Raven Press.

Jones-Owens, J. L. (1991). Prespeech assessment and treatment strategies. In M. B. Langley, & L. J. Lombardino (Eds.), *Neurodevelopmental strategies for managing communication disorders in children with severe motor dysfunction*. Austin, TX: Pro-Ed.

Kaplan, H. M. (1971). *Anatomy and physiology of speech*. New York: McGraw-Hill.

Kazarian, A. G., Sarkissian, L. S., & Isaakian, D. G. (1978). Length of the human vocal folds by age. *Zhurnal Eksperimentalnoi Klinicheskoi Meditsiny, 18*, 105–109.

Kent, R. D. (1997). *The speech sciences*. San Diego, CA: Singular Publishing Group.

Kirchner, J. A., & Suzuki, M. (1968). Laryngeal reflexes and voice production. In M. Krauss (Ed.), Sound Production in Man. *Annals of the New York Academy of Sciences, 155*, 98–109.

Kuehn, D. P., Lemme, M. L., & Baumgartner, J. M. (1989). *Neural bases of speech, hearing, and language*. Boston: Little, Brown.

Langley, M. B., & Lombardino, L. J. (1991). *Neurodevelopmental strategies for managing communication disorders in children with severe motor dysfunction*. Austin, TX: Pro-Ed.

Lieberman, P. (1968). *Intonation, perception, and language*. Research Monograph No. 38. Cambridge, MA: The MIT Press.

Lieberman, P. (1977). *Speech physiology and acoustic phonetics: An introduction*. New York: Macmillan.

Liebgott, B. (2001). *The anatomical basis of dentistry*. St. Louis, MO: Mosby.

Matteucci, M. L., Rescigno, G., Capestro, F., & Torracca, L. (2012). Aortic arch patch aoroplasty for Ortner's syndrome in the age of endovascular stented grafts. *Texas Heart Institute Journal, 39*(3), 401–404.

McMinn, R. M. H., Hutchings, R. T., & Logan, B. M. (1994). *Color atlas of head and neck anatomy.* London: Mosby-Wolfe.

McHanwell, S. (2008). Larynx. In S. Standring (Ed.), *Gray's Anatomy: The anatomical and clinical basis of practice* (40th ed.), *577–594.*

Merati, A. L., & Rieder, A. A. (2003). Normal endoscopic anatomy of the larynx and pharynx. *American Journal of Medicine, 115,* 10S–14S.

Móz, L. E., Domingues, M. A., Castilho, E. C., Branco, A., & Martins, R. H. (2013). Comparative study of the behavior of p53 immunoexpression in smoking associate lesions: Reinke's edema and laryngeal carcinoma. *Inhalation toxicology, 25*(1), 17–20.

Mu, L., & Sanders, I. (2008). Newly revealed cricothyropharyngeus muscle in the human laryngopharynx. *Anatomical Record,* June 2.

Netter, F. H. (1983). *The CIBA collection of medical illustrations. Vol. 1. Nervous system. Part I. Anatomy and physiology.* West Caldwell, NJ: CIBA Pharmaceutical.

Netter, F. H. (1983). *The CIBA collection of medical illustrations. Vol. 1. Nervous system. Part II. Neurologic and neuromuscular disorders.* West Caldwell, NJ: CIBA Pharmaceutical.

Netter, F. H. (1997). *Atlas of human anatomy.* Los Angeles: Icon Learning Systems.

Proctor, D. F. (1968). The physiologic basis of voice training. In M. Krauss (Ed.), Sound production in man. *Annals of the New York Academy of Sciences, 155,* 208–228.

Rohen, J. W., Yokochi, C., Lutjen-Drecoll, E. L., & Romrell, L. J. (2002). *Color atlas of anatomy: A photographic study of the human body* (5th ed.). Philadelphia: Lippincott Williams & Wilkins.

Rosse, C., Gaddum-Rosse, P., & Rosse, G. (1997). *Hollinshead's textbook of anatomy.* Philadelphia: Lippincott-Raven.

Shepard, T. H. (1998). *Catalog of teratogenic agents* (9th ed.). Baltimore, MD: The Johns Hopkins University Press.

Schuenke, M., & Ross, L. M., (2010). *Thieme atlas of anatomy.* New York: Thieme.

Sonninen, A. (1968). The external frame function in the control of pitch in the human voice. In M. Krauss (Ed.), Sound production in man. *Annals of the New York Academy of Sciences, 155,* 68–89.

Standring, S. (2008). *Gray's anatomy: The anatomical and clinical basis of practice* (40th ed.). London, U.K.: Churchill-Livingstone.

Storck, C., Juergens, P., Fischer, C., Wolfensberger, M., Honegger, F., Sorantin, E., Friedrich, G., & Gugatschka, M. (2012). Biomechanics of the cricoarytenoid joint: three-dimensional imaging and vector analysis. *Journal of Voice, 25*(4), 406–410.

Titze, I. R. (1994). *Principles of voice production.* Englewood Cliffs, NJ: Prentice-Hall.

Van den Berg, J. (1968). Sound production in isolated human larynges. In M. Krauss (Ed.), Sound production in man. *Annals of the New York Academy of Sciences, 155,* 18–27.

Verdolini, K., Titze, I. R., & Fennell, A. (1994). Dependence of phonatory effort on hydration level. *Journal of Speech & Hearing Research, 37,* 1001–1007.

Whillis, J. (1946). Movements of the tongue in swallowing. *Journal of anatomy, 80,* 115–116.

Weaver, E. M. (2003). Association between gastroesophageal reflux and sinusitis, otitis media, and laryngeal malignancy: A systematic review. *American Journal of Medicine, 115*(3), 81–89.

Williams, P., & Warrick, R. (1980). *Gray's anatomy* (36th ed.). Philadelphia: W. B. Saunders.

Zhang, Z. (2011). Restraining mechanisms in regulating glottal closure during phonation. *Journal of the Acoustical Society of America, 130*(6), 4010–4019.

Zemlin, W. R. (1998). *Speech and hearing science: Anatomy and physiology* (4th ed.). Needham Heights, MA: Allyn & Bacon.

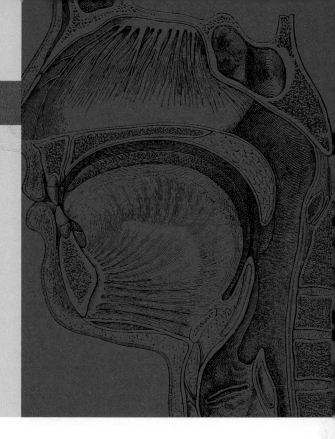

Chapter 5

PHYSIOLOGY OF PHONATION

Discussion of the function of the larynx and vocal folds revolves around the movable components and the results of that movement. We will concentrate on the nonspeech functions initially, which will help as we talk about speech and vocal functions. We use these nonspeech functions in our treatment of voice disorders, and this discussion may serve you well.

NONSPEECH LARYNGEAL FUNCTION

The protective function of the larynx is its most important role, because failure to prohibit the entry of foreign objects into the lungs is life threatening. This function is fulfilled through coughing and other associated reflexive actions.

Coughing is a response by the tissues of the respiratory passageway to an irritant or foreign object, mediated by the visceral afferent (sensory) portion of the X vagus nerve innervating the bronchial mucosa. Coughing is a violent and broadly predictable behavior, which includes deep inhalation through widely abducted vocal folds, followed by tensing and tight adduction of the vocal folds and elevation of the larynx. The axis of movement of the arytenoids guarantees that as they are rocked for adduction, they also are directed somewhat downward, providing more force in opposition to expiration. Significant positive subglottal pressure for the cough comes from tissue recoil and the muscles of expiration. The high pressure of forced expiration blows the vocal folds apart.

Anatesse Lesson

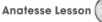

coughing: forceful evacuation of the respiratory passageway, including deep inhalation through widely abducted vocal folds, tensing and tight adduction of the vocal folds, and elevation of the larynx, followed by forceful expiration

245

The aerodynamic benefit of this is that the person coughing generates a maximal flow of air through the passageway to expel the irritating object. The negative side of the cough is the force required for its production. Chronic irritation of the respiratory system leads to vocal abuse in the form of repeated coughing.

The "near cousin" of the cough is throat clearing. It is not as violent as the full cough, but is nonetheless stressful. If you spend a moment clearing your throat and feeling its effects, you will sense increased respiratory effort that is countered by the tightening of the laryngeal musculature. You build pressure in the subglottal region and clamp the vocal folds shut to restrain the pressure. Although this clamping serves a purpose, in that it permits you to clear your respiratory passageway of mucus, it also places the delicate tissues of the vocal folds under a great deal of strain, and the result can be catastrophic to a trained voice.

There is a positive clinical side to this action, as well. If a client cannot approximate the vocal folds because of muscular weakness, the clinician has a means of achieving this closure in the cough. If you can get a client to cough voluntarily, you can very likely get the client to phonate. Both of these actions involve the muscles of adduction: lateral cricoarytenoid, arytenoids, and thyrovocalis. The medial compression generated in the cough is quite large, rivaled only by that required for abdominal fixation.

abdominal fixation: process of impounding air in thorax to stabilize the torso

Abdominal fixation is the process of capturing air within the thorax to provide the muscles with a structure on which to push or pull. The laryngeal movements in this effortful closure are one form of the Valsalva maneuver. The preparatory steps for thorax/abdomen fixation are similar to that for the cough: Take in a large inspiratory charge, followed by a tight adduction of the vocal folds. The effect is for the thorax to become a relatively rigid frame, so that the forces applied for lifting are translated to the legs. If the thorax is not fixed, those forces will act on the thorax instead, causing the rib cage to be depressed.

You may have wondered why you tend to grunt when lifting heavy objects or pushing your car. All of the components required for phonation are present. You are using force that would cause expiration, while your vocal folds are adducted. With sufficient effort, some air escapes through the adducted vocal folds, and you grunt.

Abdominal fixation plays an important role in childbirth, defecation, and vomiting. Review the Clinical Notes of Chapter 2 to refresh your memory.

So far we have dealt primarily with laryngeal functions focused on tight adduction of the vocal folds, but abduction has its place as well. Abduction dilates the larynx, an important function for respiration during physical exertion. You will recall from Chapter 3 that the physical requirements for oxygen increase significantly during work and exertion. During normal, quiet respiration, the vocal folds are abducted to provide a width of about 8 mm in the adult. During forced respiration, the need for air causes you to **dilate** or open the respiratory tract as widely as possible, doubling that width (see Figure 5-1).

dilate: to open or expand an orifice

Reflexes are involuntary, although respiratory reflexes can come under some voluntary control (e.g., you can hold your breath or stifle a yawn). We *must* eventually breathe, which requires reflexively abducting the vocal folds. In cases of drowning and near drowning, the victim may attempt to maintain adducted vocal folds, but must eventually attempt to breathe despite all logic that militates against it. Similarly, individuals rapidly immersed in cold water will reflexively gasp for air; the ability to inhibit this reflex is significantly reduced by alcohol consumption (a fact that explains one of the risks of combining drinking and boating).

We will discuss the swallowing reflex more thoroughly in Chapter 8, but it warrants a mention here. During normal deglutition, a bolus of food will trigger a swallowing reflex as it passes into the region behind the tongue and above the larynx. When the reflex

A bolus is a mass of chewed food formed into a ball in preparation for swallowing.

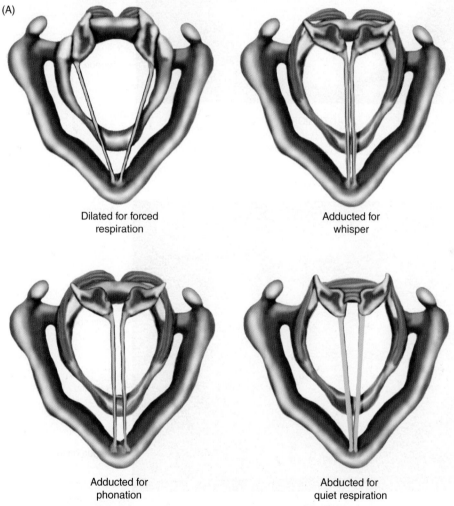

(A)

Dilated for forced
respiration

Adducted for
whisper

Adducted for
phonation

Abducted for
quiet respiration

Figure 5-1. (A) Laryngeal positions for various functions. During adduction for phonation, the vocal folds are approximated. For quiet respiration, the folds are moderately abducted, but for forced respiration, they are widely separated. Adduction for whisper involves bringing the folds close together but retaining a space between the arytenoid cartilages. Note that the view in 5-1A is a direct anatomical observation, as would be seen by fiberendoscopy. If one were to use a laryngeal mirror, the image would be reversed. (continues).

© Cengage Learning®.

(B)

POSTERIOR

Piriform sinus

Arytenoid prominence
within aryepiglottic fold

Vocal folds

False vocal folds

Epiglottis

Tongue base

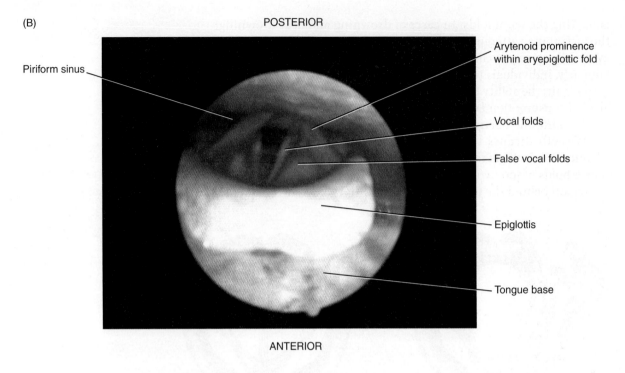

ANTERIOR

(C)

POSTERIOR

Piriform sinus

Arytenoid prominence

Vocal folds

False vocal folds

Epiglottis

Tongue base

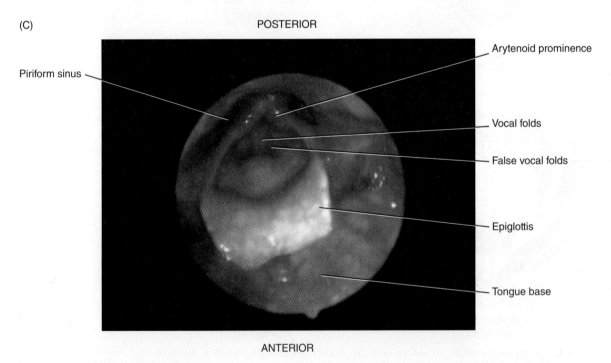

ANTERIOR

Figure 5-1 continued. (B) Fiberendoscopic view of superior larynx with abducted vocal folds. (C) Fiberendoscopic view of superior larynx with adducted vocal folds.
© Cengage Learning®.

is triggered, the larynx elevates, and the epiglottis (attached to the root of the tongue) drops down to cover the aditus. The aryepiglottic folds tense by the action of the aryepiglottic muscle, and the vocal folds are adducted. Try this: Hold your finger lightly on your thyroid notch and swallow. You may feel your larynx elevate and tense up as you swallow. That finger on the thyroid, by the way, is one component of the clinical swallowing evaluation.

✔ *To summarize:*

- We use the larynx and associated structures for many **nonspeech functions**, including coughing, throat clearing, swallowing, and abdominal fixation.
- These functions serve important biological needs and provide us with the background for useful clinical intervention techniques.

LARYNGEAL FUNCTION FOR SPEECH

Before getting into our discussion of phonation, let's review some basic concepts concerning acoustics.

A Brief Discussion of Acoustics

Frequency of Vibration

You are already familiar with the notion that things are capable of vibrating, because you have undoubtedly set a ruler into vibration on your desktop, or plucked a guitar string. When a physical body is set into vibration, it tends to continue vibrating (i.e., oscillating), and that vibration tends to continue at the same rate.

Let us examine why a body tends to oscillate. If you have a guitar, pluck one of the strings. As you listen to the twang of the string, you will notice that it continues vibrating for quite a while before finally quieting down. The tone produced remains at about the same pitch throughout the audible portion of its vibration.

The actual process of vibration is determined by a lawful interplay of the elastic restoring forces of a material, the stiffness of the material, and the inertia, a quality of its mass. **Elasticity** is that property of a material that causes it to return to its original shape after being displaced. **Stiffness** refers to the *strength* of the forces within a given material that restore it to its original shape on being distended. **Inertia** is the property of mass dictating that a body in motion tends to stay in motion. If we discuss the vibration of the guitar string in detail, the interaction of these elements may become clearer. Look at Figure 5-2 as we discuss this.

In the first panel of Figure 5-2, the guitar string is at its resting point. At this point, all forces are balanced. Next, the string is being displaced by someone's finger. This displacing force is distending the string. In the next panel, the string has been released and is moving

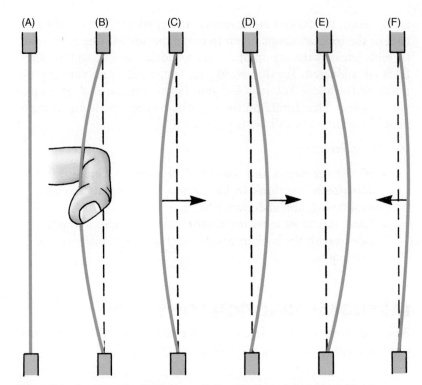

Figure 5-2. A guitar string illustrates oscillation. (A) The string is at rest. (B) A finger forces the string into displacement. (C) The string is released and its elastic elements cause it to return toward the rest position. (D) The string overshoots the rest position because of its inertia. (E) The string reaches the extreme point of its excursion past the rest position. (F) Elastic forces within the string cause the string to return toward the rest position.
© Cengage Learning®.

toward its starting point. This is a direct result of the restoring forces of the elastic material. The elastic qualities of the material from which the string is made and the stiffness of that material determine the efficiency with which the string returns.

In panel D, when the string reaches the midpoint, it is moving too fast to stop and sails on by that midpoint even though it is the point of equilibrium. This is similar to when you push someone in a swing, the swing does not simply return to the point of rest and stop, but rather overshoots that point. The reason the string travels past the point of rest is that it has mass. It takes energy to move mass and it takes energy to stop it once it has started moving. The string will not only return to its original resting position, due to elastic restoring forces, but will fly past that position due to the inertia associated with moving the mass of the object. In panel E, the string eventually stops moving because it is now being distended in the opposite direction. The energy you expended in the first distension has now been translated into an opposite distension as a result of inertia. In the final panel, the string may begin its return trip toward the starting point, but it will once again overshoot that point because of inertia.

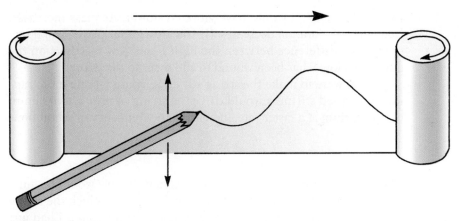

Figure 5-3. Periodic motion of a vibrating body graphically recorded.
© Cengage Learning®.

If you had set a pencil into vibration instead of a string and we had moved a sheet of paper in front of it as it vibrated, it might have drawn a picture something like that shown in Figure 5-3, which depicts the periodic motion of a vibrating body. This picture is a graphic representation of the vibration of that object. The drawing represents a waveform, which is the representation of displacement of a body over time, and displays what the pencil or string was doing as it vibrated.

This waveform is **periodic**. When we say that vibration is periodic, we mean that it repeats itself in a predictable fashion. If it took the ruler 1/100 of a second to move from the first point of distension back to that point again, it will take 1/100 of a second to repeat that cycle if it is vibrating periodically.

Moving from one point in the vibratory pattern to the same point again defines one **cycle of vibration**, and the time it takes to pass through one cycle of vibration is referred to as the **period**. In our example, the period of vibration was 1/100 second, or 0.01 second. **Frequency** refers to how often something occurs, as in the frequency with which you shop for groceries (e.g., two times per month). The frequency of vibration is how often a cycle of vibration repeats itself, which, in our example, is 100 times per second. Frequency and period are the inverse of each other, and that relationship may be stated as $f = 1/T$ or $T = 1/f$. That is, frequency (f) equals 1 divided by period (T for "time"). For our example, frequency = 1/0.01 second. If you will take a moment with your calculator, you will find that this calculation gives a result of 100.

Because frequency refers to the repetition rate of vibration, we speak of it in terms of number of cycles per second. The pencil vibrated with a frequency of 100 cycles per second, but shorthand notation for cycles per second is **Hertz** (Hz), after Heinrich Hertz. When we set the pencil into vibration, it vibrated with a period of 0.01 seconds and a frequency of 100 Hz.

We said that frequency of vibration in a body was governed by the elasticity, stiffness, and mass. If you had added a large weight to

frequency: number of cycles of vibration per second

the guitar string, it would have vibrated slower. As mass increases, frequency of vibration decreases. (If you are a guitar player, you'll recognize the difference between the high E and low E strings on the guitar: the low E has been wound to add mass to the string.)

If you were to make the string stiffer, it would vibrate more rapidly. Increased stiffness would drive the string to return to its point of equilibrium at a faster rate, increasing the frequency of vibration.

Amplitude and Intensity

There's another aspect of the acoustic signal that we would be quite remiss if we did not mention: Intensity. If I were to pluck the string with force, the string would be displaced a lot more than if I had just *lightly* plucked it. The frequency of vibration is the same whether it is plucked lightly or forcefully, but the amplitude of vibration has increased. For audible sounds, amplitude corresponds with signal intensity in a lawfully related way. The amplitude of vibration, which translates into the degree to which that waveform deviates from the zero line, correlates well with sound pressure. In fact, if this were a microphone output being recorded, the *Y*-axis would be volts, reflecting the degree to which the microphone receiver had moved when we spoke into it. Sound waves consist of oscillations of air molecules, called compressions and rarefactions. When the vibration is pushing toward the microphone, it is considered to be a compression, and it is a rarefaction when it is moving away from the microphone. These oscillations are direct correlates of the positive and negative movements you see in Figure 5-4, which is a recording of a diphthong from a microphone. These oscillations reflect small changes in pressure. When the waveform goes positive, it translates into a *positive voltage* and when it goes negative, that is a *negative voltage* change.

Voltage is the correlate of pressure, as in *sound pressure*. There are a couple of things we should say about sound pressure, and then you should seriously consider doing the worksheet on the decibel at the end of the chapter. (As you are probably aware, the decibel is one of those aspects of our field that we tend to shy away from. The activity is designed to walk you through some calculations, without leaving too bad a taste in your mouth!)

As you remember from Chapter 3, pressure is equal to force over a unit area ($P = F/A$). In this case, the area is the surface of the microphone, and the pressure is that which is generated by your voice when you say /a/. In the following sections you will learn that the vocal folds vibrate as a result of physical characteristics of the tissue that interact with airflow, but all you need to know for this discussion is that the

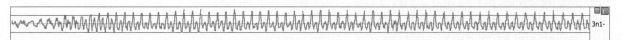

Figure 5-4. Speech waveform of the diphthong /aɪ/, as in "pie," recorded from a microphone.

vibration results in small changes in air pressure that we (as listeners) translate into sound (sound is defined as an audible disturbance in a medium). This air pressure change produces the sound waveform, and you can imagine it looking like that in Figure 5-4. The waveform represents an oscillation that moves from positive pressure (condensation; above the X-axis) to negative pressure (rarefaction; below the X-axis). Getting back to our original statement, the degree to which the waveform goes beyond the X-axis (either negative or positive) is the amplitude of the waveform. The larger the excursion there is, the louder the sound is. Now let us talk about how to measure that.

The ear is one of the true marvels of the universe, although we are admittedly a little biased. It is capable of a range of pressures that is immense, as you will remember from your audiology class. We can measure sound intensity as either power or pressure, which will change our measurement units, but not the intensity itself. If we talk of power, we are discussing intensity of a signal as related to the amount of work it is doing (the amount of energy flow per unit area), so the measurement unit will be watts per unit time. If you are dealing with pressures, you'll be discussing intensity in terms of force over unit area. These two measures are lawfully related, but we will only work with pressures for this discussion.

You can hear a sound in which the amplitude of air movement is just over the diameter of a molecule of hydrogen atom (20 micropascals = 0 dB SPL) assuming you have young, healthy ears), to a pressure that is a million times that (20,000,000 micropascals = 120 dB SPL). The 120 db SPL measure would be about the sound pressure your ears would get if you were 200 feet behind a jet engine as the plane is taking off: This is not recommended. This is an astounding range and is beyond a simple linear description. If you were to have a ruler that represented our range of hearing in micropascals, where 1 mm = 1 micropascal, the ruler to represent the range of hearing for humans would have to be 1,000 meters long, which would stretch for over 1/2 mile. Clearly, this is an ungainly way to represent intensity.

In order to account for our range of hearing, we utilize a logarithmic scale. The auditory system also functions in a logarithmic way, so the resulting scale comes close to matching our natural perception of loudness. The match is not perfect as we will see later in Chapter 10, but it comes much closer than a direct linear measurement of amplitude. Figure 5-5 shows you how logarithms compress a linear scale

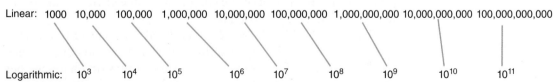

Linear: 1000   10,000   100,000   1,000,000   10,000,000   100,000,000   1,000,000,000   10,000,000,000   100,000,000,000

Logarithmic: 10^3 10^4 10^5 10^6 10^7 10^8 10^9 10^{10} 10^{11}

Figure 5-5. Relationship between linear and logarithmic scales. The top row of numbers reflects linear increases from 1,000 to 100,000,000,000. The bottom row shows what happens if you express that as the Logarithm (Base 10). The logarithmic expression makes the ungainly top row much more manageable.
© Cengage Learning®.

into a manageable framework. Basically, a logarithm is the power to which the number 10 is raised to reach that given value. (We will only talk about base 10 logarithms here, so relax.) The logarithm of 100 is 2: 10^2 is the equivalent of multiplying 10×10, = 100. So the exponent (2) is the power to which you raise 10 to get 100. If you have a calculator that will give you logarithms, enter 100 and ask for the log. The answer will be 2.

Now you might start to see the utility of the logarithm. If I have a scale, such as audible sound pressures, that ranges from 20 to 20,000,000, then expressing it using logarithms will make the scale manageable. We talk about the threshold of audibility, which has been defined as 20 micropascals. This is really somewhat arbitrary, since some ears are more sensitive than that, but it gives us the standard for sound pressure level. Sound pressure level (SPL) is defined as 20 micropascals at 1000 Hz: a Pascal is the derived measure for pressure that is the equivalent of the force of 1 newton (1 N) exerted on 1 m² (one square meter). (A newton is a measure of force defined as the amount of force required to accelerate 1 kilogram of mass 1 meter/second².) A micropascal is 1/1,000,000 of a Pascal. The reason we are forced to use such small measures is that we are sensitive to air pressures that represent displacement of molecules by only 1 billionth of a centimeter.

The decibel is actually a ratio of two pressures (or powers). If a sound has a sound pressure level of 40 dB (40 dB SPL), we are talking about the pressure of that sound wave relative to the reference for sound pressure level, 20 micropascals. The calculation is straightforward, and you can get some practice with it by doing the worksheet at the end of the chapter. The formula for the pressure-based decibel is dB = 20 log (input pressure/reference pressure).

As an example, if the input pressure 20,000,000 micropascals, and we are comparing it to the reference for dB SPL, the formula would be

dB = 20 log (20,000,000 micropascals/20 micropascals)

First divide 20,000,000 by 20 to get 1,000,000

Then take the logarithm of that (6). This is the power to which you would raise 10 to reach 1,000,000.

Now multiply that logarithm times 20 ($6 \times 20 = 120$). The answer, then, is that the signal has a sound pressure level of 120 dB.

We can also look at the decibel change from one signal to another, which can be even handier than using the SPL reference. Take a look at the activity at the end of the chapter for some examples of how to do that, and amaze your friends.

Frequency and intensity are both critical elements for our discussion in this chapter. As you read this material, don't forget your roots: Frequency is merely looking at how often something happens per unit time, and intensity is a ratio related to the amount of pressure exerted on a microphone diaphragm (or your ear, for that matter). Both of these concepts will help you as you treat clients with voice disorders.

Instruments for Voicing

Instrumentation for voicing includes tools for processing and analyzing the audio signal (frequency and intensity, mostly) and the physiology vocal folds. The standby for intensity is the sound level meter (SLM), which allows you to measure the sound pressure emanating from a source. This is a very useful tool for your work with clients in voice therapy, since inadequate or excessive vocal intensity (intensity of phonation) can arise from both physiological and psychological sources. In voice, the frequency of interest is generally the fundamental frequency (frequency of vibration of the vocal folds), and there are many tools that allow you to measure this in sustained phonation or running speech. A measure of phonatory stability is vocal jitter (or perturbation, to be discussed), which quantifies the cycle-by-cycle differences in vibration. A similar measure of cycle-by-cycle variation in intensity is vocal shimmer. Both of these measures are often bundled with instruments that measure the fundamental frequency. You're going to see that vocal intensity and fundamental frequency can be controlled separately, but also that it is difficult to do so. The phonogram (Pabon & Plomp, 1988) (also known as voice range profile or phonetogram) is a means of showing the interaction between intensity and frequency for an individual, revealing the degree of control a person can exert on his or her physiology, and as importantly, the range of intensity and frequency for an individual (Behrman, 2007).

We know that the respiratory system provides the energy for speech (see Chapter 3), and we can look at the glottal airflow and airway pressures using a number of instruments. Airflow is sensed by means of a pneumotachograph, typically placed within a face mask. Airflow measures allow researchers to examine the relationship between the phonatory and respiratory systems, such as glottal resistance related to phonemes produced, vocal intensity and airflow, and so forth. Measuring subglottal pressure is a little trickier. To get to the region below the vocal folds you must insert a hypodermic needle through the cricothyroid membrane and read the pressures generated below the level of the vocal folds. It can be estimated by examining intraoral pressure when the vocal folds are open, such as in production of /p/, which is an indirect measurement.

We can view the upper surface of the vocal folds directly using fiber endoscopy. Nasoendoscopy is a fiber-optic instrument that is inserted transnasally (through the nose, and through the velopharyngeal port) so that the fiber-optic bundle can provide an image of the vocal folds and laryngeal structures in real time. While the instrument can certainly be inserted orally and aimed toward the larynx, the view from the velopharyngeal port allows the tongue to move (so it is an excellent tool for swallowing evaluation, as well). When a stroboscopic source is used with the endoscope the examiner can actually stop the action of vibrating vocal folds. This allows close examination of vibratory function of the vocal folds and has provided great insight into the modes of vocal fold vibration, as we will discuss. Another excellent tool for examining the vibrating vocal folds is the electroglottograph (EGG). A pair of electrodes is affixed to the surface of the neck at the thyroid laminae. One electrode emits a very small current, which is read by the other electrode. The EEG trace that is recorded is the impedance (resistance to electrical flow) between the two electrodes (the patient or subject cannot feel the current, by the way). EGG provides a graphic trace that corresponds to the degree of vocal fold contact (see Figure 5-16 later in this chapter).

✔ *To summarize:*

- Vibration is governed by the interplay elastic restoring forces, stiffness, and inertia.
- **Elasticity** is the property of material that causes it to return to its original shape after being displaced.
- **Stiffness** refers to the *strength* of elastic forces.
- **Inertia** is the property of mass that causes it to stay in motion once it is placed into motion.
- Periodicity refers to a waveform that is predictable.
- Moving from one point in the vibratory pattern to the same point again defines one **cycle** of vibration.
- The time it takes to pass through one cycle of vibration is referred to as the **period**.
- **Frequency** refers to how often something occurs. Frequency of vibration in sound is measured in cycles per second, abbreviated Hz.
- The intensity of sound is lawfully related to the amplitude of the waveform.
- Sound pressure is the correlate of voltage, so measurement of the output of a microphone can be used to calculate intensity of sound.
- The decibel (dB) is a ratio of two sound pressures or powers, which is expressed logarithmically.
- Instrumentation for voicing includes tools for processing and analyzing the audio signal (frequency and intensity, mostly) and the physiology vocal folds.
- Intensity is measured using the sound level meter, and there are many tools that allow you to measure this in sustained phonation or running speech. Vocal jitter (perturbation) quantifies cycle-by-cycle differences in vibration of the vocal folds, and vocal shimmer examines cycle-by-cycle differences in intensity.
- The phonogram is a means of showing the interaction between intensity and frequency for an individual.
- Airflow is sensed using a pneumotachograph, typically placed within a face mask.
- Subglottal pressure may be measured by hypodermic needle through the cricothyroid membrane or estimated by examining intraoral pressure when the vocal folds are open.

- Nasoendoscopy involves insertion of a fiber endoscope trans-nasally to provide an image of the vocal folds and laryngeal structures in real time.
- The electroglottograph (EGG) uses a pair of electrodes affixed to the surface of the neck to provide a graphic trace that corresponds to the degree of vocal fold contact.

Now it is time to look at the primary physical principle supporting phonation: the Bernoulli effect.

The Bernoulli Effect

Vocal folds are masses that may be set into vibration. The **larynx** is the cartilaginous structure housing the two bands of tissue we call the vocal folds. The paired vocal folds are situated on both sides of the larynx so that they actually intrude into the airstream, as you can see from the schematic in Figure 5-6. This figure is a view from above and a view from behind. From above, you can see that the vocal folds are bands of tissue that are actually visible from a point immediately behind your tongue, looking down toward the lungs. From behind, you can see that the vocal folds are also a constriction in the airway, a critical concept for phonation.

You will remember from our discussion of respiratory physiology that any constriction in the airway greatly increases airway turbulence. If you are a passenger in a car and put your hand out of the window, you will feel the force of the wind dragging against your hand and you will hear the turbulence associated with it. You can rotate your hand so that the turbulence is reduced or increased; as the force on your hand increases, it becomes more difficult to keep your hand in the airstream.

The vocal folds are also a source of turbulence in the vocal tract. Without them, air would pass relatively unimpeded out of the lungs and into the oral cavity. The addition of the vocal folds results in

See Chapter 3 for a discussion of respiratory physiology.

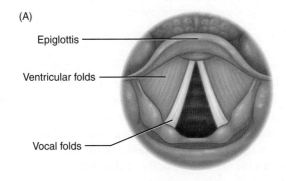

(A)

Epiglottis

Ventricular folds

Vocal folds

SUPERIOR VIEW

Figure 5-6. (A) Vocal folds from above. (continues).
© Cengage Learning®.

(B)

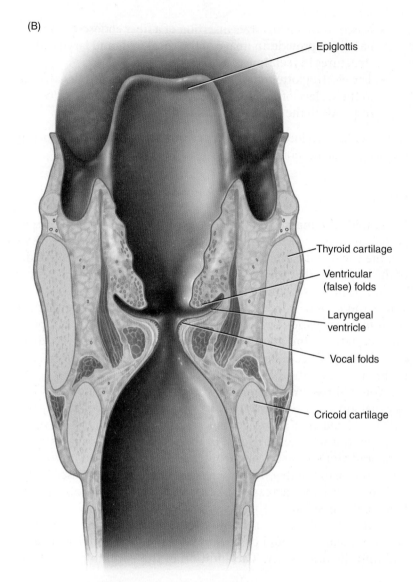

Epiglottis

Thyroid cartilage

Ventricular (false) folds

Laryngeal ventricle

Vocal folds

Cricoid cartilage

CORONAL SECTION, FROM BEHIND

Figure 5-6 continued. (B) Coronal section of larynx looking toward front, showing constriction in laryngeal space caused by the vocal folds.
© Cengage Learning®.

air having to make a detour around the folds, and the result of that detour invokes a discussion of the Bernoulli effect.

Daniel Bernoulli, a seventeenth-century Swiss scientist, recognized the effects of constricting a tube during fluid flow. The **Bernoulli effect** states that, given a constant volume flow of air or fluid, at a point of constriction there will be a decrease in pressure perpendicular to the flow and an increase in velocity of the flow. If you put a constriction in a tube, air flows faster as it passes through the constriction, and the pressure on the wall at the point of constriction will be lower than that of the surrounding area. Let us examine this statement.

The Bernoulli Effect in Everyday Life

The next time you go flying in an airplane, feel free to thank Daniel Bernoulli for the flight. While the thrust of the engines has a very large contribution to keeping the plane afloat, the configuration of the wings is critical to keeping you afloat so that you can arrive at your destination. If you viewed a wing in cross-section from the end you would note that the top surface of the wing is fatter, while the bottom is more streamlined. This configuration causes the air on the upper surface of the wing to move a little faster than that of the underbelly of the wing, which corresponds to a reduction in air pressure *above* the wing. This low pressure above "sucks" the airplane up into the sky as airflow increases, so that the net result is an airplane that rises. (This is why wings are treated for ice in winter: Ice changes the aerodynamics of the wing, destabilizing the difference between upper and lower surfaces, greatly compromising the lift that can be gained.)

For those of you who prefer fly balls to flying, realize that the pitcher in a baseball game is capitalizing on the Bernoulli effect as well. To produce a curve ball, the pitcher ensures that the ball begins its flight with the smooth surface toward the front and that the seam on the ball rotates to the side of the ball sometime during its brief flight. The seam acts as a constriction; the pressure on the seam side is lower than that on the opposite smooth side, and the ball is "sucked" toward the seam (there are other processes involved, but we will ignore them here). At least one pitcher has demonstrated the ability to "weave" the ball through a series of fence posts by putting just the right spin on the ball. For an excellent discussion of this effect, see Adair (1995).

Airflow Increase

Figure 5-7 shows a tube with a constriction in it representing the vocal folds. If you have placed your thumb over a garden hose, you know that the rate of water flow increases as a result of that constriction. Likewise, if you have ever been white-water rafting, you will immediately recognize that the white water rapids arise from constrictions in the flow of the river, in the form of boulders. As the water flows through the constriction, the rate of flow increases, giving you a thrill as you speed uncontrollably toward your fate.

Air Pressure Drop

To get an intuitive feel for the pressure drop, you must think about the flow in terms of molecules of air. Look again at Figure 5-7. We have drawn it so that you can count the number of molecules of air in the tube relative to the tube's length. In the unconstricted regions, you can count 10 molecules of air. Where the tube becomes narrower, there will be fewer air molecules because there is less space for them to occupy, and therefore, you count only five in that area. Where the constriction ends, you once again see 10 molecules.

When air is forced into a narrower tube, the same total volume of air has to squeeze through a smaller space. Because each unit mass of air becomes longer and narrower, it covers a longer stretch of the tube's walls. The pressure exerted by this mass, although the same in an overall sense, is now distributed over more of the wall. The result

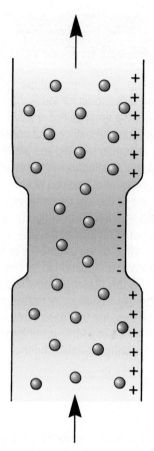

Figure 5-7. Rate of airflow through the tube will increase at the point of constriction, and air pressure will decrease at that point as well.
© Cengage Learning®.

See the Introduction of Chapter 2 for a discussion of force, pressure, and area.

is that each atom of the wall feels less force from the air molecules, and the narrow part of the tube is more likely to collapse. This effect occurs only when the air is forced to move; air without any forced movement will sooner or later equalize its pressure everywhere. If you remember that pressure is force exerted on an area ($P = F/A$), a drop in pressure makes perfect sense. Less force on the wall translates into lower pressure on the wall.

These two elements are the heart of the Bernoulli effect and help us to understand vocal fold vibration. Return to the notion of vocal folds being a constriction in a tube, as illustrated in Figure 5-8. You will want to refer to this figure as we discuss the Bernoulli principle applied to phonation.

The vocal folds are soft tissue, made up of muscle and epithelial tissue. Because of this characteristic, the folds are also capable of moving when sufficient force is exerted on them, as in the case of your hand extended out of the moving car window.

By examining panel A in Figure 5-8, you will see that the vocal folds are closed. In the next panel (B), the air pressure generated by

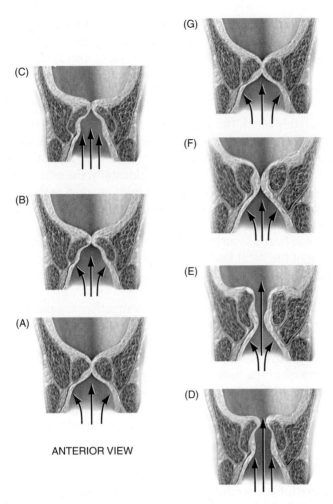

Figure 5-8. One cycle of vocal fold vibration as seen through a frontal section.
(A) Air pressure beneath the vocal folds arises from respiratory flow. (B) Air pressure causes the vocal folds to separate in the inferior. (C) The superior aspect of the vocal folds begins to open. (D) The vocal folds are blown open, the flow between the folds increases, and pressure at the folds decreases. (E) Decreased pressure and the elastic quality of vocal folds causes folds to move back toward midline. (F) The vocal folds make contact inferiorly. (G) The cycle of vibration is completed.
© Cengage Learning®.

the respiratory system is beginning to force the vocal folds open, but there is no transglottal flow because the folds are still making full contact. By panel D the vocal folds have been blown open. Because the vocal folds are elastic, they will tend to return to the point of equilibrium, which is the point of rest. They cannot return to equilibrium, however, as long as the air pressure is so great that they are blown apart. When they are in that position, however, there is a drop in pressure at the point of constriction (the Bernoulli effect), and we already know that if there is a drop in pressure, something is going to move to equalize that pressure.

In the last three panels (E, F, and G) you can see the result of the negative pressure: The vocal folds are being sucked back toward midline (E) as a result of the negative pressure and aided by tissue elasticity. The final panels (F and G) show the folds again making contact, with airflow being completely halted. When the vocal folds are pulled back toward the midline by their tissue-restoring forces, they completely block the flow of air for an instant as they make contact. At this point, the negative pressure related to flow is gone also. Instead, there is the force of respiratory charge beneath the folds ready to blow them apart once again. Incidentally, the minimum subglottal pressure that will blow the vocal folds apart to sustain phonation is approximately 3–5 cm H_2O, although much larger subglottal pressures are required for louder speech.

What you hear as voicing is the product of the repeated opening and closing of the vocal folds. The motion of the tissue and the resultant airflow disturb the molecules of air, causing the phenomenon we call sound.

The act of bringing the vocal folds together for phonation is referred to as **adduction**, and the process of drawing the vocal folds apart to terminate phonation is called **abduction**. As we shall see, both of these movements are achieved using specific muscles, but the actual vibration of the vocal folds is the product of airflow interacting with the tissue in the *absence* of repetitive muscular contraction.

If you have followed this introductory discussion of the principles governing vocal fold vibration, you are prepared to examine the structures of the larynx.

✔ *To summarize:*

- **Phonation**, or voicing, is the product of vibrating vocal folds within the larynx.
- The **vocal folds** vibrate as air flows past them; the Bernoulli phenomenon and tissue elasticity help maintain phonation.
- The **Bernoulli principle** states that, given a constant volume flow of air or fluid, at a point of **constriction** there will be a **decrease** in **pressure** perpendicular to the flow and an **increase** in **velocity** of the flow.
- The interaction of **subglottal pressure**, **tissue elasticity**, and **constriction** within the airflow caused by the vocal folds produces sustained phonation as long as pressure, flow, and vocal fold approximation are maintained.

Attack

Phonation is an extremely important component of the speech signal. To accomplish phonation we must achieve three basic laryngeal adjustments. To *start* phonation, we must adduct the vocal folds, moving them into the airstream, a process referred to as **vocal attack**. We then hold the vocal folds in a fixed position in

vocal attack: movement of vocal folds into the airstream for the purpose of initiating phonation

the airstream as the aerodynamics of phonation control the actual vibration associated with **sustained phonation**. Finally, we abduct the vocal folds to achieve **termination of phonation**.

When we are *not* phonating, the vocal folds are sufficiently abducted to prohibit air turbulence in the airway from starting audible vibration of the vocal folds. To initiate voicing, we bring the vocal folds close enough together that the forces of turbulence can cause vocal fold vibration. **Vocal attack** is the process of bringing vocal folds together to *begin* phonation, and this requires muscular action. Vocal attack occurs quite frequently in running speech. If you were to say the sentence "Anatomy is not for the faint of heart," you would have brought the vocal folds together and drawn them apart at least six times in two seconds to produce voiced and voiceless phonemes.

There are three basic types of attack. When we initiate phonation using **simultaneous vocal attack**, we coordinate adduction and onset of respiration so that they occur simultaneously. The vocal folds reach the critical degree of adduction at the same time that the respiratory flow is adequate to support phonation. Chances are you are using simultaneous attack when you say the word *zany*, because starting the flow of air before voicing would add the unvoiced /s/ to the beginning of the word, whereas adducting the vocal folds before producing the first sound would add a glottal stop to production.

Breathy vocal attack involves starting significant airflow before adducting the vocal folds. This occurs frequently during running speech, because we keep air flowing throughout the production of long strings of words. Say the following sentence while attending to the airflow over your tongue and past your lips: "Harry is my friend." If you did this, you felt the constant airflow, which indicates that some of the adductions involved had to be produced with air already flowing.

The third type of attack is **glottal attack**. In this attack, adduction of the vocal folds occurs prior to the airflow, much like a cough. Try this. Bring your vocal folds together (be gentle!) as if to cough, but instead of opening your vocal folds as you push air through the folds, keep them adducted and say /a/. That was a glottal attack. You might have felt a little tension or irritation from doing this exercise, a reminder of the delicacy of the vocal mechanism. We use glottal attack when a word begins with a stressed vowel. Say the following sentence and pay close attention to your vocal folds during the production of the first phoneme of the words: *Okay, I want the car.* If you noticed a buildup of tension and pressure for those words, you were experiencing glottal attack.

All three of these attacks are quite functional in speech and are not at all pathological. Problems occur when an attack is misused. If a glottal attack becomes a **hard glottal attack**, the speaker may damage the delicate vocal mechanism tissues. If the speaker inadequately adducts the vocal folds, air may escape between them to produce a **breathy phonation**; a much more common phenomenon is breathy voice caused by a physical tissue change that obstructs adduction.

sustained phonation: phonation that continues for long durations as a result of tonic contraction of vocal fold adductors

simultaneous vocal attack: vocal attack in which expiration and vocal fold adduction occur simultaneously

breathy vocal attack: vocal attack in which expiration occurs before the onset of vocal fold adduction

glottal attack: the vocal attack in which expiration occurs after adduction of the vocal folds

Termination

We bring the vocal folds together to begin phonation, and termination of phonation requires that we abduct them. We pull the vocal folds out of the airstream far enough to reduce the turbulence, using muscular action. When the turbulence is sufficiently reduced, the vocal folds stop vibrating. As with attack, we terminate phonation many times during running speech to accommodate voiced and voiceless speech sounds.

Both adduction and abduction occur very rapidly. Muscles controlling these functions can complete contraction within about 9 milliseconds (ms) (9/1000 seconds). In running speech, you may see periods of vibration of the vocal folds as brief as three cycles of vibration (approximately 25 ms) for unstressed vowels, which would bring the total adduction, phonation, and abduction time to only 53/1000 of a second.

Adduction is a constant in all types of attack. The arytenoid cartilages are capable of moving in three dimensions, involving movement such as **arytenoid rotation**, **rocking**, and **gliding**. It appears that the primary arytenoid movement for adduction is inward rocking. When the arytenoids are pulled medially on the convex arytenoid facet of the cricoid, the arytenoids rock down, with apices approaching each other. (You may wish to review Figure 4-11 in Chapter 4.) Some rotatory movement will occur during the adductory movement of the arytenoid, and this has been demonstrated using cadaver specimens (Storck, Juergens, Fischer, Wolfensberger, Honegger, Sorantin, Friedrich, & Gugatschka, 2012), but it appears to be greatest at the extremes of lateral movement (i.e., nearly abducted: Fink & Demarest, 1978).

Ventricular Phonation

The false or ventricular vocal folds are technically unable to vibrate for voice, but in some instances, clients may use them for this purpose. Boone (1999) cites instances in which clients used ventricular phonation as an adaptive response to severe vocal fold dysfunction, such as growths on the folds. Apparently the client forces the lateral superior walls close together during the adductory movement, permitting the folds to make contact and vibrate.

The ventricular folds are thick, and the phonation heard is deep and often raspy. The false folds may **hypertrophy** (increase in size), facilitating ventricular phonation. A study by Young, Wadie, and Sasaki (2012) has confirmed that the ventricular folds are innervated by the recurrent laryngeal nerves, and unilateral adductor vocal fold paralysis will result in unilateral paralysis of the ventricular folds.

Fans of old movies may remember the 1930s era "My Gang" series of rough-and-tumble children set against the world. If you are one of those fans you may remember "Froggy," one of the children who had such strong allegiance to Spanky. Take another listen to Froggy's voice and you will hear (and see) an excellent example of ventricular phonation. In Froggy's case, it was a claim to fame that made him a star of the silver screen.

Vocal Fold Nodules

Vocal fold nodules are aggregates of tissue arising from abuse. This condition makes up a large share of the voice disorder cases seen by school clinicians. Common forms of "vocal abuse" (a.k.a. phonotrauma) are yelling, screaming, cheerleading, or "barking" commands (such as a drill sergeant). The result of this abuse is a sequence of events that can lead to a permanent change in the vocal fold tissue. You are probably familiar with **laryngitis**, which is an inflammation of the larynx. It causes hoarseness, often with loss of voice (**aphonia**). The laryngeal effect is the swelling (**edema**) of the delicate vocal fold tissue, so that it is difficult to make the folds vibrate. In fact, they are often bowed so badly that expiratory flow will pass between them, even if you can produce phonation; we refer to this as a **breathy voice**. Laryngitis may easily be caused by **vocal hyperfunction**, which is over-adduction of the vocal folds. This is a form of vocal abuse, and you may have experienced it after a particularly thrilling football game.

The soreness is a message from your body to stop doing what made the vocal folds sore in the first place. Continued abuse results in the formation of a protective layer of epithelium that is callous-like and is not a very effective oscillator. If the vocal hyperfunction continues, the hardened tissue will increase in size until a nodule forms on one (**unilateral**) or both (**bilateral**) vocal folds. The site of abuse is usually at the juncture of the anterior and middle thirds of the vocal folds, because this is the point of greatest impact during phonation. Although untreated vocal nodules may eventually have to be removed surgically, voice therapy to reverse the vocal behavior driving the phenomenon is always recommended. If the vocal hyperfunction is not eliminated, the vocal nodules will return after surgery; however, surgery may be avoided if therapy is sought in a timely manner.

These motions are the product of the lateral cricoarytenoid muscle and the lateral portion of the thyromuscularis, facilitated by the oblique and transverse arytenoids. The arytenoid cartilages are also capable of limited gliding in the anterior–posterior dimension, which could alter the total vocal fold length. Adduction does not seem to affect the overall length of the glottis, although it tends to lengthen the membranous portion. The combined forces of the cricothyroid and posterior cricoarytenoid cause the entire glottis to lengthen (Hirano, Kiyokawa, & Kurita, 1988).

laryngitis: inflammation of the larynx

aphonia: loss of ability to produce voicing for speech

vocal hyperfunction: excessive use of vocal mechanism, for speech or nonspeech function, which has the potential to produce organic pathology

Sustained Phonation

Sustained phonation is the purpose of adduction and abduction for speech. Let us examine this closely.

Vocal attack requires muscular action, as does termination of phonation. In contrast, sustaining phonation simply requires *maintenance* of a laryngeal posture through **tonic** (sustained) contraction of musculature. This is a very important point. The vibration of the vocal folds is achieved by placing and holding the vocal folds in the airstream in a manner that permits their physical aspects to interact with the airflow, thereby causing vibration. The vocal folds are *held* in place during sustained phonation, and the vibration of the vocal folds is not the product of repeated adduction and abduction of the vocal folds. Muscle spindles embedded within the thyrovocalis and thyromuscularis serve an important function in holding the sustained posture. As you will learn in the neurophysiology section (Chapter 12), muscle spindles are responsible for the maintenance of muscle posture. These sensors provide input to the nervous system about the length of muscle in a resting (or in this case, steady-state) posture, and when that muscle moves away from the chosen posture without voluntary contraction, the muscle spindle is responsible for correcting that "accidental" movement. So, during steady-state phonation the vocal folds are in a steady-state, tonic contraction to control fundamental frequency and to stabilize intensity. The business of vocal fold vibration is purely that of aerodynamic interaction with the elastic characteristics of the vocal folds.

Phonation actually begins a few milliseconds prior to vocal fold approximation. As the vocal folds are brought together during attack, they begin vibrating as the turbulence increases, and this vibration is sustained as long as the folds are approximated and there is sufficient subglottal air pressure. Incidentally, the vocal folds need not be touching to vibrate, as you can demonstrate for yourself. Begin the word *hairy* by stretching out the /h/ sound, and then let that breathiness carry forward into the vowel. The vocal folds very likely are not touching or are making only very light contact if you hear a breathy quality.

Vocal Register

The **mode of vibration** of the vocal folds during sustained phonation refers to the pattern of activity that the vocal folds undergo during a cycle of vibration. Moving from one point in the vibratory pattern to the same point again defines one **cycle** of vibration, and within one cycle the vocal folds undergo some very significant changes. There are actually a number of modes or **vocal registers** that have been differentiated perceptually. Narrowly defined for purposes of phonatory discussion, register refers to differences in the mode of vibration of vocal folds.

The three registers most commonly referred to are modal register, glottal fry or pulse register, and falsetto. We are also interested in the variant breathy and pressed phonatory modes, as well as whispered speech.

Modal Register

The first register, known as the **modal register** or modal phonation, refers to the pattern of phonation used in daily conversation. This pattern is the most important one for the speech-language pathologist and is the most efficient.

Figure 5-9 shows the vocal folds from the sides and from above, which will let us talk about the vertical and anterior-posterior modes

Trained singers refer to combinations of thorax/oral/nasal cavity configurations, laryngeal positions, and muscular "concentrations" to define registers that are perceptually differentiable but about which there are few acoustical or physiological data. See Titze (1994) for a lively discussion of register.

The "mode" is that which occurs most often in a distribution.

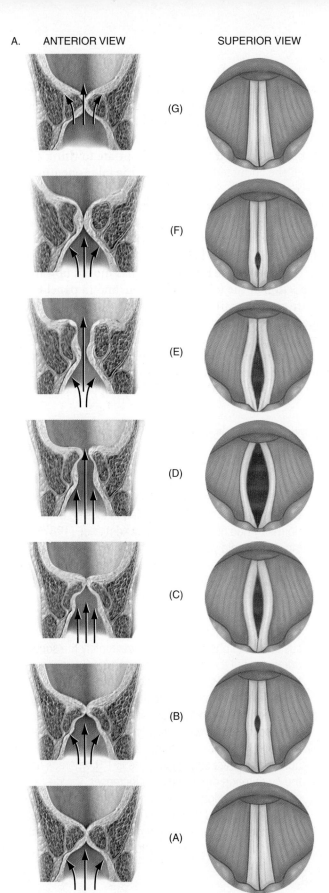

A. ANTERIOR VIEW   SUPERIOR VIEW

(G)

(F)

(E)

(D)

(C)

(B)

(A)

Figure 5-9. (A) Graphic representation of vertical and transverse phase relationships during one glottal cycle. Note that generally the vocal folds open from inferior to superior and also close from inferior to superior. Simultaneously, the glottis grows generally from posterior to anterior, but the vocal folds close from anterior to posterior.

© Cengage Learning®.

267

of phonation. In the **vertical mode** of phonation, the vocal folds *open* from inferior to superior (bottom to top) and also *close* from inferior to superior. You might suspect that they would open and close like a door swinging on a hinge, but that is not the case. The folds are an undulating wave of tissue, and it is more appropriate to think of air as bubbling through the adducted folds than of the folds opening and closing as if hinged.

You can see from the first panel of Figure 5-9 that the vocal folds are approximated at the beginning of a cycle of vibration. In the second panel, air pressure from beneath is forcing the folds apart in the inferior aspect. (This makes sense, because that is where the pressure is located.) In the third panel, the bubble of air has moved upward so that the superior portion of the folds is now open, and in panel E you can see that they are closing again. Note that they begin closing at the bottom: They open at the bottom first, and they start closing first at the bottom as well. In the final panel the cycle is complete.

Titze (1994) has demonstrated that this phase difference in the mucosal wave from inferior to superior is a result of the mass and elasticity of the vocal folds, and that these conditions support continued

Sustained and Maximum Phonation

Physical systems, such as those encompassing the mechanisms of speech, are rarely employed at maximum output and stress. For instance, we generally do not breathe in maximally or speak using our entire vital capacity, although we are capable of doing this. When clinicians wish to examine whether there is a deficit in a system, one useful technique is to ask the client to perform a test of maximal output for a given parameter. In respiration, such tests would be the examination of vital capacity, inspiratory reserve, and expiratory reserve.

This useful concept may be extended to voicing. If you ask a client to sustain a vowel for as long as he or she can, you are testing not only how well the vocal folds function but also the vital capacity and checking action ability of the person under examination. If the respiratory system is intact, on average an adult female in the 17- to 41-year-old range will be able to sustain the /a/ vowel for approximately 15 seconds, and the male will be able to sustain that vowel for 23 seconds. This function changes with age, increasing through the second decade of life. Generally you may expect the phonation time

of children to increase from about 10 seconds at 6 years, but you may be interested in looking at the norms by age as summarized by Kent et al. (1987). Incidentally, did you wonder why males are able to phonate a little longer? If you attributed it to larger vital capacity, you were right.

Another phonation-related task involves maximum duration of the sustained sibilants, /s/ and /z/. Boone (1999) states that individuals are able to sustain these phonemes for approximately the same durations, but that the addition of physical change to the vocal folds (such as vocal nodules) will cause a significant reduction in the duration of the voiced /z/. Males again produce longer fricatives, and the duration increases with age. Clinicians calculate the ratio of s:z duration to aid their decisions. If the two durations are the same, the value is 1.0, whereas as the /z/ duration drops, the ratio increases. The decline in /z/ duration arises from reduced phonatory efficiency caused by swelling (edema). Although the ratio undergoes continual examination for its clinical utility, many studies have substantiated the use of this clinical tool.

Can Elephants Purr?

There are two ways for vocal fold tissue to move: active muscle contraction (AMC) (Herbst, Stoeger, Frey, Lohscheller, Titze, Gumpenberger & Fitch, 2012) or arising from the myoelastic aerodynamic principles we've described here. For many years speech and hearing scientists fought the battle of the mechanism that drives vocal fold vibration, and the theory that is most viable is the myoelastic-aerodynamic theory, and its updated version, Titze's mucoviscoelastic-aerodynamic theory. Before we had a firm notion of the limits of the neuromuscular system, a competing theory, called the neurochronaxic theory, held that each vibratory cycle of the vocal folds was the product of neuromuscular activation. The theory posited that vibration of the vocal folds was a function governed directly by the central nervous system, which activated the X vagus recurrent laryngeal nerve, to cause each vibration of the vocal folds. It didn't take the field long to figure

out that the motor system could not respond quickly enough to control each vibration (and besides, people with paralyzed vocal folds can still make the fold vibrate if it is within the airflow). The neurochronaxic theory was proven absolutely wrong in humans.

If cats have speech scientists among their ranks they are not so quick to abandon the neurochronaxic theory. The cat's purr is the product of individual, cyclic contractions of the laryngeal muscles, which is why it is so distinctly different from their "meow." Herbst et al. (2012) wondered whether the subsonic phonations of elephants might arise from the same mechanism, and found that, using an excised larynx from a deceased elephant, they could produce the sound *without* muscular contraction. So, cats capitalize on active muscular contraction (neurochronaxic theory) to make their contentment known, but elephants rely on the myoelastic aerodynamic theory to communicate.

oscillation by the vocal folds (i.e., the tissue continues to vibrate after the energy has been removed). You can change the tension and mass per unit length to arrive at a given, relatively constant laryngeal tone.

The vocal folds have one primary frequency of vibration, called the **vocal fundamental frequency**, but they produce an extremely rich set of harmonics as well, which are whole-number multiples of the fundamental. These harmonics provide important acoustical information for identification of voiced phonemes. If the vocal folds were simple tuning forks without these harmonics, we would not be able to tell one vowel from another. The complex vibrational mode of the vocal folds is extremely important.

The second mode of vibration of the vocal folds is in the anterior-posterior dimension. Whereas the vertical phase difference appears to be consistent in modal vibration, the anterior–posterior mode is less stereotypical. Zemlin (1998) reported that the vocal folds tend to open from posterior to anterior, but that closure at the end of a cycle is made by contact of the medial edge of the vocal fold, with the posterior closing last.

Because the vocal folds offer resistance to air flow, the **minimum driving pressure** of the vocal folds in modal phonation is approximately 3–5 cm H_2O subglottal pressure. If pressure is lower than this, the folds will not be blown apart. This is clinically important, because a client who cannot generate 3–5 cm H_2O and sustain it for 5 seconds

vocal fundamental frequency: primary frequency of vibration of the vocal folds

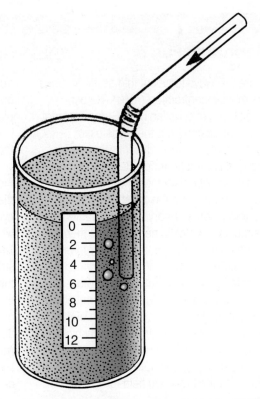

Figure 5-10. A useful clinical tool described by Hixon, Hawley, and Wilson (1982). This portable manometer gives the client feedback concerning respiratory ability and provides the clinician with a measure of function.
© Cengage Learning®.

will not be able to use the vocal folds for speech. (See the Clinical Note on measurement of subglottal pressure and Figure 5-10.)

Glottal Fry

The second register is known as **glottal fry** but is also known as **pulse register** and **Strohbass** ("straw bass"). What *fry, pulse,* and *straw bass* all allude to is the crackly, "popcorn" quality of this voice. Perceptually, this voice is extremely low in pitch and sounds rough, almost like eggs frying in a pan. Some voice scientists jokingly refer to it as the "I'm sick" voice, as it is the weak, low-pitched voice you might use to explain the reason you cannot come to work today.

Glottal fry is the product of a complex glottal configuration, and it occurs in frequencies ranging from as low as 30 Hz, to 80 or 90 Hz. This mode of vibration requires low subglottal pressure to sustain it (on the order of 2 cm H_2O), and tension of the vocalis is significantly reduced relative to modal vibration, so that the vibrating margin is flaccid and thick. The lateral portion of the vocal folds is tensed, so that there is strong medial compression with short, thick vocal folds and low subglottal pressure. If either vocalis tension or subglottal pressure is increased, the popcorn-like perception of this mode of vibration is lost.

In glottal fry the vocal folds take on a secondary, syncopated mode of vibration, such that there is a secondary beat for every cycle of the fundamental frequency. In addition to this syncopation, the vocal folds spend up to 90 percent of the cycle in approximation. Oscillographic waveforms of modal vibration and glottal fry are shown in Figure 5-11, and the presence of the extra beat may be clearly seen. This should reemphasize the notion that the vocal folds are not simply vibrating at a slower rate than in modal phonation, but are vibrating *differently*.

In music, syncopation is the change in accent arising from stressing of a weak beat. In the case of glottal fry, this definition is stretched to accommodate the notion of including a weak beat in the rhythm. Glottal fry appears to include both weak and strong beats.

Falsetto

The third and highest register of phonation, the **falsetto**, also is characterized by a vibratory pattern that varies from modal production. In falsetto, the vocal folds lengthen and become extremely thin and "reedlike." When set into vibration, they tend to vibrate along the tensed, bowed margins, in contrast to the complex pattern seen in other modes of phonation. The vocal folds make contact only briefly, as compared with modal phonation, and the degree of movement (amplitude of excursion) is reduced. The posterior portion of the vocal folds tends to be damped, so that the length of the vibrating surface is decreased to a narrow opening. Contrast this to elevated pitch in modal phonation, which involves *lengthening* the vocal folds.

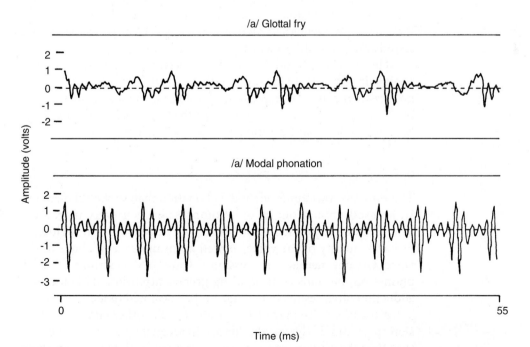

Figure 5-11. Oscillographic comparison of glottal fry (top) and modal phonation for the vowel /a/ (bottom).
© Cengage Learning®.

Clinical Measurement of Subglottal Air Pressure

Hixon, Hawley, and Wilson (1982) have provided us with an excellent and simple tool to assess the adequacy of subglottal pressure for speech. In their article, the authors recommend marking a cup of water in cm gradations (see Figure 5-10). Place a small pinhole in a flexible soda straw, and put a paper clip over the straw to hold it to the edge of the glass. Fill the glass up to the top centimeter mark.

As you push the straw deeper into the water, it becomes increasingly difficult to blow bubbles in the water through the straw. At the point where the straw is 3 cm below the water line, you must generate 3 cm H_2O of subglottal pressure to make bubbles.

When assessing a client for adequacy of subglottal pressure, you can have the individual begin blowing as you push the straw into the water. The point at which bubbles are no longer is the limit of the individual's pressure ability. This is an excellent therapy tool as well, because it provides a practice device with visual feedback of progress toward respiratory support for speech. Realize that this is a measurement of respiratory ability, which is essential for phonation.

The perception of falsetto is one of an extremely thin, high-pitched vocal production. The difference between falsetto and modal vibration is not simply one of the frequency of vibration (in the 300 to 600 Hz range). Although it is true that falsetto is the highest register, the modal and falsetto registers overlap.

Whistle Register. There is actually a register above falsetto, known as the **whistle register**, but it is not apparently a mode of vibration as much as it is the product of turbulence on the edge of the vocal fold. It occurs at frequencies as high as 2,500 Hz, typically in females, and sounds very much like a whistle.

The shift from modal register to glottal fry or falsetto is clearly audible in the untrained voice. If you perform an up-glide of a sung note, reaching up to your highest production, you may hear an audible "break" in the voice as you enter that register. Trained singers learn to smooth that transition so that it is inaudible.

Pressed and Breathy Phonation

There are two variations on modal phonation that we should mention. In **pressed** phonation, medial compression is greatly increased. The product of pressed phonation is an increase in the stridency or harsh quality of the voice, as well as an increase in abuse to the voice. Greater medial compression is translated as stronger, louder phonation, perhaps commanding greater attention. This forceful adduction often results in damage to the vocal fold tissue.

A breathy voice may be the product of the other end of this tension spectrum. If the vocal folds are inadequately approximated, so that the vibrating margins permit excessive airflow between them when in the closed phase, you will hear air escape as a **breathy**

Puberphonia

During normal development, children undergo a great deal of change during puberty, the time in a child's life when he or she becomes capable of reproduction. This occurs between 13 and 15 years of age for boys and between 9 and 16 years of age for girls. Puberty is characterized by rapid muscle development and height and weight gain. The thyroid cartilage and thyroarytenoid are not left out of development. They grow rapidly during this time, although the larynges of boys will grow considerably more than those of girls.

The result of this spurt of laryngeal growth is that the child (typically a boy) will have periods of voice change (mutation) in which his voice breaks down in pitch as he is speaking. This is, of course, a normal result of the changing tissue and the young man's attempt to control it for phonation, but it is nonetheless disturbing. **Puberphonia** refers to the maintenance of the childhood pitch despite having passed through the developmental stage of puberty. It surely represents an attempt to hold *something* constant during the roller-coaster ride of puberty, but the result is a significant mismatch between the large body of the developing teenaged boy and the high-pitched voice of the prepubescent child. Typically, the young man is speaking in falsetto but is aware of the "lower" voice. Therapy performed over the summer to help the individual alter habitual pitch, in the absence of peer pressures associated with the classroom regimen, is quite effective.

phonation. Breathiness is inefficient and causes air wastage, but is not a condition that will damage the phonatory mechanism.

There is a potential danger in the breathy voice, however. The underlying factor keeping the vocal folds from approximating could be any of a number of organic conditions, so that even when the speaker pushes the vocal folds tightly together, air escapes. In this case, a breathy voice may signal the presence of vocal nodules, or even benign or malignant growths such as polyps or laryngeal cancer. In addition, if an individual attempts to overcome the breathy quality caused by nodules or other obstructing pathology, the vocal hyperfunction will result in abuse.

Whispering

Whispering is not really a phonatory mode, because no voicing occurs. This does *not* mean that there are no laryngeal adjustments, but rather that they do not produce vibration in the vocal folds. Prove this to yourself. Exhale forcefully and attend to your larynx, and then on the next forceful exhalation *whisper* the word *Ha!* You probably felt the tension in your larynx increased during whispering. In respiration the vocal folds are abducted, but when whispering they must be partially adducted and tensed to develop turbulence in the airstream, and that turbulence is the noise you use to make speech. The arytenoid cartilages are rotated slightly in but are separated posteriorly, so that there is an enlarged "chink" in the cartilaginous larynx. A whisper is *not* voiced, but is strenuous and can cause vocal fatigue. Whispering is not economical, as you can prove to yourself by sustaining production

Electroglottography

The electroglottograph (EGG) is a useful and nonintrusive instrument for the examination of vocal function. A pair of surface electrodes is placed on the thyroid lamina, typically held in place by an elastic band. An extremely small and imperceptible current is introduced through one electrode, and the impedance (resistance to current flow) is measured at the other electrode. When the vocal folds are approximated during phonation, there is less resistance to flow. The less contact the vocal folds make, the greater the impedance.

This nice arrangement permits researchers to examine at least some aspects of vocal fold function with ease. As you can see from the EGG trace of Figure 5-16, there are marked differences in the duration of vocal fold contact for quiet (A) versus loud (B) speech. For further reading, you may want to review Childers, Hicks, Moore, Eskenazi, and Lalwani (1990).

intensity: magnitude of sound, expressed as the relationship between two pressures or powers

vocal intensity: sound pressure level associated with a given speech production

of an /a/ in modal phonation and again in whispered production. You should see quite a difference in maximum duration.

In Chapter 4 we discussed the notion of frequency of vibration. As mentioned earlier in this chapter, the primary frequency of vibration of the vocal folds is called the *fundamental frequency*. This is the number of cycles the vocal folds go through per second, and it is audible. The movement of the vocal folds in air produces an audible disturbance in the medium of air known as **sound**. That sound is transmitted through the air as a wave, with molecules being compressed by movement of the vocal folds.

The interplay of the elasticity and mass of the vocal folds leads them to vibrate in a periodic fashion. However, we have not yet mentioned a final element of phonation, intensity. **Intensity** refers to the relative power or pressure of an acoustic signal, measured in decibels (abbreviated **dB**). In phonation, we may refer to the intensity of voice as **vocal intensity**. Intensity is a direct function of the amount of pressure exerted by the *sound wave* (as opposed to air pressure, as generated by the respiratory system). As molecules vibrate from movement of the vocal folds, the molecular movement exerts an extremely small but measurable force over an area, and that is defined as pressure. The larger the excursion of the vibrating body, the greater the intensity of the signal produced, because air will be displaced with greater force. The next two sections deal with frequency and intensity of vocal fold vibration.

✔ *To summarize:*

- We must adduct the vocal folds to **initiate phonation**. This adduction may take several forms, including **breathy, simultaneous**, and **glottal attacks**.
- Conversational speech naturally encompasses all of these, although overuse of glottal attack in inappropriate contexts may be problematic.

- **Termination** of **phonation** requires abduction of the vocal folds, a process that must occur with the transition of voiced to voiceless speech sounds.
- **Sustained phonation** may take several forms, depending on the laryngeal configuration.
- **Modal phonation** will, by definition, characterize most speech.
- **Falsetto** occupies the upper range of laryngeal function, while **glottal fry** is found in the lower range.
- Vocal fold vibration varies for each of these phonatory modes, and the differences are governed by **laryngeal tension, medial compression**, and **subglottal pressure**.
- **Breathy phonation** occurs when there is inadequate medial compression to approximate the vocal folds. **Whispering** arises from tensing the vocal fold margins while holding the folds in a partially adducted position.

Frequency, Pitch, and Pitch Change

Pitch is the psychological correlate of frequency and is closely related to it: As frequency increases, pitch increases, and as frequency decreases, so does pitch. It is an important element in speech perception. Therefore, we should closely examine the mechanism of pitch change.

The vocal folds are made up of masses and elastic elements that tend to promote oscillation or repeated vibration at a particular frequency. Because of these qualities, the vocal folds will tend to vibrate at the same frequency when mass and elastic elements remain constant. However, the frequency of vibration will change when these characteristics are altered.

There are several important terms with which we should become familiar. Unfortunately, most of these terms refer to perceived pitch when they really should refer to physical **frequency**. Let us take a look at terms *optimal and habitual pitch*, *average fundamental frequency*, and *range of fundamental frequency*.

Optimal Pitch

The term **optimal pitch** is used to refer to the pitch (actually, the *frequency*) of vocal fold vibration that is optimal or most appropriate for an individual. This frequency of vibration will be the most efficient for a given pair of vocal folds and is a function of the mass and elasticity of the vocal folds. Some voice scientists and clinicians estimate optimal pitch directly from the individual's range of phonation, because it is considered to be approximately one-fourth octave above the lowest frequency of vibration of an individual. Others will estimate it from a cough or throat clearing, because the frequency of the vibrating vocal folds during throat clearing will

pitch: the psychological (perceptual) correlate of frequency of vibration

optimal pitch: the perceptual characteristic representing the ideal or most efficient frequency of vibration of the vocal folds

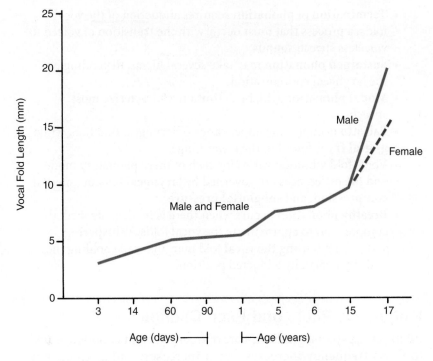

Figure 5-12. Changes in vocal fold length for males and females as a function of age. Note that males and females have essentially the same length of vocal folds until puberty, at which time both genders undergo marked physical development.
Source: (Data of Kaplan, 1971.)

An octave is a doubling of frequency, so that the octave beginning at 120 Hz will end at 240 Hz, the octave beginning at 203 Hz will end at 406 Hz, and so forth.

approximate conditions associated with conversational frequency, but without the psychological conditions associated with the use of phonation for communication.

Optimal pitch varies as a function of gender and age. You can expect an adult female to have a fundamental frequency of approximately 212 Hz during a reading task, whereas the optimal fundamental frequency for an adult male will be much lower, around 132 Hz, for the same task. The mean fundamental frequency will tend to be lower for spontaneous speech, and it tends to increase with each decade of life.

The reason for the difference in fundamental frequency between males and females has everything to do with tissue mass and length of the vocal folds. During puberty, males undergo a significant growth of muscles and cartilages, resulting in greater muscle mass in males than in females. The laryngeal product of this growth is the prominent Adam's apple you can see in boys that comes from the thyroid laminae joining at a more acute angle than that of the female larynx, as well as a significant drop in fundamental frequency arising from the increased mass of the folds (see Figure 5-12). Children will have a fundamental frequency in the vicinity of 300 Hz, but that rapidly changes in both boys and girls during puberty. Take a look at the Clinical Note on puberphonia to see what may occur when the fundamental frequency *does not* change with puberty.

Habitual Pitch

We use the term **habitual pitch** to refer to the frequency of vibration of vocal folds that is habitually used during speech. In the ideal condition, this would be the same as optimal pitch. For some individuals, there are compelling reasons to alter their everyday pitch in speech beyond the range expected for their age, size, or gender. Although the choice to use an abnormally higher or lower fundamental frequency is often not a conscious decision, it will have an effect on phonatory efficiency and effort. When the vocal folds are forced into the extremes of their range of ability, greater effort is required to sustain phonation, and this will result in vocal and physical fatigue. Many different techniques are used to estimate this from a speech sample, including asking the individual to sustain a vowel or sustain a vowel in a spoken word.

Average Fundamental Frequency

The **average fundamental frequency** of vibration of the vocal folds during phonation may reflect the frequency of vibration of *sustained phonation*, or some other condition, such as conversational speech. This actually reflects habitual pitch over a longer averaging period, and the use of conversational speech or reading of passages probably more accurately reflects an individual's true average rate of vocal fold vibration than a single vowel sample.

Pitch Range

Pitch range refers to the range of fundamental frequency for an individual and is calculated as the difference between the highest and lowest frequencies. The vocal mechanism is quite flexible and is capable of approximately two octaves of change in fundamental frequency from the lowest possible frequency to the highest. An individual with a low fundamental frequency of 90 Hz will be able to reach a high of about 360 Hz (octave 1 = 90 Hz to 180 Hz; octave 2 = 180 to 360 Hz). This range is often reduced by laryngeal pathology, such as, for example, vocal nodules. The normal range can be expanded through voice training. Let us examine how we make changes in vocal fundamental frequency, hence in perceived pitch.

Pitch-Changing Mechanism

Fundamental frequency increase comes from stretching and tensing the vocal folds using the cricothyroid and thyrovocalis muscles. Here is the mechanism of this change.

Laryngeal development

In Chapter 8 we will discuss the development of the larynx in the context of swallowing, but let us discuss some specific laryngeal changes that arise from birth to puberty. At birth, the vocal folds are approximately 4 mm long, as opposed to the adult length of between 12 and 15 mm. If you look at Figure 5-12, you can see the steady progression of vocal fold length as the individual develops. If you look now at the data of Kazarian et al. (1978), you can see the life-span development

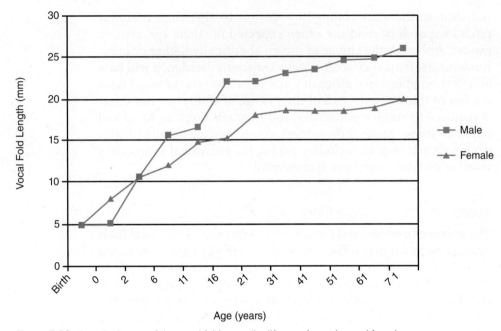

Figure 5-13. Length change of the vocal folds over the lifespan for males and females.

Source: (Drawn from the data of Kazarian, A. G., Sarkissian, L. S., & Isaakian, D. G. (1978). Length of the human vocal folds by age. Zhurnal Eksperimentalnoi Klinicheskoi Meditsiny, 18, 105–109.)

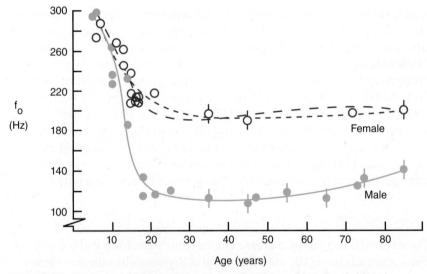

Figure 5-14. Fundamental frequency change over the lifespan for males and females.

Source: Adapted from Reference Manual for Communicative Sciences and Disorders: Speech and Language (p. 160), by R.D. Kent, 1994, Austin, TX: PRO-ED. Copyright 1994 by PRO-ED, Inc. Adapted with permission.

(Figure 5-13). Pay special attention to changes that occur between 11 and 16 years, when puberty begins. The vocal folds of both males and females increase in length but that of males become much longer. Take a look at Kent's (1976) plot of the vocal fundamental frequency of males and females from birth to adulthood (Figure 5-14), and you can clearly see the effect of this change. The fundamental frequency (denoted as f_0) tends to stabilize in adulthood. As you can see from this figure, when you spread out the adult range, males undergo a gradual increase in f_0 after age 50 or so, while females hold quite steady throughout life. You will also see that the average male f_0 is around 130 Hz at 20 years, increasing to about 140 Hz at 80 years of age. Females, on the other hand, hold steady at around 190 Hz throughout adult life.

In Chapter 4 we discussed the importance of a viable respiratory source for phonation. It should not surprise you, then, to know that as our respiratory function matures our ability to sustain phonation increases as well. Kent (1994) demonstrated that males and females both show a rather steady increase in the ability to sustain phonation. At 3 years of age a child can sustain a vowel for around 7 seconds, but that ability climbs by about 1.4 seconds per year through young adulthood (till around 17 years of age). By 17, an adolescent should be able to sustain a vowel for 26 seconds or so, although the variability in function is quite large at all ranges.

Tension, Length, and Mass. The changeable elements of the vocal folds are tension, length, and mass. We cannot actually change the mass of the vocal folds, but we can change the mass per unit length by spreading the muscle, mucosa, and ligament out over more distance. We can also change the tension of the vocal folds by stretching them tighter or relaxing them. Both of these changes arise from elongation.

When the cricothyroid muscle is contracted, the thyroid tilts down, lengthening the vocal folds and increasing the fundamental frequency. When the tension on the vocal folds is increased, the natural frequency of vibration will increase.

The thyrovocalis is a tenser of the vocal folds as well, because contraction of this muscle will pull both cricoid and thyroid closer together, an action opposed by the simultaneously contracted cricothyroid. This tensing process must be opposed by contraction of the posterior cricoarytenoid, although it is not classified as a tenser of the vocal folds. The posterior cricoarytenoid is invested with **muscle spindles**, structures responsible for monitoring and maintaining tonic muscle length. As the length of this muscle changes, its length may be reflexively controlled to compensate for the stretching force on the vocal folds.

These tensers tend to operate together, but for slightly different functions. It is currently believed that the cricothyroid contracts to approximate the degree of tension required for a given frequency of vibration. The thyrovocalis appears to fine-tune this adjustment. That is, the cricothyroid makes the gross adjustment, and the thyrovocalis causes the fine movement.

We have still not dealt with mass changes. As the mass of a vibrating body decreases, frequency of vibration will increase. The mass of the vocal folds is constant, because to actually increase or decrease mass would require growth of tissue or atrophy, and neither of which occurs quickly. Instead, the mass is rearranged by lengthening. When the vocal folds are stretched by contraction of the tensers, the mass of the folds will be distributed over a greater distance, thus reducing mass per unit length.

The natural frequency of vibration refers to the frequency at which a body vibrates given the mass, tension, and elastic properties of the body.

See Chapter 12 for a discussion of the muscle spindle.

The effect of the lengthening and tensing actions is to make vocal folds longer and thinner in appearance. Interestingly, there is evidence that the vocal folds do not lengthen continuously as fundamental frequency increases, but rather that, at some point near or in the falsetto range, the vocal folds again begin to shorten as frequency increases (Nishizawa, Sawashima, & Yonemoto, 1988). Others have found that increased medial compression may effectively shorten the vibrating surface, increasing frequency (Van den Berg & Tan, 1959).

Lowering fundamental frequency requires the opposite manipulation. As mass per unit length increases and tension decreases, fundamental frequency will decrease. We relax the vocal folds by shortening them, moving the cricoid and thyroid closer together in front. This process is achieved by contraction of the thyromuscularis. When it contracts, the vocal folds are relaxed and shortened so that they become more massive and less tense. It appears that there is help from some of the suprahyoid musculature that indirectly pulls up on the thyroid cartilage, shortening the vocal folds by distancing the thyroid from the cricoid.

Subglottal Pressure and Fundamental Frequency. There are also changes in subglottal pressure that must be reckoned with. Increasing pitch requires increasing the tension of the system, thereby increasing the glottal resistance to airflow. If airflow is to remain constant through the glottis, pressure must increase. It appears, however, that the increases in subglottal pressure are a *response* to the increased tension required for frequency change rather than its *cause*. Subglottal pressure does increase, but the primary influence on fundamental frequency change is muscular tension (Titze, 1994). It is a delicate balancing act that we perform. It appears that the cricothyroid and posterior cricoarytenoid tense the vocal folds, while the thyroarytenoid (thyromuscularis + thyrovocalis) increased medial contact of the vocal folds (Chhetri, Neurbauer, & Berry, 2012).

✔ *To summarize:*

- **Pitch** is the psychological correlate of frequency of vibration, although the term has come into common usage when referring to phenomena associated with the physical vibration of the vocal folds.
- **Optimal pitch** refers to the frequency of vibration that is most efficient for a given pair of vocal folds, and **habitual pitch** is the frequency of vibration habitually used by an individual.
- The **pitch range** of an individual will span approximately two octaves, although it will be reduced by pathology and may be increased through vocal training.
- Changes in **vocal fundamental frequency** are governed by the tension of the vocal folds and their mass per unit length.
- Increasing the length of the vocal folds will increase vocal fold tension as well as decrease the mass per unit area. This will increase the fundamental frequency.

- The **respiratory system** will respond to increased vocal fold tension with **increased subglottal pressure**, so that pitch and subglottal pressure tend to covary.
- Increased subglottal pressure is a response to increased vocal fold tension.

Intensity and Intensity Change

Just as pitch is the psychological correlate of frequency, **loudness** is the psychological correlate of intensity. **Intensity** (or its correlate, sound pressure level) is the physical measure of power (or pressure) ratios, but loudness is how we perceive power or pressure differences. As with pitch, there is a close relationship between loudness and intensity.

To increase vocal intensity of the vibrating vocal folds, one must somehow increase the vigor with which the vocal folds open and close. In sustained phonation, the vocal folds move only as a result of the air pressure beneath them and the flow between them. Subglottal pressure and flow provide the energy for this vocal engine, so to increase the intensity or strength of the phonatory product we will have to increase the energy that drives it. We increase subglottal pressure to increase vocal intensity. To prove this to yourself, do the following. You need to feel what you do to produce loud speech. You may be in a quiet setting right now and you really may not want to yell, but that is fine. Pay attention to your lungs and larynx as you *prepare to yell as loudly as you can* to someone across the room. Without even yelling, you should have been able to feel your lungs take in a large charge of air, and you should have also felt your vocal folds tighten up. These are the two steps of significance for increasing vocal intensity: increased subglottal pressure and medial compression.

Subglottal pressure and increased medial compression vary together, but the causal relationship is better established for vocal intensity than for the tension–pressure relationship for pitch. For intensity to increase, the energy source must also increase, so subglottal pressure must rise. To explain the effect that medial compression has on vocal intensity requires a return to the discussion of a cycle of vocal fold vibration.

We can break a cycle of vibration into stages, such as an **opening stage**, in which the vocal folds are opening up; a **closing stage**, in which the vocal folds are returning to the point of approximation; and a **closed stage**, in which there is no air escaping between the vocal folds (see Figure 5-15 and Figure 5-16). In modal phonation at conversational intensities, it has been found that the vocal folds spend about 50 percent of their time in the opening phase, 37 percent of the time in the closing phase, and 13 percent of the cycle completely closed. When the vocal folds are tightly adducted for increased vocal intensity, they tend to return to the closed position more quickly and to stay closed for a longer period of time. The opening phase reduces to approximately 33 percent, while the closed phase increases to more than 30 percent, depending on the intensity increase.

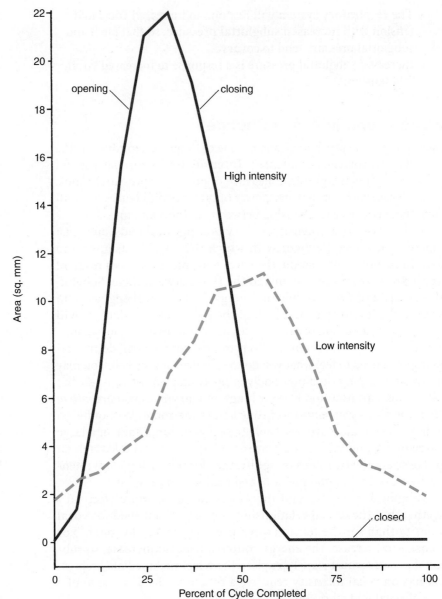

Figure 5-15. Effect of vocal intensity on vocal fold vibration. During low-intensity speech the opening and closing phases occupy most of the vibratory cycle, as revealed in the area of the glottis. During high-intensity speech the opening phase is greatly compressed, as is the closing phase, while the time spent in the closed phase is greatly increased.
Source: (Data from Fletcher, 1950.)

The concept you should retain is this: To increase vocal intensity, the vocal folds are tightly compressed, it takes more force to blow them open, they close more rapidly, and they tend to stay closed because they are tightly compressed. This is the *cause* side of the equation. The *effect* portion is that, because so much energy is required to hold the folds in compression, the release of the folds from this condition is markedly stronger. Each time the folds open, they do so with vigor, producing an explosive compression of the air medium. The harder that eruption of the vocal folds is, the greater is the amplitude of the cycle of vibration. Remembering that as the amplitude of the

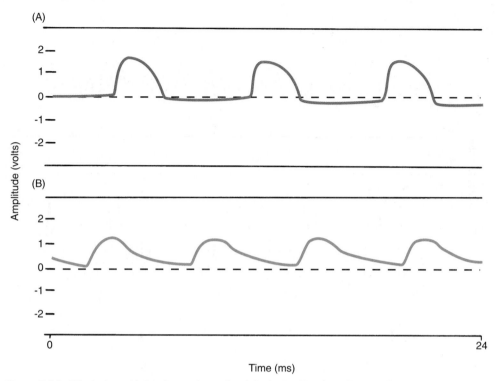

Figure 5-16. Effect of vocal intensity, as shown through electroglottographic trace. The electroglottograph measures impedance across the vocal folds, and the peak represents the closed phase of the glottal cycle. (A) Conversational-level sustained vowel. (B) High-level sustained vowel.
© Cengage Learning®.

signal increases, so does the intensity, you will recognize the increase in intensity between the two panels of Figure 5-17.

The two waveforms in Figure 5-17 are different in intensity, but not in frequency. The time between the cycles is exactly the same, so the frequency must be the same. From this comes a very important point: Intensity and frequency are controlled independently, and you can increase intensity without increasing frequency. Here is the paradox. Increases in intensity and fundamental frequency depend upon the same basic mechanism (tension/compression and subglottal pressure), so it is difficult to increase intensity without increasing pitch, but trained or well-controlled speakers can do this. The tendency is for frequency and intensity to increase together, which is a natural process that you can demonstrate to yourself. Find a place where you can shout, and then say a word before shouting it. Your pitch will most certainly go up when you shout, unless you try very hard to avoid it.

The relationship between subglottal pressure and the actual sound pressure level output of the vocal folds depends on the speaker. However, it appears that for every doubling of subglottal pressure, there is an increase of between 8 and 12 decibels in vocal intensity. Plant and Younger (2000) found that this relationship breaks down for some individuals, with marked changes in intensity without

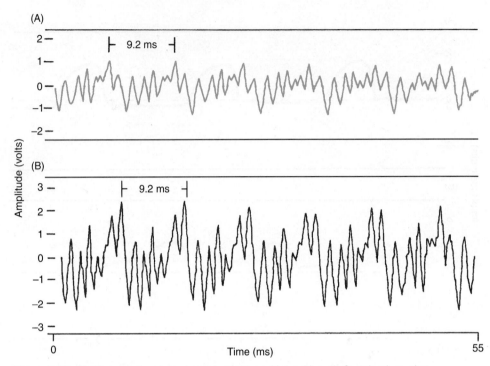

Figure 5-17. Oscillogram of sustained vowel at two vocal intensities. (A) Sustained vowel at conversational level. (B) Sustained vowel at increased vocal intensity. Although the vocal intensity increases, the period of each cycle of vibration remains constant at 9.2 milliseconds.
© Cengage Learning®.

corresponding subglottal pressure changes, dependent upon the fundamental frequency. It would appear that we, as humans, are capable of solving physical problems in multiple ways. Don't despair for lack of simple answers to complex questions: This represents what many refer to as the "degree of freedom" problem. Given multiple degrees of flexibility in a system (in this case, the ability to simultaneously manipulate subglottal pressure, muscular tension, and adductory force), the "problem" of intensity control can be "solved" through various combinations of the tools at hand.

✔ *To summarize:*

- **Vocal intensity** refers to the increase in sound pressure of the speech signal.
- To increase vocal intensity of phonation, a speaker must increase **medial compression** through the muscles of adduction.
- This increased adductory force requires greater **subglottal pressure** to produce phonation and forces the vocal folds to remain in the closed portion of the phonatory cycle for a longer period of time.
- The increased **laryngeal tension** required for increasing intensity can also increase the vocal fundamental frequency, although the trained voice is quite capable of controlling fundamental frequency and vocal intensity independently.

CLINICAL CONSIDERATIONS

The phonatory mechanism is extraordinarily sensitive to the physical well-being of a speaker. When individuals are ill, their voices often get weak and, in the case of upper respiratory problems, "rough." Diseases that weaken individuals also tend to compromise phonatory effort, so that the voice weakens in intensity, and pitch range is reduced. Increasing muscle tension for pitch and intensity variation requires work, and illness tends to reduce the ability to exert such forces. A number of neuromuscular diseases have been shown to affect phonation, and many methods of measuring phonatory stability and ability have gained clinical acceptance.

Frequency perturbation is a measure of cycle-by-cycle variability in phonation. Perturbation, or **vocal jitter**, provides an exquisite index of muscle tone and stability but requires instrumentation for measurement. The client is asked to sustain a vowel as steadily as possible while it is recorded on computer. Following this, the computer program measures each cycle of vibration and calculates how closely each cycle corresponds to the next in duration. The computer measures the duration of the first cycle (e.g., 10.2 ms), and subtracts it from that of the next cycle (e.g., 10.4 ms) and stores that number. It performs this for all succeeding cycles of vibration and calculates the average of the (unsigned) differences as compared with the average period of vibration. The resulting percent of perturbation (or percent jitter) is an indication of how perfectly this imperfect system is oscillating. The broad rule of thumb is that variation in excess of 1–2 percent will be perceived as hoarse. This is a good measure of client change over time and a less effective means of comparing between clients.

This measure has been shown to be sensitive to a number of characteristics. Individuals who are more physically fit will have lower perturbation values than those who are not. Individuals with **neuromotor dysfunction** (neurological conditions that affect motor function) will have higher perturbation than healthy individuals. Increased mass (such as vocal nodules and laryngeal polyps) will increase perturbation (Jiang, Zhang, MacCallum, Sprecher, & Zhou, 2009), while therapy to reduce the mass will result in a decrease in the jitter.

More prosaic measures do not require this degree of instrumentation, but nonetheless provide insight into the phonatory function. The process of assessment often requires us to stress the system under examination so that its weakness can be seen with relation to normal abilities. Kent, Kent, and Rosenbek (1987) provided an excellent overview of methods of stressing the phonatory system.) As mentioned earlier, **maximum phonation time** refers to the duration an individual is capable of sustaining a phonation. Sustained phonation provides an index of phonatory-plus-respiratory efficiency. You can examine the respiratory system by itself, to determine the ability of your client to sustain expiration in the absence of voicing, and have some confidence that length and steadiness of a sustained vowel are an indicator of laryngeal function (Kurtz & Cielo, 2010).

vocal jitter: cycle-by-cycle variation in fundamental frequency of vibration

Another time-honored measure is the diadochokinetic rate. **Oral diadochokinesis** refers to the alternation of articulators (you may hear it referred to as *alternating motor rate* as well). Specifically, it is the number of productions of a single or multiple syllables an individual produces per second. This is an excellent tool for assessing the articulators (the topic of Chapter 6 and Chapter 7), but also helps the assessment of the coordination of phonatory and articulatory systems.

As mentioned earlier, pathological conditions often have an impact on vocal range and vocal intensity. For instance, the presence of vocal nodules may reduce an individual's vocal range from two octaves to one-half octave or less, and the breathy component will have a real impact on vocal intensity. Similarly, physical weakness may limit a client's ability to exert effort for either pitch or vocal intensity change.

The exquisitely sensitive vocal mechanism is an excellent window to the health and well-being of a client, as you will find in your advanced studies of voice.

LINGUISTIC ASPECTS OF PITCH AND INTENSITY

suprasegmental: parameters of speech that include prosody, pitch, and loudness changes for meaning

prosody: the system of stress used to vary the meaning in speech

Pitch and intensity play significant roles in the suprasegmental aspects of communication. **Suprasegmental** elements are the parameters of speech that are above the segment (phonetic) level. This term generally refers to elements of **prosody**, the system of stress used to vary meaning in speech. The prosodic elements include pitch, intonation, loudness, stress, duration, and rhythm; these elements not only convey a great deal of information concerning emotion and intent but also provide information that can disambiguate meaning.

Prosody and Neuromuscular Disorder

The prosodic element of speech can be a window to speech physiology in neuropathology. *Prosody* is the combination of changes in fundamental frequency, vocal intensity, and duration that produce linguistically relevant intonation and stress characteristics. When the neuromuscular system is compromised, prosody may be affected. When muscle tone increases (hypertonus) due to spasticity, the individual may demonstrate prosody characterized by even and equal stress with inappropriately high vocal intensity on each syllable or word, in combination with a harsh phonatory quality.

When an individual has ataxic signs from cerebellar damage, she will have disrupted prosody from the discoordination of respiratory, phonatory, and articulatory systems. Speech syllable timing will be defective, and the control of phonatory elements will be seriously deficient.

In many of the hyperkinetic dysarthrias, the element of speech control is overridden by movements of speech structures that are involuntary and uncontrollable. In these cases, prosody will be serious.

Even though it is not the purpose of an anatomy text to delve into these suprasegmental elements, pitch and intensity play such a heavy role that we should at least glance at them.

Intonation refers to the changes in pitch during speech, whereas **stress** refers to syllable or word emphasis relative to an entire utterance. For example, say the following sentence out loud: "That's a cat." You end it with a falling *intonation* and put more *stress* on "that's" than on "a" or "cat." To a large extent, these elements both arise out of variation in vocal intensity and fundamental frequency. Intonation may be considered the melodic envelope that contains the sentence and may serve to mark the sentence type. Generally, statements tend to have falling intonation at the end; questions tend to have rising intonation. Figure 5-18 shows traces of the fundamental frequency for the productions of "Bev bombed Bob." and "Bev bombed Bob?" If you say these two sentences, you can hear for yourself the changes that are so strong in the second sentence. Hirano, Ohala, and Vennard (1969) used this sentence contrast to show that the lateral cricoarytenoid, thyrovocalis, and cricothyroid were all quite active in making these rapid laryngeal adjustments.

Stress helps punctuate speech, providing emphasis to syllables or words through both intensity and frequency changes. To increase stress, we increase the fundamental frequency and intensity by increasing subglottal pressure, medial compression, and laryngeal tension. As you will remember from our earlier discussion, changes in both frequency and intensity involve adjustments of these variables. We capitalize on the fact that both intensity and fundamental frequency vary together, so stressed syllables or words will show changes in both. If you look at the pitch and intensity traces of Figure 5-19, you can see how they vary together.

The musculature involved in stress is not unlike that of intonation, although we must factor in the increase in subglottal pressure. The changes in fundamental frequency will be to the order of 50 Hz

intonation: the melody of speech, provided by variation of the fundamental frequency during speech

stress: the product of relative increase in fundamental frequency, vocal intensity, and duration

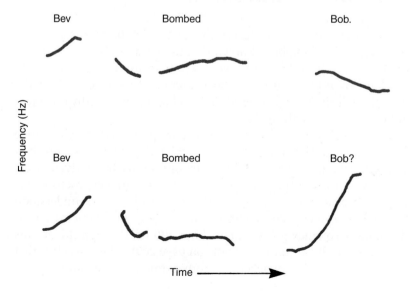

Figure 5-18. Fundamental frequency fluctuation for declarative statement and question form. Note the difference in falling and rising intonation between these two sentence forms.

© Cengage Learning®.

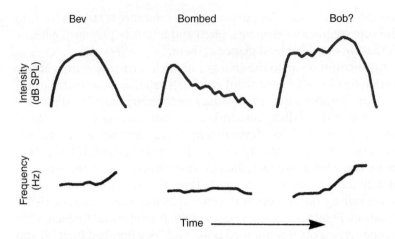

Figure 5-19. Fundamental frequency and intensity changes during production of a question form.
© Cengage Learning®.

(Netsell, 1973), governed by the lateral cricoarytenoid, the thyrovocalis, and the cricothyroid. The changes in subglottal pressure will be small but rapid, or pulsatile (Hixon, 1973). Because they require bursts of increased expiratory force, they will be driven by expiratory muscles.

Although stress and intonation are not *essential* for communication, they *are* essential for naturalness. Clearly you can speak in a **monopitch** (unvarying vocal pitch) or **monoloud** voice (unvarying vocal loudness), but the effect is so distracting that it certainly interferes with communication. You may find individuals with neurological impairments who show both of these characteristics. Treatment directed toward increasing muscular effort at points requiring stress will greatly enhance the naturalness of speech, because increasing vocal effort at these points will inevitably increase both fundamental frequency and vocal intensity.

monopitch: without variation in vocal pitch (the perception of frequency)

monoloud: without variation in vocal loudness (the perception of vocal intensity)

THEORIES OF PHONATION

The history of theories of vocal fold vibration is long and colorful, leading certainly from Helmholtz of the 1800s to the present. Although it has long been known that the vocal folds are the source of voicing, only recently did we develop an understanding of the mechanism of phonation, and refinements continue. Certainly, the underlying principles discussed in this chapter are broadly accepted, although it has not always been so.

An early battle arose within the field of speech science when some researchers questioned whether the vocal folds vibrated as a result of direct stimulation of the intrinsic laryngeal muscles (active muscle contraction). The theory that proposed this view (the neurochronaxic theory of vocal fold vibration) was abandoned when it was understood that the neuromuscular system was not capable of producing a fundamental frequency greater than about 200 Hz through this means (Herbst et al., 2012) (see boxed note on page 269). It became clear that some version of the myoelastic-aerodynamic theory would explain vocal fold dynamics. As discussed earlier, the myoelastic-aerodynamic theory of phonation states that vibration of the vocal folds depends on the elements embodied in the name of the theory. The myoelastic element is the elastic component of muscle (*myo* = muscle) and the associated soft tissues of the larynx, and the aerodynamic component is that of the airflow and pressure through this constricted tube. Van den Berg (1958) recognized that the combination of tissue elasticity, which causes the vocal folds to return to their original position after being distended, and the Bernoulli effect, which helps promote this return by dropping the pressure at the constriction, could account for the sustained vibration shown in even a cadaverous specimen provided with an artificial source of expiratory charge.

Work by Hirano and Kakita (1983) and expanded by Titze (1994) has sought to explain how complex acoustic output can come from a simple oscillator such as the vocal folds. We have long recognized that the vocal folds are not simple oscillators, but rather undulate in the modes discussed earlier. Titze recognized that this complex vibration arises from the loosely bound masses associated with the membranous **cover** of the vocal folds (the epithelium and superficial layer of the lamina propria) and the **body** of the vocal folds (the intermediate and deep layers of lamina propria and thyrovocalis muscle). The loosely bound elastic tissue supports oscillation, and viewing the soft tissue as an infinite (or at least uncountable) number of masses reveals that a very large number of modes of vibration is possible. This discussion in no way does justice to the elegance of this theory, and we recommend that you take time for the exceptionally readable work of Titze.

The phonatory mechanism is an important component of the speaking mechanism, providing the voiced source for speech. It is time for us to see what happens to the voice source after it leaves the larynx. See Chapter 6 for a continuation of this story.

Laryngeal Stridor

aryngeal stridor refers to a harsh sound produced during respiration. The sound is associated with some obstruction in the respiratory passageway and is always a sign of dysfunction. Stridor may arise from a growth in the larynx or trachea causing turbulence during respiration, or it may arise from the vocal folds. If the vocal folds are paralyzed in the adducted position (**abductor paralysis**), they will not only obstruct the airway but will also vibrate as the air of inspiration passes by them. In this case, the harsh sound will be referred to as **inhalatory stridor**. You may want to imitate this in yourself so that you will come to recognize this sign of obstruction. Phonate while breathing out, and then, without abducting your vocal folds, force your inspiration through the closed vocal folds. You will notice not only a harsh sound but also the extreme difficulty of inhaling through an obstruction, pressure to produce phonation, and this forces the vocal folds to remain in the closed portion of the phonatory cycle for a longer time. The increased laryngeal tension will increase the vocal fundamental frequency as well, although the fundamental frequency and vocal intensity may be controlled independently.

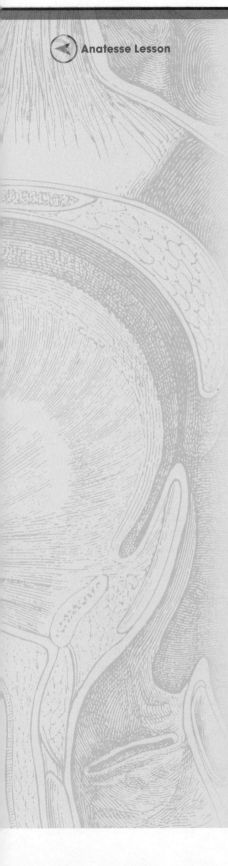

Anatesse Lesson

CHAPTER SUMMARY

Frequency of vibration of sound is measured in cycles per second, abbreviated Hz. The intensity of sound is measured in decibels, which represent a ratio of pressures or powers, expressed logarithmically. Instrumentation for phonation includes the sound level meter for intensity, various instruments for measurement of fundamental frequency, as well as vocal jitter and vocal shimmer. The phonetogram shows the interaction of intensity and frequency in an individual's speech. The electroglottograph is a useful tool for estimating vocal fold contact during phonation, while the nasoendoscope allows viewing the vocal folds during phonation.

Phonation is the product of vibrating vocal folds within the larynx. The vocal folds vibrate as air flows past them, capitalizing on the Bernoulli phenomenon and tissue elasticity to maintain phonation. The interaction of subglottal pressure, tissue elasticity, and constriction within the airflow caused by the vocal folds produces sustained phonation as long as pressure, flow, and vocal fold approximation are maintained.

The larynx is an important structure for a number of non-speech functions as well, including coughing, throat clearing, and abdominal fixation. The degree of muscle control during phonation is greatly increased, however, because the successful use of voice requires careful attention to vocal fold tension and length.

Adduction takes several forms, including breathy, simultaneous, and glottal attacks, and termination of phonation requires abduction of the vocal folds. Sustained phonation depends on the laryngeal configuration. The modal pattern of phonation is most efficient, capitalizing on the optimal combination of muscular tension and respiratory support for the vocal folds. The falsetto requires increased vocal fold tension, and glottal fry demands a unique glottal and respiratory configuration. Each of these modes of vocal fold vibration is different, and the variations are governed by laryngeal tension, medial compression, and subglottal pressure. Breathy phonation occurs when there is inadequate medial compression to approximate the vocal folds, and whispering results from tensing the vocal fold margins while holding the folds partially adducted.

Pitch is the psychological correlate of the frequency of vibration, and loudness is the correlate of intensity, although both of the terms *pitch* and *intensity* have been used to represent physical phenomena. Optimal pitch is the most efficient frequency of vibration for a given pair of vocal folds, and habitual pitch is the frequency of vibration used by an individual habitually. The pitch range of an individual will span approximately two octaves but can be reduced by pathology or increased through vocal training.

Vocal fundamental frequency changes are governed by vocal fold tension and mass per unit length. To increase the fundamental

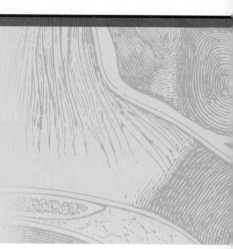

frequency, we increase the length of the vocal folds, which will increase the tension of the vocal folds and decrease the mass per unit length. To compensate for increased tension, subglottal pressure will increase.

Medial compression is increased to produce an increase in vocal intensity of phonation, and this is performed largely through the muscles of adduction. Increased adductory force requires greater subglottal pressure to produce phonation, and this forces the vocal folds to remain in the closed portion of the phonatory cycle for a longer time. The increased laryngeal tension will increase the vocal fundamental frequency as well, although the fundamental frequency and vocal intensity may be controlled independently.

Media Connection

Go to the accompanying online resources at CengageBrain.com and have fun learning! Study with the Anatesse software program, play games, view animations and videos, and take practice tests to help reinforce the key concepts you learned in this chapter.

Decibel practice activity

This was produced through a grant funded by the Fund for Improvement of Postsecondary Education (FIPSE), No. P116B90965-90. Seikel, J. A. (1990–1992). Project to Enhance Graduate and Undergraduate Education in Speech and Hearing Sciences. Department of Education: Fund for the Improvement of Postsecondary Education (FIPSE; $93,234).

This activity involves practice working with exponents, logarithms, and finally figuring the decibel.

A. **EXPONENTS AND LOGARITHMS:**

If you are comfortable with exponents and logarithms, go directly to the next page and do the problems marked "FIGURING EXPONENTS AND LOGARITHMS." Otherwise, continue reading.

An exponent is the power to which a number is raised. For instance, 2 is the exponent in 4^2 (4 squared, which is 4×4, which $= 16$)

1. What are the exponents and answers below?

exponent	answer		exponent	answer
$4^2 =$ _____	_____		$10^3 =$ _____	_____
$2^3 =$ _____	_____		$10^2 =$ _____	_____
$3^3 =$ _____	_____		$10^5 =$ _____	_____
$4^6 =$ _____	_____		$10^1 =$ _____	_____

The exponent tells the number of times you will multiply an item times itself:

$3^2 = 3 \times 3 = 9$

$4^2 = 4 \times 4 = 16$

$3^3 = 3 \times 3 \times 3 = 27$

$5^3 = 5 \times 5 \times 5 = 125$

Logarithms (LOGS) are exponents (in our work we will only talk about logarithms to the base 10, so relax. It will be presented as log10, which means to take the base 10 logarithm of a number).

I know that $10^3 = 10 \times 10 \times 10 = 1000$

So, the Log_{10} of 1000 = 3: That is, the "exponent for 10" to give me 1000 is 3. Or I could say, the "power to which I must raise 10 to get 1000 is 3."

Figure the logarithms$_{10}$ (log_{10}) for the following:

$log_{10} (1000) = $ _____ $log_{10} (10,000) = $ _____

$log_{10} (100) = $ _____ $log_{10} (100,000) = $ _____

$log_{10} (100,000) = $ _____ $log_{10} (1,000,000) = $ _____

So, by now you should see that if the exponent is a whole number, the log_{10} will be the number of zeroes after the "1."

Figure a few more:

$log_{10} (10,000,000) = $ _____

$log_{10} (100,000,000) = $ _____

$log_{10} (10) = $ _____

If you have a logarithm key on your calculator, you are all set. If not, you may count zeroes.
"FIGURING EXPONENTS AND LOGARITHMS"

What are the exponents in the following?

$2^2 = $ $9^4 = $

$3^4 = $ $6^3 = $

$6^{10} = $ $10^1 = $

$7^5 = $ $41^2 = $

$8^1 = $ $15^6 = $

Determine the logarithms (log_{10}) in the following statements:

$log_{10} (1000) = $ _____ $log_{10} (10) = $ _____

$log_{10} (100) = $ _____ $log_{10} (1,000,000) = $ _____

$log_{10} (100,000) = $ _____ $log_{10} (10,000) = $ _____

II. dB SPL Problems

　A. Figure dB SPL in the following examples. If you have a calculator that will figure Logarithms, this could be fun. If your group does not have a calculator, do those which marked "no calculator" until you can flag me down and I will loan you mine.

　　Note: If your calculator only calculates natural logarithms (ln), then simply multiply the result times .4343: that is, log10 = ln * .4343

　　Example for figuring dB SPL

　　　dB SPL = 20 log10 (Pressure$_{out}$/Pressure$_{ref}$)

　　　Given a pressure output = 2,000,000 micropascals

　　　dB SPL = 20 log10 (2,000,000 micropascals / 20 micropascals)

　　　　　= 20 log10 (100,000)

　　　　　　(*Note*: count zeroes to get log10)

　　　　　= 20(5)

　　　　　= 100 dB SPL

1. No calculator: Given pressure output = 200 micropascals. Figure dB SPL
   (Answer: 20 dB SPL)

2. No Calculator: Given pressure output = 2,000 micropascals. Figure dB SPL
   (Answer: 40 dB SPL)

3. No Calculator: Given pressure output = 20,000 micropascals. Figure dB SPL
   (Answer: 60 dB SPL)

4. Given pressure output = 200,000,000 micropascals. Figure dB SPL
   (Answer: 140 dB SPL)

B. **SPL: More Complex Examples**

   Given 12,000,000 micropascals as output. Figure dB SPL

   $$x \text{ dB SPL} = 20 \log 10 \, (\text{PRESSURE}_{out}/\text{PRESSURE}_{ref})$$
   $$= 20 \log 10 \, (12{,}000{,}000 \text{ micropascals} / 20 \text{ micropascals})$$
   $$= 20 \log 10 \, (600{,}000)$$
   $$= 20 \times 5.778$$
   $$= 115.56 \text{ db SPL}$$

   1. Calculator: Figure dB SPL with Pressure$_{out}$ = 346,000 micropascals
      (Answer = 84.7 dB SPL)

   2. No Calculator: Figure dB SPL with Pressure$_{out}$ = 200,000 micropascals
      (Answer = 80 dB SPL)

   3. Calculator: Figure dB SPL with Pressure$_{out}$ = 25,000 micropascals
      (Answer = 61.9 dB SPL)

   4. No Calculator: Figure dB SPL with Pressure$_{out}$ = 20,000 micropascals
      (Answer = 60 dB SPL)

   5. Calculator: Figure dB SPL with Pressure$_{out}$ = 486,000 micropascals
      (Answer = 87.71 dB SPL)

   6. No Calculator: Figure dB SPL with Pressure$_{out}$ = 2,000,000 micropascals
      (Answer = 100 dB SPL)

   7. Calculator: output = 17,022 micropascals. Figure dB SPL.
      (Answer = 58.59 dB SPL)

   8. No Calculator: output = 2,000 micropascals. Figure dB SPL.
      (Answer = 40 dB SPL)

II. dB Increase and decrease (a really useful thing to learn! e.g., reading from an oscilloscope trace)

A. **Example: You measure a sine wave, = 3 volts, zero-to-peak.**

B. **After raising the volume control (or lowering attenuation) you measure the output voltage to be 96 V.**

C. **What is the change in dB?**

   $$x \text{ dB} = 20 \log 10 \, (\text{volts}_{output}/\text{volts}_{reference}) = 20 \log 10 (96 \text{ volts}/3 \text{ volts})$$
   $$= 20 \log 10 \, (32 \text{ volts})$$
   $$= 20 \, (1.505)$$
   $$= 30.1 \text{ dB re: 3 volt reference (or dB increase)}$$

So if your original signal was 10 dB SPL, this new output signal is 40 dB SPL (assuming a perfect world).

1. Given an initial reading of 11.3 V (your reference) you raise the sound output and get a reading of 431 V. What is dB change?
   (Answer: 31.62 dB re: 11.3 V)

2. Given an initial reading of 640 V, you turn the loudness control down and get an output of 21 V. How many dB did you drop?
   (Answer: –29.68 dB re: 640 V)

3. You measure a sine wave from an audiometer. The dial says 20 dB (which you know is HL), and you read a voltage on your oscilloscope of 46 V at 20 dB. What is the voltage if you turn the audiometer up 6 dB? (hint: remember that voltage is the correlate of pressure. What happens to dB when you double pressure?).
   (Answer: 92 V)

4. Given an initial voltage of 3 volts. You increase the volume control and now read 300 V. What is the dB difference?
   (Answer: 40 dB re: 3 V)

5. You turn on the radio and measure .006 volts. After cranking it up until it parts your hair you measure output as 600 volts. How many dB have you increased the signal?
   (Answer: 100 dB re: .006 V)

6. Your upstairs neighbor has his stereo set to a mind-boggling level. After verbally assaulting him, you slap an oscilloscope on the speaker leads and get a reading of 43 volts. After he turns it down under protest it reads .00043 volts. How many dB did you drop the intensity? (hint: 43 volts is your reference).
   (Answer: –100 dB re: 43 V)

   FINISHED!

Study Questions

1. _____ is the process of capturing air within the thorax to provide the muscles with a structure against which to push or pull.

2. In _____ attack, the vocal folds are adducted prior to initiation of expiratory flow.

3. In _____ attack, the vocal folds are adducted after the initiation of expiratory flow.

4. In _____ attack, the vocal folds are adducted simultaneous with the initiation of expiratory flow.

5. During modal phonation, the vocal folds will open from _____ (inferior/superior) to (inferior/superior). The folds will close from _____ (inferior/superior) to _____ (inferior/superior).

6. The minimum subglottal driving pressure for speech is _____ cm H_2O.

7. In the mode of vibration known as _____, the vocal folds vibrate at a much lower rate than in modal phonation, and the folds exhibit a syncopated vibratory pattern.

8. In the mode of vibration known as _____, the vocal folds lengthen and become extremely thin and "reedlike."

9. Presence of vocal nodules or other space-occupying laryngeal pathology may result in _____ phonation.

10. To increase vocal intensity, one must _____ (increase/decrease) subglottal pressure and _____ (increase/decrease) medial compression.

11. To increase vocal fundamental frequency, one must _____ vocal fold tension by _____ (lengthening/shortening) the vocal folds.

12. _____ refers to the pitch of phonation that is most appropriate for an individual.

13. _____ refers to the vocal pitch that is habitually used during speech.

14. As vocal intensity increases, the closed phase of the vibratory cycle _____ (increases/decreases).

15. We had occasion to record the speech of an individual with a maxillary fistula secondary to squamous cell carcinoma. The cancerous condition had required removal of part of her maxilla, which meant that the oral cavity was continuous with the nasal cavity. While working with the physician who was fitting her for an oral prosthesis, we recorded her speech, only to find that when speech was produced with the open fistula, the fundamental frequency was highly irregular, but became regular again when the oral prosthesis was in place. What could be the link between the vocal folds and the oral-nasal communication?

Study Question Answers

1. **ABDOMINAL** or **THORACIC FIXATION** is the process of capturing air within the thorax to provide the muscles with a structure against which to push or pull.

2. In **GLOTTAL** attack, the vocal folds are adducted prior to initiation of expiratory flow.

3. In **BREATHY** attack, the vocal folds are adducted after the initiation of expiratory flow.

4. In **SIMULTANEOUS** attack, the vocal folds are adducted simultaneous with the initiation of expiratory flow.

5. During modal phonation, the vocal folds will open from **INFERIOR** to **SUPERIOR**. The folds will close from **INFERIOR** to **SUPERIOR**.

6. The minimum subglottal driving pressure for speech is **3–5** cm H_2O.

7. In the mode of vibration known as **GLOTTAL FRY**, the vocal folds vibrate at a much lower rate than in modal phonation, and the folds exhibit a syncopated vibratory pattern.

8. In the mode of vibration known as **FALSETTO**, the vocal folds lengthen and become extremely thin and "reedlike."

9. Presence of vocal nodules or other space-occupying laryngeal pathology may result in **BREATHY** phonation.

10. To increase vocal intensity, one must **INCREASE** subglottal pressure and **INCREASE** medial compression.

11. To increase vocal fundamental frequency, one must **INCREASE** vocal fold tension by **LENGTHENING** the vocal folds.

12. **OPTIMAL PITCH** refers to the pitch of phonation that is most appropriate for an individual.

13. **HABITUAL PITCH** refers to the vocal pitch that is habitually used during speech.

14. As vocal intensity increases, the closed phase of the vibratory cycle **INCREASES**.

15. The vocal folds vibrate as a function of the transglottal pressure drop: The subglottal pressure is higher than the supraglottal (oral) pressure, so air flows through the glottis and the vocal folds vibrate. When the fistula was unoccluded, the transglottal pressure drop increased markedly, making control of the vocal folds difficult and causing the aperiodicity we saw. We have seen the same phenomenon in individuals with neurological diseases such as multiple sclerosis. In that case, we saw increased aperiodicity as a function of open vowel position, but the principle still holds.

Bibliography

Adair, R. K. (1995). The physics of baseball. *Physics Today, 48* (5), 26–31.

Adair, R. K. (2002). *The physics of baseball* (3rd ed.). New York: HarperCollins.

Aronson, A. E., & Bless, D. M. (2009). *Clinical voice disorders* (4th ed.). New York: Thieme.

Baer, T., Sasaki, C., & Harris, K. (1985). *Laryngeal function in phonation and respiration.* Boston: College-Hill Press.

Baken, R. J., & Orlikoff, R. F. (1999). *Clinical measurement of speech and voice* (2nd ed.). San Diego, CA: Singular Publishing Group.

Bateman, H. E., & Mason, R. M. (1984). *Applied anatomy and physiology of the speech and hearing mechanism.* Springfield, IL: Charles C. Thomas.

Behrman, A. (2007). *Speech and voice science.* San Diego, CA: Plural Publishing.

Bless, D. M., & Abbs, J. H. (1995). *Vocal fold physiology* (2nd ed.). San Diego, CA: Singular Publishing Group.

Boone, D. R. (1999). *The voice and voice therapy* (6th ed.). Boston: Allyn & Bacon.

Boone, D. R., McFarlane, S. C., Von Berg, S. L., & Zraick, R. I. (2009). *The voice and voice therapy, 8e.* Upper Saddle River, NJ: Pearson.

Broad, D. J. (1973). Phonation. In F. D. Minifie, T. J. Hixon, & F. Williams (Eds.), *Normal aspects of speech, hearing, and language* (pp. 127–168). Englewood Cliffs, NJ: Prentice-Hall.

Chhetri, D. K., Neurbauer, J., & Berry, D. A. (2012). Neuromuscular control of fundamental frequency at phonation onset. *Journal of the Acoustical Society of America, 131*(2), 1401–1412.

Childers, D. G., Hicks, D. M., Moore, G. P., Eskenazi, L., & Lalwani, A. L. (1990). Electroglottography and vocal fold physiology. *Journal of Speech and Hearing Research, 33,* 245–254.

Daniloff, R. G. *Speech science.* San Diego, CA: College-Hill Press.

Eckel, F., & Boone, D. (1981). The S/Z ratio as an indicator of laryngeal pathology. *Journal of Speech and Hearing Disorders, 46,* 147–149.

Fink, B. R., & Demarest, R. J. (1978). *Laryngeal biomechanics.* Cambridge, MA: Harvard University Press.

Fletcher, W. W. (1950). *A study of internal laryngeal activity in relation to vocal intensity.* Doctoral dissertation, Northwestern University, Evanston, IL.

Fucci, D. J., & Lass, N. J. (1999). *Fundamentals of speech science.* Boston: Allyn & Bacon.

Fujimura, O. (1988). *Vocal fold physiology: Vol. 2. Vocal physiology.* New York: Raven Press.

Ganong, W. F. (2003). *Review of medical physiology* (21st ed.). New York: McGraw-Hill/Appleton & Lange.

Gilroy, A. M., MacPherson, B. R., & Ross, L.M. (2012). *Atlas of anatomy* (2nd ed.). New York: Thieme.

Gosling, J. A., Harris, P. F., Humpherson, J. R., Whitmore, I., & Willan, P. L. T. (1985). *Atlas of human anatomy.* Philadelphia: J. B. Lippincott.

Gray, H., Bannister, L. H., Berry, M. M., & Williams, P. L. (Eds.) (1995). *Gray's anatomy.* London: Churchill Livingstone.

Grobler, N. J. (1977). *Textbook of clinical anatomy* (Vol. 1). Amsterdam: Elsevier Scientific.

Herbst, C. T., Stoeger, A. S., Frey, R., Lohscheller, J., Titze, I. R., Gumpenberger, M., & Fitch, W. T. (2012). How low can you go? Physical production mechanisms of elephant infrasonic vocalization. *Science, 337,* 595–598.

Hirano, M. (1974). Morphological structure of the vocal cord as a vibrator and its variations. *Folia Phoniatrica, 26*, 89–94.

Hirano, M., Kiyokawa, K., & Kurita, S. (1988). Laryngeal muscles and glottic shaping. In O. Fujimura (Ed.), *Vocal physiology: Voice production, mechanisms, and functions* (pp. 49–65). New York: Raven Press.

Hirano, M., Ohala, J., & Vennard, W. (1969). The function of laryngeal muscles in regulation of fundamental frequency and intensity of phonation. *Journal of Speech and Hearing Research, 12*, 616–628.

Hirano, M., & Kakita, Y. (1985). Cover-body theory of vocal fold vibration. In R. G. Daniloff (Ed.). *Speech science.* San Diego, CA: Singular Publishing Group.

Hixon, T. J. (1973). Respiratory function in speech. In F. D. Minifie, T. J. Hixon, & F. Williams (Eds.), *Normal aspects of speech, hearing, and language* (pp. 73–126). Englewood Cliffs, NJ: Prentice-Hall.

Hixon, T. J. (1982). Speech breathing kinematics and mechanism inferences therefrom. In S. Grillner, A. Persson, B. Lindblom, & J. Lubker (Eds.), *Speech motor control* (pp. 75–94). New York: Pergamon Press.

Hixon, T. J., Hawley, J. L., & Wilson, K. J. (1982). An around-the-house device for the clinical determination of respiratory driving pressure: A note on making simple even simpler. *Journal of Speech and Hearing Disorders, 47*, 413–415.

Hufnagle, J., & Hufnagle, K. K. (1988). S/Z ratio in dysphonic children with and without vocal cord nodules. *Language, Speech, and Hearing Services in Schools, 19*, 418–422.

Husson, R. (1953). Sur la physiologie vocale. *Annals of Otolaryngology, 69,* 124–137.

Isshiki, N. (1964). Regulatory mechanisms of voice intensity variation. *Journal of Speech and Hearing Research, 7*, 17–29.

Jiang, J. J., Zhang, Y., MacCallum, J., Sprecher, A., & Zhou, L (2009). Objective analysis of pathological voices with vocal nodules and polyps. *Folia phoniatrica et logopedica, 61*, 342–349.

Kaplan, H. M. (1971). *Anatomy and physiology of speech.* New York: McGraw-Hill.

Kazarian, A. G., Sarkissian, L. S., & Isaakian, D. G. (1978). Length of human vocal cords by age. (Russian). *Zhurnal Eksperimentalnoi I Klinicheskoi Meditsiny, 18*, 105–109.

Kent, R. (1976). Anatomical and neuromuscular maturation of the speech mechanism: Evidence from acoustic studies. *Journal of Speech and Hearing Research, 19*, 421–447.

Kent, R. (1994). *Reference manual for communication sciences & disorders.* Austin: Pro-Ed.

Kent, R. D. (1997). *The speech sciences.* San Diego, CA: Singular Publishing Group.

Kent, R. D., Kent, J. F., & Rosenbek, J. C. (1987). Maximum performance tests of speech production. *Journal of Speech and Hearing Disorders, 52*, 367–387.

Kirchner, J. A., & Suzuki, M. (1968). Laryngeal reflexes and voice production. In M. Krauss (Ed.), Sound production in man. *Annals of the New York Academy of Sciences, 155*, 98–109.

Kuehn, D. P., Lemme, M. L., & Baumgartner, J. M. (1989). *Neural bases of speech, hearing, and language.* Boston: Little, Brown.

Kurtz, L. O. & Cielo, C. A. (2010). Maximum phonation time of vowels in adult women with vocal nodules. *Pro Fono, 22*(4), 451-454.

Lieberman, P. (1968a). *Intonation, perception, and language.* Research monograph No. 38. Cambridge, MA: The MIT Press.

Lieberman, P. (1968b). Vocal cord motion in man. *Annals of the New York Academy of Sciences, 155*, 28–38.

Lieberman, P. (1977). *Speech science and acoustic phonetics: An introduction.* New York: Macmillan.

Logemann, J. (1997). *Evaluation and treatment of swallowing disorders.* Austin: Pro-Ed.

McHanwell, S. (2008). Larynx. In Standring, S. (Ed.), *Gray's Anatomy: The anatomical and clinical basis of practice* (40th ed., 577–594). London: Churchill Livingstone.

Netsell, R. (1973). Speech physiology. In F. D. Minifie, T. J. Hixon, & F. Williams (Eds.), *Normal aspects of speech, hearing, and language* (pp. 134–211). Englewood Cliffs, NJ: Prentice-Hall.

Netsell, R., & Hixon, T. J. (1978). A noninvasive method for clinically estimating subglottal air pressure. *Journal of Speech and Hearing Disorders, 43*, 326–330.

Nishizawa, N., Sawashima, M., & Yonemoto, K. (1988). Vocal fold length in vocal pitch change. In O. Fujimua (Ed.), *Vocal physiology: Voice production, mechanisms and functions* (pp. 49–65). New York: Raven Press.

Pabon, J. P. H. & Plomp, R. (1988). Automatic phonetogram recording supplemented with acoustical voice-quality parameters. *Journal of speech and hearing research, 31*, 710–722.

Plant, R. L., & Younger, R. M. (2000). The interrelationship of subglottal pressure, fundamental frequency, and vocal intensity during speech. *Journal of Voice, 14*(2), 170–177.

Proctor, D. F. (1968). The physiologic basis of voice training. In M. Krauss (Ed.), Sound production in man. *Annals of the New York Academy of Sciences, 155*, 208–228.

Ptacek, P. H., & Sander, E. K. (1963). Maximum duration of phonation. *Journal of Speech and Hearing Disorders, 28*(2), 171–182.

Ramig, L. A., & Ringel, R. L. (1983). Effects of physiological aging on selected acoustic characteristics of voice. *Journal of Speech and Hearing Research, 26*, 22–30.

Rastatter, M. P., & Hyman, M. (1982). Maximum phoneme duration of /s/ and /z/ by children with vocal nodules. *Language, Speech, and Hearing Services in Schools, 13*, 197–199.

Rosse, C., Gaddum-Rosse, P., & Rosse, G. (1997). *Hollinshead's textbook of anatomy*. Philadelphia: Lippincott-Raven.

Sapienza, C. M., & Stathopoulos, E. T. (1994). Respiratory and laryngeal measures of children and women with bilateral vocal fold nodules. *Journal of Speech and Hearing Research, 37*, 1229–1243.

Schuenke, M., & Ross, L. M., (2010). *Thieme atlas of anatomy*. New York: Thieme.

Sonninen, A. (1968). The external frame function in the control of pitch in the human voice. In M. Krauss (Ed.), Sound production in man. *Annals of the New York Academy of Sciences, 155*, 68–89.

Sorensen, D. N., & Parker, P. A. (1992). The voiced/voiceless phonation time in children with and without laryngeal pathology. *Language, Speech, and Hearing Services in Schools, 23*, 163–168.

Storck, C., Juergens, P., Fischer, C., Wolfensberger, M., Honegger, F., Sorantin, E. Friedrich, G., & Gugatschka, M. (2012). Biomechanics of the cricoarytenoid joint: Three-dimensional imaging and vector analysis. *Journal of Voice, 25*(4), 406–410.

Standring, S. (2008). *Gray's anatomy: The anatomical and clinical basis of practice* (40th ed.). London: Churchill Livingstone.

Tait, N. A., Michel, J. F., & Carpenter, M. A. (1980). Maximum duration of sustained /s/ and /z/ in children. *Journal of Speech and Hearing Disorders, 15*, 239–246.

Timcke, R., Von Leden, H., & Moore, G. P. (1958). Laryngeal vibrations: Measurements of the glottic wave I: The normal vibratory cycle. *Archives of Otolaryngology, 68*, 1–19.

Titze, I. (1973). The human vocal cords: A mathematical model, Part I. *Phonetica, 28*, 129–170.

Titze, I. R. (1988). The physics of small amplitude oscillation of the vocal folds. *Journal of the Acoustical Society of America, 83*(4), 1536–1552.

Titze, I. R. (1994). *Principles of voice production*. Englewood Cliffs, NJ: Prentice-Hall.

Van den Berg, J. W. (1958). Myoelastic-aerodynamic theory of voice production. *Journal of Speech and Hearing Research, 1*, 227–244.

Van den Berg, J. W. (1968). Sound production in isolated human larynges. In M. Krauss (Ed.), Sound production in man. *Annals of the New York Academy of Sciences, 155*, 18–27.

Van den Berg, J. W., & Tan, T. S. (1959). Results of experiments with human larynxes. *Practica Oto-Rhino-Laryngologica, 21*, 425–450.

Verdolini, K., Titze, I. R., & Fennell, A. (1994). Dependence of phonatory effort on hydration level. *Journal of Speech and Hearing Research, 37*, 1001–1007.

Whillis, J. (1946). Movements of the tongue in swallowing. *Journal of Anatomy, 80*, 115–116.

Young, N., Wadie, M., & Sasaki, C. T. (2012). Neuromuscular basis for ventricular fold function. *Annals of Otorhinolaryngology, 121*(5), 317–321.

Zemlin, W. R. (1998). *Speech and hearing science. Anatomy and physiology* (4th ed.). Needham Heights, MA: Allyn & Bacon.

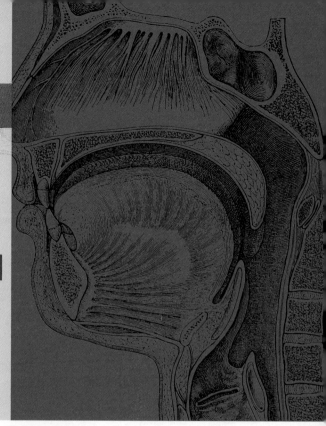

Chapter 6

ANATOMY OF ARTICULATION AND RESONATION

When a layperson thinks of the process of speaking, it is more than likely that he or she is actually thinking about articulation. You, of course, now know that there is much more to speech than moving the lips, tongue, mandible, and so forth. Nonetheless, the articulatory system is an extremely important element in our communication system.

Articulation is the process of joining two elements, and the **articulatory system** is the system of mobile and immobile articulators brought into contact for the purpose of shaping the sounds of speech. As you will remember from Chapters 4 and 5, laryngeal vibration produces the sound required for voicing in speech. We are capable of rapidly starting and stopping phonation, depending on whether we want voiced or voiceless production. This chapter focuses on what happens after that sound reaches the oral cavity. In this cavity, the undifferentiated buzz produced by the vocal folds is shaped into the sounds we call *phonemes*. Let us present an overview of how the oral cavity is capable of creating phonemes.

articulation: the process of joining two elements

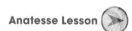

Anatesse Lesson

SOURCE-FILTER THEORY OF VOWEL PRODUCTION

A widely accepted description of how the oral cavity shapes speech sounds is the **source-filter theory** of vowel production. In general terms, the theory states that a voicing source is generated by the vocal folds and routed through the vocal tract where it is shaped into the sounds of speech. Changes in the shape and configuration of the tongue, mandible, soft palate, and other articulators govern the resonance characteristics of the vocal tract, and the resonances of the tract determine the sound of a given vowel. Here is how that works.

The **vocal tract**, consisting of the mouth (oral cavity), the region behind the mouth (pharynx), and the nasal cavity, may be thought of as a series of linked tubes (see Figure 6-1). From your experience you

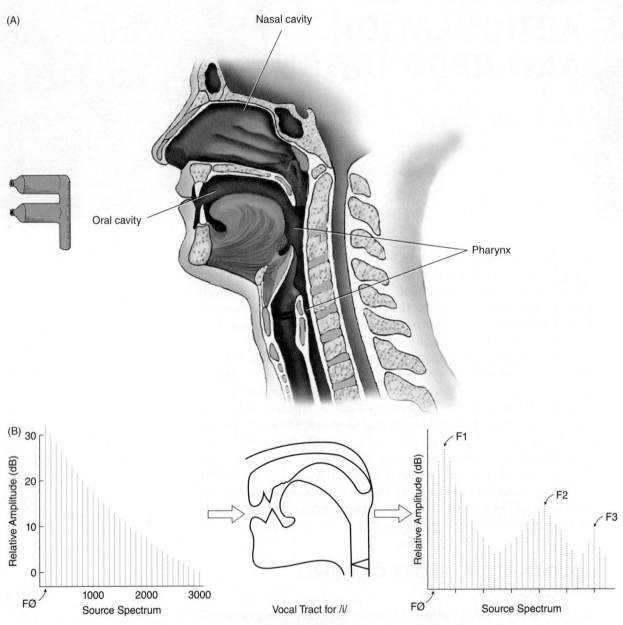

Figure 6-1. (A) Visualization of the oral, nasal, and pharyngeal cavities as a series of linked tubes. This linkage provides the variable resonating cavity that produces speech. (B) Relationship among source (spectrum of output from vocal folds), filter (vocal tract transfer function), and filtered output of the vocal tract (formants).

© Cengage Learning®.

know that if you blow carefully across the top of a soda bottle, you will hear a tone. If you decrease the volume of the air in the bottle by adding fluid to it, the frequency of vibration of the tone increases. Likewise, if you blow across the top of a bottle with larger volume, the tone decreases in frequency. As the volume of the air in the bottle increases, the frequency of the tone decreases. As the volume decreases, the frequency increases. You are experimenting with the **resonant frequency** of a cavity, which is the frequency of sound to which the cavity most effectively responds. You might think of the bottle as a filter that lets only one frequency of sound through and rejects the other frequencies, much as a coffee filter lets the liquid through but traps the grounds. The airstream blowing across the top of the bottle is actually producing a very broad-spectrum signal, but the bottle selects the frequency components that are at its resonant frequency. The resonant frequency of a cavity is largely governed by its volume and length. Now, if you were somehow able to blow across two bottles (one low-resonant frequency and one high-resonant frequency), the two tones would combine.

When you move your tongue around in your mouth, you are changing the shape of your oral cavity, making it smaller or larger, lengthening or shortening it. It is as if you had a series of bottles that you could manipulate in your mouth, changing their shape at will. When you change the shape of the oral cavity, you are changing the resonant frequencies, and therefore you are changing the sound that comes out of the mouth. This, then, is the source-filter theory view of speech production. The vocal folds produce a quasi-periodic tone (see Chapters 4 and 5), which is passed through the filter of your vocal tract. The vocal tract filter is manipulable, so that you can change its shape and therefore change the sound.

The resonant frequencies govern our perception of vowels. To prove that vocal folds do not govern the nature of a vowel, whisper the words *he* and *who*. Could you tell the difference? The vocal folds were not vibrating, but you excited the oral cavity filter through the turbulence of your whispered production, and the vowels were quite intelligible.

The source-filter theory can be easily expanded to other phonemes as well. The source of the sound may vary. With vowels, the source will always be phonation in normal speech. With consonants, other sources will include the turbulence of frication or combinations of voicing and turbulence. In all cases, you produce a noise source and pass it through the filter of the oral cavity that has been configured to meet your acoustic needs. Now look at Figure 6-1A. On the left is the spectrum output of the vocal folds before the sound has filtered through the vocal tract. Notice that the spectrum is made up of a fundamental frequency (lowest bar in the graph) and whole-number multiples, known as harmonics. These harmonics are evenly spaced, and diminish in intensity by about 12 dB per octave. In the middle of that figure is the filter

resonant frequency:
frequency of stimulation to which a resonant system responds most vigorously

itself: the vocal tract through which the sound source is being fed. We have drawn this so the shape of the articulators is making the /i/ vowel. The /i/ vowel is a high-front vowel, which means its constriction is forward in the mouth, near the alveolar ridge, behind the upper teeth. This means that the space in front of the constriction is very small. Now look at the right-most part of that figure. The spectrum that entered the vocal tract filter on the left has been shaped into the output spectrum on the right, which is the spectrum for the vowel /i/. We identify that vowel by the second formant (F2), which is produced by the space anterior to the constriction. That F2 frequency, by the way, is approximately 2,500 Hz, while the F1 frequency is about 300 Hz.

Look at Figure 6-2, and notice the difference between production of the /s/ and /ʃ/ phonemes. Sustain an /s/ and realize that when you produce it, your tongue is high, forward, and tense. You pass a compact stream of air over the surface of the tongue, and then between the tongue tip and the upper front teeth. Now produce the /ʃ/ and recognize that the tongue is farther back in your mouth, much as in the figure. The source in both cases is the turbulence associated with the airstream escaping from its course between your tongue and an immobile structure of your mouth (front teeth or roof of your mouth). The turbulence excites the cavity in front of the constriction and you have a recognizable sound. Which of the two phonemes has the larger cavity distal to the constriction? The /ʃ/ has a larger resonant cavity than the /s/, so its resonant frequency will be lower, following our discussion of bottles. Now make the /s/ again, but without stopping, slide your tongue back in your mouth until you reach the /ʃ/ position. As you do this, you will hear the noise drop in frequency because the cavity is increasing in size. The source-filter theory dictates this change.

✔ *To summarize:*

- The source-filter theory states that speech is the product of sending an acoustic source, such as the sound produced by the vibrating vocal folds, through the filter of the vocal tract that shapes the output.
- The ever-changing speech signal is the product of moving articulators.
- Sources may be voicing, as in the case of vowels, or the product of turbulence, as in fricatives. Articulators may be moveable (such as the tongue, lips, pharynx, and mandible) or immobile (such as the teeth and hard palate).

Let us now examine the structures of the articulatory system. As with the phonatory system, we must examine the support structures (the skull and bones of the face) and the muscles that move the articulators. Before we begin, we will define the articulators used in speech production.

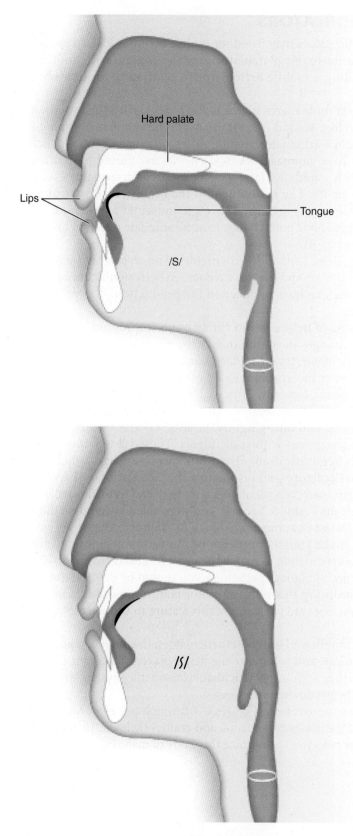

SAGITTAL VIEW

Figure 6-2. Comparison of the articulatory posture used for production of /s/ and /ʃ/.
Source: (After the data and view of Shriberg & Kent, 2002.)

THE ARTICULATORS

As noted, articulators may be either mobile or immobile. In speech we will often move one articulator to make contact with another, thus positioning a mobile articulator in relation to an immobile articulator.

The largest mobile articulator is the *tongue*, with the lower jaw (*mandible*) a close second (see Figure 6-3). The *velum* or *soft palate* is another mobile articulator, used to differentiate nasal sounds such as /m/ or /n/ from nonnasal sounds. The *lips* are moved to produce different speech sounds, and the *cheeks* play a role in changes of resonance of the cavity. The region behind the oral cavity (the **fauces** and the *pharynx*) may be moved through muscular action, and the *larynx* and *hyoid bone* both change to accommodate different articulatory postures.

There are three immobile articulators. The *alveolar ridge* of the upper jaw (*maxillae*) and the *hard palate* are both significant articulatory surfaces. The *teeth* are used in the production of a variety of speech sounds.

The process of **articulation for speech** is quite automatic. To get a feel for changes in speech that occur when you alter the function of an articulator, try this. Place a small stack of tongue depressors between your molars on one side of your mouth and bite lightly (this is a *bite block*). Now say, "You wish to know all about my grandfather." Now say the same sentence after placing your tongue between your front teeth, and biting lightly. Finally, say the sentence while pulling your cheeks out with your fingers. There are two important points to this demonstration. First, your speech changed when you altered the articulatory and resonatory characteristics of the vocal tract. You restrained the articulators, and they had to work harder to make yourself understood. Second, you were able to overcome these difficulties. Despite having a bite block or clamped tongue tip, you were able to make yourself understood. In fact, you automatically adjusted your articulation to match the new physical constraints. As a student in speech-language pathology, you should be quite heartened by the extraordinary flexibility of motor planning exhibited in this demonstration, because you can use this feature to your advantage in treatment.

Of these mobile and immobile articulators, the tongue, mandible, teeth, hard palate, and velum are the major players, although all surfaces and cavities within the articulatory/resonatory system are contributors to the production of speech.

You may wish to refer to Figures 6-4 through 6-9 as we begin our discussion of the bones of the facial and cranial skeleton. In addition, Table 6-1 may help you to organize this body of material.

fauces: the pillars at the posterior margin of the oral cavity

articulation for speech: the process of bringing two or more moveable speech structures together to form the sounds of speech

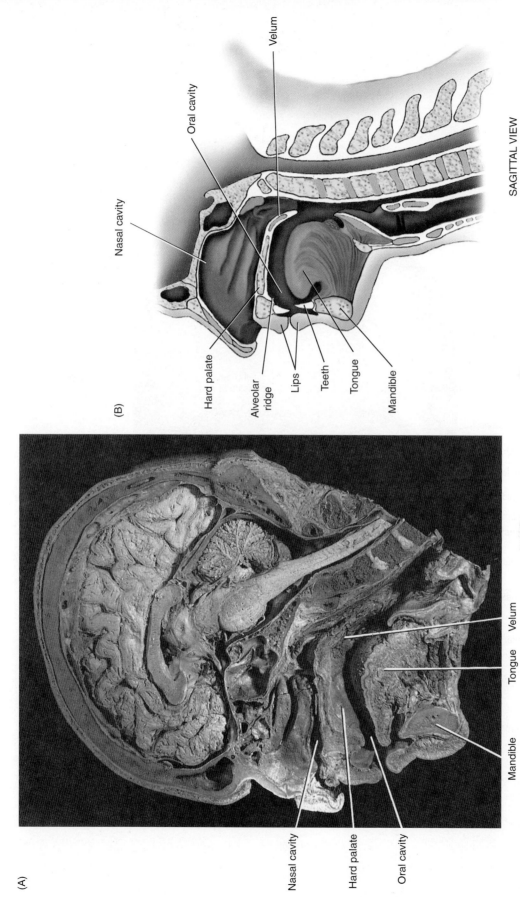

Figure 6-3. (A) Photograph of articulators seen through sagittal section. (B) Relationships among the articulators.

© Cengage Learning®.

(A)

ANTERIOR VIEW

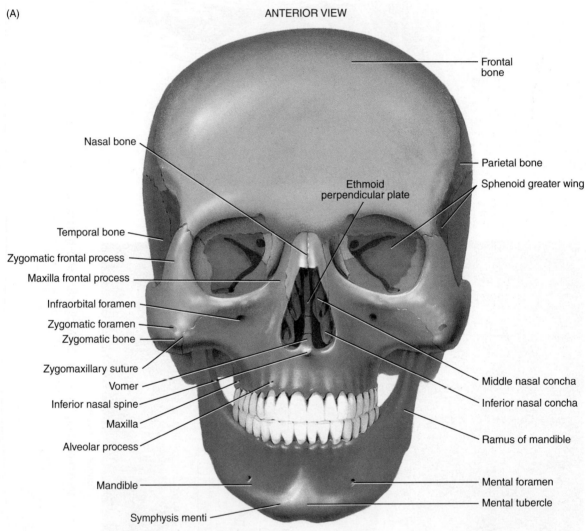

Frontal bone

Nasal bone

Parietal bone

Sphenoid greater wing

Ethmoid perpendicular plate

Temporal bone

Zygomatic frontal process

Maxilla frontal process

Infraorbital foramen

Zygomatic foramen

Zygomatic bone

Zygomaxillary suture

Vomer

Inferior nasal spine

Maxilla

Alveolar process

Middle nasal concha

Inferior nasal concha

Ramus of mandible

Mandible

Mental foramen

Mental tubercle

Symphysis menti

Figure 6-4. (A) Anterior view of the skull. (continues).

(B)

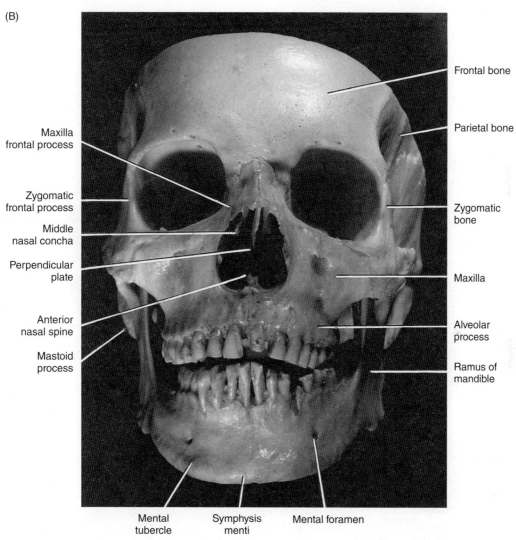

Figure 6-4 continued. (B) Photograph of the anterior skull.

(A)

LATERAL VIEW

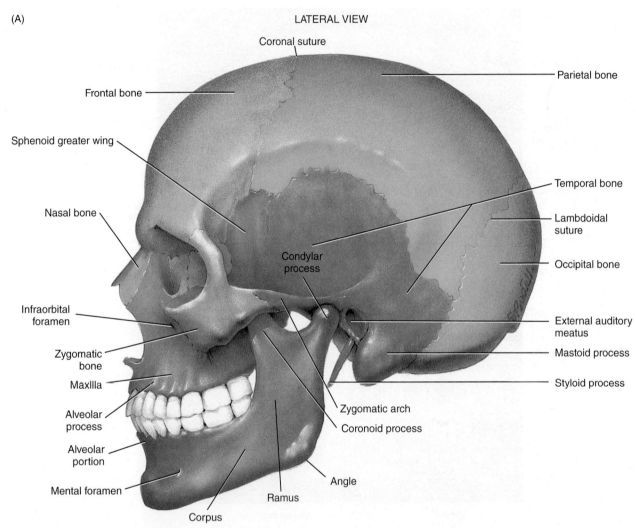

Figure 6-5. (A) Lateral view of the skull. (continues).
© Cengage Learning®.

(B)

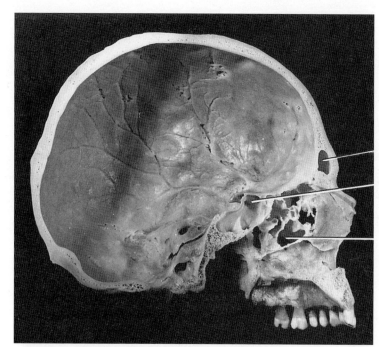

Frontal sinus

Sphenoid sinus

Maxillary sinus

(C)

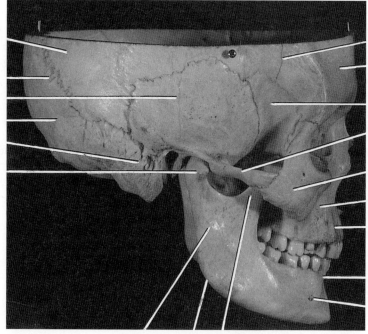

Parietal bone

Lambdoidal suture

Temporal bone

Occipital bone

Mastoid process

Condylar process

Coronal suture

Frontal bone

Sphenoid greater wing

Zygomatic arch

Zygomatic bone

Maxilla

Alveolar process

Alveolar portion

Mental foramen

Ramus   Angle   Coronoid process

Figure 6-5 continued. (B) Medial surface of the skull. (C) Photo of the lateral skull.

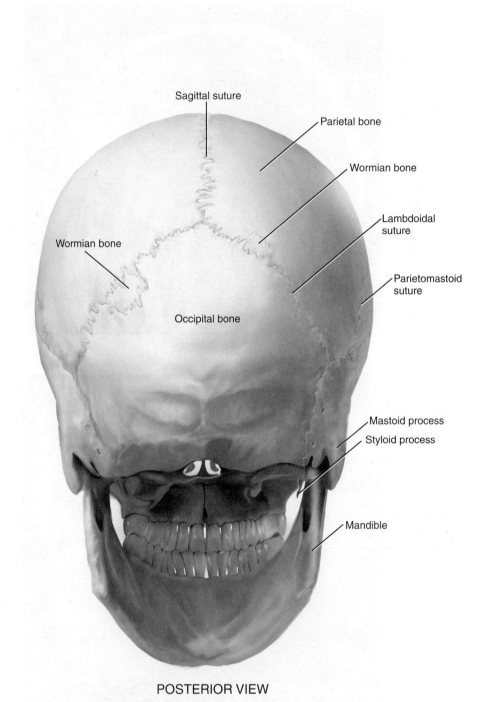

Sagittal suture

Parietal bone

Wormian bone

Lambdoidal suture

Parietomastoid suture

Wormian bone

Occipital bone

Mastoid process

Styloid process

Mandible

POSTERIOR VIEW

Figure 6-6. Posterior view of the skull.

© Cengage Learning®.

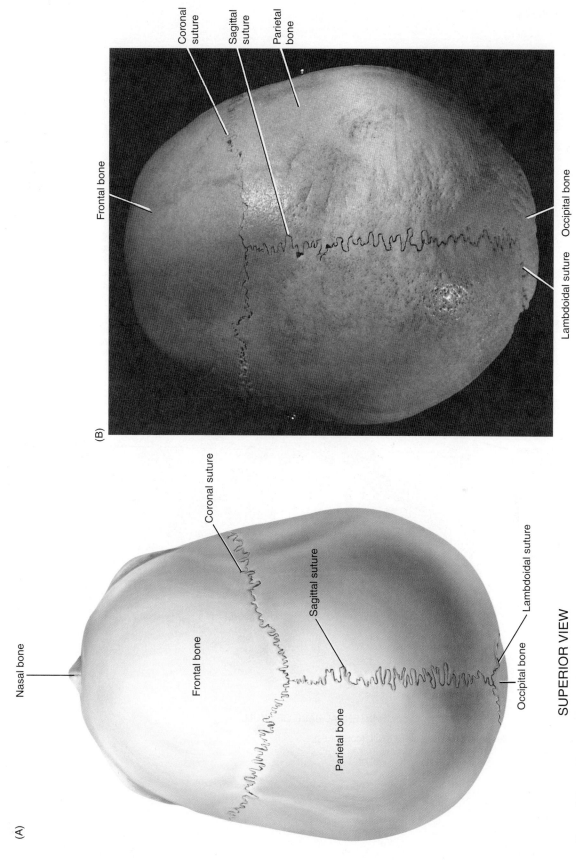

Figure 6-7. (A) Superior view of the skull. (B) Superior view photo of the skull.

© Cengage Learning®.

SUPERIOR VIEW

(A)

Nasal bone

Coronal suture

Frontal bone

Sagittal suture

Parietal bone

Lambdoidal suture

Occipital bone

(B)

Frontal bone

Coronal suture

Sagittal suture

Parietal bone

Occipital bone

Lambdoidal suture

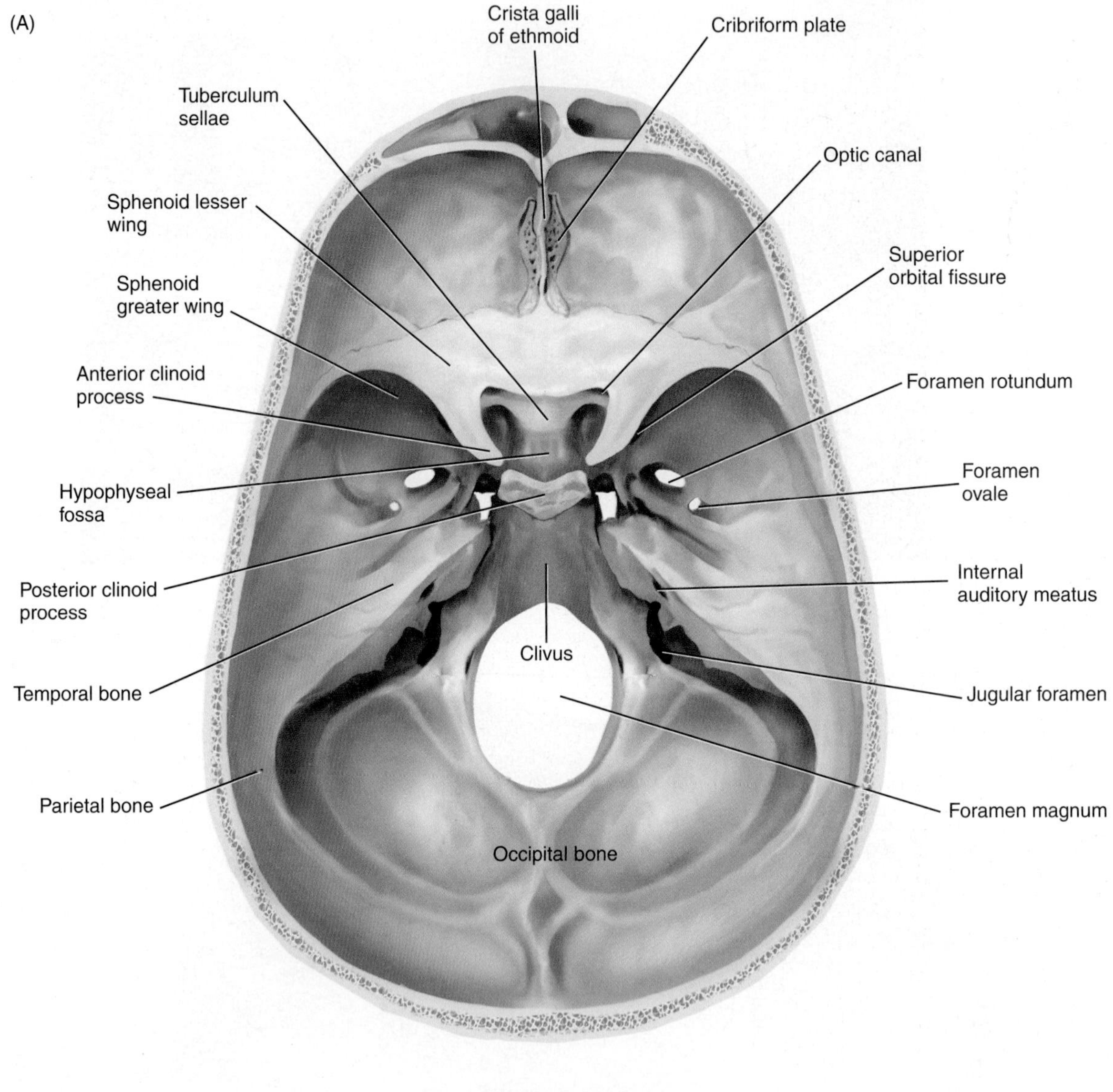

(A)

INTERNAL BASE OF SKULL

Figure 6-8. (A) Internal view of base of the skull. (continues).

© Cengage Learning®.

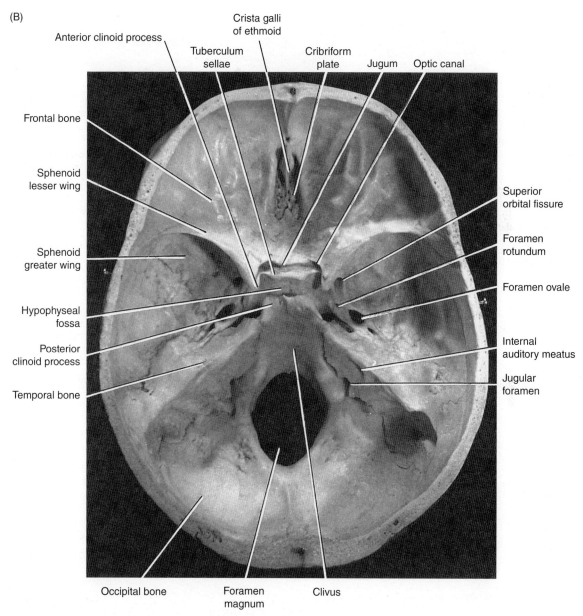

Figure 6-8 continued. (B) Photo of the internal skull.

© Cengage Learning®.

(A)

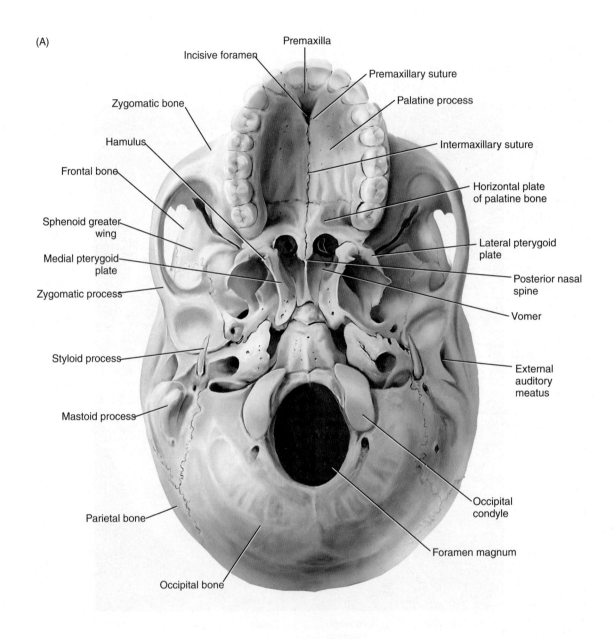

INFERIOR VIEW

Figure 6-9. (A) Inferior view of the skull. (continues).

© Cengage Learning®.

(B)

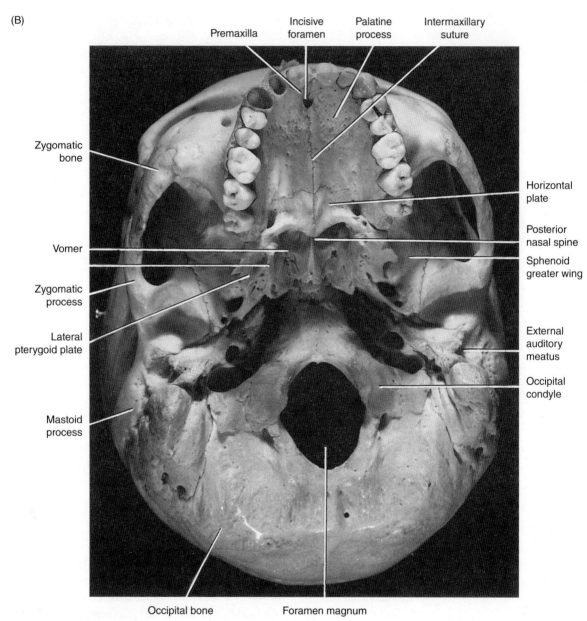

Figure 6-9 continued. (B) Photo of inferior view of the skull.

Table 6-1 **Bones of the face and cranial skeleton**	
Bones of the Face	**Bones of the Cranial Skeleton**
Mandible	Ethmoid bone
Maxillae	Sphenoid bone
Nasal bone	Frontal bone
Palatine bone and nasal conchae	Parietal bone
Vomer	Occipital bone
Zygomatic bone	Temporal bone
Lacrimal Bone	
Hyoid bone	

© Cengage Learning®.

BONES OF THE FACE AND CRANIAL SKELETON
Bones of the Face

- **Mandible**
- **Maxillae**
- **Nasal bone**
- **Palatine bone and nasal conchae**
- **Vomer**
- **Zygomatic bone**
- **Lacrimal bone**
- **Hyoid bone**

There are numerous bones of the face with which you should become familiar. As with the respiratory and phonatory systems, learning the landmarks will serve you well as you identify the course and function of the muscles of articulation.

Mandible

The mandible is the massive unpaired bone making up the lower jaw of the face. It begins as a paired bone but fuses at the midline by the child's first birthday. As you can see from Figure 6-10, there are several landmarks of interest on both outer and inner surfaces. The point of fusion of the two halves of the mandible is the **symphysis menti** or **mental symphysis**, marking the midline mental **protuberance** and separating the paired mental **tubercles**. Lateral to the tubercles on either side is the mental **foramen**, the hole through which the mental nerve of V trigeminal passes in life. The lateral mass of bone is the **corpus** or body, and the point at which the mandible angles upward is the **angle**. The rhomboidal plate rising up from the mandible is the **ramus**. The **condylar** and **coronoid** processes are

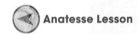

Anatesse Lesson

mental: L., mentum, chin

symphysis: Gr., growing together

protuberance: Gr., pro, before + tuber, bulge

tubercles: little swelling

foramen: L., a passage, opening, orifice

corpus: body

ramus: L., branch

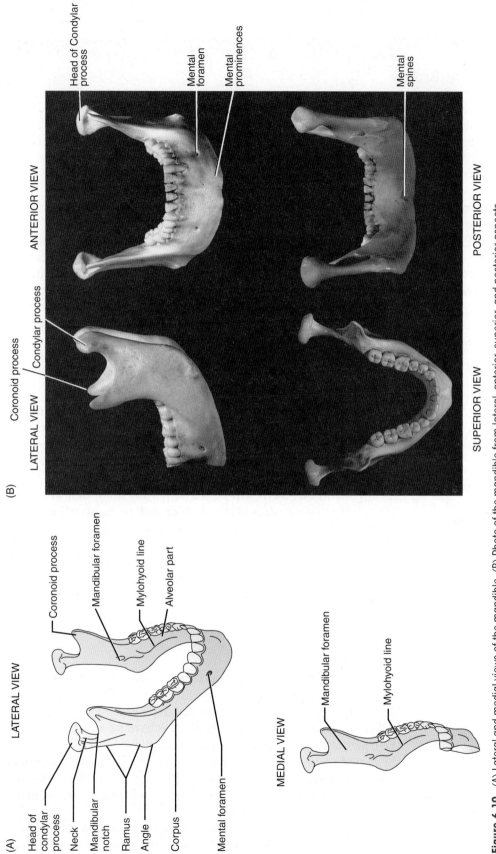

Figure 6-10. (A) Lateral and medial views of the mandible. (B) Photo of the mandible from lateral, anterior, superior, and posterior aspects.
© Cengage Learning®.

(A)

LATERAL VIEW

Coronoid process
Mandibular foramen
Mylohyoid line
Alveolar part

Head of
condylar
process
Neck
Mandibular
notch
Ramus
Angle
Corpus
Mental foramen

MEDIAL VIEW

Mandibular
foramen
Mylohyoid line

(B)

Coronoid process

LATERAL VIEW   Condylar process

Head of Condylar
process

Mental
foramen
Mental
prominences

ANTERIOR VIEW

Mental
spines

SUPERIOR VIEW   POSTERIOR VIEW

On Use of the Bite Block

A bite block is a device used to stabilize the mandible so that other articulators can be evaluated or exercised. Bite blocks come in many shapes, sizes, and textures, ranging from acrylic blocks about 1 cm square to bite blocks that are created from dental impression material. The softer, more pliable dental impression bite block provides a better surface for sustained use and is particularly good for clients who have limited motor control.

A bite block is used when you cannot differentiate the contribution of the mandible from that of the lips or tongue during articulation. For instance, if you say /ta ta ta ta/ repeatedly while lightly holding your mandible, you will feel the mandible move, even though the dominant articulator is the tongue. If you wanted to strengthen the tongue, such as having it push toward the roof of the mouth against a resistance, you could place a bite block between the molars and have your client push up against a tongue depressor.

Needless to say, having your client perform oral motor activities such as the one mentioned here requires that you have a firm understanding of the anatomy and physiology of articulation, as well as a deep knowledge of motor development. Oral motor therapy focuses on remediating muscle imbalance, and inappropriate application of oral motor activities can create even greater problems. For an excellent discussion, see Langley and Lombardino (1991).

---

pterygoid: Gr., pterygodes, wing, referring to one of two prominent processes arising from the base of the sphenoid bone

fovea: L., a pit

important landmarks and are separated by the **mandibular notch**. The prominent **head** of the condylar process articulates with the skull, permitting the rotation of the mandible. The **pterygoid fovea** on the anterior surface of the condylar process marks the point of attachment of the lateral pterygoid muscle, which will be discussed later. In the healthy mandible, teeth will be found within small **dental alveoli** (sacs) on the upper surface of the **alveolar arch** of the mandible.

On the inner surface of the mandible are prominent midline **superior** and inferior **mental spines** and the laterally placed **mylohyoid line**, landmarks that will figure prominently as we attach muscles to this structure. The **mandibular foramen** is the conduit for the inferior alveolar nerve of V trigeminal, providing sensory innervation for the teeth and gums.

Maxillae

Maxilla is the singular of maxillae.

The paired maxillae (singular, **maxilla**) are the bones making up the upper jaw. These bones deserve careful study, for they make up most of the roof of the mouth (**hard palate**), nose, and upper dental ridge and are involved in clefting of the lip and hard palate. As you study the landmarks of this complex bone, it might help you to realize that the various processes are logically named. For example, the *frontal* process of maxilla articulates with the *frontal* bone. Thus, learning the names of the larger structures early on will facilitate learning the processes and attachments later.

In Figure 6-11 you can see the significant landmarks of the maxillae. As you can see, the **frontal process** is the superior-most point

(A)

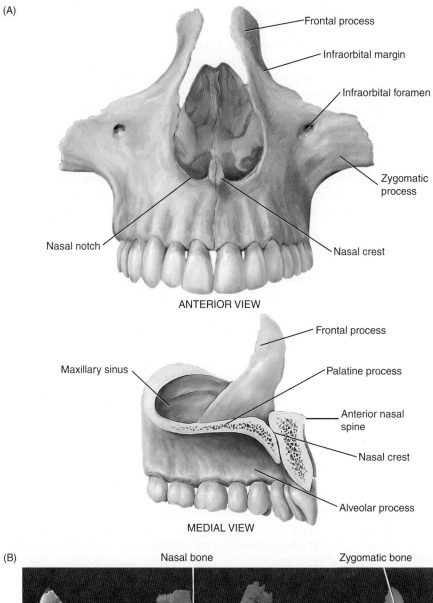

ANTERIOR VIEW

MEDIAL VIEW

(B)

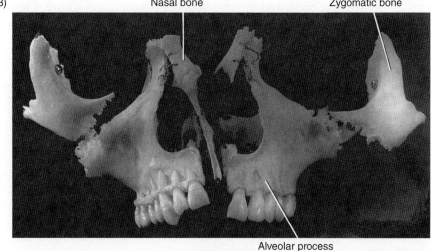

ANTERIOR VIEW

Figure 6-11. (A) Anterior and medial views of the maxilla. (B) Anterior view of maxillae, showing the relationship with nasal and zygomatic bones.

© Cengage Learning®.

orbital: L., orbita, orbit

canine: L., caninus, related to dog

suture: L., sutura, seam; the fibrous union of skull bones

micrognathia: Gr., micro, small + gnathos, jaw

of this bone. You can palpate this process on yourself by placing your finger on your nose at the nasal side of your eye. You could run your finger down the **infraorbital margin** from there to the lower mid-point of your eye. The **orbital** process projects into the eye socket, providing support for the eye ball. Just below your finger is the **infraorbital foramen**, the conduit for the infraorbital nerve arising from the maxillary nerve of the V trigeminal, providing sensory innervation of the lower eyelid, upper lip, and nasal alae. Lateral to your finger is the **zygomatic process** of the maxilla bone, which articulates with the zygomatic bone.

At the midline you can see the **anterior nasal spine (nasal crest)**, and lateral to this is the **nasal notch**. The lower tooth-bearing ridge, the **alveolar process**, contains alveoli that hold teeth in the intact adult maxilla. The region between the **canine eminence** and the **incisive foramen** will become important as we discuss cleft lip.

A medial view requires disarticulation of left and right maxillae. This view reveals the **maxillary sinus**, the **palatine process**, and the important inner margin of the alveolar process.

Figure 6-12 shows an inferior view of the maxillae. As you can see from this view, the two palatine processes of the maxilla articulate at the **intermaxillary suture** (also known as the **median palatine suture**). This **suture** marks the point of a cleft of the hard palate. The palatine process makes up three-fourths of the hard palate, with the other one-fourth being the horizontal plate of the palatine bone, to be discussed.

The incisive foramen in the anterior aspect of the hard palate serves as a conduit for the nasopalatine nerve serving the nasal mucosa. Trace the **premaxillary suture** forward from the incisive foramen to the alveolar process and you have identified the borders of the **premaxilla**. The premaxilla is difficult to see on the adult skull but is nonetheless an important topic of discussion. Note that the premaxillary suture neatly separates the lateral incisors from the cuspids. A cleft of the lip will occur at this location and may include lip, alveolar bone, and the region of the premaxillary suture. Cleft lip may be either unilateral or bilateral, but in virtually all cases it will occur at this suture (there is very rarely a midline cleft lip).

Mandibular Hypoplasia and Micrognathia

Congenital mandibular hypoplasia is a condition in which there is inadequate development of the mandible. Although some specific genetic syndromes have this as a trait (e.g., Robin syndrome), **micrognathia** (small jaw) may occur without any known mediating condition. The misalignment of the mandibular and maxillary arches may be corrected through surgery to extend the mandible. It is hypothesized that, during development, micrognathia may lead to cleft palate: The mandible may not develop adequately to accommodate the tongue, which, in turn, blocks the extension of the palatine processes of the maxillae.

Nasal Bones

The nasal bones are small, making up the superior nasal surface. As you can see from Figure 6-4, the nasal bones articulate with the frontal bones superiorly, the maxillae laterally, and the perpendicular plate of the ethmoid bone and the nasal septal cartilage, all to be discussed.

(A)

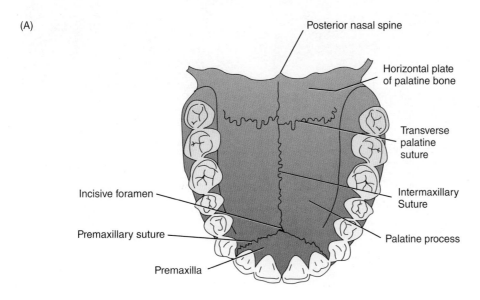

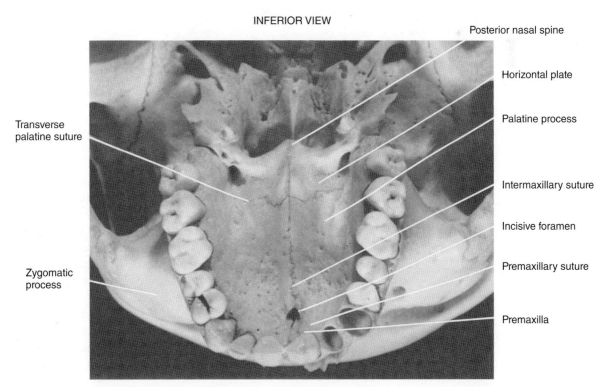

Figure 6-12. (A) Schematic and photo of inferior view of hard palate. (continues).
© Cengage Learning®.

(B)

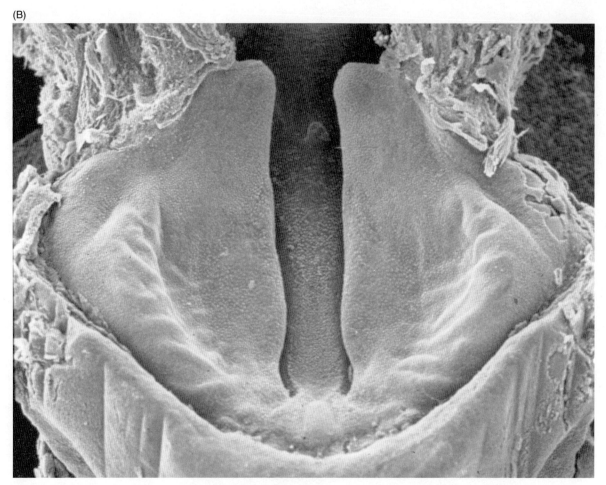

Figure 6-12 continued. (B) Experimentally induced cleft palate in mouse.

Source: Photograph courtesy of Marilyn Russell, PhD.

Palatine Bones and Nasal Conchae

You will recall that the posterior one-fourth of the hard palate is made up of the horizontal plate of the palatine bone. Let us now examine this small but complex bone (see Figure 6-13).

When viewed from the front, you can see that the articulated palatine bones echo the nasal cavity defined by the maxillae. The **posterior nasal spine** and **nasal crest** provide midline correlates to the anterior nasal spine and nasal crest of the maxillae, while the **horizontal plate** parallels the palatine process of the maxilla. When viewing from the side, you can note the **perpendicular plate** that makes up the posterior wall of the nasal cavity. The **orbital process** makes up a small portion of the orbit cavity.

The **inferior nasal conchae** (**inferior turbinates**) are small, scroll-like bones located on the lateral surface of the nasal cavity (see Figure 6-4). These small but significant bones articulate with the maxilla, palatine, and ethmoid bones. The **middle** and

turbinate: L., turbo, whirl; turbine-like bone of the nasal cavity

Nasoendoscopy

Endoscopy is a visualization technology that utilizes fiber optics. The endoscope is a long, flexible or rigid scope that is passed into a cavity or space that would otherwise not be visible. Nasoendoscopy involves using a flexible scope to enter the nasal passageway, typically passing under the inferior turbinates but sometimes between the middle and superior turbinates. From this vantage the scope can be maneuvered through the opened velopharyngeal port to permit viewing of the laryngeal structures. If the scope is used to examine the lungs and bronchi, it will be termed *bronchoscopy*.

The flexible endoscope is rapidly becoming one of the "tools of the trade" for speech-language pathologists working in practice with otorhinolaryngologists, or in hospital settings. The device can be used to view not only the structures of the nasal, oral, laryngeal, and pharyngeal spaces but can be also used to watch swallow function. The scope is passed through the nasal cavity, typically above the inferior nasal concha. It now serves as a valued adjunct to the radiologic procedure known as the modified barium swallow. This procedure has the added benefit of not exposing a patient to radiation, which means that a clinician can spend much more time examining the structures without fear of damaging tissues through overexposure.

(A)

RIGHT PALATINE BONE

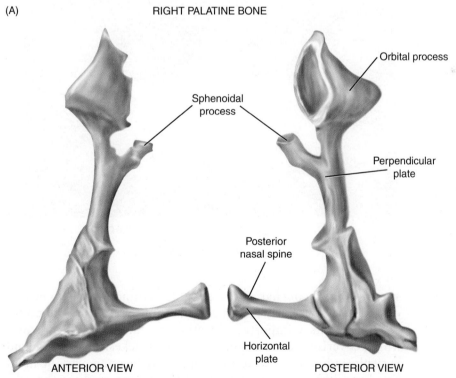

Orbital process

Sphenoidal process

Perpendicular plate

Posterior nasal spine

Horizontal plate

ANTERIOR VIEW

POSTERIOR VIEW

Figure 6-13. (A) Anterior and posterior views of palatine bones. (continues).
© Cengage Learning®.

(B)   ANTERIOR VIEW

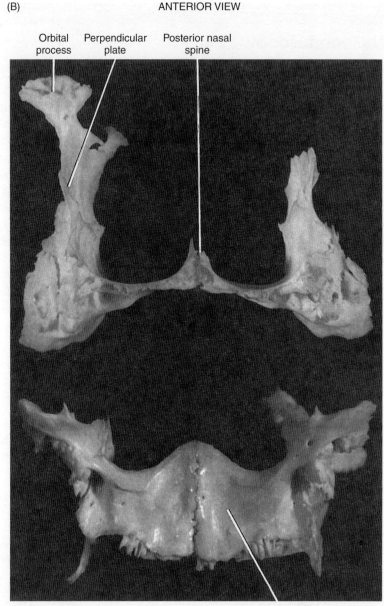

Orbital   Perpendicular   Posterior nasal
process   plate   spine

Horizontal plate

INFERIOR VIEW

Figure 6-13 continued.
(B) Articulated palatine bones from
front and beneath. Note that the left
perpendicular plate is incomplete.
(continues).
© Cengage Learning®.

conchae: Gr., konche, small
scroll-like bones of the nasal
cavity

superior nasal conchae, processes of the ethmoid bone (to be discussed), are superiorly placed correlates of the inferior **conchae**,
all of which have important function in mammals. The mucosal
lining covering the nasal conchae is the thickest of the nose and
is richly endowed with vascular supply. Air passing over the nasal
conchae will be warmed and humidified before reaching the delicate tissues of the lower respiratory system. The shape of the conchae greatly increases the surface area available, promoting rapid
heat exchange.

(C)

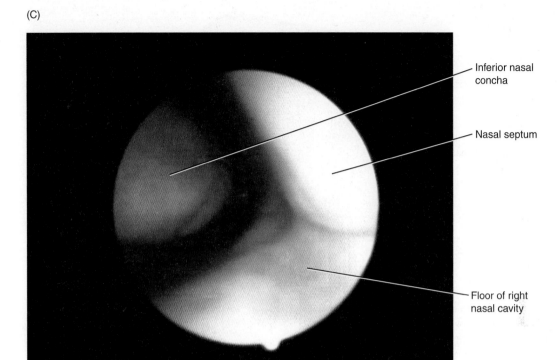

Inferior nasal concha

Nasal septum

Floor of right nasal cavity

(D)

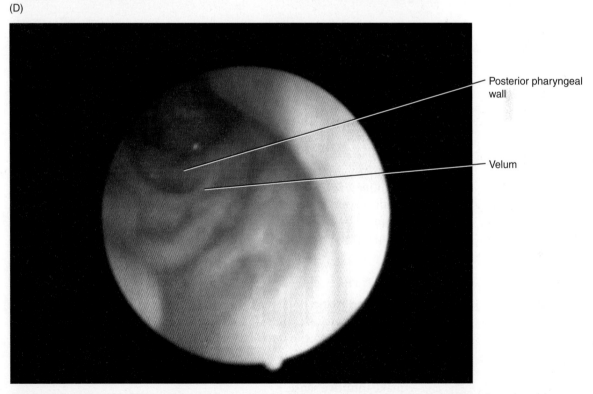

Posterior pharyngeal wall

Velum

Figure 6-13 continued. (C) Nasoendoscopic view of entry to right naris. Note the prominent inferior nasal concha arising from the left side (medial wall of nasal cavity). (D) Nasoendoscopic view of nasopharynx as seen from the right naris, showing superior surface of velum and posterior pharyngeal wall. (continues).

(E)

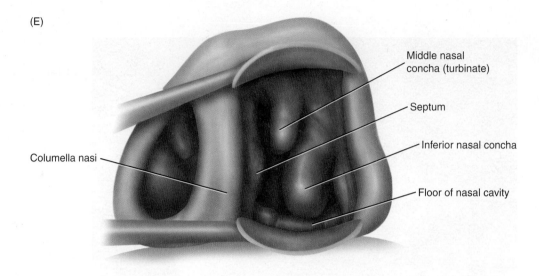

Columella nasi

Middle nasal concha (turbinate)

Septum

Inferior nasal concha

Floor of nasal cavity

SPECULUM VIEW

Figure 6-13 continued. (E) View of left nares opened using speculum for visualization, showing inferior and middle conchae.

© Cengage Learning®.

Vomer

The vomer (see Figure 6-14) is an unpaired, midline bone making up the inferior and posterior **nasal septum**, the dividing plate between the two nasal cavities (see Figure 6-15). The vomer has the appearance of a knife blade or a plowshare, with its point aimed toward the front. It articulates with the sphenoid **rostrum** and perpendicular plate of the ethmoid bone in the posterior-superior margin, and with the maxillae and palatine bones on the inferior margin. The posterior **ala** of the vomer marks the midline terminus of the nasal cavities. As you examine Figure 6-15, attend to the fact that the bony nasal **septum** is made up of two elements: the vomer and the perpendicular plate of the ethmoid bone. With the addition of the midline **septal cartilage**, the nasal septum is complete.

rostrum: L., beak or beaklike

ala: L., wing

septum: L., partition

Zygomatic Bone

zygomatic: zygoma, yoke

The **zygomatic** bone makes up the prominent structure we identify as cheekbones. As you can see from Figure 6-16, the zygomatic bone articulates with the maxillae, frontal bone, and temporal bone (you cannot see the articulation with the sphenoid bone), and makes up the lateral orbit. Fortunately, the landmarks of the zygomatic bone make intuitive sense.

At the base of the **orbital margin** is the **maxillary process**, the point of articulation of the zygomatic bone and maxilla.

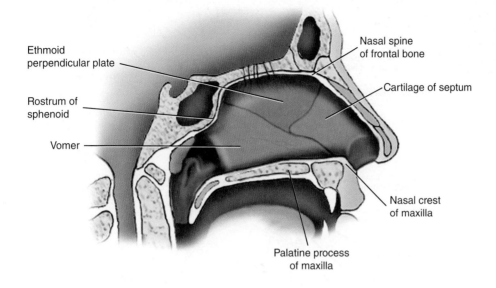

Ethmoid
perpendicular plate

Rostrum of
sphenoid

Vomer

Nasal spine
of frontal bone

Cartilage of septum

Nasal crest
of maxilla

Palatine process
of maxilla

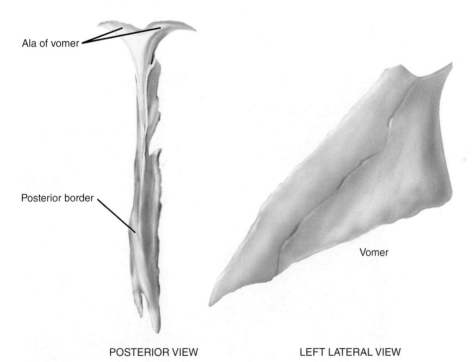

Ala of vomer

Posterior border

Vomer

POSTERIOR VIEW

LEFT LATERAL VIEW

Figure 6-14. Lateral view of the vomer.
© Cengage Learning®.

The **temporal process** seen in the lateral aspect projects back, forming half of the **zygomatic arch**. (The zygomatic arch consists of the
temporal process of the zygomatic bone and the zygomatic process of
the temporal bone.) The **frontal process** forms the articulation with
the frontal and sphenoid bones.

Figure 6-15. (A) Medial view of the nasal septum. Note that the septum is composed of the perpendicular plate of the ethmoid, the vomer, and the septal cartilage. (B) Sagittal section through the nasal septum. (continues).

© Cengage Learning®.

(A)

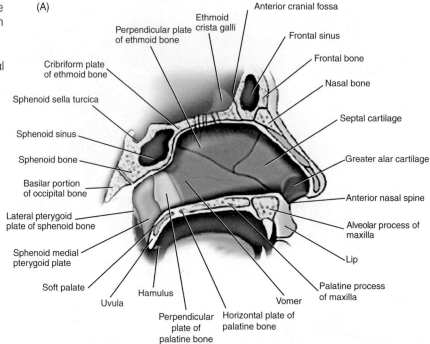

(B)

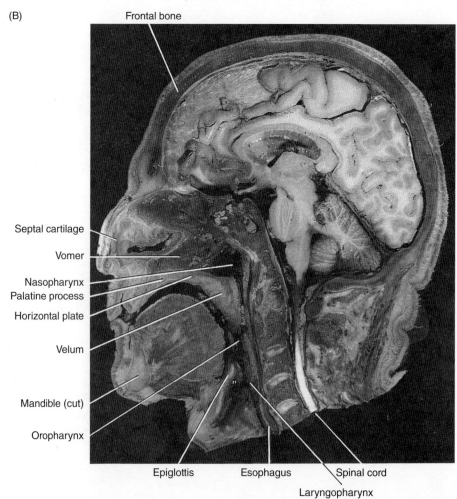

(C)

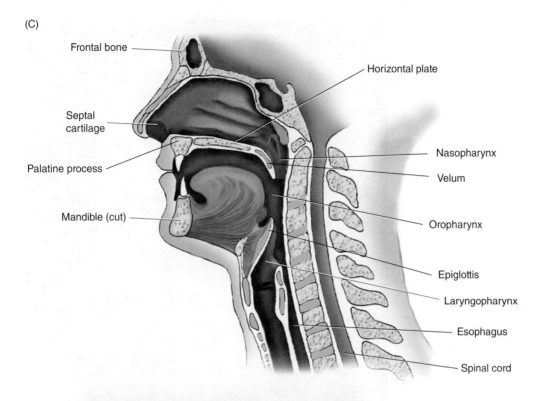

Frontal bone

Horizontal plate

Septal
cartilage

Nasopharynx

Velum

Palatine process

Mandible (cut)

Oropharynx

Epiglottis

Laryngopharynx

Esophagus

Spinal cord

(D)

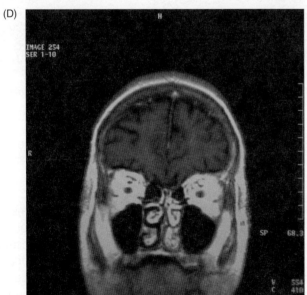

Figure 6-15 continued. (C) Drawing of the sagittal section through the nasal septum. (D) Frontal magnetic resonance image showing deviated nasal septum and hypertrophied nasal mucosa and turbinate. (continues).

Source: John Foster.

(E)

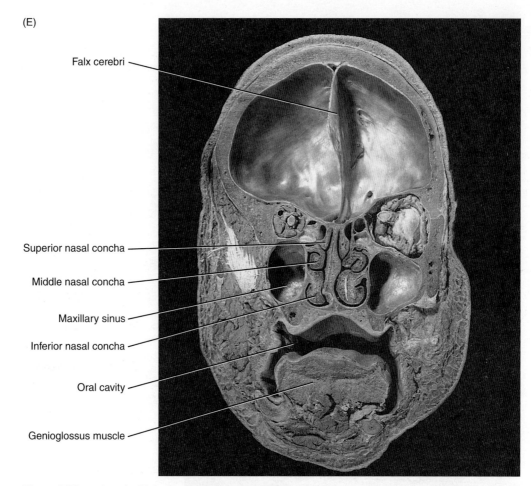

Falx cerebri

Superior nasal concha

Middle nasal concha

Maxillary sinus

Inferior nasal concha

Oral cavity

Genioglossus muscle

Figure 6-15 continued. (E) Frontal section revealing maxillary sinuses, nasal cavities, and the relationship of oral articulators. (continues).
© Cengage Learning®.

Cleft Lip and Cleft Palate

Cleft lip and cleft palate arise during early development. Cleft lip may be either unilateral or bilateral, occurring along the premaxillary suture. Cleft lip will almost never be midline, but may involve soft tissue alone or include a cleft of the maxilla up to the incisive foramen. Cleft palate may involve both hard and soft palates.

Cleft lip appears to result from a failure of embryonic facial and labial tissue to fuse during development. It looks as though tissues migrate and develop normally but, for some reason, either fail to fuse or the fusion of the migrating medial nasal, maxillary, and lateral nasal processes breaks down. Cleft palate apparently arises from some mechanical intervention in development. Prior to the seventh embryonic week the palatine processes of the maxillae have been resting alongside the tongue so that the tongue separates the processes. As the oral cavity and mandible grow, the tongue drops away from the processes, and the processes can extend, make midline contact, and fuse. If something (such as micrognathia) blocks the movement of the tongue, the palatine processes will not move in time to make contact. The head grows rapidly, and the plates will have missed their chance to become an intact palate.

(F)

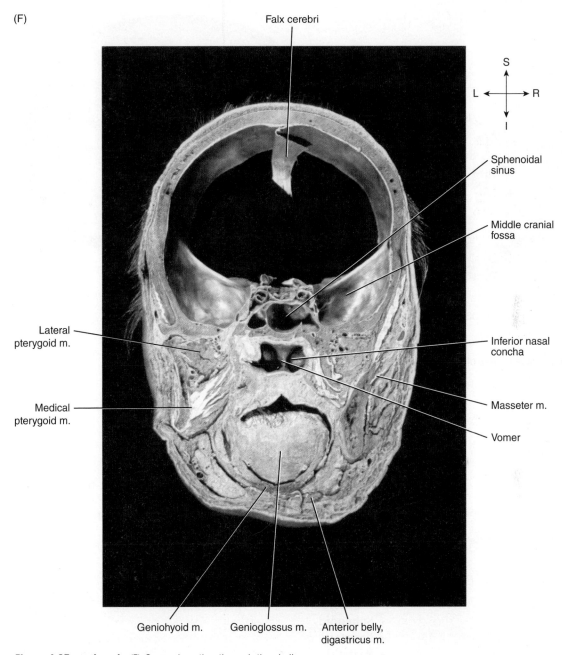

Falx cerebri

S

L ← → R

I

Sphenoidal sinus

Middle cranial fossa

Lateral pterygoid m.

Medical pterygoid m.

Inferior nasal concha

Masseter m.

Vomer

Geniohyoid m.   Genioglossus m.   Anterior belly, digastricus m.

Figure 6-15 continued. (F) Coronal section through the skull.
© Cengage Learning®.

Lacrimal Bones

The small **lacrimal** bones are almost completely hidden in the intact skull. They articulate with the maxillae, frontal bone, nasal bone, and inferior conchae. They constitute a small portion of the lateral nasal wall and form a small portion of the medial orbit as well.

lacrimal: L., lacrima, tear

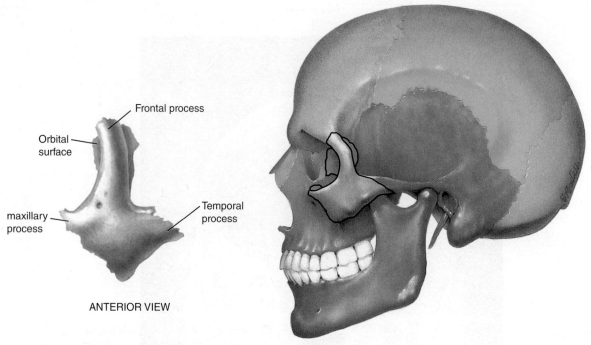

Figure 6-16. Anterior view of the zygomatic bone.
© Cengage Learning®.

Hyoid Bone

The hyoid bone was discussed in Chapters 4 and 5, but rightfully belongs in this chapter as well. Its presence in this listing should remind you of the interconnectedness of the phonatory and articulatory systems.

Bones of the Cranial Skeleton

- **Ethmoid**
- **Sphenoid**
- **Frontal**
- **Parietal**
- **Occipital**
- **Temporal**

The bones of the cranium include those involved in the creation of the cranial cavity.

Ethmoid Bone

ethmoid: Gr., ethmos, sieve + eidos, like

The **ethmoid** bone is a complex, delicate structure with a presence in the cranial, nasal, and orbital spaces. If the cranium and facial skeleton were an apple, the ethmoid would be the core (Figure 6-17).

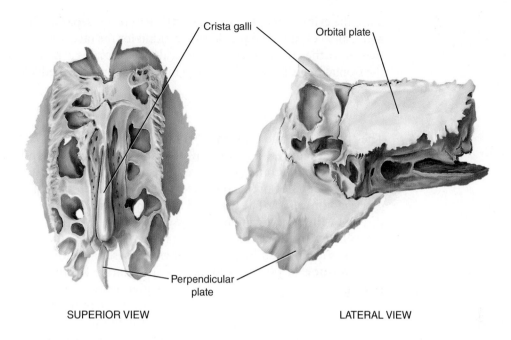

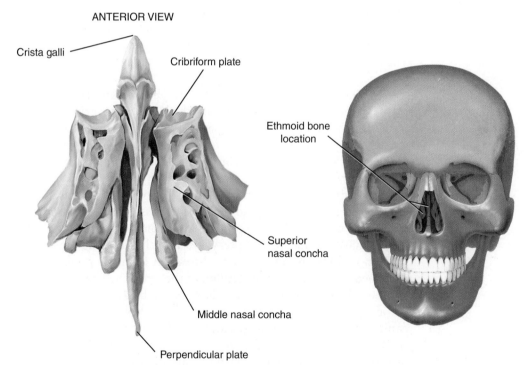

Figure 6-17. Views of the ethmoid bone.
© Cengage Learning®.

When viewed from the front, the superior surface is dominated by the **crista galli**, which protrudes into the cranial space. Projecting down is the perpendicular plate, making up the superior nasal septum, and lateral to this plate are the middle and superior nasal conchae. On both sides of the perpendicular plate and perpendicular to

cribriform: L., cribum, sieve + forma, the porous component of the ethmoid bone

sphenoid: Gr., spheno, wedge + eidos, like

sella turcica: L., Turkish saddle

chiasma: Gr., khiasma, cross; an X-shaped crossing

fossa: L., furrow or depression

tuberculum: L., little swelling

clivus: L., slope

it are the **cribriform plates**. The **cribriform** plates separate the nasal and cranial cavities and provide the conduit for the olfactory nerves as they enter the cranial space. The lateral **orbital plates** articulate with the frontal bone, lacrimal bone, and maxilla to form the medial orbit.

Sphenoid Bone

The **sphenoid** bone is much more complex than the ethmoid bone. A glance at Figure 6-18 will show that the sphenoid is a significant contributor to the cranial structure. The sphenoid consists of a corpus and three pairs of processes, the greater wings, lesser wings, and pterygoid processes. The sphenoid also contains numerous foramina through which nerves and blood vessels pass.

When viewed from above, you can see that the medially placed **corpus** is dominated by the **hypophyseal fossa** (also known as the **sella turcica** or **pituitary fossa**), the indentation holding the pituitary gland (hypophysis) in life. This gland projects down from the hypothalamus and is placed at the point where the optic nerve decussates, the **chiasma**. The anterior portion of the **fossa** is the **tuberculum sellae**, and the posterior aspect is the **dorsum sellae**. The **anterior clinoid processes** project from the lesser wing of the sphenoid, lateral to the **tuberculum** sellae. The optic nerve passes under these processes, having passed through the optic foramen anteriorly. The **clivus** forms the union with the foramen magnum of the occipital bone. Within the corpus are the air-filled **sphenoid sinuses**.

The **lesser** and **greater wings** of the sphenoid are striking landmarks, likened to the wings of a bat. The lesser wings arise from the corpus and clinoid process and partially cover the optic canal. The greater wings arise from the posterior corpus, making up a portion of the orbit. The greater wing comprises a portion of the anterolateral skull and articulates with the frontal and temporal bones.

Projecting downward from the greater wing and corpus are the **lateral** and **medial pterygoid plates**. The fossa between the medial and lateral plates will be the point of attachment for one of the muscles of mastication (medial pterygoid muscle), and the tensor veli palatini will attach to the **scaphoid fossa**. A hamulus projects from each medial lamina, and the tendon of the tensor veli palatini passes around this on its course to the velum, as will be discussed.

The openings of the superior sphenoid are particularly significant. For example, the **optic canal** carries the II optic nerve, and the **foramen ovale** provides the conduit for the mandibular nerve of V trigeminal. The maxillary nerve arising from the V trigeminal passes through the **foramen rotundum**, and the **superior orbital fissure** conveys the III oculomotor, IV trochlear, several branches of the ophthalmic nerve of V trigeminal, and VI abducens nerves. The **body** of the sphenoid includes the anteriorly placed **jugum** and the **chiasmatic groove**, which accommodates the optic chiasm.

jugum: L., a yoke

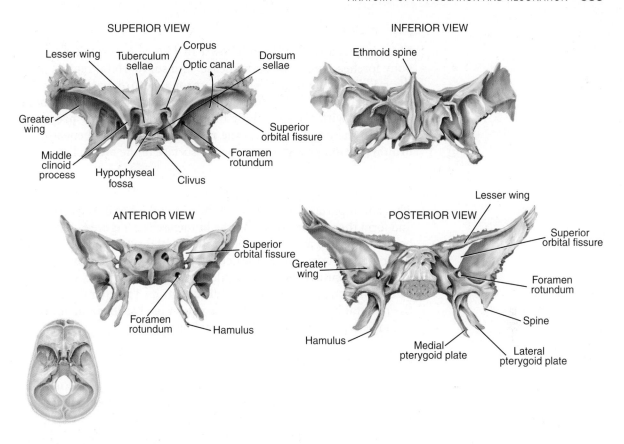

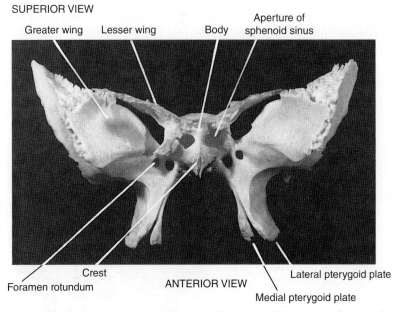

Figure 6-18. Photograph of the anterior view of the sphenoid bone and schematic drawings of the sphenoid from four views.
© Cengage Learning®.

Frontal Bone

The unpaired frontal bone shown in Figure 6-19 makes up the bony forehead, anterior cranial case, and supraorbital region. Near the middle of the intact skull, the coronal suture marks the point of articulation of the frontal and parietal bones. The frontal bone articulates with the zygomatic bones via the **zygomatic processes** and with the nasal bones via the **nasal portion**. From beneath, the **orbital portion** provides the superior surface of the eye socket.

Parietal Bones

The paired parietal bones overlie the parietal lobes of the cerebrum and form the middle portion of the braincase (see Figure 6-20). These bones are united at the midline by the sagittal suture, running from the frontal bone in front to the occipital bone in back, separated by the **lambdoidal suture**. Small, irregular **wormian bones** may be formed by the bifurcations of the **lambdoidal** suture. The lateral margin of the parietal bone is marked by the **squamosal suture**, forming the union between parietal and temporal bones.

lambdoidal: Gr., "L"-like, refers to the suture separating occipital and parietal bones

Occipital Bone

The unpaired occipital bone is deceptively simple in appearance (see Figure 6-21). It overlies the occipital lobe of the brain and makes up the posterior braincase. It articulates with the temporal, parietal, and sphenoid bones. The **external occipital protuberance** is a midline prominence visible from behind. The **cerebral** and **cerebellar fossa** of the inner superior surface mark the locations of the occipital lobe and cerebellum, respectively, in the intact braincase.

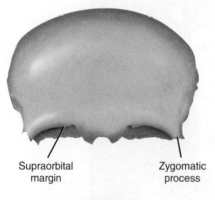

Supraorbital
margin

Zygomatic
process

ANTERIOR VIEW

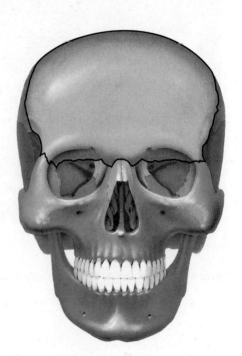

Figure 6-19. Anterior view of the frontal bone.

© Cengage Learning®.

(A)

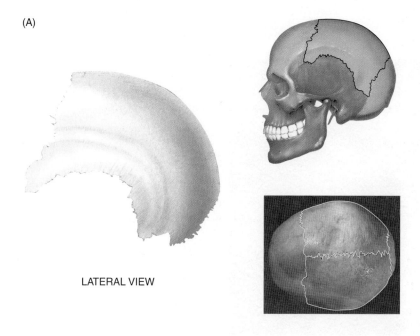

LATERAL VIEW

(B)

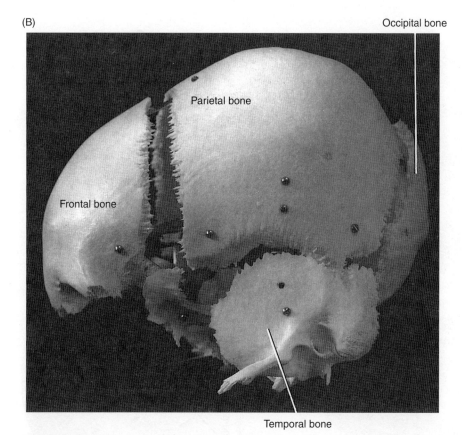

Figure 6-20. (A) Lateral view of the parietal bone. (B) Photo of disarticulated parietal, frontal, temporal, and occipital bones.

© Cengage Learning®.

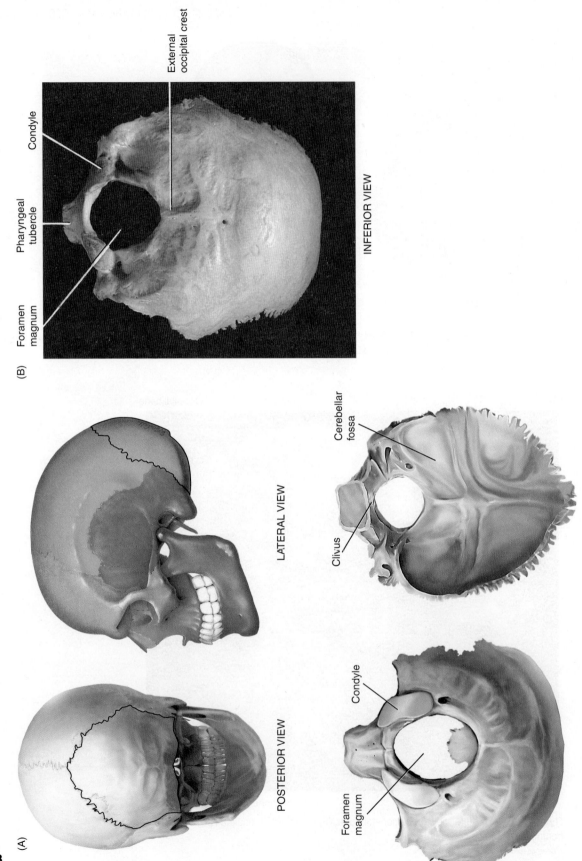

Figure 6-21. (A) Occipital bone seen from inferior and superior aspects. (B) Photo of occipital bone, inferior view.

© Cengage Learning®.

(B)

Condyle

Pharyngeal tubercle

Foramen magnum

External occipital crest

INFERIOR VIEW

(A)

LATERAL VIEW

POSTERIOR VIEW

Cerebellar fossa

Clivus

SUPERIOR VIEW

Condyle

Foramen magnum

INFERIOR VIEW

Synostosis and Craniostenosis

Synostosis refers to the articulation of adjacent bones by means of ossification of a suture. The suture, such as the coronal suture of the skull, undergoes ossification, during which it is converted to bone and the joint is immobilized. Craniostenosis (also known as **craniosynostosis**) is a rare condition affecting 1 out of 2,000 live births, which arises from premature ossification or closing of cranial sutures. At birth these sutures are pliable, being made up of sutural membrane, a fibrous connective tissue. The process of ossification occurs well into adulthood, but premature closure (craniosynostosis) apparently begins during prenatal development. The result of premature closure is that the pressure of the developing brain will cause deformation of the skull and, if left uncorrected, damage to the brain. The good news is that surgical procedures have been developed to completely correct the problem if identified in a timely fashion.

The most significant landmarks are those visible from beneath. From this vantage point, you can see that the occipital bone forms the base of the skull, wrapping beneath the brain. The **foramen magnum** provides the opening for the spinal cord and beginning of the medulla oblongata, and the **condyles** mark the resting point for the first cervical vertebra. The **basilar part** articulates with the corpus of the sphenoid.

Temporal Bone

The temporal bone is an important structure for students of speech pathology and audiology. On gross examination of the lateral skull, you can see that the temporal bone is separated from the parietal bone by the **squamosal** suture (also known as the *parietomastoid suture*) and from the occipital bone by the **occipitomastoid suture** (see Figure 6-22).

The temporal bone seen from the side is extremely dense and is remarkably rich in important landmarks. This complex bone is divided into four segments: the squamous, tympanic, mastoid, and petrous portions.

The **squamous portion**, which abuts the squamosal suture, is fan-shaped and thin. The lower margin includes the roof of the **external auditory meatus**, the conduit for sound energy to the middle ear. The anteriorly directed zygomatic process also arises from the squamous portion, articulating with the temporal process of the zygomatic bone to form the **zygomatic arch** (see Figure 6-5A). Beneath the base of the zygomatic process is the **mandibular fossa** of the temporal bone with which the condyloid process of the mandible articulates to form the temporomandibular joint.

The **tympanic portion** includes the anterior and inferior walls of the external auditory meatus. The prominent **styloid process** protrudes beneath the external auditory meatus and medial to the

squamosal: referring the squamous portion of the temporal bone

meatus: L., opening

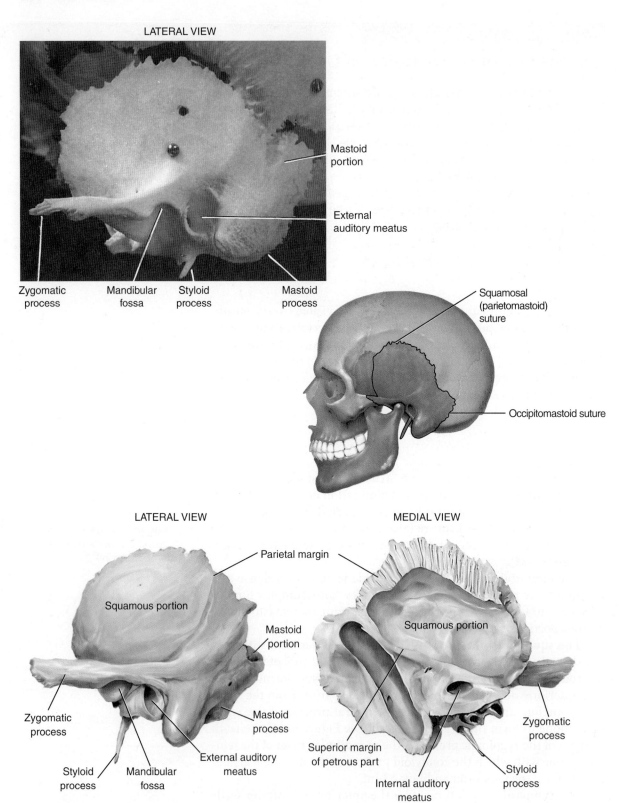

LATERAL VIEW

Mastoid portion

External auditory meatus

Zygomatic process

Mandibular fossa

Styloid process

Mastoid process

Squamosal (parietomastoid) suture

Occipitomastoid suture

LATERAL VIEW

Parietal margin

Squamous portion

Mastoid portion

Zygomatic process

Mastoid process

Styloid process

Mandibular fossa

External auditory meatus

MEDIAL VIEW

Squamous portion

Zygomatic process

Superior margin of petrous part

Internal auditory meatus

Styloid process

Figure 6-22. Schematic and photo of the lateral and medial view of the temporal bone.

© Cengage Learning®.

mastoid process. The **petrous portion** includes the cochlea and semi-circular canals in life. The **mastoid portion** makes up the posterior part of the temporal bone. Air cells in the mastoid portion communicate with the **tympanic antrum**. Above the antrum is the **tegmen tympani**, a thin plate of bone, and medial to it is the lateral semicircular canal. The **mastoid process**, a structure you can easily palpate by feeling behind your ear, arises from this portion.

The **temporal fossa** is a region including a portion of the temporal, parietal, and occipital bones. The temporal portion is the large region near the parietal and occipital bones. A band including the squamosal suture on the parietal bone and the superior portion of the occipitotemporal suture are included in the temporal fossa as well, with the entire region marking the point of origin of the fan-shaped temporalis muscle (to be discussed). The medial surface of the temporal bone reveals the **internal auditory meatus** through which the VIII cranial nerve will pass on its way to the brain stem.

> **tympanic antrum:** L., drum cavity
>
> **tegmen tympani:** L., drum covering

✔ *To summarize:*

- The bones of the **face** and **skull** work together in a complex fashion to produce the structures of **articulation**.
- The **mandible** provides the lower **dental arch** (lower set of teeth), **alveolar region**, and the resting location for the tongue.
- The **maxillae** provide the **hard palate**, point of attachment for the **soft palate**, **alveolar ridge**, upper **dental arch**, and dominant structures of the **nasal cavities**.
- The midline **vomer** articulates with the perpendicular plate of the **ethmoid** and the **cartilaginous septum** to form the **nasal septum**.
- The **zygomatic bone** articulates with the **frontal bone** and **maxillae** to form the cheekbone. The small **nasal bones** provide the upper margin of the nasal cavity.
- The **ethmoid bone** serves as the core of the skull and face, with the prominent **crista galli** protruding into the **cranium** and the **perpendicular plate** dividing the nasal cavities.
- The **frontal, parietal, temporal**, and **occipital** bones of the skull overlie the lobes of the brain of the same names.
- The **sphenoid bone** has a marked presence within the braincase, with the prominent **greater** and **lesser wings** of the sphenoid being found lateral to the **corpus**. The **hypophyseal fossa** houses the pituitary gland. The **clivus** joins the **occipital** bone near the **foramen magnum**.

DENTITION

Anatesse Lesson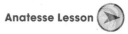

The teeth are vital components of the speech mechanism. Housed within the alveoli of the maxillae and mandible, teeth provide the mechanism for mastication, as well as articulatory surfaces for several speech sounds.

Before we discuss the specific teeth, let us begin with an orientation to the dental arch itself. The upper and lower dental arches contain equal numbers of teeth of four types: incisors, cuspids, bicuspids, and molars. It is convenient to think of half-arches, knowing that left and right sides will have equal distribution of teeth (see Figure 6-23).

Generally, teeth in the upper arch are larger than those in the lower arch, and the upper arch typically overlaps the lower arch in front. Each tooth has a **root**, hidden beneath the protective **gingival** or

gingival: L., gingiva, gum

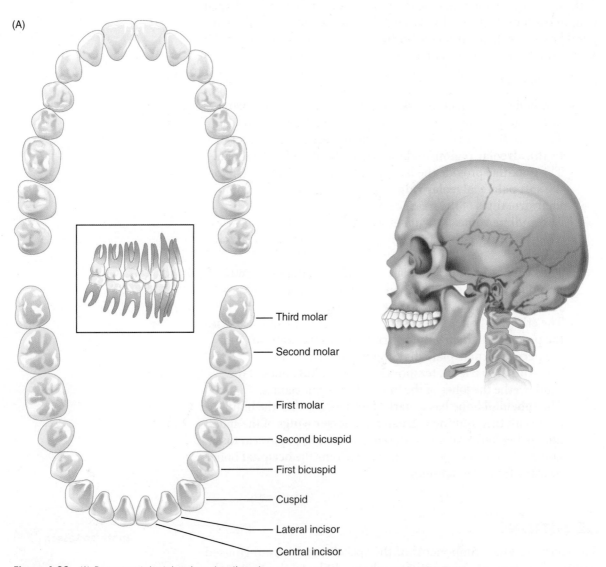

(A)

— Third molar

— Second molar

— First molar

— Second bicuspid

— First bicuspid

— Cuspid

— Lateral incisor

— Central incisor

Figure 6-23. (A) Permanent dental arches. (continues).
© Cengage Learning®.

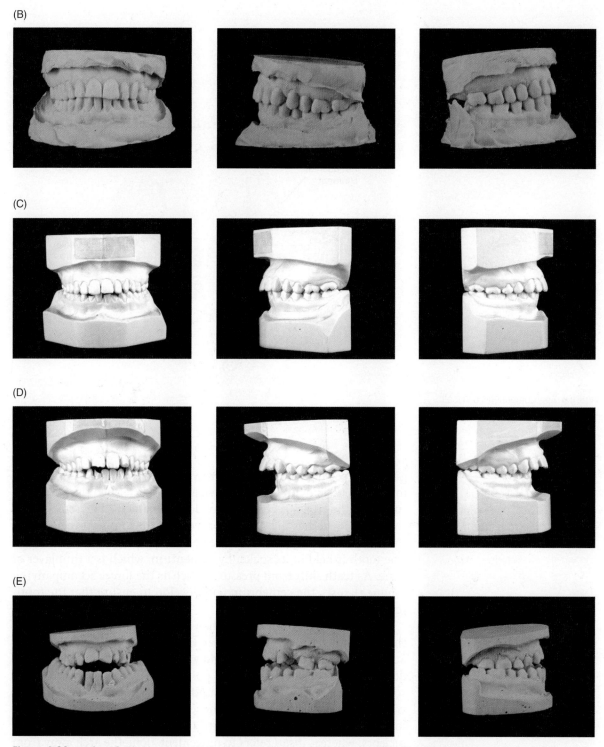

Figure 6-23 continued. (B) Anterior and lateral views of a normal adult dental arch. (C) Anterior and lateral views of the deciduous dental arch. (D) The dental arch of a child with significant oromyofunctional disorder. Note the marked labioversion of the incisors. (E) The deciduous dental arch of a child with significant oromyofunctional disorder. Note significant cross-bite, open bite, and malocclusion.

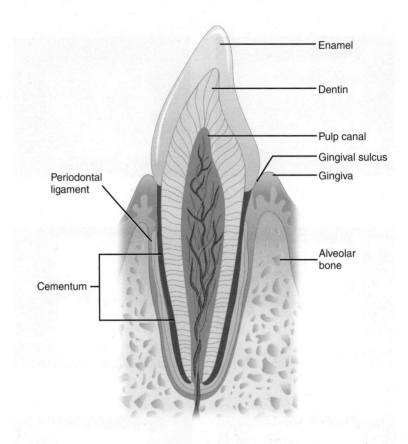

Figure 6-24. Components of a tooth.
© Cengage Learning®.

dentin: L., dens, tooth

gum line (see Figure 6-24). The **crown** is the visible one-third of the tooth, and the juncture of the crown and root is termed the **neck**. The surface of the crown is composed of dental **enamel**, an extremely hard surface that overlies the **dentin**, or ivory, of the tooth. At the heart of the tooth is the **pulp**, in which the nerve supplying the tooth resides. The tooth is held in its socket by **cementum**, which is a thin layer of bone. As teeth shift from pressures (such as the forces accompanying tongue thrust), the cementum will develop to ensure that the tooth remains firmly in its socket.

Five surfaces are important when discussing teeth. To understand the terminology, you need to alter your thinking about the dental arch a bit. Examine Figure 6-25 and you will see that the center of the dental arch is considered to be the point between the two central incisors, in front. Follow the arch around toward the molars in back and you have traced a path distal to those incisors. That is, *medial* refers to movement along the arch toward the midline between the central incisors, whereas *distal* refers to movement along the arch away from that midpoint. From this you can see that the **medial surface** (or **mesial**) of any tooth is the surface looking along the arch toward the midpoint between the central incisors. The **distal surface** is the surface of any tooth that is farthest from that midline point. Every tooth

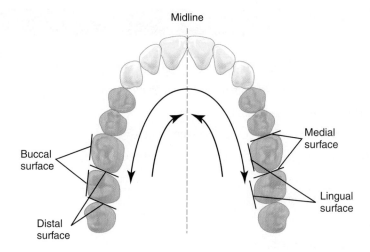

Figure 6-25. Surface referents of teeth and the dental arch.
© Cengage Learning®.

has a medial and a distal surface. Table 6-2 provides descriptions of terms related to dentition.

The **buccal surface** of a tooth is that which could come in contact with the **buccal** wall (cheek), and the **lingual surface** is the surface facing the tongue. The **occlusal surface** is the contact surface between teeth of the upper and lower arches. Not surprisingly, the thickest enamel overlies the occlusal surface, because it receives the most abrasion. However, the habit of chewing ice can undo this plan of nature causing premature **attrition** or wearing away of the dental enamel.

Incisors clearly are designed for cutting, as their name implies (see Figure 6-26). The **central incisors** of the upper dental arch present a large, spade-like surface with a thin cutting surface. The **lateral incisors** present a smaller but similar surface. If you feel your superior incisors with your tongue, you will feel a prominent ridge or **cingulum**. The lower incisors are markedly smaller than the upper incisors, resting within the upper arch, and you must slightly open and protrude your mandible to make contact between the occlusal surfaces of the incisors.

The **cuspid** (also **canine; eye tooth**) is well named. It has a single cusp or point that is used for tearing. In carnivores this tooth is particularly well suited for separating the fibers of muscle to support meat eating. Lateral to the cuspids are the **first** and **second bicuspids** or **premolars**. These teeth have two cusps on the occlusal surface and are absent in the deciduous dental arch.

Molars are large teeth with great occlusal surfaces designed to grind material, and their placement in the posterior arch capitalizes on the significant force available in the muscles of mastication. This mix of cutting teeth (incisors, cuspids, and bicuspids) and grinding teeth (molars) is just right for omnivorous humans: We can eat virtually anything.

buccal: L., bucca, cheek

incisor: L., cutter, referring to either lateral or central incisors of the upper or lower dental arch

cingulum: L., girdle

cuspid: L., cuspis, point

molars: L., molaris, grinding, referring to the posterior 6 teeth in either upper or lower adult dental arch

Table 6-2 **Terms related to dentition**	
Surfaces:	
Medial/mesial	Surface of an individual tooth closest to midline point on arch between central incisors.
Distal	Surface of an individual tooth farthest from midline point on arch between central incisors.
Buccal	Surface of a tooth that could come in contact with the buccal wall.
Lingual	Surface of a tooth that could come in contact with the tongue.
Occlusal	The contact surface between teeth of the upper and lower arches.
Development:	
Intraosseous eruption	Eruption of teeth through the alveolar process.
Clinical eruption	Eruption of teeth into the oral cavity.
Successional teeth	Teeth that replace deciduous teeth.
Superadded teeth	Teeth in the adult arch not present within the deciduous arch.
Supernumerary	Teeth in excess of the normal number for an arch.
Dental Occlusion:	
Overjet	Normal projection of upper incisors beyond lower incisors in transverse plane.
Overbite	Normal overlap of upper incisors relative to lower incisors.
Class I occlusal relationship	Relationship between upper and lower teeth in which the first molar of the mandibular arch is one-half tooth advanced of the maxillary molar.
Class I malocclusion	Occlusal relationship in which there is normal orientation of the molars, but an abnormal orientation of the incisors.
Class II malocclusion	Relationship of upper and lower arches in which the first mandibular molars are retracted at least one tooth from the first maxillary molars.
Class III malocclusion	Relationship of upper and lower arches in which the first mandibular molar is advanced more than one tooth beyond the first maxillary molar.
Relative micrognathia	Condition in which mandible is small in relation to the maxillae.
Axial Orientation:	
Torsiversion	Condition in which an individual tooth is rotated or twisted on its long axis.
Labioverted	Condition in which an individual tooth tilts toward the lips.
Linguaverted	Condition in which an individual tooth tilts toward the tongue.
Buccoversion	Condition in which an individual tooth tilts toward cheek.
Distoverted	Condition in which an individual tooth tilts away from midline of dental arch.
Mesioverted	Condition in which an individual tooth tilts toward the midline of the dental arch.
Infraverted	Condition in which a tooth is inadequately erupted.
Supraverted	Condition in which a tooth protrudes excessively into the oral cavity, causing inadequate occlusion of other dentition.
Persistent open bite	Condition in which the front teeth do not occlude because of excessive eruption of posterior teeth.
Persistent closed bite	Condition in which the posterior teeth do not occlude because of excessive eruption of anterior dentition.

UPPER ARCH

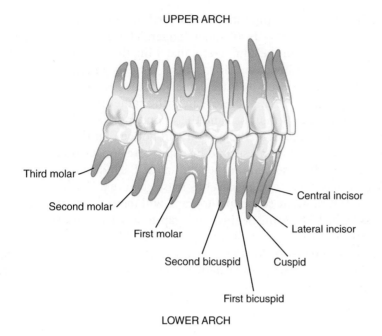

Third molar

Second molar

First molar

Second bicuspid

First bicuspid

Central incisor

Lateral incisor

Cuspid

LOWER ARCH

Figure 6-26. Types of teeth.
© Cengage Learning®.

There are three molars in each half of the adult dental arch. The medial-most **first molar** is the largest of the group, with the **second** and **third molars** descending in size. The first molar has four cusps, the second molar may have three or four, and the third molar has three. The third molar is sometimes known as the **wisdom tooth**, often erupting well into adulthood. The third molar is very likely a safeguard against losing teeth. In days before dental hygiene, it was not uncommon to lose many teeth to **caries**. A late-emerging set of molars, useful for grinding grain and pulverizing fibers, would be just the item to extend the life of our ancestors. Now those wisdom teeth seem less "wise," as they tend to crowd the other teeth and often develop with an orientation that makes them not only useless but also a threat to the healthy teeth.

The roots of the teeth reflect the forces applied to the teeth. The incisors and cuspids have a single long root, with the cuspid, which has a great deal of force on it from tearing, having the longest root. The bicuspids have variously one or two roots, and the molars have two or three roots to help anchor them against the massive forces of grinding.

Dental Development

Dental development clearly parallels that of the individual. Infants develop **deciduous** or **shedding teeth** (also known as **milk teeth**) that give way to the **permanent teeth** that must last a lifetime. Deciduous teeth actually begin development quite early in prenatal development, but start erupting through the bone (**intraosseous eruption**) and the gum (**clinical eruption**) when the child is between six and nine months of age. Tooth buds form when the developing mandible and

deciduous: L., deciduus, falling off

maxillae are only 1 mm long, but by birth the buds have spread out to match the jaw that is 40 times longer. These teeth are not only much smaller than the adult teeth, matching the size of the arch, but are fewer in number. Generally, central incisors emerge first (lower, then upper), followed by lateral incisors (upper, then lower). The first molars emerge at approximately the same time as the cuspids (between 15 and 20 months), and the second molars will have erupted by the child's second birthday. You will notice that there is no third molar, and the first and second bicuspids are conspicuously absent. These teeth are reserved for the adult arch. Each deciduous arch has 10 teeth, whereas the adult arch has 16 (see Figure 6-27 and Table 6-3).

Your first-grade school photograph will remind you of the period during which shedding begins. That gap-toothed grin of the six-year-old child comes from the shedding of the deciduous arch, beginning with the incisors (6 through 9 years), followed by first molars and cuspids (9 to 12 years), and finally second molars (beginning around 10 years of age).

(A)

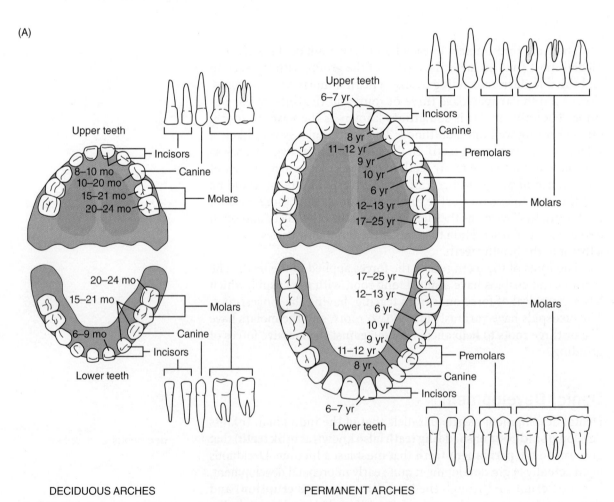

DECIDUOUS ARCHES   PERMANENT ARCHES

Figure 6-27. (A) Age of eruption of teeth in the permanent and deciduous arches. (continues).
© Cengage Learning®.

(B)

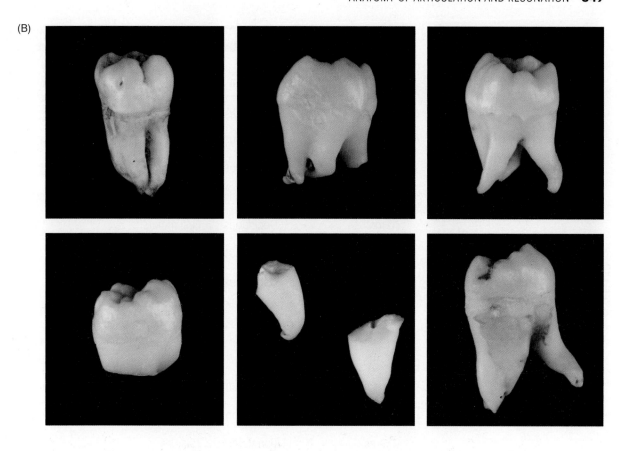

(C)

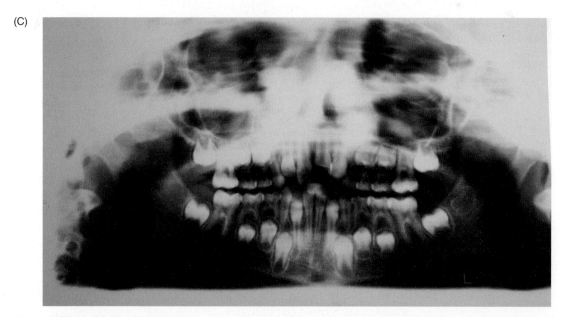

Figure 6-27 continued. (B) Individual deciduous and permanent teeth: Top row: adults 3rd molars; Bottom, left to right: deciduous molar, deciduous cuspids, deciduous molar. (C) Pantomagraph of mixed dentition. Note the presence of unerupted permanent teeth within the maxilla and mandible.

Source: Photograph courtesy of Dr. P. Chad Ellis, D.D.S.

Table 6-3 **Timeline for eruption of mandibular and maxillary dentition**			
Earliest Age of Expected Eruption	**TYPE of Dentition**	**Mandibular Dentition**	**Maxillary Dentition**
5 mo.	Deciduous	Central incisors	
6 mo.	Deciduous		Central incisors
7 mo.	Deciduous	Lateral incisors	
8 mo.	Deciduous		Lateral incisors
10 mo.	Deciduous	First molars	
16 mo.	Deciduous	Cuspids	Cuspids
20 mo.	Deciduous	Second molars	
36 mo.			Second molars
6 years	Permanent	Central incisors First molars	First molars
7 years	Permanent	Lateral incisors	Central incisors
8 years	Permanent		Lateral incisors
9 years	Permanent	Cuspids	
10 years	Permanent	First bicuspids	First bicuspids Second bicuspids
11 years	Permanent	Second bicuspids	Cuspids
12 years	Permanent	Second molars	Second molars
17 years	Permanent	Third molars	Third molars

Source: Based on data of Behrman, Vaughan, & Nelson, 1987.

periodontal: Gr., peri, around + odous, referring to the gum ridge surrounding a tooth

Shedding is not a passive process. If you have an occasion to view a tooth shed by a child, you will see very little of the root. The deciduous tooth is suspended in the socket by means of a **periodontal ligament** that serves as a pressure sensor. As the permanent tooth migrates toward the surface, its proximity stimulates the conversion of the deciduous **periodontal** ligament into osteoclasts that promote resorption of the root and enamel. Thus, by the time the permanent tooth is ready to erupt, the deciduous tooth has lost its anchor in the alveolus and comes out easily.

The permanent teeth that replace deciduous teeth are called **successional teeth**. The third molar and bicuspids erupt in addition to the original constellation and thus are referred to as **superadded**.

Dental Occlusion

The primary purpose of dentition is mastication, and this fact makes the orientation of teeth of the utmost importance. **Occlusion** is the process of bringing the upper and lower teeth into contact, and proper occlusion is essential for successful mastication. Clearly, if the upper molars do not make contact with the lower molars, no grinding will occur. We will discuss the orientation of the upper and lower dental arches, as well as orientation that the individual teeth can take within the arches. These terms of orientation will serve you well as you prepare for your clinical work, because they are central to the oral-peripheral examination of teeth.

To discuss this orientation, first examine your own dental arch relationship. Lightly tap your molars, and then bite down lightly and leave them occluded. This sets the orientation of the arches. With your teeth making contact in this manner, open your lips so that you can see the front teeth while looking at a mirror. If you have a **Class I occlusal relationship** between your upper and lower teeth, the first molar of the mandibular arch is one-half tooth advanced of the maxillary molar. Your upper incisors project beyond the lower incisors vertically by a few millimeters (termed **overjet**), and the upper incisors naturally hide the lower incisors (termed **overbite**) so that only a little of the lower teeth will show. This Class I occlusion (also known as **neutroclusion**) (see Figure 6-28) is considered the normal relationship between the molars of the dental arches.

In **Class II malocclusion**, the first mandibular molars are retracted at least one tooth from the first maxillary molars. This is sometimes the product of **relative micrognathia**, a condition in which the mandible is small in relation to the maxillae (see Figure 6-29).

A **Class III malocclusion** is identified if the first mandibular molar is advanced farther than one tooth beyond the first maxillary molar. Thus, in Class II malocclusion the mandible is retracted, whereas in Class III the mandible is protruded. There is a **Class I malocclusion**, as well. This is defined as an occlusion in which there is normal orientation of the molars, but an abnormal orientation of the incisors.

Individual teeth may be misaligned as well. If a tooth is rotated or twisted on its long axis, it has undergone **torsiversion**. If it tilts toward the lips, it is referred to as **labioverted**, whereas tilting toward

Dental Anomalies

There are numerous developmental dental anomalies. Children may be born with **supernumerary teeth** (teeth in addition to the normal number), or teeth may be smaller than appropriate for the dental arch (**microdontia**). Teeth may **fuse** together at the root or crown. In addition to this, enamel may be extremely thin or even missing from the surface of the tooth (**amelogenesis imperfecta**), or the enamel may be stained by use of the antibiotic tetracycline or fluoride.

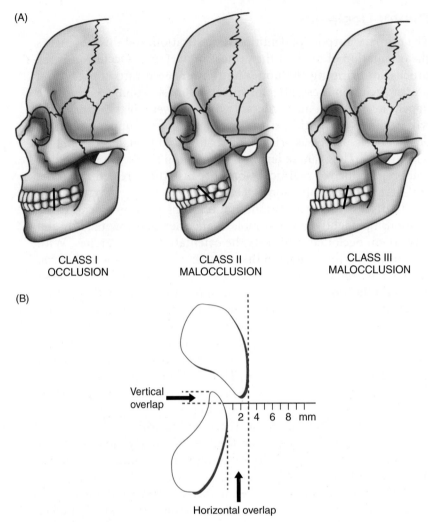

(A)

CLASS I
OCCLUSION

CLASS II
MALOCCLUSION

CLASS III
MALOCCLUSION

(B)

Vertical overlap

2 4 6 8 mm

Horizontal overlap

Figure 6-28. (A) Types of malocclusion. (B) Normal occlusal relationship between upper and lower central incisors.
© Cengage Learning®.

the tongue is **linguaverted** (see Figure 6-29A). When molars tilt toward the cheeks, it is called *buccoversion*. A tooth that tilts away from the midline along the arch is said to be **distoverted**, whereas one tilting toward that midline between the two central incisors is **mesioverted**. When a tooth does not erupt sufficiently to make occlusal contact with its pair in the opposite arch, it is said to be **infraverted**; the tooth that erupts too far is said to be **supraverted**. In some cases the front teeth may not demonstrate the proper occlusion because teeth in the posterior arch prohibit anterior contact, a condition that is termed **persistent open bite**. If supraversion prohibits the posterior teeth from occlusion, it is called **persistent closed bite**. As you examine the dental orientation of the photographs in Figure 6-29B and 6-29C, attend closely to the variety of misalignments in this dentition. The cast in Figure 6-29C was made from the teeth of a young person who had low muscle tone as well as marked and uncorrected tongue thrust.

✔ *To summarize:*

- The **teeth** are housed within the **alveoli** of the **maxillae** and **mandible** and consist of **incisors, cuspids, bicuspids,** and **molars**.
- Each tooth has a **root** and **crown**, with the surface of the crown composed of **enamel** overlying **dentin**.
- Each tooth has a **medial, distal, lingual, buccal** (or labial), and **occlusal** surface; the occlusal surface reflects the function of the teeth in the omnivorous human dental arch.

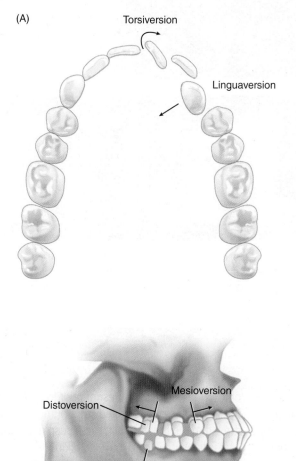

Figure 6-29. (A) Graphic representation of torsiversion, linguaversion, infraversion, distoversion, and mesioversion. (continues).

(B)

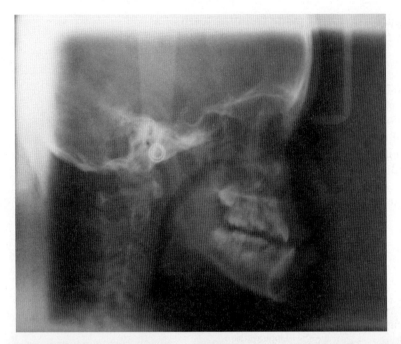

(C)

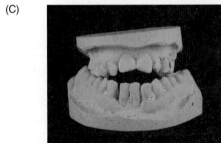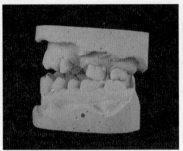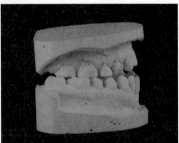

Figure 6-29 continued. (B) Radiograph of prognathic mandible that was later surgically corrected. (C) Dental impression of young adult with significant oromyofunctional disorder, revealing extreme palatal arch, distoversion, torsiversion, linguaversion, and labioversion secondary to tongue thrust. Note the evidence of gingival lesion (gum recession) secondary to retained tongue thrust.
Source: (B) Tanis Knopp.

Supernumerary Teeth

Supernumerary teeth arise from a developmental anomaly in which the embryonic dental lamina produces excessive numbers of tooth buds. When this occurs, the individual will be born with more teeth than predicted, often resulting in "twinning" of incisors. Below is a report from J. M. Harris, D.D.S., of a child he saw in his dental practice in Idaho Falls, Idaho.

An eight-year-old girl was brought to Dr. Harris's clinic with the complaint that one of her deciduous teeth needed to be extracted due to her age. Dr. Harris performed panelipse radiography to verify that the permanent teeth were present prior to the extraction, but the radiograph revealed supernumerary teeth in the left mandibular arch in the bicuspid region.

Extraction of the decayed deciduous tooth revealed a pocket of 15 supernumerary teeth: Some were simply tooth buds, but some had developed small roots and looked like fully formed molars. In an arch built ultimately for 16 teeth, that would be a significant addition!

The cluster was removed, Gelfoam was placed in the cavity, and sutures closed the space. There were no further complications.

- **Clinical eruption** of the **deciduous** arch begins between six and nine months of age, while the **permanent arch** emerges between six and nine years.
- **Class I occlusion** refers to normal orientation of mandible and maxillae, while **Class II malocclusion** refers to a relatively retracted mandible. **Class III malocclusion** refers to a relatively protruded mandible.
- Individual teeth may have aberrant orientation within the alveolus, including **torsiversion, labioversion, linguaversion, distoversion**, and **mesioversion**.
- Inadequately erupted or hypererupted teeth are referred to as **infraverted** and **supraverted**.

CAVITIES OF THE VOCAL TRACT

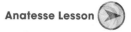
Anatesse Lesson

We mentioned that the source-filter theory depends upon cavities to shape the acoustic output. Before we show you the muscles associated with articulation, let us discuss how the cavities are shaped by the movements of those muscles. These are the oral, buccal, nasal, and pharyngeal cavities (see Figure 6-30).

(A)

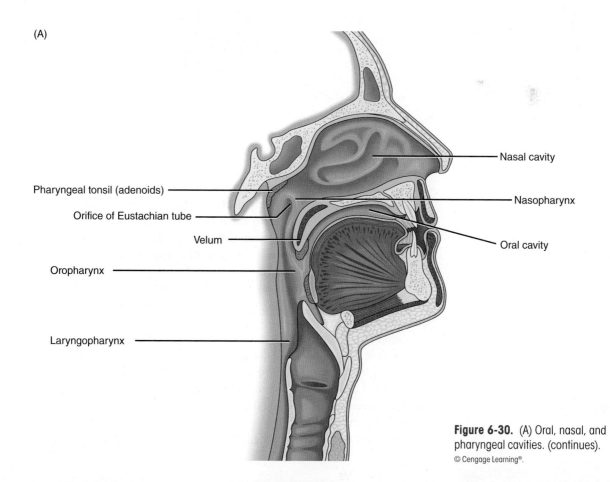

Pharyngeal tonsil (adenoids)

Orifice of Eustachian tube

Velum

Oropharynx

Laryngopharynx

Nasal cavity

Nasopharynx

Oral cavity

Figure 6-30. (A) Oral, nasal, and pharyngeal cavities. (continues).
© Cengage Learning®.

(B)

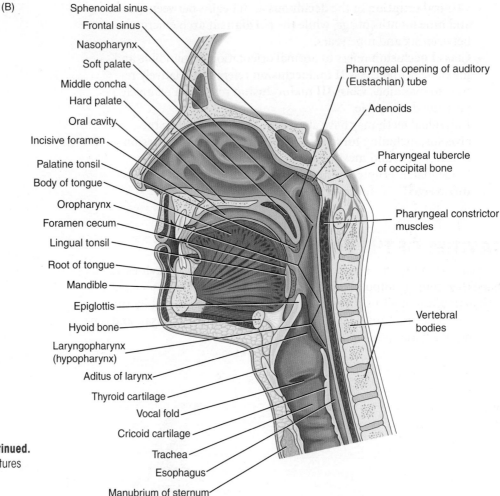

Sphenoidal sinus
Frontal sinus
Nasopharynx
Soft palate
Middle concha
Hard palate
Oral cavity
Incisive foramen
Palatine tonsil
Body of tongue
Oropharynx
Foramen cecum
Lingual tonsil
Root of tongue
Mandible
Epiglottis
Hyoid bone
Laryngopharynx
(hypopharynx)
Aditus of larynx
Thyroid cartilage
Vocal fold
Cricoid cartilage
Trachea
Esophagus
Manubrium of sternum

Pharyngeal opening of auditory
(Eustachian) tube
Adenoids
Pharyngeal tubercle
of occipital bone
Pharyngeal constrictor
muscles
Vertebral
bodies

Figure 6-30 continued.
(B) Detail of structures
and cavities.
© Cengage Learning®.

rugae: Gr., crease

The **oral cavity** is the most significant cavity of the speech mechanism, as it undergoes the most change during the speech act. Its shape can be altered by the movement of the tongue or mandible.

The oral cavity extends from the oral opening, or mouth, in front to the faucial pillars in back. The oral opening is strongly involved in articulation, being the point of exit of sound for all orally emitted phonemes (i.e., all sounds except those emitted nasally). The lips of the mouth are quite important for the articulation of a number of consonants and vowels.

This is a good opportunity to take a guided tour of your own mouth (see Figure 6-31). Palpate the roof of your mouth (you can use your tongue to feel this if you wish). The hard roof of your mouth is the **hard palate**. The prominent ridges running laterally are the **rugae**, potentially useful structures in the formation of the bolus of food during deglutition and serving as a landmark in articulation. The **median raphe** divides the hard palate into two equal halves.

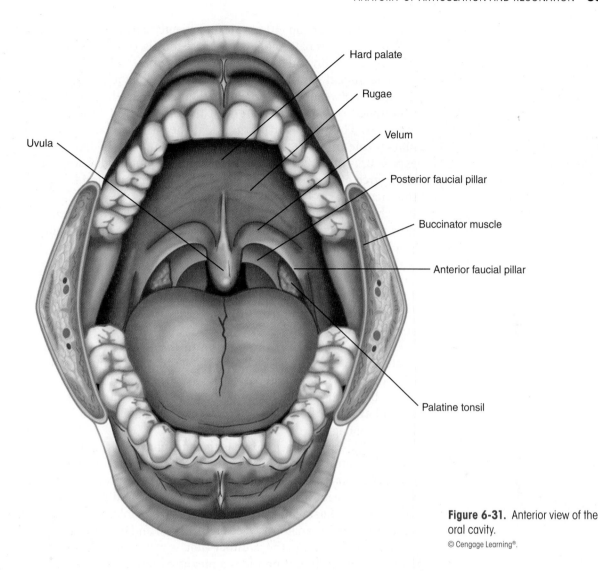

Figure 6-31. Anterior view of the oral cavity.
© Cengage Learning®.

As you run your tongue or finger back along the roof of your mouth, you can feel the point at which the hard palate suddenly becomes soft. This is the juncture of the hard and soft palates, and the soft portion is the **soft palate** or **velum**, with the **uvula** marking the terminus of the velum. The velum is the movable muscle mass separating the oral and nasal cavities (or more technically, the oropharynx and nasopharynx, as you shall see). The velum is attached in front to the palatine bone and is thus a muscular extension of the hard palate.

On either side of the soft palate and continuous with it are two prominent bands of tissue. These are the **anterior** and **posterior faucial pillars**, and they mark the posterior margin of the oral cavity. The teeth and alveolar ridge of the maxillae make up the lateral margins of the oral cavity. The tongue occupies most of the lower mouth.

Between the anterior and posterior faucial pillars you may see the **palatine tonsils**. These masses of lymphoid tissue are situated

velum: L., veil

between the pillars on either side and even invade the lateral under-surface of the soft palate. Medial to these tonsils, on the surface of the tongue, are the lingual tonsils (to be discussed).

The **buccal cavity** lies lateral to the oral cavity, composed of the space between the posterior teeth and the cheeks of the face. It is bounded by the cheeks laterally, the lips in front, and the teeth medially. The posterior margin is at the third molar. This space plays a role in oral resonance when the mandible is depressed to expose it, is involved in high-pressure consonant production, and is the source of the distortion heard in the misarticulation known as the lateral /s/.

The **pharyngeal cavity**, or **pharynx**, is broken into three logi-cally named regions. You can envision the pharynx as a tube approxi-mately 12 cm in length, extending from the vocal folds, below, to the region behind the nasal cavities, above. This tube is lined with muscle capable of constricting the size of the tube to facilitate deglutition, and this musculature plays an important role in effecting the closure of the **velopharyngeal port**, the opening between the oropharynx and the nasopharynx.

The **oropharynx** is the portion of the pharynx immediately posterior to the fauces, bounded above by the velum. The lower boundary of the oropharynx is the hyoid bone, which marks the upper boundary of the laryngopharynx. The **laryngopharynx** (or **hypopharynx**) is bounded anteriorly by the epiglottis and inferiorly by the esophagus.

The third pharyngeal space is the **nasopharynx**, the space above the soft palate, bounded posteriorly by the pharyngeal protuberance of the occipital bone and by the nasal **choanae** in front. The lateral nasopharyngeal wall contains the **orifice** of the **auditory tube** (also known as the **Eustachian tube**, named after Bortolomeo Eustachi, a sixteenth-century anatomist; see Figures 6-30 and 6-32).

Although minute, the auditory tube serves an extremely impor-tant function in that it provides a means of aerating the middle ear cavity. Recognize that the nasopharynx is on a level with the ears, so that the tube connecting the nasopharynx with the middle ear space must course slightly up, back, and out to reach that cavity. The audi-tory tube is actively opened through contraction of the tensor veli palatini muscle, as discussed later in this chapter. The bulge of tis-sue partially encircling the orifice of the auditory tube is the **torus tubarius**, and the ridge of tissue coursing down from the orifice is the **salpingopharyngeal fold**—actually the salpingopharyngeus muscle covered with mucous membrane.

Also within the nasopharynx are the **pharyngeal tonsils** (also known as **adenoids**). This mass of lymphoid tissue is typically found to arise from the base of the posterior nasopharynx. By virtue of its proximity to the velopharyngeal port, the tissue of the pharyn-geal tonsil may provide support for velar function. Removal of the adenoids from children with short or hypotrophied soft palates may result in persistent hypernasality.

choanae: Gr., funnel, posterior entry of the nasal cavities

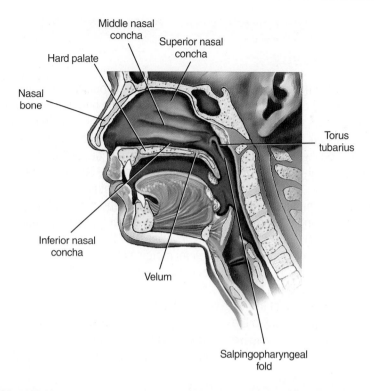

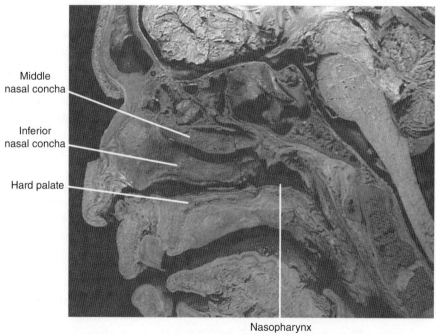

Figure 6-32. Nasal cavity and nasopharynx.
© Cengage Learning®.

The final cavities of concern to articulation are the nasal cavities (see Figure 6-32). The nasal cavities are produced by the paired maxillae, palatine, and nasal bones, and are divided by the nasal septum, made up of the singular vomer bone, perpendicular plate of the ethmoid, and the cartilaginous septum (as discussed in section the

Palpation of the Oral Cavity

This palpation exercise is best performed with one of your friends and requires aseptic procedures. You will want to perform it under the guidance of your instructor, as this will be a procedure that will carry into the oral peripheral examination in your clinical practice. A flashlight will help you identify structures.

Have your friend open his or her mouth as you look inside. Ensure that your nondominant hand (e.g., left hand if you are right-handed) is the only hand that holds the flashlight, as the other hand is gloved and must not touch anything but your friend. Ask your friend to say *ah* and watch the velum in back elevate. Look for presence or absence of the palatine tonsils between the faucial pillars. Shine the light on the hard palate and note the median **raphe** and rugae. Now palpate both of these structures,

running your finger back along both sides of the median raphe of the hard palate. Palpate the margin of the hard and soft palate, being sensitive to the fact that this may elicit a gag reflex in some people. As you palpate the hard palate, be sensitive to the potential presence of occult (hidden; submucous) clefts of the hard palate.

Have your friend bite lightly on his or her molars and hold his or her teeth closed but lips open for an /i/ vowel. With the gloved finger, palpate the lateral margins of the teeth and gums. With a tongue depressor, move the cheeks away from the teeth and examine the relationship between the upper and lower teeth for occlusion.

Pull the lower lip down gently and examine the labial frenulum. Ask your friend to open the mouth and elevate the tongue, and examine the lingual frenulum.

---

raphe: L., folds or creases, midline prominence on hard palate

"Bones of the Face and Cranial Skeleton"). The nasal cavities and turbinates are covered with mucous membrane endowed with beating and secreting epithelia, as well as a rich vascular supply. The moisture inherent in the nasal mucosa, combined with the rich vascular supply of the nasal tissue, serves to humidify and warm the air as it enters the passageway. Beating epithelia propel encapsulated pollutants toward the nasopharynx, from whence they slowly work their way toward the esophagus, to be swallowed (a much better fate than being deposited in the lungs).

The **nares** or nostrils mark the anterior boundaries of the nasal cavities, while the **nasal choanae** are the posterior portals connecting the nasopharynx and nasal cavities. The floor of the nasal cavity is the hard palate of the oral cavity, specifically the palatine processes of the maxillae and horizontal plates of the palatine bones.

✔ *To summarize:*

- The **cavities** of the articulatory system can be likened to a series of linked tubes.
- The most posterior of the tubes is the vertically directed **pharynx**, made up of the **laryngopharynx**, **oropharynx**, and **nasopharynx**.
- The horizontally coursing tube representing the nasal cavities arises from the nasopharynx, with the nasal and nasopharyngeal regions entirely separated from the oral cavity by elevation of the **soft palate**.

Auditory Tube Development

The Eustachian tube is the communicative port between the nasopharynx and middle ear cavity. It is opened during deglutition and yawning and provides a means of aeration of the middle ear cavity. In the adult, the auditory tube courses down at an angle of about 45°. In the infant, the tube is more horizontal, with the shift in the angle of descent brought about by head growth. It is felt that this horizontal course in the infant contributes to middle ear disease, with the assumption being that liquids and bacteria have a low-resistance path to the middle ear from the nasopharynx of an infant being bottle-fed in the supine position.

- The large tube representing the **oral cavity** is flanked by the small **buccal cavities**.
- The shape and size of the oral cavity is altered through movements of the tongue and mandible, and the nasal cavity may be coupled with the oral/pharyngeal cavities by means of the **velum**.

Let us examine the muscles involved in the articulatory system. Appendix E may assist you in your study of these muscles.

MUSCLES OF THE FACE AND MOUTH

The articulatory system is dominated by three significant structures: the lips, the tongue, and the velum. Movement of the lips for speech is a product of the muscles of the face, while the tongue capitalizes on its own musculature and that of the mandible and hyoid for its movement. The muscles of the velum elevate that structure to completely separate the oral and nasal regions. Table 6-4 may assist you in organizing the muscles of the face and mouth, while Figure 6-33 will help you recognize their functions.

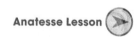 **Anatesse Lesson**

Muscles of the Face
- **Orbicularis oris**
- **Risorius**
- **Buccinator**
- **Levator labii superioris**
- **Zygomatic minor**
- **Levator labii superioris alaeque nasi**
- **Levator anguli oris**
- **Zygomatic major**
- **Depressor labii inferioris**
- **Depressor anguli oris**
- **Mentalis**
- **Platysma**

Table 6-4 Muscles of articulation

Muscles of the Face

Orbicularis oris	Levator anguli oris
Risorius	Zygomatic major
Buccinator	Depressor labii inferioris
Levator labii superioris	Depressor anguli oris
Zygomatic minor	Mentalis
Levator labii superioris alaeque nasi	Platysma

Intrinsic Tongue Muscles

Superior longitudinal

Inferior longitudinal

Transverse

Vertical

Extrinsic Tongue Muscles

Genioglossus

Hyoglossus

Styloglossus

Chondroglossus

Palatoglossus

Mandibular Elevators and Depressors

Masseter	Digastricus muscle
Temporalis muscle	Mylohyoid muscle
Medial pterygoid muscle	Geniohyoid muscle
Lateral pterygoid muscle	Platysma

Muscles of the Velum

Levator veli palatini

Musculus uvulae

Tensor veli palatini

Palatoglossus

Palatopharyngeus

Pharyngeal Musculature

Superior pharyngeal constrictor	Thyropharyngeus muscle
Middle pharyngeal constrictor	Salpingopharyngeus muscle
Inferior pharyngeal constrictor	Stylopharyngeus muscle
Cricopharyngeal muscle	

© Cengage Learning®.

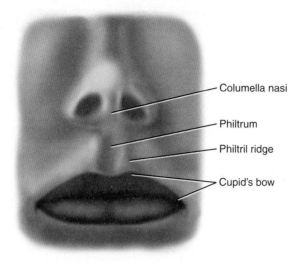

Columella nasi

Philtrum

Philtril ridge

Cupid's bow

Figure 6-33. Landmarks of the lips.
© Cengage Learning®.

Orbicularis Oris. The lips form the focus of the facial muscles, as their movement largely determines their function in both facial expression and speech (see Figure 6-33). The lips consist of muscle and mucous membrane that is richly invested with vascular supply, a trait made apparent by the translucent superficial epithelia. Although the lips serve a significant articulatory function, their social, cultural, and esthetic values as a central feature of the face are quite important. In cases where symmetry and morphology of the lips are compromised, as in clefting of the lip, the plastic surgeon will perform precise examination and measurement of the structure prior to performing exacting procedures to restore aesthetic balance.

To the plastic surgeon, the fine points of the **cupid's bow** are extremely important. The symmetry of this region is judged by the grace of its curve and its relationship to the **columella** and **philtrum**.

The **orbicularis oris** has been characterized as both a single muscle encircling the mouth opening (see Figure 6-34) and paired upper and lower muscles (**orbicularis oris superior** and **orbicularis oris inferior**). As we shall see in Chapter 7, there is ample evidence for *functional* differentiation of the upper and lower orbicularis oris. The upper and lower orbicularis oris act much like a drawstring to pull the lips closer together and effect a labial seal. The orbicularis oris is innervated by the mandibular marginal and lower buccal branches of the VII facial nerve.

The orbicularis oris serves as the point of insertion for many other muscles and interacts with the muscles of the face to produce the wide variety of facial gestures, of which we are capable. The muscles inserting into the orbicularis oris have different effects, based on their course and point of insertion into the lips. The **risorius** and buccinator muscles insert into the corners of the mouth and retract

risorius: L., laughing, most superficial of the buccal muscles

Muscle:	Orbicularis oris inferior and superior
Origin:	Corner of lips
Course:	Laterally within lips
Insertion:	Opposite corner of lips
Innervation:	VII facial nerve
Function:	Constrict oral opening

(A)

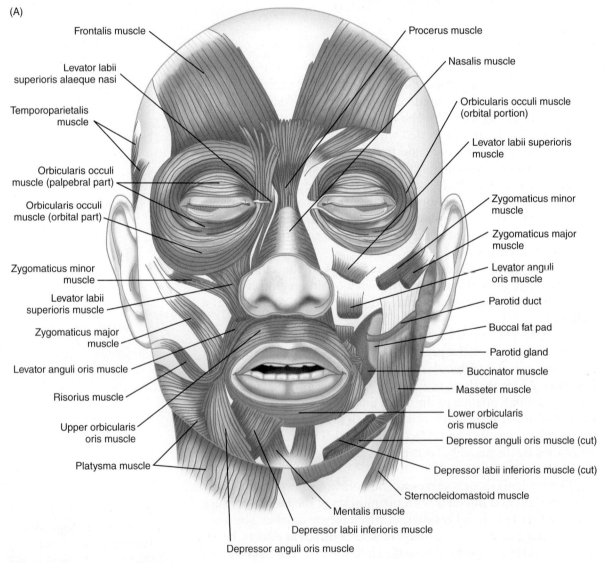

Figure 6-34. (A) Muscles of the face. (continues).

(B)

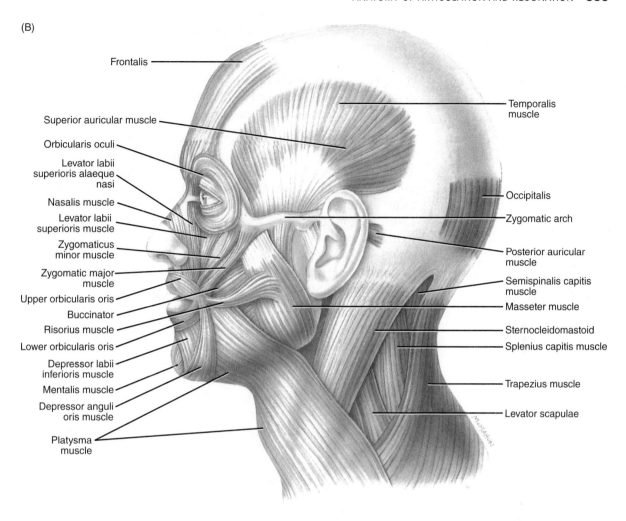

Frontalis

Superior auricular muscle

Orbicularis oculi

Levator labii superioris alaeque nasi

Nasalis muscle

Levator labii superioris muscle

Zygomaticus minor muscle

Zygomatic major muscle

Upper orbicularis oris

Buccinator

Risorius muscle

Lower orbicularis oris

Depressor labii inferioris muscle

Mentalis muscle

Depressor anguli oris muscle

Platysma muscle

Temporalis muscle

Occipitalis

Zygomatic arch

Posterior auricular muscle

Semispinalis capitis muscle

Masseter muscle

Sternocleidomastoid

Splenius capitis muscle

Trapezius muscle

Levator scapulae

(C)

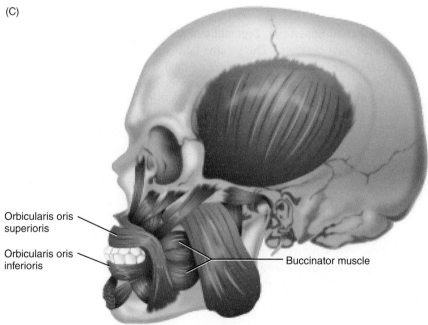

Orbicularis oris superioris

Orbicularis oris inferioris

Buccinator muscle

Figure 6-34 continued.
(B) The lateral view of facial muscles. (C) The relationship among facial muscles and pharyngeal constrictor muscles. Note that the orbicularis oris are continuous with the buccinator muscle, and ultimately with the superior pharyngeal constrictor.
© Cengage Learning®.

the lips. The depressor labii inferioris depresses the lower lip, and the **levator** labii superioris, zygomatic minor, and levator labii superioris alaeque nasi muscles elevate the upper lip. The zygomatic major muscle elevates and retracts the lips, whereas the depressor anguli oris depresses the corner of the mouth. The levator anguli oris pulls the corner of the mouth up and medially.

Risorius Muscle. It is evident from the course of the buccinator and risorius that they retract the corners of the mouth (see Figure 6-34). The buccinator is the dominant muscle of the cheeks. The **risorius muscle** is the most superficial of the pair, originating from the posterior region of the face along the fascia of the masseter muscle. The risorius is considerably smaller than the buccinator, coursing forward to insert into the corners of the mouth. The function of the risorius muscles is to retract the lips at the corners, facilitating smiling and grinning. Innervation of the risorius is by means of the buccal branch of the VII facial nerve.

Buccinator Muscle. The **buccinator muscle** ("bugler's muscle") lies deep to the risorius, following a parallel course. It originates at the pterygomandibular ligament, a tendinous slip running from the hamulus of the internal pterygoid plate of the sphenoid to the posterior mylohyoid line of the inner mandible. Fibers of the buccinator also arise from the posterior alveolar portion of the mandible and maxillae, while the posterior fibers appear to be continuous with those of the superior pharyngeal constrictor. The buccinator courses forward to insert into the upper and lower orbicularis oris.

The buccinator, like the risorius, is primarily involved in mastication. The buccinator is used to move food onto the grinding surfaces of the molars, and contraction of this muscle tends to constrict the oropharynx. The buccinator is innervated by the buccal branch of the VII facial nerve.

Levator Labii Superioris, Zygomatic Minor, and Levator Labii Superioris Alaeque Nasi Muscles. The levator labii superioris, zygomatic minor, and levator labii superioris alaeque nasi share a common insertion into the mid-lateral region of the upper lip, such that some anatomists refer to them as heads of the same muscle. The three hold the major responsibility for the elevation of the upper lip.

The medial-most **levator labii superioris alaeque nasi** courses nearly vertically along the lateral margin of the nose, arising from the frontal process of the maxilla. The intermediate **levator labii superioris** originates from the infraorbital margin of the maxilla, coursing down and in to the upper lip. The **zygomatic minor** begins its downward course from the facial surface of the zygomatic bone.

Together, these three muscles are the dominant forces in lip elevation. Working in conjunction, these muscles readily dilate the oral opening, and fibers from the levator labii superioris alaeque nasi that insert into the wing (ala) of the nostril will flare the nasal opening.

Muscle:	Risorius
Origin:	Posterior region of the face along the fascia of the masseter
Course:	Forward
Insertion:	Orbicularis oris at the corners of mouth
Innervation:	Buccal branch of the VII facial nerve
Function:	Retracts lips at the corners
Muscle:	Buccinator
Origin:	Pterygomandibular ligament
Course:	Forward
Insertion:	Orbicularis oris at the corners of mouth
Innervation:	Buccal branch of the VII facial nerve
Function:	Moves food onto the grinding surfaces of the molars; constricts oropharynx

The levator labii superioris, zygomatic minor, and levator labii superioris alaeque nasi are innervated by the buccal branches of the VII facial nerve.

Levator Anguli Oris. The **levator anguli oris** arises from the canine fossa of the maxilla, coursing to insert into the upper and lower lips. This muscle is obscured by the levator labii superioris. The levator anguli oris draws the corner of the mouth up and medially. The levator anguli oris is innervated by the superior buccal branch of the VII facial nerve.

Zygomatic Major. The **zygomatic major muscle** (zygomaticus) arises lateral to the zygomatic minor on the zygomatic bone. It takes a more oblique course than the minor, inserting into the corner of the orbicularis oris. The zygomatic major elevates and retracts the angle of

Muscle:	Levator labii superioris
Origin:	Infraorbital margin of the maxilla
Course:	Down and in to the upper lip
Insertion:	Mid-lateral region of the upper lip
Innervation:	Buccal branches of the VII facial nerve
Function:	Elevates the upper lip

Muscle:	Zygomatic minor
Origin:	Facial surface of the zygomatic bone
Course:	Downward
Insertion:	Mid-lateral region of upper lip
Innervation:	Buccal branches of the VII facial nerve
Function:	Elevates the upper lip

Muscle:	Levator labii alaeque nasi superioris
Origin:	Frontal process of maxilla
Course:	Vertically along the lateral margin of the nose
Insertion:	Mid-lateral region of the upper lip
Innervation:	Buccal branches of the VII facial nerve
Function:	Elevates the upper lip

Muscle:	Levator anguli oris
Origin:	Canine fossa of maxilla
Course:	Down
Insertion:	Corners of upper and lower lips
Innervation:	Superior buccal branches of VII facial nerve
Function:	Draws corner of mouth up and medially

the mouth, as in the gesture of smiling. The zygomatic major muscle is innervated by the buccal branches of the VII facial nerve.

Depressor Labii Inferioris. The **depressor labii inferioris** is the counterpart to the levator triad listed previously. It originates from the mandible at the oblique line, coursing up and in to insert into the lower lip. Contraction of the depressor labii inferioris dilates the orifice of the mouth by pulling the lips down and out. The depressor labii inferioris is innervated by the mandibular marginal branches of the VII facial nerve.

Depressor Anguli Oris. The **depressor anguli oris** (triangularis) originates along the lateral margins of the mandible on the oblique line. Its fanlike fibers converge on the orbicularis oris and upper lip at the corner. Contraction of the depressor anguli oris will depress the corners of the mouth and, by virtue of attachment to upper lip, help compress the upper lip against the lower lip, as well as help produce a frown. The depressor anguli oris is innervated by the mandibular marginal branch of the VII facial nerve.

Muscle:	Zygomatic major (zygomaticus)
Origin:	Lateral to the zygomatic minor on zygomatic bone
Course:	Obliquely down
Insertion:	Corner of the orbicularis oris
Innervation:	Buccal branches of the VII facial nerve
Function:	Elevates and retracts the angle of mouth
Muscle:	Depressor labii inferioris
Origin:	Mandible at the oblique line
Course:	Up and in to the lower lip
Insertion:	Lower lip
Innervation:	Mandibular marginal branch of the VII facial nerve
Function:	Dilates the orifice by pulling the lips down and out

Mentalis Muscle. The **mentalis muscle** arises from the region of the incisive fossa of the mandible, coursing down to insert into the skin of the chin below. Contraction of the mentalis elevates and wrinkles the chin and pulls the lower lip out, as in pouting. The mentalis receives its innervation via the mandibular marginal branch of the VII facial nerve.

Platysma. The **platysma** is more typically considered a muscle of the neck, but it is discussed here because of its function as a mandibular depressor. The platysma arises from the fascia overlying the pectoralis major and deltoid, coursing up to insert into the corner of the mouth, the region below the symphysis menti, and the lower margin of the mandible, fanning as well to insert into the skin near the masseter. The platysma is highly variable, but assists in the depression of the mandible. The platysma is innervated by the cervical branch of the VII facial nerve.

platysma: Gr., plate

✔ *To summarize:*

- The muscles of **facial expression** are important for articulation involving the lips.
- Numerous muscles insert into the **orbicularis oris** inferior and superior muscles, providing a flexible system for lip **protrusion**, **closure**, **retraction**, **elevation**, and **depression**.
- The **risorius** and **buccinator** muscles assist in the retraction of the lips, as well as supporting entrapment of air within the oral cavity.

Muscle:	Depressor anguli oris (triangularis)
Origin:	Lateral margins of the mandible on the oblique line
Course:	Fanlike upward
Insertion:	Orbicularis oris and upper lip corner
Innervation:	Mandibular branch of the VII facial nerve
Function:	Depresses corners of mouth and helps compress the upper lip against the lower lip

Muscle:	Mentalis
Origin:	Region of the incisive fossa of mandible
Course:	Down
Insertion:	Skin of the chin below
Innervation:	Mandibular marginal branch of the VII facial nerve
Function:	Elevates and wrinkles the chin and pulls the lower lip out

Muscle:	Platysma
Origin:	Fascia overlaying pectoralis major and deltoid
Course:	Up
Insertion:	Corner of the mouth, region below symphysis menti, lower margin of mandible, and skin near masseter
Innervation:	Cervical branch of the VII facial nerve
Function:	Depresses the mandible

- The contraction of the **levator labii superioris**, **zygomatic minor**, and **levator labii superioris alaeque nasi** elevates the upper lip, and the contraction of the **depressor labii inferioris** depresses the lower lip.
- The contraction of the **zygomatic major** muscle elevates and retracts the angle of the mouth, while the **depressor labii inferioris** pulls the lips down and out.
- The **depressor anguli oris** muscle depresses the corner of the mouth, the **mentalis** muscle elevates and wrinkles chin and pulls the lower lip out, and the **platysma** depresses the mandible.

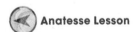 **Anatesse Lesson**

Muscles of the Mouth

Musculature of the mouth is dominated by intrinsic and extrinsic muscles of the tongue, as well as those responsible for the elevation of the soft palate. The movement of the tongue is an interesting engineering feat, as you shall see.

The Tongue

The tongue is a massive structure occupying the floor of the mouth. If you take a moment to examine Figure 6-35, you can get some notion of the magnitude of this organ. When a child uses the tongue as an expressive instrument, he or she protrudes only a small portion of it, leaving the bulk of the tongue within the mouth. We divide the muscles of the tongue into intrinsic and extrinsic musculature, a division that proves to be both anatomical and functional. The extrinsic muscles tend to move the tongue into the general region desired, while the intrinsic muscles tend to provide the fine, graded control of the articulatory gesture. The tongue is primarily involved in mastication and deglutition, being responsible for the movement of food within the oral cavity to position it for chewing and to propel it backward for swallowing.

The tongue is divided longitudinally by the **median fibrous septum**, a dividing wall between right and left halves that serves as the point of origin for the transverse muscle of the tongue (see Figure 6-38). The septum originates at the body of the hyoid bone via the hyoglossal membrane, forming the tongue attachment with the hyoid. The septum courses the length of the tongue.

It is useful to divide the tongue into regions as we discuss its characteristics (see Figure 6-35). The superior surface is referred to as the **dorsum**, and the anterior-most portion is the **tip** or **apex**. The **base** of the tongue is the portion of the tongue that resides in the oropharynx (also known as the **pharyngeal portion**). The portion of the tongue surface within the oral cavity, referred to as the **oral** or **palatine surface**, makes up about two-thirds of the surface of the tongue. The other third of the tongue surface lies within the oropharynx and is referred to as the **pharyngeal surface**. The **root** has variable definition by anatomists. Some refer to the pharyngeal portion as the root and call the palatine surface the body, while others view the base of the tongue as the root, as we have indicated in

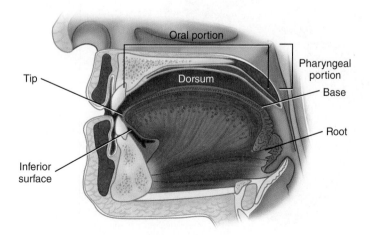

Figure 6-35. Demarcation of the regions of the tongue.

© Cengage Learning®.

Figure 6-36. Phoneticians will use the palatine definition, such that "advancement of the root" results in "fronting" of a sound (Cooper, personal communication; Edmonson & Esling, 2006).

The mucous membrane covering the tongue dorsum has numerous landmarks (see Figures 6-36 and 6-37). The prominent central or **median sulcus** divides the tongue into left and right sides. The posterior of the tongue is invested with **lingual papillae**, small, irregular prominences on the surface of the tongue. The **terminal sulcus** marks the posterior palatine surface, and the center of this groove is the **foramen cecum**, a deep recess in the tongue.

Beneath the membranous lining of the pharyngeal surface of the tongue are **lingual tonsils**, groups of lymphoid tissue. Working in conjunction with the pharyngeal and palatine tonsils, the lingual tonsils form the final portion of the ring of lymphatic tissue in the oral and pharyngeal cavities. Tonsils tend to atrophy over time. Although the pharyngeal and palatine tonsils may be quite prominent during childhood, they are markedly diminished in size by puberty.

The tongue is invested with taste buds to convey the gustatory sense. Sensors for all types of tastes are found throughout the oral cavity, although there are regions of concentration of receptor types. The anterior tongue has receptors that are primarily sensitive to both sweet and sour tastes, and the sides of the tongue are primarily sensitive to sour tastes. Bitter tastes are generally sensed near the terminal sulcus. The sensors, or "taste buds," are located in the various **papillae** found on the tongue, as will be discussed in detail in Chapter 8.

papillae: L., nipple, small prominences on the tongue that hold taste sensors

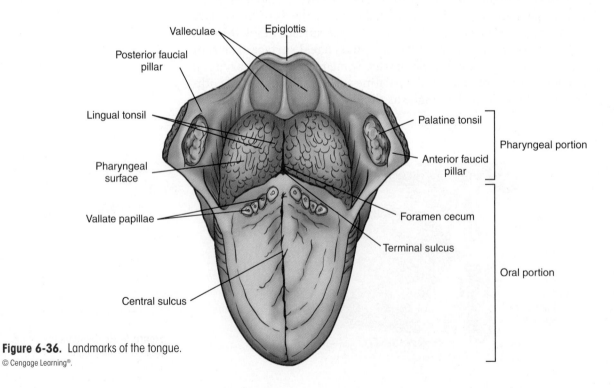

Figure 6-36. Landmarks of the tongue.
© Cengage Learning®.

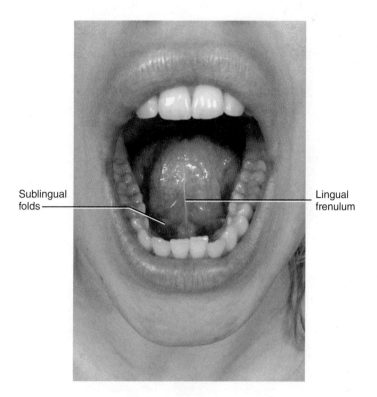

Sublingual folds

Lingual frenulum

Figure 6-37. Inferior surface of the tongue.
© Cengage Learning®.

If you examine the inferior surface of your tongue in a mirror, you will see three important landmarks (see Figure 6-37). Notice the rich vascular supply on that undersurface: Medications administered under the tongue will be very quickly absorbed into the bloodstream. You will see a prominent band of tissue running from the inner mandibular mucosa to the underside of the tongue. The **lingual frenulum (or lingual frenum)** joins the inferior tongue and the mandible, perhaps stabilizing the tongue during the movement. Also notice the transverse band of tissue on either side of the tongue (the **sublingual fold**). At this point are the ducts for the sublingual salivary glands. Lateral to the lingual frenulum are the ducts for the submandibular salivary glands that are hidden under the mucosa on the inner surface of the mandible. These salivary glands and their functions are discussed in detail in Chapter 8.

Intrinsic Tongue Muscles

The intrinsic muscles of the tongue include two pairs of muscles running longitudinally, as well as muscles coursing transversely and vertically. At the outset we should note that the intrinsic muscles interact in a complex fashion to produce the rapid, delicate articulations needed for speech and nonspeech activities. As we discuss each muscle, we will provide you with the basic function, but will deal thoroughly with the integration of these muscles in

LATERAL VIEW

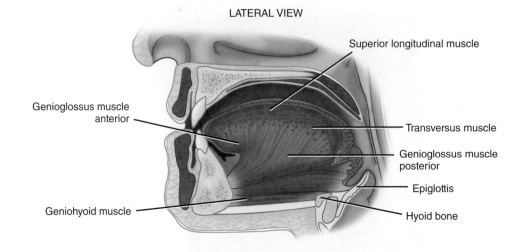

ANTERIOR VIEW
FRONTAL SECTION

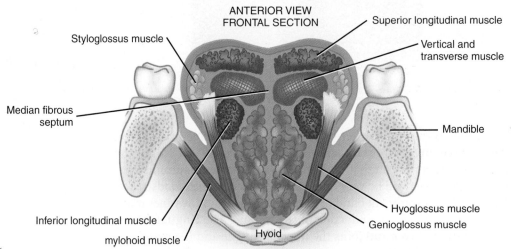

Figure 6-38.
Intrinsic muscles
of the tongue.
Source: (From the data of
Netter, 1997).

Chapter 7. Figure 6-38 will assist you in our discussion of these very important lingual muscles.

- **Superior longitudinal**
- **Inferior longitudinal**
- **Transverse**
- **Vertical**

Superior Longitudinal Muscle of the Tongue. The **superior longitudinal muscle** courses along the length of the tongue, comprising the upper layer of the tongue. This muscle originates from the fibrous submucous layer near the epiglottis, from the hyoid, and from the median fibrous septum. Its fibers fan forward and outward to insert into the lateral margins of the tongue and region of the apex. By virtue of their course and insertions, fibers of the superior longitudinal muscle tend to elevate the tip of the tongue. If one superior longitudinal muscle is contracted without the other, it will tend to pull the tongue toward the

Ankyloglossia (Tongue Tie)

The *lingual frenulum* is a band of tissue connecting the tongue to the floor of the mouth. It appears to assist in stabilizing the tongue during the movement but occasionally may be too short for proper lingual function. This condition is known as ankyloglossia ("ankyl" = stiffness or immobility, "glossia" = tongue), colloquially referred to as **tongue tie**, will result in difficulty elevating the tongue for phonemes requiring palatal or alveolar contact. The tongue may appear heart-shaped when protruded, resulting from the excessive tension on the midline by the short frenulum. A surgical procedure to correct the condition may be useful, although such surgery is not minor.

Muscle:	Superior longitudinal
Origin:	Fibrous submucous layer near the epiglottis, the hyoid, and the median fibrous septum
Course:	Fans forward and outward
Insertion:	Lateral margins of the tongue and region of apex
Innervation:	XII hypoglossal nerve
Function:	Elevates, assists in retraction, or deviates the tip of the tongue

side of contraction. Innervation of all intrinsic muscles of the tongue is by means of the XII hypoglossal nerve.

Inferior Longitudinal Muscle of the Tongue. The **inferior longitudinal muscle** originates at the root of the tongue and corpus hyoid, with fibers coursing to the apex of the tongue. This muscle occupies the lower sides of the tongue but is absent in the medial tongue base, which is occupied by the extrinsic genioglossus muscle (to be described in a later section). The inferior longitudinal muscle pulls the tip of the tongue downward and assists in the retraction of the tongue if co-contracted with the superior longitudinal. As with the superior longitudinal, unilateral contraction of the inferior longitudinal will cause the tongue to turn toward the contracted side and downward. Innervation of all intrinsic muscles of the tongue is by means of the contralateral XII hypoglossal nerve.

Transverse Muscles of the Tongue. The **transverse muscles of the tongue** provide a mechanism for narrowing the tongue. Fibers of these muscles originate at the median fibrous septum and course laterally to insert into the side of the tongue in the submucous tissue. Some fibers of the transverse muscle continue as the palatopharyngeus muscle, to be described in a later section. The transverse muscle of the tongue pulls the edges of the tongue toward the midline, effectively narrowing the tongue. Innervation of all intrinsic muscles of the tongue is by means of the XII hypoglossal nerve.

Muscle:	Inferior longitudinal
Origin:	Root of the tongue and corpus hyoid
Course:	Forward
Insertion:	Apex of the tongue
Innervation:	XII hypoglossal nerve
Function:	Pulls tip of the tongue downward, assists in retraction, and deviates the tongue
Muscle:	Transverse muscles of the tongue
Origin:	Median fibrous septum
Course:	Laterally
Insertion:	Side of the tongue in the submucous tissue
Innervation:	XII hypoglossal nerve
Function:	Provide a mechanism for narrowing the tongue

Vertical Muscles of the Tongue. The **vertical muscles of the tongue** run at right angles to the transverse muscles and flatten the tongue. Fibers of the vertical muscle course from the base of the tongue and insert into the membranous cover. The fibers of the transverse and vertical muscles interweave. Contraction of the vertical muscles pulls the tongue down into the floor of the mouth. Innervation of all intrinsic muscles of the tongue is by means of the XII hypoglossal nerve.

Extrinsic Tongue Muscles

- **Genioglossus**
- **Hyoglossus**
- **Styloglossus**
- **Chondroglossus**

Palatoglossus

The intrinsic muscles of the tongue are responsible for precise articulatory performance, and the extrinsic muscles of the tongue tend to move the tongue as a unit. It appears that they set the general posture for articulation, with the intrinsic muscles performing the refined perfection of that action.

Genioglossus Muscle. The **genioglossus** is the prime mover of the tongue, making up most of its deeper bulk. As you can see from Figure 6-39, the genioglossus arises from the inner mandibular surface at the symphysis and fans to insert into the tip and dorsum of the tongue, as well as to the corpus of the hyoid bone.

The genioglossus muscle occupies a medial position in the tongue, with the inferior longitudinal muscle, hyoglossus, and styloglossus being lateral to it. Fibers of the genioglossus insert into the entire surface of the tongue but are sparse to absent in the tip. Contraction of the anterior fibers of the genioglossus muscle results in the retraction of the tongue, whereas contraction of the posterior fibers draws the tongue forward to aid protrusion of the apex. If both anterior and

Muscle:	Vertical muscles of the tongue
Origin:	Base of the tongue
Course:	Vertically
Insertion:	Membranous cover
Innervation:	XII hypoglossal nerve
Function:	Pull the tongue down into the floor of the mouth
Muscle:	Genioglossus
Origin:	Inner mandibular surface at the symphysis
Course:	Fans up, back, and forward
Insertion:	Tip and dorsum of tongue and corpus hyoid
Innervation:	XII hypoglossal nerve
Function:	Anterior fibers retract the tongue; posterior fibers protrude the tongue; together, anterior and posterior fibers depress the tongue

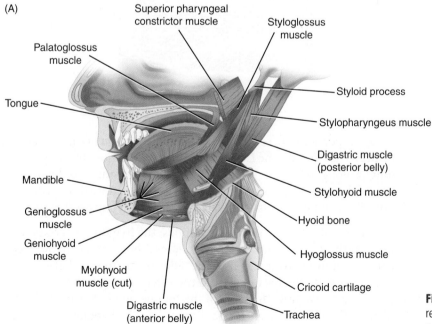

(A)

Superior pharyngeal constrictor muscle

Styloglossus muscle

Palatoglossus muscle

Tongue

Styloid process

Stylopharyngeus muscle

Digastric muscle (posterior belly)

Mandible

Stylohyoid muscle

Genioglossus muscle

Geniohyoid muscle

Hyoid bone

Hyoglossus muscle

Mylohyoid muscle (cut)

Cricoid cartilage

Digastric muscle (anterior belly)

Trachea

Figure 6-39. (A) Genioglossus and related muscles. (continues).
© Cengage Learning®.

(B)

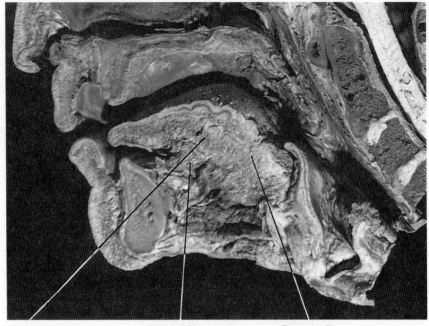

Genioglossus   Anterior fibers   Posterior fibers

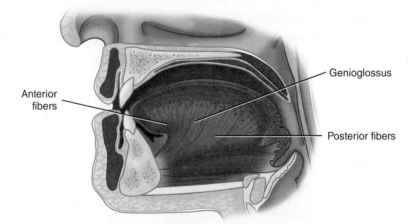

Figure 6-39 continued.
(B) Photograph showing
genioglossus muscle, with drawing
showing landmarks.
© Cengage Learning®.

posterior portions are contracted, the middle portion of the tongue will be drawn down into the floor of the mouth, functionally cupping the tongue along its length. Needless to say, we will return to the interaction of the genioglossus and intrinsic muscles when we discuss deglutition. The genioglossus is innervated by the XII hypoglossal nerve.

Hyoglossus Muscle. As the name implies, the **hyoglossus** arises from the length of the greater cornu and lateral body of the hyoid bone, coursing upward to insert into the sides of the tongue between the styloglossus (to be discussed) and the inferior longitudinal muscles. The hyoglossus pulls the sides of the tongue down, in direct antagonism to the palatoglossus (to be discussed). The hyoglossus is innervated by the XII hypoglossal nerve.

Muscle:	Hyoglossus
Origin:	Length of greater cornu and lateral body of hyoid
Course:	Upward
Insertion:	Sides of the tongue between styloglossus and inferior longitudinal muscles
Innervation:	XII hypoglossal nerve
Function:	Pulls sides of the tongue down

Styloglossus. If you examine Figure 6-39 again, you will see that the **styloglossus** originates from the anterolateral margin of the styloid process of the temporal bone, coursing forward and down to insert into the inferior sides of the tongue. It divides into two portions: one interdigitates with the inferior longitudinal muscle, and the other with the fibers of the hyoglossus. As you can guess from the examination of the course and insertion of this muscle, contraction of the paired styloglossi will draw the tongue back and up. The styloglossus is innervated by the XII hypoglossal nerve.

Chondroglossus. The **chondroglossus** muscle is often considered to be part of the hyoglossus muscle. As with the hyoglossus, the chondroglossus arises from the hyoid (lesser cornu), coursing up to interdigitate with the intrinsic muscles of the tongue medial to the point of insertion of the hyoglossus. The chondroglossus is a depressor of the tongue. The chondroglossus is innervated by the XII hypoglossal nerve.

chondroglossus: Gr., chondros, cartilage + glossus, tongue

Palatoglossus. The **palatoglossus** may be functionally defined as a muscle of the tongue or of the velum, although it is more closely allied with palatal architecture and origin (see Figures 6-43 and 6-45). It will be described in a later section, but you should realize that it serves the dual purpose of depressing the soft palate or elevating the back of the tongue. The palatoglossus makes up the anterior faucial pillar.

Muscle:	Styloglossus
Origin:	Anterolateral margin of styloid process
Course:	Forward and down
Insertion:	Inferior sides of the tongue
Innervation:	XII hypoglossal nerve
Function:	Draws the tongue back and up

Muscle:	Chondroglossus
Origin:	Lesser cornu hyoid
Course:	Up
Insertion:	Interdigitates with intrinsic muscles of the tongue medial to the point of insertion of hyoglossus
Innervation:	XII hypoglossal nerve
Function:	Depresses the tongue

Muscle:	Palatoglossus
Origin:	Anterolateral palatal aponeurosis
Course:	Down
Insertion:	Sides of posterior tongue
Innervation:	Pharyngeal plexus from the XI accessory and X vagus nerves
Function:	Elevates the tongue or depresses the soft palate

✔ *To summarize:*

- The **tongue** is a massive structure occupying the floor of the mouth. It is divided by a **median fibrous septum** from where the transverse intrinsic muscle of the tongue originates.
- The tongue is divided into **dorsum**, **apex** (tip), and **base**.
- Fine movements of the tongue are produced by the contraction of the intrinsic musculature (**transverse, vertical, inferior longitudinal**, and **superior longitudinal** muscles of the tongue).
- Larger adjustments of lingual movement are completed through the use of **extrinsic muscles**. The **genioglossus** retracts, protrudes, or depresses the tongue. The **hyoglossus** and **chondroglossus** depress the tongue, while the **styloglossus** and **palatoglossus** elevate the posterior tongue.

Muscles of Mastication: Mandibular Elevators and Depressors

mastication: L., masticare, chewing

The process of chewing food, or **mastication**, requires the movement of the mandible so that the molars can make a solid, grinding contact. The muscles of mastication are among the strongest of the body, and the coordinated contraction of these muscles is required for proper food preparation. The muscles of mastication include the mandibular elevators (masseter, temporalis, and medial pterygoid), muscles of protrusion (lateral pterygoid), and depressors (digastricus, mylohyoid, geniohyoid, and platysma).

- **Masseter**
- **Temporalis**

- **Medial pterygoid**
- **Lateral pterygoid**
- **Digastricus**
- **Mylohyoid**
- **Geniohyoid**
- **Platysma**

Masseter. As you may see from Figure 6-40, the **masseter** is the most superficial of the muscles of mastication. This massive quadrilateral muscle originates on the lateral, inferior, and medial surfaces of the zygomatic arch, coursing down to insert primarily into the ramus of the mandible, but with some of the deeper fibers terminating on the coronoid process. The course and attachments of the masseter make it ideally suited for placing maximum force on the molars. Contraction of this muscle elevates the mandible, and when the teeth are clenched, the prominent muscular belly is clearly visible. The masseter is innervated by the anterior trunk of the mandibular nerve arising from the V trigeminal.

Temporalis Muscle. The **temporalis muscle** is deep to the masseter, arising from a region of the temporal and parietal bones known as the **temporal fossa**. As you can see in Figure 6-41, it arises from a broad region of the lateral skull, converging as it courses down and forward. The terminal tendon of the temporalis passes deep to the zygomatic arch and inserts into the coronoid process and ramus of the mandible. The temporalis elevates the mandible and draws it back if protruded. It appears to be capable of more rapid contraction than the masseter. The temporalis is innervated by the temporal branches arising from the mandibular nerve of V trigeminal.

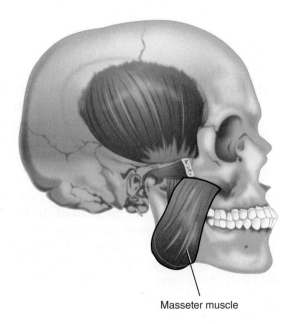

Masseter muscle

Figure 6-40. Graphic representation of masseter.
© Cengage Learning®.

Muscle:	Masseter
Origin:	Zygomatic arch
Course:	Down
Insertion:	Ramus of the mandible and coronoid process
Innervation:	Anterior trunk of mandibular nerve arising from the V trigeminal
Function:	Elevates the mandible

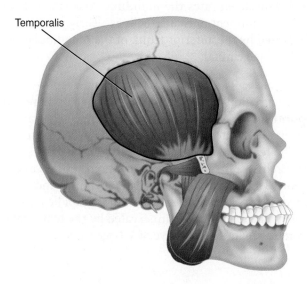

Temporalis

Figure 6-41. Graphic representation of the temporalis.
© Cengage Learning®.

Medial Pterygoid Muscle. The **medial pterygoid muscle** (also known as the **internal pterygoid muscle**) originates from the medial pterygoid plate and fossa lateral to it (see Figure 6-42). Fibers from the muscle course down and back to insert into the mandibular ramus. The medial pterygoid muscle elevates the mandible, acting in conjunction with the masseter. The medial pterygoid muscle is innervated by the mandibular division of the V trigeminal nerve.

Lateral Pterygoid Muscle. The **lateral** (or external) **pterygoid muscle** arises from the sphenoid bone. One head of the lateral pterygoid arises from the lateral pterygoid plate (hence the name of the muscle); another head attaches to the greater wing of the sphenoid. Fibers course back to insert into the pterygoid fovea of the mandible, the lower inner margin of the condyloid process of the mandible (see Figure 6-42). Contraction of the lateral pterygoid muscle protrudes the mandible, and it works in contrast with the mandibular elevators for grinding action at the molars. The lateral pterygoid muscle is innervated by the mandibular branch of the V trigeminal nerve.

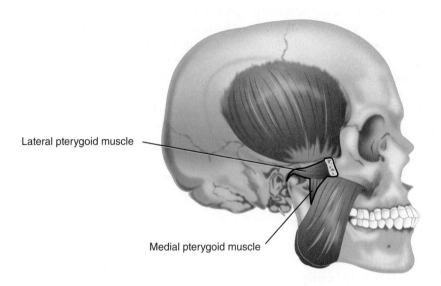

Lateral pterygoid muscle

Medial pterygoid muscle

Figure 6-42. Lateral and medial pterygoid muscles.
© Cengage Learning®.

Muscle:	Temporalis
Origin:	Temporal fossa of temporal and parietal bones
Course:	Converging downward and forward, through the zygomatic arch
Insertion:	Coronoid process and ramus
Innervation:	Temporal branches arising from the mandibular nerve of V trigeminal
Function:	Elevates the mandible and draws it back if protruded

Muscle:	Medial pterygoid
Origin:	Medial pterygoid plate and fossa
Course:	Down and back
Insertion:	Mandibular ramus
Innervation:	Mandibular division of the V trigeminal nerve
Function:	Elevates the mandible

Tongue Thrust

As with other motor functions, swallowing develops from immature to mature forms. The immature swallow capitalizes on the needs of the moment: An infant needs to compress his or her mother's nipple to stimulate release of milk, so the tongue moves forward naturally during this process. As the infant develops teeth, anterior movement of the tongue is blocked even as the need for it diminishes. The child begins eating semi-solid and solid food, and chewing becomes more important than sucking. The mature swallow propels a bolus back toward the oropharynx, a maneuver requiring posterior direction of the tongue.

If the child fails to develop the mature swallow, he or she has a condition known as **tongue thrust**. The anterior force of the tongue in its rest posture will cause labioversion of the incisors. This child may have flaccid oral musculature, weak masseter action during swallow, and a disorganized approach to generation of the bolus. Considering that we swallow between 400 and 600 times per day, the immature swallow is difficult (but far from impossible) to reorganize into a mature swallow. Many speech-language pathologists specialize in **orofacial myofunctional therapy** directed toward remediation of such problems, a rich and rewarding practice that results in (literally) smiling clients (see Zickefoose, 1989). Chapter 9 discusses issues related to tongue thrust.

digastric: L., two + belly, refers to the two-bellied muscle, digastricus

Digastricus. The dual-bellied digastricus was described in Chapter 4, so it is only briefly discussed here. The **digastricus anterior** originates at the inner surface of the mandible at the digastricus fossa, near the symphysis, while the **digastricus posterior** originates at the mastoid process of the temporal bone. The anterior fibers course medially and down to the hyoid, where they join with the posterior digastricus by means of an intermediate tendon that inserts into the hyoid at the juncture of the hyoid corpus and greater cornu. If the hyoid bone is fixed by infrahyoid musculature, contraction of the anterior component will result in the depression of the mandible. The anterior belly is innervated by the mandibular branch of the V trigeminal nerve via the mylohyoid branch of the inferior alveolar nerve. The posterior belly is supplied by the **digastric** branch of the VII facial nerve.

Mylohyoid Muscle. This muscle was described in Chapter 4. The **mylohyoid** originates at the underside of the mandible and courses to the corpus hyoid. This fanlike muscle courses from the **mylohyoid line** of the mandible to the median fibrous raphe and inferiorly to the hyoid, forming the floor of the mouth. With the hyoid fixed in position, the mylohyoid will depress the mandible. The mylohyoid is innervated by the alveolar nerve, arising from the V trigeminal nerve, mandibular branch.

Geniohyoid Muscle. Also described in Chapter 4, the **geniohyoid muscle** originates at the mental spines of the mandible and projects

Muscle:	Lateral pterygoid (external pterygoid)
Origin:	Lateral pterygoid plate and the greater wing of sphenoid
Course:	Back
Insertion:	Pterygoid fovea of the mandible
Innervation:	Mandibular branch of the V trigeminal nerve
Function:	Protrudes the mandible

Muscle:	Digastricus anterior
Origin:	Inner surface of the mandible at digastricus fossa, near the symphysis
Course:	Medially and down
Insertion:	Intermediate tendon to juncture of hyoid corpus and greater cornu
Innervation:	Mandibular branch of V trigeminal nerve via the mylohyoid branch of the inferior alveolar nerve
Function:	Pulls the hyoid forward; depresses the mandible if in conjunction with digastricus posterior

Muscle:	Digastricus posterior
Origin:	Mastoid process of temporal bone
Course:	Medially and down
Insertion:	Intermediate tendon to juncture of hyoid corpus and greater cornu
Innervation:	Digastric branch of the VII facial nerve
Function:	Pulls the hyoid back; depresses mandible if in conjunction with anterior digastricus

parallel to the anterior digastricus from the inner mandibular surface to insert into the corpus hyoid. Contraction of the geniohyoid depresses the mandible if the hyoid is fixed. Innervation of the geniohyoid is by means of the XII hypoglossal nerve.

Platysma. The platysma was discussed in the "Muscles of the Face" section.

✔ *To summarize:*

- The muscles of **mastication** include mandibular **elevators** and **depressors**, as well as muscles to **protrude** the mandible.
- Mandibular elevators include the **masseter, temporalis,** and **medial pterygoid** muscles, while the **lateral pterygoid** protrudes the mandible.
- Depression of the mandible is performed by the **mylohyoid, geniohyoid,** and **platysma** muscles. The grinding action of the molars requires coordinated and synchronized contraction of the muscles of mastication.

Muscle:	Mylohyoid
Origin:	Mylohyoid line, inner mandible
Course:	Back and down
Insertion:	Median fibrous raphe and inferiorly to hyoid
Innervation:	Alveolar nerve, arising from the V trigeminal nerve, mandibular branch
Function:	Depresses the mandible
Muscle:	Geniohyoid
Origin:	Mental spines of the mandible
Course:	Medially
Insertion:	Corpus hyoid
Innervation:	XII hypoglossal nerve
Function:	Depresses the mandible

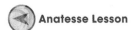 **Anatesse Lesson**

Muscles of the Velum

Only three speech sounds in English require that the soft palate be depressed (/m/, /ŋ/, and /n/). During most speaking time and swallowing, the soft palate is actively elevated. We will discuss the general configuration of the soft palate and then discuss how we go about elevating and depressing this important structure.

The **soft palate** or **velum** is actually a combination of muscle, aponeurosis, nerves, and blood supply covered by the mucous membrane lining. The **palatal aponeurosis** makes up the mid-front portion of the soft palate, being an extension of an aponeurosis arising from the tensor veli palatini (to be described). The palatal aponeurosis divides around the musculus uvulae but serves as the point of insertion for other muscles of the soft palate. The mucous membrane lining is invested with lymph and mucous glands, and the oral side of the lining also has taste buds.

- **Levator veli palatini**
- **Musculus uvulae**
- **Tensor veli palatini**
- **Palatoglossus**

Palatopharyngeus

Muscles of the soft palate include elevators (levator veli palatini and musculus uvulae), an auditory tube dilator (tensor veli palatini), and depressors (palatoglossus and palatopharyngeus). Although the superior constrictor muscle is a pharyngeal muscle, we should note that it is an important muscle for the function of the soft palate.

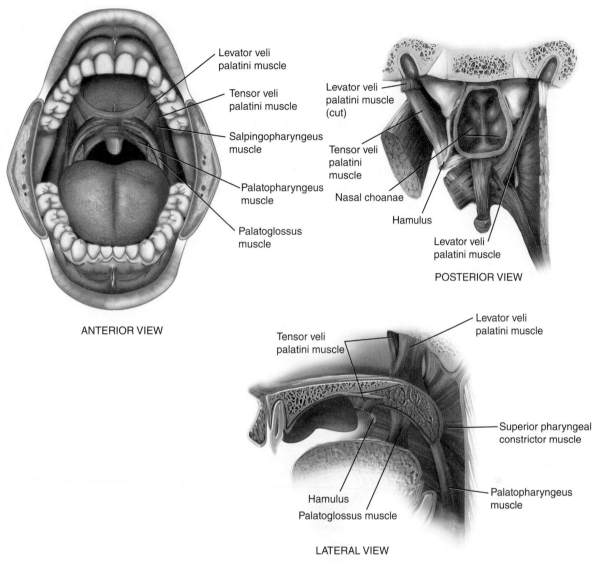

Figure 6-43. Muscles of the soft palate from superior-posterior (*left*), posterior (*right*), and the side (*lower figure*).
Source: (From the data of Schprintzen & Bardach, 1995; Langley, Telford, & Christensen, 1969; and Williams & Warrick, 1980.)

We will discuss the muscles of the pharynx following the discussion of the muscles of the soft palate. Figure 6-43 will assist you in the following discussion.

Levator Veli Palatini Muscle. The **levator veli palatini** (or **levator palati**) is the palatal elevator, making up the bulk of the soft palate (see Figure 6-44). This muscle arises from the apex of the petrous portion of the temporal bone, as well as from the medial wall of the auditory tube cartilage. The levator veli palatini courses down and forward to insert into the palatal aponeurosis of the soft palate, lateral to the musculus uvulae. The levator veli palatini is the primary elevator of the soft palate. Contraction elevates and retracts the posterior velum. The levator veli palatini is innervated by the pharyngeal plexus, arising from the XI accessory and X vagus nerves (Keller, Saunders, Loveren, & Shipley, 1984), although there is evidence of co-innervation by the IX glossopharyngeal nerve (Furusawa, Yamaoka, Kogo & Matsuya, 1991).

Musculus Uvulae. A casual examination of the inner workings of your own mouth reveals the structure of the **musculus uvulae**. The uvula makes up the medial and posterior portions of the soft palate, and the musculus uvulae is the muscle embodied within this structure. This paired muscle arises from the posterior nasal spines of the palatine bones and from the palatal aponeurosis. Fibers run the length of the soft palate on either side of the midline, inserting into the mucous membrane cover of the velum. Contraction of the uvula shortens the soft palate, effectively bunching it up. The musculus uvulae is innervated by the pharyngeal plexus, arising from the XI accessory and X vagus nerves.

(A)

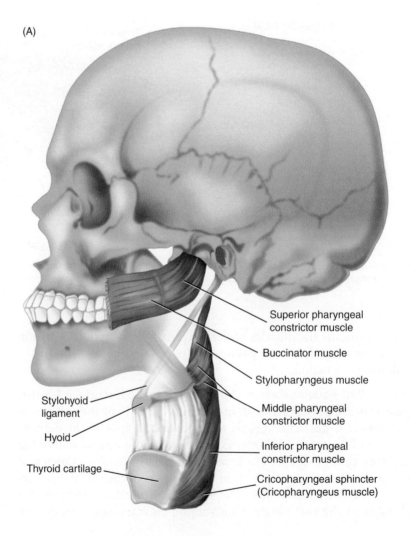

Figure 6-44. (A) The lateral view of pharyngeal constrictor muscles. (continues).
© Cengage Learning®.

(B)

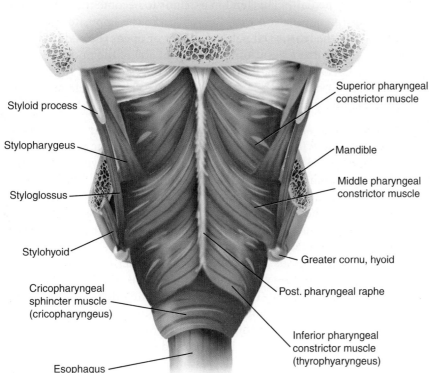

Styloid process

Stylopharygeus

Styloglossus

Stylohyoid

Cricopharyngeal
sphincter muscle
(cricopharyngeus)

Esophagus

Superior pharyngeal
constrictor muscle

Mandible

Middle pharyngeal
constrictor muscle

Greater cornu, hyoid

Post. pharyngeal raphe

Inferior pharyngeal
constrictor muscle
(thyrophyaryngeus)

Figure 6-44 continued.
(B) The posterior view of
pharyngeal constrictor
musculature.
© Cengage Learning®.

Muscle:	Levator veli palatini (levator palati)
Origin:	Apex of petrous portion of temporal bone and medial wall of the auditory tube cartilage
Course:	Down and forward
Insertion:	Palatal aponeurosis of the soft palate, lateral to musculus uvulae
Innervation:	Pharyngeal plexus from the XI accessory and X vagus nerves
Function:	Elevates and retracts the posterior velum

Tensor Veli Palatini Muscle. The **tensor veli palatini** (tensor veli palati)
has long been viewed as a tensor of the soft palate, as well as the dilator
of the auditory tube. In reality, the tensor veli palatini appears only to
function as a dilator of the auditory tube. This muscle arises from the
sphenoid bone (scaphoid fossa between lateral and medial pterygoid
plates, and sphenoid spine) as well as from the lateral auditory tube

wall. The fibers converge to course down to terminate in a tendon. The tendon, in turn, passes around the pterygoid hamulus and then is directed medially. This tendon expands to become the palatal aponeurosis in conjunction with the tendon of the opposite side. Contraction of the tensor veli palatini dilates or opens the auditory tube, thereby permitting **aeration** (exchange of air) of the middle ear cavity. The tensor veli palatini muscle is the only muscle of the soft palate not innervated by the XI accessory nerve. This muscle receives its innervation by means of the mandibular nerve of the V trigeminal.

Palatoglossus Muscle. If you again look into your mouth using a mirror, you will be able to see the structure of the **palatoglossus** (see Figure 6-43). At the posterior of the oral cavity you will see two prominent arches that mark the entry to the pharynx. The arch closest to you is the anterior **faucial pillar**, and the muscle of which it is comprised is the palatoglossus. (While you are in there, take a look at the posterior faucial pillar, just behind it. That is the palatopharyngeus, to be discussed shortly.)

The palatoglossus muscle was discussed briefly as a muscle of the tongue, because it serves a dual purpose. This muscle originates at the anterolateral palatal aponeurosis, coursing down to insert into the sides of the posterior tongue. This muscle will either help to elevate the tongue, as mentioned earlier, or depress the soft palate. The fact that the soft palate, in its relaxed state, is depressed does not mean that we do not actively depress it, especially during speech. The palatoglossus is innervated by the pharyngeal plexus, arising from the XI accessory and X vagus nerves.

Muscle:	Musculus uvulae
Origin:	Posterior nasal spines of the palatine bones and palatal aponeurosis
Course:	Runs the length of the soft palate
Insertion:	Mucous membrane cover of the velum
Innervation:	Pharyngeal plexus of XI accessory and X vagus nerves
Function:	Shortens the soft palate
Muscle:	Tensor veli palatini (tensor veli palati)
Origin:	Scaphoid fossa of sphenoid, sphenoid spine, and lateral auditory tube wall
Course:	Courses down, terminates in tendon that passes around pterygoid hamulus, then is directed medially
Insertion:	Palatal aponeurosis
Innervation:	Mandibular nerve of V trigeminal
Function:	Dilates the auditory tube

Muscle:	Palatoglossus
Origin:	Anterolateral palatal aponeurosis
Course:	Down
Insertion:	Sides of posterior tongue
Innervation:	Pharyngeal plexus from the XI accessory and X vagus nerves
Function:	Elevates the tongue or depresses the soft palate

Muscle:	Palatopharyngeus
Origin:	Anterior hard palate and midline of the soft palate
Course:	Laterally and down
Insertion:	Posterior margin of the thyroid cartilage
Innervation:	Pharyngeal plexus from XI accessory and pharyngeal branch of X vagus nerve
Function:	Narrows the pharynx; lowers the soft palate

Palatopharyngeus Muscle. Although classically considered a pharyngeal muscle, the **palatopharyngeus** is included in this discussion because of its role in velar function (see Figure 6-43). Anterior fibers of the palatopharyngeus originate from the anterior hard palate, and posterior fibers arise from the midline of the soft palate posterior to the fibers of the levator veli palatini, attached to the palatal aponeurosis. Fibers of each muscle course laterally and down, forming the posterior faucial pillar and inserting into the posterior thyroid cartilage. This muscle has wide variability, mingling with fibers of the stylopharyngeus and salpingopharyngeus muscles prior to its ultimate insertion into the posterior margin of the thyroid cartilage. This muscle will assist in narrowing the pharyngeal cavity, as well as lowering the soft palate. It may also help to elevate the larynx. The palatopharyngeus is innervated by the pharyngeal plexus, arising from the XI accessory and pharyngeal branch of the X vagus nerve.

Pharyngeal Musculature

- **Superior pharyngeal constrictor**
- **Middle pharyngeal constrictor**
- **Inferior pharyngeal constrictor**
- **Cricopharyngeus muscle**
- **Thyropharyngeus muscle**
- **Salpingopharyngeus**
- **Stylopharyngeus muscle**

Muscles of the pharynx are closely allied with the tongue, muscles of the face, and laryngeal musculature. It will help if you imagine the pharynx as a vertical tube. This tube is made of muscles wrapping more or less horizontally from the front to a midline point in the back, as well as by muscles and connective tissue running from skull structures. Thus, the pharynx is composed of a complex of muscles that, when contracted, will constrict the pharynx to assist in deglutition.

Pharyngeal Constrictor Muscles. The superior, middle, and inferior **constrictor muscles** are the means by which the pharyngeal space is reduced in diameter. Of these, the superior constrictor is an important muscle of velopharyngeal function (see Figure 6-45).

Superior Pharyngeal Constrictor. Conceptually, the **superior pharyngeal constrictor** forms a tube beginning at the pterygomandibular raphe (the term "raphe" refers to a seam in a structure, and in this case it is the point of attachment of the buccinator muscles). The superior constrictor projects back from this structure on both sides to attach to the **median pharyngeal raphe**, the posterior midline tendinous component of the pharyngeal aponeurosis. This aponeurosis arises from the pharyngeal tubercle of the occipital bone (immediately anterior to the foramen magnum) and forms the superior sleeve of the pharyngeal wall by attaching to the temporal bone (petrous portion), medial pterygoid plate, and auditory tube. The median pharyngeal raphe is the posterior midline portion of this structure, descending along the back wall of the pharynx and providing the points of insertion for pharyngeal muscles. The superior constrictor muscle forms the sides

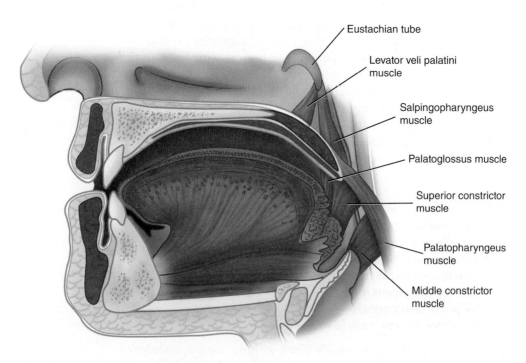

Figure 6-45. Salpingopharyngeus muscle.
© Cengage Learning®.

Muscle:	Superior pharyngeal constrictor
Origin:	Pterygomandibular raphe
Course:	Posteriorly
Insertion:	Median raphe of pharyngeal aponeurosis
Innervation:	XI accessory nerve and X vagus via pharyngeal plexus
Function:	Pulls pharyngeal wall forward; constricts pharyngeal diameter

and back wall of the nasopharynx and part of the back wall of the oropharynx, a function requiring a variety of points of attachment.

The median pterygoid plate gives rise to the uppermost fibers of the muscle, and these fibers are the "landing pad" for the soft palate, known as **Passavant's pad**. When present, this pad of muscle at the posterior pharyngeal wall appears as a ridge at the point of articulation of the soft palate with the wall. Clearly, the addition of tissue at this point can only assist in effecting a seal with the soft palate, and in fact, this pad appears to develop most markedly in individuals with palatal insufficiency, perhaps from compensatory activity.

The fibers from the pterygomandibular raphe are parallel to those of the buccinator, coursing back to insert into the median raphe of the posterior pharynx. Beneath these fibers, another portion of the superior constrictor arises from the mylohyoid line on the inner mandibular surface, while some other fibers arise from the sides of the tongue. Contraction of the superior pharyngeal constrictor muscle pulls the pharyngeal wall forward and constricts the pharyngeal diameter, an especially prominent movement during swallowing. It assists in effecting the velopharyngeal seal and thereby prevents the bolus from entering the nasopharynx. The superior pharyngeal constrictor is innervated by the XI accessory nerve in conjunction with the X vagus, via the pharyngeal plexus.

Middle Pharyngeal Constrictor. The **middle pharyngeal constrictor** arises from the horns of the hyoid bone, as well as from the **stylohyoid ligament** that runs from the styloid process to the lesser horn of the hyoid. The middle constrictor courses up and back, inserting into the median pharyngeal raphe. The middle constrictor narrows the diameter of the pharynx. The middle pharyngeal constrictor is innervated by the XI accessory nerve in conjunction with the X vagus, via the pharyngeal plexus.

Inferior Pharyngeal Constrictor. The **inferior pharyngeal constrictor** makes up the inferior pharynx. The portion arising from the sides of the cricoid cartilage forms the cricopharyngeal portion, frequently referred to as a separate muscle, the **cricopharyngeal muscle** (or

Muscle:	Middle pharyngeal constrictor
Origin:	Horns of the hyoid and stylohyoid ligament
Course:	Up and back
Insertion:	Median pharyngeal raphe
Innervation:	XI accessory nerve and X vagus via pharyngeal plexus
Function:	Narrows diameter of the pharynx

cricopharyngeus). This portion, which courses back to form the muscular orifice of the esophagus, is an important muscle for swallowing and is the structure set into vibration during esophageal speech, as will discussed in Chapter 8. The upper thyropharyngeal portion (or **thyropharyngeus muscle**) arises from the oblique line of the thyroid lamina, coursing up and back to insert into the median pharyngeal raphe. Contraction of the inferior constrictor reduces the diameter of the lower pharynx. The inferior pharyngeal constrictor is innervated by the XI accessory nerve in conjunction with the X vagus, via the pharyngeal plexus.

Salpingopharyngeus. The **salpingopharyngeus muscle** arises from the lower margin of the auditory tube, descending the lateral pharynx to join the palatopharyngeus muscle (see Figure 6-45). The **salpingopharyngeal fold** is a crease in the lateral nasopharynx formed by the mucosa covering this muscle. The salpingopharyngeus assists in the elevation of the lateral pharyngeal wall. The salpingopharyngeus is innervated by the X vagus and XI spinal accessory nerve via the pharyngeal plexus.

Stylopharyngeus Muscle. As the name implies, the **stylopharyngeus** arises from the styloid process of the temporal bone, coursing down between the superior and middle pharyngeal constrictors (see Figure 6-44). Some fibers insert into the constrictors; others insert into the posterior thyroid cartilage in concert with the palatopharyngeus muscle. The stylopharyngeus elevates and opens the pharynx, particularly during deglutition. The stylopharyngeus muscle is innervated by the muscular branch of the IX glossopharyngeal nerve.

✔ *To summarize:*

- The **soft palate** is a structure attached to the posterior hard palate and is comprised of muscle and aponeuroses.
- The **levator veli palatini** muscle elevates the soft palate, while the **musculus uvulae** shortens it. The **tensor veli palatini** dilates the auditory tube.
- The soft palate is depressed by means of the **palatoglossus** and **palatopharyngeus**.

Muscle:	Inferior pharyngeal constrictor; cricopharyngeus
Origin:	Cricoid cartilage
Course:	Back
Insertion:	Orifice of the esophagus
Innervation:	XI accessory nerve and X vagus, recurrent laryngeal nerve, via pharyngeal plexus
Function:	Constricts superior orifice of esophagus

Muscle:	Inferior pharyngeal constrictor; thyropharyngeus
Origin:	Oblique line of thyroid lamina
Course:	Up and back
Insertion:	Median pharyngeal raphe
Innervation:	XI accessory nerve and X vagus via pharyngeal plexus
Function:	Reduces the diameter of the lower pharynx

Muscle:	Salpingopharyngeus
Origin:	Lower margin of the auditory tube
Course:	Down
Insertion:	Converges with the palatopharyngeus muscle
Innervation:	X vagus and XI spinal accessory nerve via the pharyngeal plexus
Function:	Elevates the lateral pharyngeal wall

- The **superior pharyngeal constrictor** assists in gaining velopharyngeal closure, while peristaltic movement of food is facilitated by the **middle** and **inferior pharyngeal constrictors**.
- The **cricopharyngeal muscle**, a component of the inferior constrictor, forms the muscular orifice of the **esophagus**.
- Fibers of the **salpingopharyngeus** intermingle with those of the superior constrictor, providing assistance in elevation of the pharyngeal wall.
- The **stylopharyngeus** assists in elevation of the pharynx.

Muscle:	Stylopharyngeus
Origin:	Styloid process
Course:	Down
Insertion:	Into pharyngeal constrictors and posterior thyroid cartilage
Innervation:	Muscular branch of IX glossopharyngeal nerve
Function:	Elevates and opens the pharynx

As you can tell from this chapter, the structures of the articulatory system are extremely complex and mobile. We are capable of myriad movements that are incorporated into nonspeech and speech functions. Let us move on to Chapter 7.

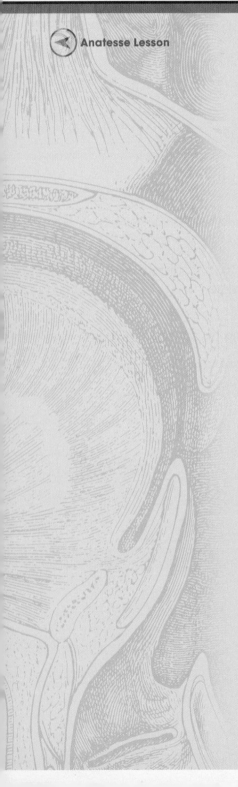

Anatesse Lesson

CHAPTER SUMMARY

The source-filter theory states that speech is the product of sending an acoustic source, such as the sound produced by the vibrating vocal folds, through the filter of the vocal tract that shapes the output. Sources may be voicing, as in the case of vowels, or the product of turbulence, as in fricatives. Articulators may be movable (such as the tongue, lips, pharynx, mandible, and velum) or immobile (such as the teeth, hard palate, and alveolar ridge).

Facial bones and those of the skull work together in a complex fashion to produce the structures of articulation. The mandible provides the lower dental arch, alveolar regions, and the resting location for the tongue. The maxillae provide the bulk of the hard palate, alveolar ridge, upper dental arch, and dominant structures of the nasal cavities, and the palatine bones provide the rest of the hard palate and the point of attachment for the velum. The midline vomer articulates with the perpendicular plate of the ethmoid and the cartilaginous septum to form the nasal septum. The zygomatic bone articulates with the frontal bone and maxillae to form the cheekbone. The small nasal bones form the upper margin of the nasal cavity. The ethmoid bone serves as the core of the skull and face, with the prominent crista galli protruding into the cranium and the perpendicular plate dividing the nasal cavities. The frontal, parietal, temporal, and occipital bones of the skull overlie the lobes of the brain of the same name. The sphenoid bone has a marked presence within the braincase, with the prominent greater and lesser wings of the sphenoid located lateral to the corpus. The hypophyseal fossa houses the pituitary gland. The clivus joins the occipital bone near the foramen magnum.

Incisors, cuspids, bicuspids, and molars are housed within the alveoli of the maxillae and mandible. Teeth have roots and crowns, and the exposed tooth surface is covered with enamel. Each tooth has a medial, lateral, lingual, buccal (or labial), and occlusal surface. Clinical eruption of the deciduous arch begins between six and nine months, and eruption of the permanent arch begins at six years. Class I occlusion refers to normal orientation of mandible and maxillae. Class II malocclusion refers to a relatively retracted mandible, and Class III malocclusion refers to a relatively protruded mandible. Individual teeth may have aberrant orientations within the alveolus, including torsiversion, labioversion, linguaversion, distoversion, and mesioversion. Inadequately erupted or hypererupted teeth are referred to as infraverted and supraverted, respectively.

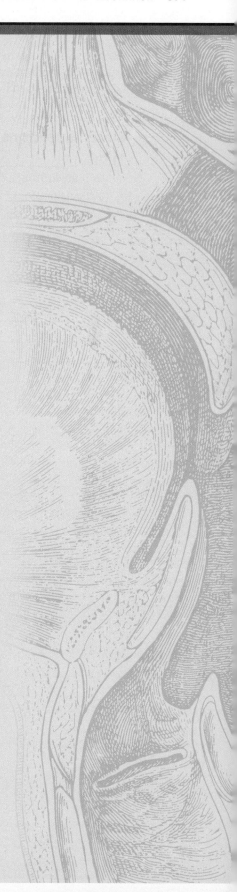

The cavities of the articulatory and resonatory system can be envisioned as a series of linked tubes. The vertically directed pharynx consists of the laryngopharynx, oropharynx, and nasopharynx. The nasal cavities arise from the nasopharynx, with the nasal and nasopharyngeal regions entirely separated from the oral cavity by the soft palate or velum. The oral cavity is flanked by the small buccal cavities. The shape and size of the oral cavity are altered through the movements of the tongue and mandible, and the nasal cavity may be coupled with the oral and pharyngeal cavities by means of the soft palate. The shape of the pharyngeal cavity is altered by the pharyngeal constrictor muscles but is secondarily changed by the elevation or depression of the larynx.

Facial muscles are important for articulations involving the lips. Numerous muscles insert into the orbicularis oris inferior and superior muscles, permitting lip protrusion, closure, retraction, elevation, and depression. The risorius and buccinator muscles retract the lips and support entrapment of air within the oral cavity. The levator labii superioris, zygomatic minor, levator labii superioris alaeque nasi, and levator anguli oris elevate the upper lip, and the depressor labii inferioris depresses the lower lip. The zygomatic major muscle elevates and retracts the corner of the mouth. The depressor labii inferioris pulls the lips down and out. The depressor anguli oris muscle depresses the corner of the mouth, and the mentalis muscle pulls the lower lip out. The platysma depresses the mandible.

The tongue, which occupies the floor of the mouth, is divided into dorsum, apex (tip), and base. Fine movements are the product of the intrinsic musculature (transverse, vertical, inferior longitudinal, and superior longitudinal muscles of the tongue). Larger adjustments of lingual movement require extrinsic muscles. The genioglossus retracts, protrudes, or depresses the tongue, and the hyoglossus and chondroglossus depress the tongue. The styloglossus and palatoglossus elevate the posterior tongue.

Muscles of mastication include mandibular elevators and depressors, as well as muscles to protrude the mandible. The masseter, temporalis, and medial pterygoid muscles elevate the mandible, and the lateral pterygoids protrude it. Mandibular depression is achieved by the mylohyoid, geniohyoid, and platysma muscles.

The velum or soft palate is attached to the posterior hard palate. The levator veli palatini muscle elevates and retracts the posterior velum and the musculus uvulae bunches it. The tensor veli palatini dilates the auditory tube. The velum is depressed by the palatoglossus and palatopharyngeus. The superior pharyngeal constrictor assists in gaining velopharyngeal closure, while peristaltic movement of food is facilitated by the middle and inferior pharyngeal constrictors. The cricopharyngeus forms the muscular orifice of the esophagus. The salpingopharyngeus elevates the pharyngeal wall, and the stylopharyngeus assists in elevation of the pharynx.

Media Connection

Go to the accompanying online resources at CengageBrain.com and have fun learning! Study with the Anatesse software program, play games, view animations and videos, and take practice tests to help reinforce the key concepts you learned in this chapter.

Study Questions

1. The _____ theory of vowel production states that the voicing source is routed through the vocal tract, where it is shaped into the sounds of speech by the articulators.

2. In the following figure, identify the bones and landmarks indicated.

   a. _____ (bone)
   b. _____ (bone)
   c. _____ bone
   d. _____ bone
   e. _____ bone
   f. _____ process
   g. _____ process
   h. _____

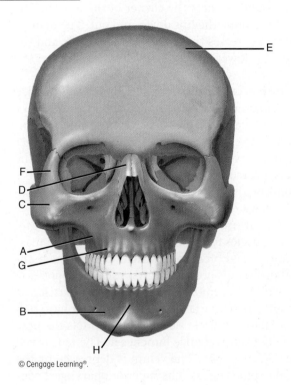

© Cengage Learning®.

3. In the following figure, identify the bones and landmarks indicated.

   a. _____ (bone)

   b. _____ bone

   c. _____ bone

   d. _____

   e. _____

   f. _____

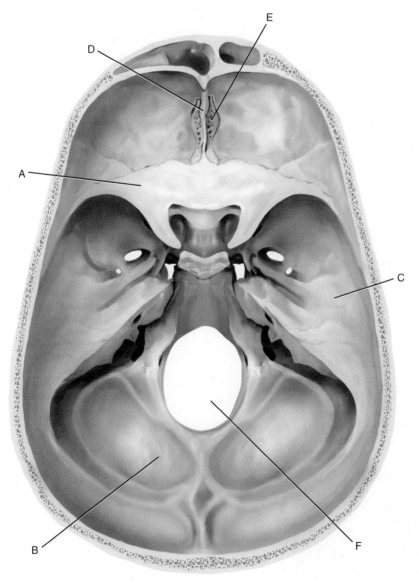

4. In the following figure, identify the bones and landmarks indicated.

a. _____ bone

b. _____ bone

c. _____ (bone)

d. _____ (bone)

e. _____ bone

f. _____ bone

g. _____ bone

h. _____ bone

i. _____

j. _____

k. _____ process

l. _____ process

m. _____ process

n. _____

o. _____ process

p. _____ process

q. _____

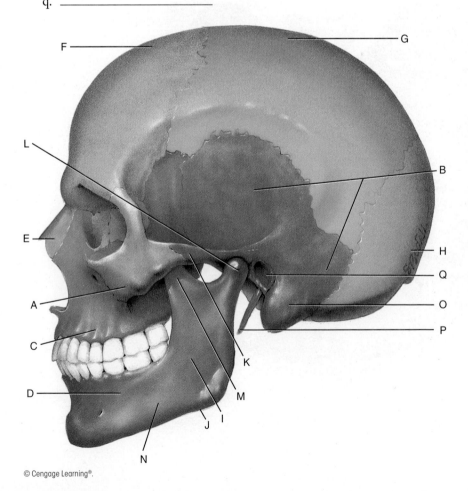

© Cengage Learning®.

5. In the following figure, identify the structures indicated.

a. _____ process

b. _____ (bone)

c. _____ bone

d. _____

e. _____ foramen

f. _____ suture

g. _____ process

h. _____ plate

i. _____ plate

j. _____ process

k. _____

l. _____

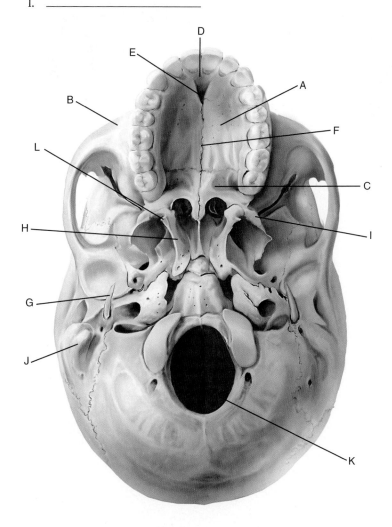

INFERIOR VIEW

6. In the following figure, identify the muscles indicated.

a. _____

b. _____

c. _____

d. _____

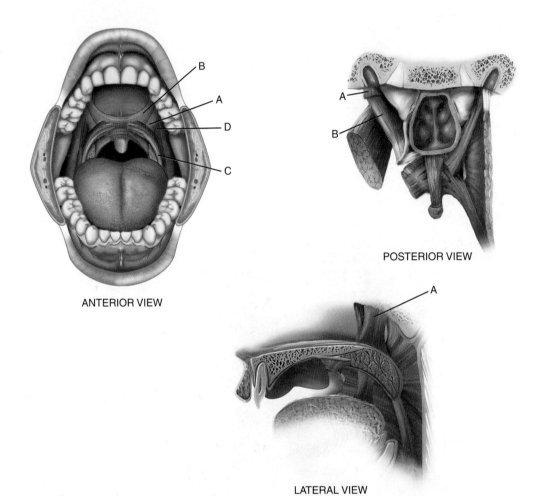

ANTERIOR VIEW

POSTERIOR VIEW

LATERAL VIEW

7. In the following figure, identify the muscles indicated.

a. _____

b. _____

c. _____

d. _____

e. _____

f. _____

g. _____

h. _____

i. _____

j. _____

k. _____

l. _____

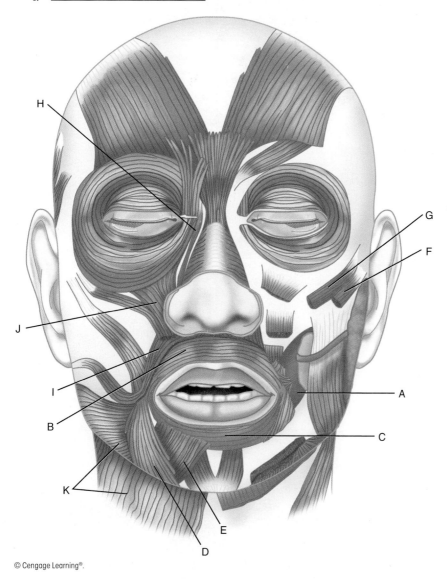

8. In the following figure, identify the muscles indicated.

a. _____

b. _____

c. _____

d. _____

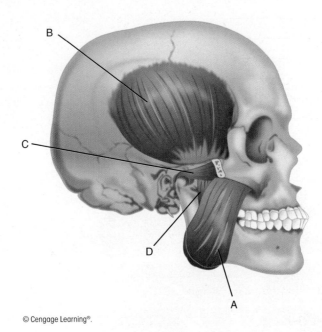

© Cengage Learning®.

9. In the following figure, identify the muscles indicated.

a. _____

b. _____

c. _____

d. _____

e. _____

f. _____

g. _____

h. _____

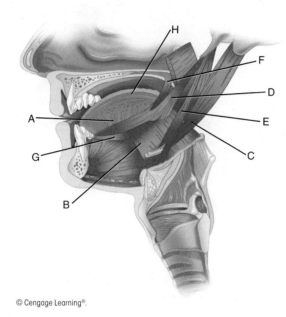

© Cengage Learning®.

10. In the following figure, identify the structures indicated.

a. _____ (bone)

b. _____ process

c. _____ process

d. _____ plate

e. _____

f. _____ bone

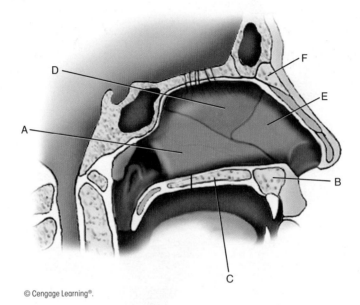

11. The soft palate is a diverse structure that typically serves us well, in that it separates the oropharynx and nasopharynx to protect against nasal regurgitation, not to mention keeping nonnasal phonemes from becoming nasalized. In our clinical practice, we have seen that low-back vowels tend to become nasalized more frequently in neurologically compromised clients than other vowels. What could be the cause for this?

Study Question Answers

1. The **SOURCE-FILTER** theory of vowel production states that the voicing source is routed through the vocal tract, where it is shaped into the sounds of speech by the articulators.

2. On the following figure, identify the bones and landmarks indicated.
   a. **MAXILLA** (bone)
   b. **MANDIBLE** (bone)
   c. **ZYGOMATIC** bone
   d. **NASAL** bone
   e. **FRONTAL** bone
   f. **FRONTAL** process
   g. **ALVEOLAR** process
   h. **SYMPHYSIS MENTI**

3. In the following figure, identify the bones and landmarks indicated.
   a. **SPHENOID** bone
   b. **OCCIPITAL** bone
   c. **TEMPORAL** bone
   d. **CRISTA GALLI**
   e. **CRIBRIFORM PLATE**
   f. **FORAMEN MAGNUM**

4. In the following figure, identify the bones and landmarks indicated.
   a. **ZYGOMATIC** bone
   b. **TEMPORAL** bone
   c. **MAXILLA** (bone)
   d. **MANDIBLE** (bone)
   e. **NASAL** bone
   f. **FRONTAL** bone
   g. **PARIETAL** bone
   h. **OCCIPITAL** bone
   i. **RAMUS**
   j. **ANGLE**
   k. **ZYGOMATIC** process
   l. **CONDYLAR** process
   m. **CORONOID** process
   n. **CORPUS**
   o. **MASTOID** process
   p. **STYLOID** process
   q. **EXTERNAL AUDITORY MEATUS**

5. In the following figure, identify the structures indicated.
   a. **PALATINE** process
   b. **MAXILLA** (bone)
   c. **PALATINE** bone

    d. **PREMAXILLA**

    e. **INCISIVE** foramen

    f. **INTERMAXILLARY** suture

    g. **STYLOID** process

    h. **MEDIAL PTERYGOID** plate

    i. **LATERAL PTERYGOID** plate

    j. **MASTOID** process

    k. **FORAMEN MAGNUM**

    l. **PTERYGOID HAMULUS**

6. In the following figure, identify the muscles indicated.

    a. **LEVATOR VELI PALATINI**

    b. **TENSOR VELI PALATINI**

    c. **PALATOGLOSSUS**

    d. **SALPINGOPHARYNGEUS**

7. In the following figure, identify the muscles indicated.

    a. **BUCCINATOR**

    b. **ORBICULARIS ORIS SUPERIORIS**

    c. **ORBICULARIS ORIS INFERIORIS**

    d. **DEPRESSOR ANGULI ORIS**

    e. **DEPRESSOR LABII INFERIORIS**

    f. **ZYGOMATIC MAJOR**

    g. **ZYGOMATIC MINOR**

    h. **LEVATOR LABII SUPERIORIS ALAEQUE NASI**

    i. **LEVATOR ANGULI ORIS**

    j. **LEVATOR LABII SUPERIORIS**

    k. **PLATYSMA**

8. In the following figure, identify the muscles indicated.

    a. **MASSETER**

    b. **TEMPORALIS**

    c. **LATERAL PTERYGOID**

    d. **MEDIAL PTERYGOID**

9. In the following figure, identify the muscles indicated.

    a. **GENIOGLOSSUS**

    b. **HYOGLOSSUS**

    c. **DIGASTRICUS POSTERIOR**

    d. **STYLOGLOSSUS**

    e. **STYLOHYOID**

    f. **PALATOGLOSSUS**

    g. **INFERIOR LONGITUDINAL**

    h. **SUPERIOR LONGITUDINAL**

10. In the following figure, identify the structures indicated.

    a. **VOMER** (bone)

    b. **ALVEOLAR** process

    c. **PALATINE PROCESS**

    d. **PERPENDICULAR** plate

    e. **CARTILAGINOUS SEPTUM**

    f. **NASAL** bone

11. You remember that the palatoglossus (glossopalatine) is a shared muscle of the tongue and of the soft palate. When it contracts, either the soft palate is depressed or the back and sides of the tongue are elevated, depending on whether the tongue is anchored or the soft palate is anchored. In the case of neurological deficit resulting in muscular weakness, when the tongue is depressed for the low-back vowels, the soft palate may be pulled down due to inadequate resistance by the levator veli palatini and tensor veli palatini.

Bibliography

Abrahams, P. H., McMinn, R. M. H., Hutchings, R. T., Sandy, C., & Mark, S. (2003). *McMinn's color atlas of human anatomy* (5th ed.). Philadelphia: Mosby.

Baken, R. J., & Orlikoff, R. F. (1999). *Clinical measurement of speech and voice* (2nd ed.). San Diego, CA: Singular Publishing Group.

Basmajian, J. V. (1975). *Grant's method of anatomy.* Baltimore, MD: Williams & Wilkins.

Bateman, H. E., & Mason, R. M. (1984). *Applied anatomy and physiology of the speech and hearing mechanism.* Springfield, IL: Charles C. Thomas.

Beck, E. W., Monson, H., & Groer, M. (1982). *Mosby's atlas of functional human anatomy.* St. Louis, MO: C. V. Mosby.

Black, S. M. (2008). Head and neck: External skull. In S. Strandring (Ed.) *Gray's anatomy: The anatomical and clinical basis of practice* (40th ed., pp. 409–422). London: Churchill Livingstone.

Bly, L. (1983). *The components of normal movement during the first year of life and abnormal motor movement.* Chicago, IL: Neuro-Developmental Treatment Association.

Bly, L. (1994). *Motor skills acquisition in the first year.* Tucson, AZ: Therapy Skill Builders.

Chusid, J. G. (1985). *Correlative neuroanatomy and functional neurology* (17th ed.). Los Altos, CA: Lange Medical Publications.

Clark, H. (2005). Clinical decision making and oral motor treatments. *ASHA Leader,* June 14, 8–9, 34–35.

Edmonson, J. A. & Esling, J. H. (2006). The valves of the throat and their functioning in tone, vocal register, and stress: Laryngoscopic case studies. *Phonology, 23,* 157–191.

Ettema, S. L., & Kuehn, D. P. (1994). A quantitative histologic study of the normal human adult soft palate. *Journal of Speech and Hearing Research, 37,* 303–313.

Furusawa, K., Yamaoka, M., Kogo, M. & Matsuya, T. (1991). The innervation of the levator veli palatini muscle by the glossopharyngeal nerve. *Brain Research Bulletin, 26*(4), 599–604.

Gelb, H. (1985). *Clinical management of head, neck and TMJ pain and dysfunction.* Philadelphia: W. B. Saunders.

Gilroy, A. M., MacPherson, B. R., Ross, L.M. (2012). *Atlas of anatomy* (2nd ed.). New York: Thieme.

Gosling, J. A., Harris, P. F., Humpherson, J. R., Whitmore, I., & Willan, P. L. T. (1985). *Atlas of human anatomy.* Philadelphia: J. B. Lippincott.

Gray, H., Bannister, L. H., Berry, M. M., & Williams, P. L. (Eds.). (1995). *Gray's anatomy.* London: Churchill Livingstone.

Grobler, N. J. (1977). *Textbook of clinical anatomy* (Vol. 1). Amsterdam: Elsevier Scientific.

Hauser, G., Daponte, A., & Roberts, M. J. (1989). Palatal rugae. *Journal of Anatomy, 124,* 237–249.

Kahane, J. C., & Folkins, J. F. (1984). *Atlas of speech and hearing anatomy.* Columbus, OH: Charles E. Merrill.

Kapetansky, D. I. (1987). *Cleft lip, nose, and palate reconstruction.* Philadelphia: J. B. Lippincott.

Kandel, E. R., Schwartz, J. H., Jessell, T. M., Siegelbaum, S. A. & Hudspeth, A. J. (2013). *Principles of neural science* (5th ed.). New York: McGraw Hill.

Kaplan, H. (1960). *Anatomy and physiology of speech.* New York: McGraw-Hill.

Keller, J. T., Saunders, M. C., Van Loveren, H., & Shipley, M. T. (1984). Neuroanatomical considerations of palatal muscles: Tensor and levator veli palatini. *Cleft Palate Journal, 21*(2), 70–75.

Kent, R. D. (1997). *The speech sciences.* San Diego, CA: Singular Publishing Group.

Kuehn, D. P., Lemme, M. L., & Baumgartner, J. M. (1989). *Neural bases of speech, hearing, and language.* Boston: Little, Brown.

Kuehn, D. P., Templeton, P. J., & Maynard, J. A. (1990). Muscle spindles in the velopharyngeal musculature of humans. *Journal of Speech and Hearing Research, 33,* 488–493.

Langley, L. L., Telford, I. R., & Christensen, J. B. (1969). *Dynamic anatomy and physiology.* New York: McGraw-Hill.

Langley, M. B., & Lombardino, L. J. (1991). *Neurodevelopmental strategies for managing communication disorders in children with severe motor dysfunction.* Austin, TX: Pro-Ed.

Lieberman, P. (1977). *Speech physiology and acoustic phonetics: An introduction.* New York: Macmillan.

Liss, J. M. (1990). Muscle spindles in the human levator veli palatini and palatoglossus muscles. *Journal of Speech and Hearing Research, 33,* 736–746.

McMinn, R. M. H., Hutchings, R. T., & Logan, B. M. (1994). *Color atlas of head and neck anatomy.* London: Mosby-Wolfe.

Minifie, F. (1973). Speech acoustics. In F. D. Minifie, T. J. Hixon, & F. Williams (Eds.), *Normal aspects of speech, hearing, and language* (pp. 11–72). Englewood Cliffs, NJ: Prentice-Hall.

Moore, K. L. (1988). *The developing human.* Philadelphia: W. B. Saunders.

Netter, F. H. (1983). *The CIBA collection of medical illustrations. Vol. 1. Nervous system. Part I. Anatomy and physiology.* West Caldwell, NJ: CIBA Pharmaceutical Company.

Netter, F. H. (1997). *Atlas of human anatomy.* CIBA-Geigy, Summit.

Pickett, J. M. (1980). *The sounds of speech communication.* Baltimore, MD: University Park Press.

Rohen, J. W., Yokochi, C., Lutjen-Drecoll, E., & Romrell, L. J. (2002). *Color atlas of anatomy* (5th ed.). Philadelphia: Williams & Wilkins.

Rosse, C., Gaddum-Rosse, P., & Rosse, G. (1997). *Hollinshead's textbook of anatomy.* Philadelphia: Lippincott-Raven.

Sawashima, M., & Cooper, F. S. (1977). *Dynamic aspects of speech production.* Tokyo: University of Tokyo Press.

Schuenke, M., & Ross, L. M., (2010). Thieme Atlas of Anatomy. New York: Thieme.

Shprintzen, R. J., & Bardach, J. (1995). *Cleft palate speech management*: a multidisciplinary approach. St. Louis, Mosby Inc.

Shriberg, L. D., & Kent, R. D. (2002). *Clinical phonetics* Upper Saddle River, NJ: Allyn & Bacon.

Small, A. M. (1973). Acoustics. In F. D. Minifie, T. J. Hixon, & F. Williams (Eds.), *Normal aspects of speech, hearing, and language.* Englewood Cliffs, NJ: Prentice-Hall.

Snell, R. S. (1978). *Gross anatomy dissector.* Boston: Little, Brown.

Strandring, S. (2008). Head and neck: Overview and surface anatomy. In Strandring, S. (Ed.) *Gray's anatomy: The anatomical and clinical basis of practice* (40th ed., pp. 397–408). London: Churchill Livingstone.

Standring, S. (2008). *Gray's anatomy: The anatomical and clinical basis of practice* (40th ed.). London: Churchill Livingstone.

Williams, P. L., & Warrick, R. (1980). *Gray's anatomy* (36th ed.). Edinburgh: Churchill Livingstone.

Zhang, M. (2008). Head and neck: Neck. In Strandring, S. (Ed.) *Gray's anatomy: The anatomical and clinical basis of practice* (40th ed., pp. 435–466). London: Churchill Livingstone.

Zemlin, W. R. (1998). *Speech and hearing science: Anatomy and physiology* (4th ed.). Needham Heights, MA: Allyn & Bacon.

Zickefoose, W. (1989). *Techniques of oral myofunctional therapy.* Sacramento, CA: O.M.T. Materials, Inc.

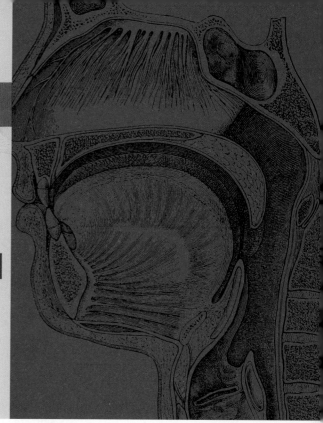

Chapter 7

PHYSIOLOGY OF ARTICULATION AND RESONATION

Clearly, the function of the articulatory system is of paramount importance in speech production. Although a review of acoustic phonetics is beyond the scope of an anatomy text, the source-filter theory of speech production discussed in Chapter 6 nonetheless provides the framework for our discussion. Intrinsic to that explanation of speech production is the notion that the movement of articulators shapes the resonant cavities of the vocal tract, and altered resonances give the acoustic output we call speech. We begin our discussion of the physiology of articulation and resonation by discussing speech function and its measurement, and we follow in Chapter 8 with our investigation of the biological function associated with swallowing.

Anatesse Lesson ➤

INSTRUMENTATION IN ARTICULATION

The measurement of articulatory function takes several forms. We can image the articulators themselves, plot their movement in space, examine muscle activity, or look at the acoustical output of the articulatory gesture itself.

Imaging the articulators in motion is ideally accomplished through cineradiography (moving X-ray), but this exposes the individual to unreasonable radiation (you may run across some old videos that were made prior to our clear understanding of the risks of radiation on the body). Better low-hazard alternatives are ultrasound imaging, which has made great strides in image resolution. A limitation of ultrasound is that it is best for viewing soft tissue, and bone is opaque (you can't see through it with ultrasound). Still imaging can be accomplished through functional magnetic resonance imaging (fMRI), but that does not allow scientists to see the movement of the articulators.

Plotting the movement of the articulators in space can be accomplished by placing sensors on structures, such as the tongue surface or on the mandible, and sensing their locations as they move over time using magnetometers. Alternately, electropalatography involves placing a set of sensors (usually in the form of a pseudopalate prosthesis) on the palate and recording tongue contact on those sensors as it moves from articulatory point to point. Optopalatography provides similar information using optical sensors within the pseudopalate. The electrostatic articulograph (EMA) allows three-dimensional measurement of articulators in space over time, allowing researchers to examine movements during speech. In this system, a sensor is placed on articulators (e.g., tongue tip, tongue dorsum, mandible, velum) and the EMA senses movement and tracks it over time. Similarly, the axiograph is used by dentists and orthodontists to plot movement of the mandible in space mechanically.

Muscle activity can be measured through surface electromyography (sEMG), or intramuscular EMG (also known as needle EMG or hook-wire EMG). sEMG involves placing electrodes on the skin surface, which allows gross motor potentials to be read as muscles move (see Figure 7-1). There is a growing literature on placement of electrodes to differentiate muscles that are being read, and this technique has provided valuable information about muscle activity over time. Needle electrodes provide a much finer resolution, allowing researchers to precisely localize muscle activity.

Acoustical measurement has a long and illustrious history in plotting articulatory function. The sound spectrogram, originally a cumbersome and expensive tool, remains a powerful tool for measurement of speech. The spectrograph is a plot of the speech spectrum over time, allowing researchers to see the formant tracks associated

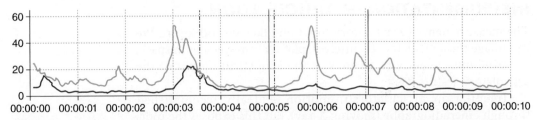

Figure 7-1. Surface electromyographic trace during swallow of a small pudding bolus. The blue trace represents submental placement (undersurface of the mouth). The vertical mark around 3.5 seconds marks the perception of swallow initiation (spacebar press), and the large blue peak is the initial movement of the tongue measured submentally. Termination of the swallow indicated by the second vertical line was perceived about 5 seconds into the trace. The second electrode (red) was recording the thyrohyoid muscle region, and you can see the elevation of the larynx shortly after initiation of the swallow, at around the 3.5 second mark.
© Cengage Learning®.

with articulator movements. Spectrum analyzers, now readily available as software applications, allow the display of the speech spectrum in time as well. The nasometer is a means of measuring the acoustical output of the nasal system, compared to the orally emitted signal. This tool allows one to identify excessive (or inadequate) nasal resonance by calculating a nasalence ratio between oral and nasal acoustic energy. In the same vein, oral and nasal airflow can be recorded by means of a pneumotachograph. Aerodynamic transducers provide elaboration of the interaction of articulation, phonation, and airflow.

No single measure captures the totality of the articulatory gestures that occur in speech, but combining methods moves us closer to understanding this complex process.

✔ *To summarize:*

- Measurement of articulatory function can be done by directly imaging the articulators, plotting their movement in space, examining muscle activity, and looking at the acoustical output of the articulatory gesture itself.
- Imaging may be accomplished by ultrasound technology, as well as static imaging methods such as functional magnetic resonance imaging (fMRI).
- Electropalatography and optopalatography allow researchers to plot contact of the tongue with the palate during articulation, while magnetometers can track sensors placed on articulators to map their movements during speech.
- Muscle activity can be measured through surface electromyography or intramuscular EMG.
- There are many tools used for acoustical measurement, with the sound spectrograph being among the earliest to develop. Similarly, spectrum analyzers allow fine-grained analysis of the acoustics of speech.

SPEECH FUNCTION

Speech production requires the execution of an extremely well-organized and integrated sequence of neuromotor events. Say the word *tube* and pay attention to the sequence of articulations. Ignoring respiratory preparation for the moment, your tongue must elevate to the alveolar ridge simultaneously with the elevation and tensing of the velum. Air pressure builds behind your tongue, and then your tongue actively drops to release the pressure and produce the /t/. Even as it releases, your tongue must quickly draw back to produce the /u/, assisted by the rounding of your lips. Your lips must then clamp together to permit the buildup of air pressure for the final /b/. All this happens in less than three-tenth of a second, and quite easily for most of us.

As you can see, thinking about the interaction of articulators and the articulatory plan can get complex if rushed. Let us begin with function of the individual movable articulators.

Lips

The lips are deceptively simple articulators. As discussed in Chapter 6, the orbicularis is primarily responsible for ensuring a labial seal, but numerous facial muscles insert into it. Those muscles, often in combination with other muscles, are capable of exerting a distinct force on the lips. Contraction of these muscles becomes an exercise in physics and force vectors: The direction of lip movement is the result of adding the directional forces of these muscles.

The lips are deceptive in another sense as well. At first glance, one might assume that the upper and lower lips have very similar qualities. In reality, however, the lower lip achieves a greater velocity and force than the upper lip and seems to do most of the work in lip closure (Folkins & Canty, 1986). The extra force is a function of the mentalis muscle, for which there is no parallel in the upper lip, and the doubled velocity is facilitated by the variable movement and placement of the mandible. The lower lip is attached to a movable articulator (the mandible), and it must quickly adapt to being closer or farther from the maxillary upper lip. That is, for sound to be accurately perceived as a chosen phoneme, the lips must make contact within closely timed tolerances. The lower lip is capable of rapidly altering its rate of closure to accommodate a variety of jaw positions, unflinchingly.

The notion of variable mandible position reinforces another fine point of labial function. The lips (as with the other articulators) are amazingly resistant to interference. We can easily adjust to perturbations of our articulators, or to even gross malformation (e.g., Folkins & Abbs, 1975). As an example, you could ask a friend to recite a poem with his or her eyes closed. At an unpredictable point, you could briefly pull down on his or her lip, and he or she would quickly adjust to the distorted articulatory position and continue talking with the new configuration (within limits, of course).

Similarly, you are able to adapt to other restrictions on supportive articulators. Try this. Repeat the syllable *puh* as rapidly as you can, counting the number of syllables you can produce in five seconds. Note that your mandible was helping, and it moved when you closed your lips. Now bite lightly on a pencil using your incisors and perform the same task. Your rate of repetition was probably very similar, despite the fact that your mandible was no longer able to help your lips close.

We are amazingly resistant to interference with the articulatory mechanism. This resistance, by the way, is evidence that the plan for an articulatory movement (e.g., Ostry, Vatikiotis-Bateson, & Gribble, 1997; Steeve & Moore, 2006) is not micromanaged by central cortical control, but rather that the details of motor execution are left to be worked out by some type of coordinative structures, as will be discussed. If the neural command, for instance, said simply to elevate the lower lip by 1.3 cm, either of the distortions mentioned previously would have resulted in a faulty articulation.

This does not mean that we do not use the proprioceptive information provided by sensors in our facial muscles to help us note muscle tone and position. As we mentioned in our introduction to neuroanatomy and neurophysiology in Chapter 1, muscle spindles are a powerful means of maintaining a specific articulatory posture, particularly when faced with the forces of gravity that are attempting to passively move elements of the anatomy. For instance, the mandible would tend to hang open as a result of the pull of gravity, but when gravity pulls on the mandible, the muscle spindles tell the muscles that elevate the mandible (especially the masseter and temporalis) to contract, thereby counteracting the forces of gravity.

Although we do not have spindles (Blair & Muller, 1987; Folkins & Larson, 1978; Seibel & Barlow, 2007) in facial muscles to assist in this process, we do have other sensors (such as those for pressure and touch) that provide feedback on the condition of facial muscles. Reflexive contraction of the orbicularis oris occurs with increased intraoral pressure, such as that produced during production of a bilabial stop or plosive. The oral mucosa and lips have sensors for light mechanical stimulation such as would occur during lingua-dental articulation. There are mechanoreceptors in the lips, and the periorial reflex can be elicited through the mechanical deformation of the angles of the mouth (Wohlert, 1996).

Evidence that you *do* use this type of information to control muscles may be found in the recollection of your last trip to the dentist. You may remember accidentally biting it while chewing or talking, if the dentist's anesthetic deadened your lip. Your unconscious perception of its position generally keeps that from happening. Mechanical stimulation of the lips affects other articulators as well. When the lower lip is stimulated, reflexive excitation in both the masseter and genioglossus can be recorded. The *degree* to which this information is *required* for speech accuracy is still a lively topic of debate. That having been said, Abbs (1973) provided solid evidence that the muscle spindle system involved in mandibular movement is also used in control of the lips and mandible for speech.

Mandible

The mandible is something of an unsung hero among articulators. It quietly and unceremoniously does its business, assisting the lips, changing its position for tongue movement, and tightly closing when necessary. It *does* move, however, and you can remind yourself of that movement by placing one finger of your right hand on your upper lip, and another finger on your chin. Close your eyes and count to 20 quickly, paying attention to the degree of movement you feel. You probably felt very little movement, but the mandible *did* move. Now clamp your mandible and count to 20. Were you still intelligible? (Yes.) Now do the opposite: Let your mouth hang absolutely slack-jaw open, and count to 20.

If you really relaxed your jaw and refused to elevate it for your speech, you probably noticed that you were largely unintelligible. The mandible is an extremely important articulator (e.g., Tasko & Greilik, 2010) in its supportive role of carrying the lips, tongue, and teeth to their targets in the maxilla (lips, teeth, alveolar ridge, and hard palate), but its adjustments are rather minute in normal speech. For this reason, paralysis of the muscles of mastication can be devastating to speech intelligibility.

The muscles of mandibular elevation (temporalis, masseter, and medial pterygoid) are endowed with muscle spindles, although those of mandibular depression (digastricus, mylohyoid, geniohyoid, and lateral pterygoid) are not. You can easily see the effects of muscle spindles on yourself. Relax your jaw while looking into a mirror. Now apply a firm rubbing pressure on the masseter in a downward-pulling direction. You will see your mandible elevate slightly as you trigger the mandibular reflex. There are also sensors of joint position within the temporomandibular joint that permit extremely accurate positioning of the jaw (within 1 mm). If these sensors are anesthetized, the speaker's accuracy diminishes markedly.

The mandible is, of course, quite important for mastication, and the function of the muscles of mastication is distinctly different for speech and for chewing. It appears that there is a central pattern generator within the brain stem that produces the rhythmic muscular contraction needed for chewing (Ostry et al., 1997; Wilson, Green & Weismer, 2012). The mandible must elevate, grind laterally, and depress, requiring coordinated activation of the elevators and depressors in a synergistic, rhythmic fashion. We will discuss this pattern further in Chapter 8.

For speech, in contrast, the mandibular elevators and depressors stay in dynamic balance, so that a slight modification in muscle activation (and inhibition by antagonists) permits a quick adjustment of the mandible (Moore, 1993). Indeed, depression of the mandible seems to be not only a function of the classically defined mandibular depressors (digastricus, mylohyoid, geniohyoid, and lateral pterygoid) but, to a significant extent, of the infrahyoid musculature as well (Westbury, 1988). The hyoid undergoes a great deal of movement during depression of the mandible.

Tongue

Arguably, the tongue is the most important of the articulators. It is involved in the production of the majority of phonemes in English. Let us look at how we achieve the individual movements of the tongue.

As a first approximation, you can think of the tongue as a group of highly organized (intrinsic) muscles being carried on the "shoulders" of the extrinsic muscles. Much as the muscles of the legs and trunk move your upper body to a position where your arms and head can interact with the environment, the extrinsic muscles set the basic posture of the tongue, whereas the intrinsic muscles have a great

Table 7-1 **Muscles of tongue movement**	
Movement	**Muscle**
Elevate tongue tip	Superior longitudinal muscles
Depress tongue tip	Inferior longitudinal muscles
Deviate tongue tip	Left and right superior and inferior longitudinal muscles for left and right deviation, respectively
Relax lateral margin	Posterior genioglossus for protrusion; superior longitudinal for tip elevation; transverse intrinsic for pulling sides medially
Narrow tongue	Transverse intrinsic
Deep central groove	Genioglossus for depression of the tongue body; vertical intrinsic for depression of central dorsum
Broad central groove	Moderate genioglossus for depression of the tongue body; vertical intrinsic for depression of dorsum; superior longitudinal for elevation of margins
Protrude tongue	Posterior genioglossus for advancement of the tougue body; vertical muscles to narrow tongue; superior and inferior longitudinal to balance and point tongue
Retract tongue	Anterior genioglossus for retraction of tongue into the oral cavity; superior and inferior longitudinal for shortening of tongue; styloglossus for retraction of tongue into the pharyngeal cavity
Elevate posterior tongue	Palatoglossus for elevation of sides; transverse intrinsic to bunch tongue
Depress tongue body	Genioglossus for depression of medial tongue; hyoglossus and chondroglossus for depression of sides if hyoid is fixed by infrahyoid muscles

© Cengage Learning®.

deal of responsibility for the microstructure of articulation. The two groups of muscles work closely together to achieve the target articulatory motion. Let us examine each of the basic actions required for speech (see Table 7-1).

Tongue Tip Elevation

Elevation of the tongue is the primary responsibility of the superior longitudinal muscles of the tongue. When these fibers are shortened, the tip and lateral margins of the tongue are pulled up.

Tongue Tip Depression

Depression of the tongue is the primary responsibility of the inferior longitudinal muscles. Their course along the lateral margins of the lower tongue makes them perfectly suited to pull the tip and sides of the tongue down.

Unilateral Tongue Weakness

One element of an **oral-peripheral examination** is the examination for relative tongue strength. When you ask a client to push forcefully with his or her tongue sideways against a resistance, you are interested in identifying whether the client has adequate and symmetrical strength. If there appears to be greater force in one direction than the other, you will consider activities to strengthen the musculature. Improving muscle strength will improve tone and muscle control.

Tongue Tip Deviation, Left and Right

Deviation of the tongue tip to the left requires the simultaneous contraction of the left superior and inferior longitudinal muscles. This asymmetrical contraction will have the desired result, which is asymmetrical movement of the tongue tip.

Lateral Margins Relaxation

The lateral margins of the tongue must be relaxed to produce the /l/ phoneme even as the tongue is protruded into the anterior alveolar ridge and slightly elevated. This complex movement is accomplished by the slight contraction of the posterior genioglossus, which helps to move the tongue forward, and the superior longitudinal, which elevates the tip. Contraction of the transverse intrinsic muscles of the tongue will pull the sides medially away from the lateral gum ridge, opening the lateral sulcus for resonation.

Tongue Narrowing

The transverse fibers coursing from the median fibrous septum to the lateral margins of the tongue are required for this action.

Central Tongue Grooving

The degree of tongue grooving determines the magnitude of muscle involvement in this action. Wholesale depression of the medial tongue is accomplished by the contraction of the entire genioglossus in conjunction with the vertical fibers. A more moderate groove will involve the genioglossus to a lesser degree but will still use the vertical muscles. A broadened groove could be accomplished by the co-contraction of the superior longitudinal muscle, elevating the sides of the tongue as well.

Tongue Protrusion

Tongue protrusion requires the use of the posterior genioglossus (Bailey, Rice & Fuglevand, 2007), and at least two of the intrinsic muscles. Contraction of the posterior genioglossus will draw the tongue forward but will not let you point your tongue. To make a proper "statement" with your tongue, however, you will need assistance from the vertical and transverse intrinsic muscles, and deviation (up, down, or to the sides) will require the use of superior and inferior longitudinal intrinsics. The genioglossus posterior by itself would leave the tongue hanging down from your opened mouth.

Tongue Retraction

Retraction of the body of the tongue involves both the intrinsic and extrinsic muscles. The anterior genioglossus will draw the protruded tongue into the oral cavity, and co-contraction of the superior and inferior longitudinal muscles will shorten the tongue. To retract the tongue into the pharyngeal space, as in the swallowing action, the styloglossus must be engaged.

Posterior Tongue Elevation

The palatoglossi insert into the sides of the tongue, and their contraction elevates the sides. Contraction of the transverse muscles in the posterior tongue would assist in bunching the tongue up in that region.

Tongue Body Depression

Contraction of the genioglossus as a unit depresses the medial tongue. The addition of the hyoglossus and chondroglossus will depress the sides of the tongue, assuming that the hyoid is fixed by the infrahyoid muscles.

Although the tongue is capable of generating a great deal of force through contraction, we typically use only about 20 percent of its potential force for speech activities. The tongue is endowed with muscle spindles, golgi tendon organs, and tactile sensors. Muscle spindles have been found in the tongue muscles, and golgi tendon organs have been found in the transverse intrinsic muscles. Passive movement of the tongue (pulling outward) will result in a reflexive retraction of

Tongue Deviation on Protrusion

Tongue musculature is paired, and unilateral weakness will produce asymmetry on protrusion. When the tongue is protruded, the bilateral musculature of the genioglossus must contract with equal force. If the left genioglossus is weak, it will not contribute equally to the protrusion, and the right genioglossus will overcome the left's effort. As a result, left genioglossus weakness will result in deviation toward the left side. Put another way, with lower motor neuron damage the tongue "points toward the lesion."

the tongue, and mechanical stimulation of the tongue dorsum will cause excitation of the genioglossus muscle. Stimulation of the tongue dorsum has an effect on other articulators as well, causing excitation of the masseter and lower orbicularis oris.

The tongue is also remarkably sensitive to touch. We can differentiate two points on the tongue tip separated by only about 1.5 mm. Another extremely sensitive region of the mouth is the periodontal ligament of the dental arch, which can sense movement of particles as slight as 10 microns (if you have ever had a strawberry seed wedged between your teeth, you can verify this sensitivity). It is likely that this sensitivity is used to monitor production of dental consonants.

Velum

Early in the history of speech-language pathology, audiology, and speech and hearing science we found it tempting to treat the velum as a binary element: It was either opened or closed. We have since realized that it is unsafe to deal with such a complex structure in so simple a fashion. The velum is capable of a range of motion and rate of movement that, in the normally endowed individual, matches the needs of rapid speech and nonspeech functions.

The velum generally is closed for nonnasal speech, and this is the result of contraction of the levator veli palatini, a direct antagonist to the palatoglossus muscle. In speech, the opening and closing of the velar port must occur precisely and rapidly, or the result will be hyper- or hyponasality. Failure to open the port will turn a 70 ms nasal phoneme into a voiced stop consonant, an unacceptable result. The soft palate opens and closes in coordination with the other articulators, thus avoiding the effect of nasal resonance on other phonemes, which is called nasal **assimilation**. In reality, some nasal assimilation is inevitable; acceptable; and in some geographic regions, dialectically appropriate.

Production of high-pressure consonants (such as fricatives and stops) requires greater velopharyngeal effort. To accomplish this seal, additional help is needed from the superior pharyngeal constrictor and uvular muscles. Even then, the pressures for speech are far less than those for, say, playing a wind instrument. Individuals may have difficulty avoiding nasal air escape when playing in the brass section but otherwise have perfectly normal speech.

The hard and soft palates are richly endowed with receptors that provide feedback concerning pressure, and it appears that these sensors facilitate or inhibit motor lingual activity. Indeed, the tensor veli palatini, palatoglossus, and levator veli palatini muscles have been found to have muscle spindles, and the input from these sensors may be important to the initiation of the pharyngeal swallowing reflex (Kuehn, Templeton, & Maynard, 1990; Liss, 1990). In cats, when the soft palate is stimulated electrically, extrinsic tongue movement is inhibited. In contrast, when the hard palate is stimulated (as it would

Hypernasality refers to excessive, linguistically inappropriate nasal resonance arising from failure to adequately close the velopharyngeal port during nonnasal speech sound production. In contrast, hyponasality refers to the absence of appropriately nasalized speech sounds, such that the velopharyngeal port is inadequately opened for the /n/, /m/, and /ŋ/ phonemes.

be by food crushed during oral preparation), the extrinsic lingual muscles are excited, producing a rhythmic movement of the tongue. Stretching the faucial pillars by pulling on the tongue or the pillars themselves also inhibits the activity of the extrinsic tongue muscles. It appears that the interaction of the soft palate, fauces, and tongue is a well-organized and integrated system. Palatal, laryngeal, and pharyngeal stimulation activates protrusion of the tongue, whereas stimulation of the anterior oral region appears to stimulate retraction of the tongue.

✔ *To summarize:*

- Each of the articulators has both speech and nonspeech functions that do not necessarily share the same patterns.
- The lower lip is much faster and stronger than the upper lip and responds reflexively to increases of pressure. This added responsiveness makes it quite effective at overcoming incidental **perturbations** while performing its assigned tasks.
- Movement of the **mandible** for speech is slight when compared with its movement for chewing. In addition, the mandibular posture for speech is one of sustained dynamic tension between antagonists.
- The **tongue** is an extremely versatile organ, with the **extrinsic muscles** providing the major movement of the tongue, and the **intrinsic muscles** providing the shaping of the tongue.
- The **velum** must be maintained in a reasonably elevated position for most speech sounds, although it is capable of a range of movements.

Development of Articulatory Ability

Infants are faced with an enormous task during development. They begin life with no knowledge of the universe and with a motor system in which movement is governed by reflexes that are out of their control. They will spend the next several years (perhaps the rest of their lives!) making sense of the world around them and learning to manipulate their environment. Fortunately, they are born with an innate "desire" to acquire information and learn about their environment, and it appears that this desire drives the often-painful process of development.

The primitive human motor system is actually an extremely complex network of protective reflexes. Reflexes provide the means for an immature infant to respond to the environment in a stereotyped manner, without volition. This is not to argue that infants have no will, but rather to point out that they cannot express it voluntarily. If a breast touches the lips of an infant, the infant will orient to the breast and start sucking reflexively (you can stimulate this reflex with a stroke of your fingers). The infant does not need to think, "Gee, I'm hungry. I wonder if there is anything to eat around here?" Rather, nature has hardwired the infant to meet its needs.

This reflexive condition results in what Langley and Lombardino (1991) refer to as "primitive mass patterns of movement." Movements are gross responses to environmental stimuli that help the infant meet its basic needs. Development is a process of gaining cortical control of the motor patterns for volitional purposes, and the development of the articulatory system has its roots in learning to walk.

The most pervasive postnatal experience an infant has is gravity. Always present, gravity provides the ultimate challenge to an infant who wants to experience a universe that is out of reach. Reflexive movement against gravity provides the child with information about the effects of movement. Infants can see their hands as they move them and learn that there is a relationship between the sensation and the hands they see. These are the essential elements of motor development: reflexive response to environmental stimuli, providing *feedback* to an intact neuromotor system. Motor development is a process of refining gross movements, and this refinement will occur **cephalocaudally** (from head to tail) and **proximodistally** (from medial structures to distal structures). Infants will develop gross mandibular movements before developing fine mandibular movements and will have head control before they develop trunk control. They will develop posterior tongue control before developing anterior tongue control. Four vital elements of basic motor control support later-speech development: experience with gravity, flexor–extensor balance, trunk control, and differentiation.

During the reflexive period (roughly birth to six months), the infant's vestibular system is being stimulated by parental handling. Vestibular stimulation causes changes in muscle tone relative to gravity, setting the stage for the tonic activity of the postural muscles.

Effects of Neuromuscular Disease on Velopharyngeal Function

A deficit associated with the velopharyngeal port can have significant effects on speech. In neuromuscular disorders, such as amyotrophic lateral sclerosis or multiple sclerosis, muscular weakness arises from damage to the motor neurons. When the weakness involves the muscles of the velum, the nasal cavity resonance is added to that of the oral cavity for nonnasal sounds. This "anti-resonance," as it is called, pulls energy out of the speech signal in the 1500 to 2500 Hz range, causing a marked loss of clarity in the speech signal. Speech of the affected individual sounds muffled, monotonous, and low in vocal intensity.

It is not uncommon for the speech-language pathologist to be the first person approached by an individual with early signs of neuromuscular disease. The velopharyngeal port requires constant elevation for nonnasal sounds and is an early indicator of progressive muscular weakness. An individual may come to the clinician with the complaint that people say his or her speech sounds muffled. Your oral-peripheral examination will reveal slow velar activity, and your referral to a physician will be most helpful to the client at that point.

The baby begins life in a general state of flexion, and the advent of extension heralds an infant's ability to engage actively with his or her environment. When the newborn is placed on his or her stomach, the infant's weight will shift to the infant's face. When pulled up from supine, the infant's head will flop back with no control. The three-month-old has a great deal of extensor balance and can now control his or her head when pulled from the supine position. The sitting position is a stable platform from which the infant can now use head rotation to view the environment. Soon the trunk muscles will be under sufficient control that the infant can rotate the trunk and reach for objects in the environment.

The combination of trunk stability and extensor–flexor balance gives the infant the tools for standing and walking—and talking. It is no surprise that the infant's speech begins to develop in concert with his or her locomotor skills. If you remember that the tongue is intimately related to the hyoid and larynx, you will realize that it is unreasonable to expect a child to control the complex, refined movements of the tongue until the trunk and neck muscles are stabilized.

Following stabilization, the infant must develop differential motor control. In the articulatory system, the manifestations of this control are evident in the rapidly increasing complexity of speech production. The simple consonant–vowel (CV) syllable represents the most basic valving of the articulatory system. All the child must do to produce this syllable is to begin phonation and open and close the mouth repeatedly. Tongue contact will bring about a velar or alveolar stop, or lip contact will produce a bilabial plosive. In any case, this infant has babbled, much to the delight of his or her parents.

The simple valving gives way to refined control of the tongue. With mandible stability accomplished, a child can begin the process of differentiating the tongue movements from those of the mandible. Following this, the infant differentiates between tongue body and tip movements, as well as lateralization.

This development is hierarchical. The infant must balance muscle activation and muscle tone before being able to sit, and must sit before she can establish independent head and neck control. With the control of neck muscles comes the freedom to move the mandible and tongue independently, and with that freedom comes the ability to differentially move the articulators.

Use of a Palatal Lift

A **palatal lift prosthesis** is a device, typically anchored to the teeth, used to elevate the soft palate to more closely approximate the velum for closure. The device looks like an orthodontic appliance with a projection in the back. This prosthesis is useful for individuals with muscular weakness, perhaps arising as a result of **hypoplasia** (inadequate muscle development) or a **neurogenic** condition (deficit arising from neurological cause).

Does this mean that a child with deficits of motor development will never develop speech? The answer, fortunately, is "no." The task is doubly difficult, however, and still depends on gaining the voluntary control and differentiation of those muscles. This is where you, the clinician, take your cue.

Development of the Vocal Tract

The vocal tract of an infant is clearly shorter than that of an adult, but the infant is not merely a "small adult." Proportional changes occur during development that have an impact on swallowing and speech function. The nasopharynx of the infant enlarges markedly and becomes more sharply angled relative to the oropharynx. The oral cavity grows, the tongue descends, and the oropharyngeal space increases. As Vorparian et al. (2005) note, the growth of the various oral and pharyngeal tissues has differing rates, and these differences necessarily cause changes in the relationships of the structures over time. Generally, a child reaches adult oral cavity size between 7 and 18 years (Kent & Vorperian, 1995; Vorperian, et al., 2009).

Vocal tract length, from vocal folds to lips, is approximately 6–8 cm at birth, but grows to 15–18 cm in adulthood (see Figure 7-2). As you can see from these three figures, vocal tract length (VTL) and nasopharyngeal lengths (vocal tract vertical [VTV]) undergo rapid

(A)

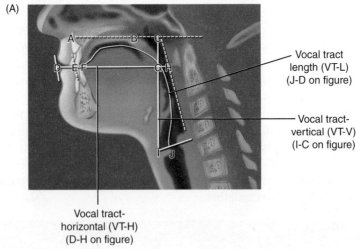

Vocal tract length (VT-L) (J-D on figure)

Vocal tract-vertical (VT-V) (I-C on figure)

Vocal tract-horizontal (VT-H) (D-H on figure)

Figure 7-2. (A) Vocal tract measurements: Vocal Fold Length (VTL) is the distance from J (plane of vocal folds) to anterior lips. Vocal Tract Vertical dimension (VTV, pharyngeal space) from anterior vocal fold to plane of posterior nasal spine. Vocal tract horizontal length (VT-H), from anterior lips to pharyngeal wall. From Vorperian, H. K., Wang, S., Chung, M. K., Schimek, E. M., Durtschi, R. B., Kent, R. D., Ziergert, A. J., & Gentry, L. R. (2009). Anatomic development of the oral and pharyngeal portions of the vocal tract: An imaging study. *Journal of the Acoustical Society of America*, 125(3), 1666-1678. (continues).
© Cengage Learning®.

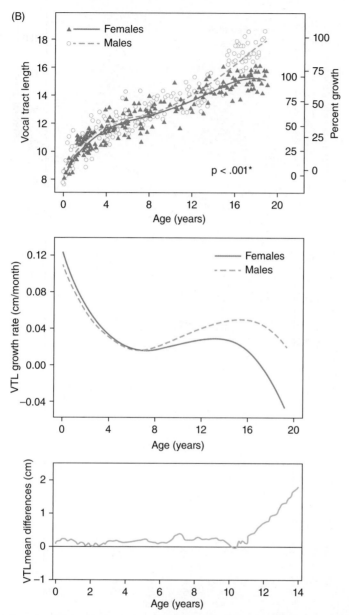

Figure 7-2 continued. (B) Top: Vocal tract length growth by age. Males are represented by the open circles and dark dashed trend line, females by the triangles and solid trend line. Middle: Rate of growth by month of vocal tract length for males and females. Notice that the most rapid growth occurs between birth and 4 years, with another increase in the 12 to 16 year range. From Vorperian, H. K., Wang, S., Chung, M. K., Schimek, E. M., Durtschi, R. B., Kent, R. D., Ziergert, A. J., & Gentry, L. R. (2009). Anatomic development of the oral and pharyngeal portions of the vocal tract: An imaging study. *Journal of the Acoustical Society of America*, 125(3), 1666-1678. Bottom: Difference between males and females, by year. Notice the rapid increase in vocal tract length difference starting at puberty (around 11 years). From Vorperian, H. K., Wang, S., Schimek, E. M., Durtschi, R. B., Kent, R. D., Gentry, L. R. & Chung, M. K. (2011). Developmental sexual dimorphism of the oral and pharyngeal portions of the vocal tract: An imaging study. *Journal of speech-language-hearing research*, 54(4), 995-1010. (continues).

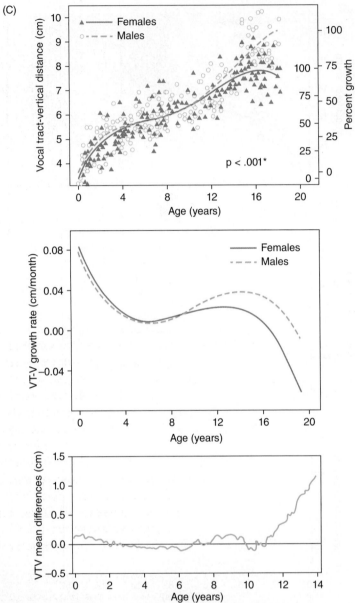

Figure 7-2 continued. (C) Top: Growth of the pharyngeal space by age in years (vocal tract-vertical, VT-V). Males are represented by the open circles and dashed trend line, while females are represented by the triangles and solid trend line. Middle: Rate of growth of pharyngeal space by years. Note that the rate of growth plateaus at around 4 years of age, but increase again between 12 and 16 years. This is a significant contributor to total vocal tract length. From Vorperian, H. K., Wang, S., Chung, M. K., Schimek, E. M., Durtschi, R. B., Kent, R. D., Ziergert, A. J., & Gentry, L. R. (2009). Anatomic development of the oral and pharyngeal portions of the vocal tract: An imaging study. *Journal of the Acoustical Society of America*, 125(3), 1666-1678. Bottom: Difference between males and females in pharyngeal space length, by years. Note that males show a marked increase relative to females around 11 years. From Vorperian, H. K., Wang, S., Schimek, E. M., Durtschi, R. B., Kent, R. D., Gentry, L. R. & Chung, M. K. (2011). Developmental sexual dimorphism of the oral and pharyngeal portions of the vocal tract: An imaging study. *Journal of speech-language-hearing research*, 54(4), 995-1010. (continues).

© Cengage Learning®.

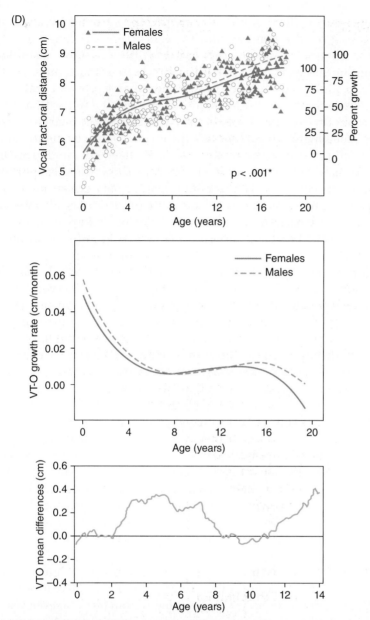

Figure 7-2 continued. (D) Top: Length of the horizontal vocal tract (lips to pharyngeal wall) as a function of age. Males are represented by the open circles and dashed trend line, and females are represented by the triangles and solid trend line. Notice that growth patterns for the vocal tract are essentially the same for males and females, with the greatest growth between birth and 4 years. The middle image shows that the rate of growth shows no significant increase after 4 years. From Vorperian, H. K., Wang, S., Chung, M. K., Schimek, E. M., Durtschi, R. B., Kent, R. D., Ziergert, A. J., & Gentry, L. R. (2009). Anatomic development of the oral and pharyngeal portions of the vocal tract: An imaging study. *Journal of the Acoustical Society of America, 125*(3), 1666–1678 Bottom: Difference between males and females as a function of age. Notice that males have greater growth than females between 4 and 6 years, and then show the pubertal increase over females beginning around 11 years. From Vorperian, H. K., Wang, S., Schimek, E. M., Durtschi, R. B., Kent, R. D., Gentry, L. R. & Chung, M. K. (2011). Developmental sexual dimorphism of the oral and pharyngeal portions of the vocal tract: An imaging study. *Journal of speech-language-hearing research, 54*(4), 995-1010.

changes during the first year of life, plateauing around 4 years, and increasing rapidly again around 12 years of age. The length of the oral cavity (including the oropharynx: VTH) undergoes a similar change until 4 years, but after that the increase is much more gradual into adulthood. In other words, both pharyngeal and oral cavity growth contribute to the rapid increase in VTL in the first four years, but the greatest change after that occurs in the pharynx. The plots beneath growth curves show the rate of change by month, and really tell the story: The first 4 years are extremely rapid growth, but that tapers off in all cases. The pharynx shows another spurt of growth between 8 and 12 years but the oral cavity dimension (VT-V) growth rate flattens out. As you study these figures, also notice the *difference* between males and females in this growth: There is a striking divergence between vocal tracts at puberty (around 11 years).

VTL is not a trivial measure since this length is a dominant determinant of the first formant in vowel production. This vocal tract increase is attributable mostly to the growth of the pharynx. During the first 24 months of life, the hard palate will increase almost 1 cm in length, while the velum will increase only about 0.5 cm in the same length of time. The mandible undergoes similar changes during development. The length of the mandible increases from 2 cm to more than 4 cm in the first two years, ultimately reaching a length of 5 cm by seven years of age. The depth of the mandible increases to accommodate the tongue, producing a steady increase in the oral cavity size. As you can see from Figure 7-3, mandible depth and length show a steady growth during the first seven years of life, achieving between 80 and 90 percent of adult size by that age. The tongue undergoes a similar growth, filling the space created by the expansion of the mandible, and achieving about 75 percent of adult size by seven years. We see a corresponding rate of descent of the larynx (about 3 cm of drop over the seven-year period), as well as of the hyoid (about 2 cm).

One more thing that you can see by examining Figure 7-3 is the presence of breakpoints that occur in the 12- to 24-year period. These breakpoints indicate that the growth from birth to seven years of age is not linear, but rather two different prediction lines must be used to describe the progression. The first line characterizes the rapid growth between birth and 1–2 years of age, while the second line characterizes the more stable development during the subsequent period. The authors note that the variation in breakpoint from structure to structure (e.g., between tongue length and hard palate length) indicates different rates of growth for the various structures. Needless to say, these changes will have a significant impact upon the resonant characteristics of the vocal tract during speech, and (as we shall see in Chapter 8) a real impact on mastication and deglutition.

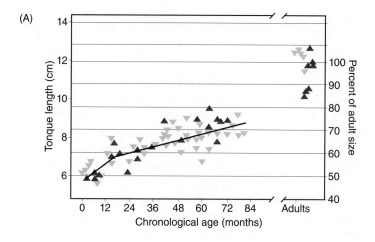

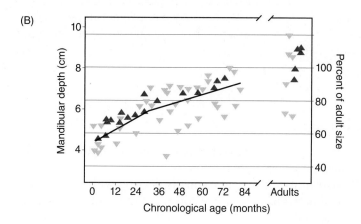

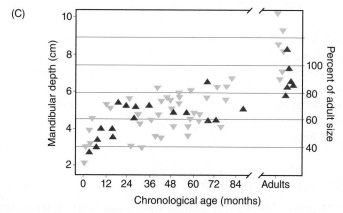

Figure 7-3. Mandibular length and depth, and related tongue length. (A) Tongue length shows a rapid increase during the first 12 months of life and then reaches 70% of adult size by 7 years. Mandibular depth (B) and length (C) show a more steady increase in size over the same time period, achieving 90% of adult size by seven years (from Vorparian et al. (2005). Development of vocal tract length during early childhood: A magnetic resonance imaging study).

Source: Reused with permission from Houri K. Vorperian, Ray D. Kent, Mary J. Lindstrom, Cliff M. Kalina, Lindell R. Gentry, and Brian S. Yandell, The *Journal of the Acoustical Society of America*, 117, 338 (2005). Copyright 2005, Acoustical Society of America.

Phonological Development and Motor Control

The development of a child's phonology is indeed a marvel. It should now be fairly clear that the maturation of the motor speech system governs, in large part, the speech sounds a child is capable of making. The stops (/p,t,k,b,d,g/) are present in the child's repertoire fairly early in development, although mastery will occur later than emergence. The reason for this is apparently motoric. A child of two or three years of age is quite capable of the basic "valving" movement of opening and closing the mouth (/ba/) raising and lowering the tongue on the alveolar ridge (/da/) or near the velum (/ga/). However, controlled production of the stops requires the ability to differentiate labial, mandibular, and lingual movements, and thus, mastery of the stops may occur as late as six years.

As the child develops greater motor control, he or she gains the ability to make graded movements with the tongue so that he or she can sustain one articulator against the other with a constant pressure. The "raspberry" you hear in the preverbal child is very likely the precursor to the fricatives that will develop later. With graded control of lingual pressure comes the ability to make minute adjustments of an articulatory posture, such as those made with the dorsum of the tongue to differentiate /s/ and /ʃ/ through widening of the tongue groove and tongue tip elevation.

✔ *To summarize:*

- A neonate depends on **reflexive responses** for protection and to meet his or her needs.
- These primitive patterns gradually develop with **voluntary control patterns** to facilitate control of the trunk, the neck, and the limbs.
- With this control comes the ability to make graded movements of the mandible and, subsequently, differentiated lingual movements.
- The vocal tract undergoes radical changes during development.
- Vocal tract length and nasopharyngeal lengths undergo rapid changes during the first year of life, plateauing around 4 years. The growth accelerates again around 12 years of age.
- The length of the oral cavity, including the oropharynx, increases rapidly to 4 years of age, and then the rate of growth slows down.

Coordinated Articulation

Theories of motor control for speech have undergone a great deal of evolution but are centered generally around the notions of locus of control, the need for consistency for the motor act, and task specification. Speech is arguably the most complex sequential motor task performed by humans. Consider the following hierarchical elements of speech, as implied by MacKay (1982).

Within the initial, conceptual system, we must first develop the proposition, or idea to be expressed, and that idea represents the sentence to be spoken. This idea or proposition must be mapped into a syntactical system to establish the language forms acceptable to match the concept, and appropriate words must be selected to match the syntax and to fit the proposition. Thus, if the idea "Tomorrow is Monday" is the chosen proposition, the syntax for that proposition must be selected, and the words chosen to fit the syntax and the proposition.

In the **phonological system**, syllable structure is parsed from the lexical selections. Phonological rules are applied to establish the correct phoneme combinations to meet the needs of the words chosen previously, and the individual features of those phonemes are parsed from the phonological specifications. Thus, at the phonological system level, the selected words ("Tomorrow" "is" "Monday") will be further broken into syllables, selected phonemes, and features for the phonemes. For instance, the /t/ in "tomorrow" will be defined as lingua-alveolar, stop, and voiceless. Note that, throughout all of this, there has been no mention of muscles of articulation.

In the muscle movement system, muscles are activated to meet the needs of the feature selection process. The /t/ of the phonological system was broken into features, such as lingua-alveolar, and this is now translated into the movement of the muscles of the tongue that will produce that lingua-alveolar gesture (such as the superior longitudinal and genioglossus muscles).

Subsequent speech proceeds from the assumption that we have developed an idea that we wish to express and that we can somehow map that idea into muscle movements that change the three-dimensional space of the oral cavity. Those changes result in an acoustical output that is an acceptable representation of our goal.

In the early twentieth century, researchers recognized that the learning of sequential acts could be easily explained if one assumed that we linked a series of basic movements, like beads on a string. By this theory, the **associated chain theory**, the production of /t/ required only that the speaker learn all of the motor sequences leading up to elevation of the tongue to the alveolar ridge, and so forth. We could link a series of reflexive movements and entrain them in a sequential activation pattern. Once the motor act was learned, the speaker would forever be prepared to produce a word with /t/ in it. Lashley (1951) argued that the articulatory system is not a set of "sleeping" muscles waiting to be activated but is rather a set of dynamic structures under continuous activation. In addition, the associative chain theories could not begin to account for variability in speech, much less the overlapping effect of one articulatory pattern on another (**coarticulation**). Future theories would have to account for the fluidity of speech production, the inherent variability of articulation based on context, and the ability of the articulators to achieve their phonetic target despite unpredictable alteration of the context of the production. Two major theoretical frameworks emerged from Lashley's concerns: the central control theory and the dynamic systems perspective.

Central Control Theory

The various forms of central control theory hold that there is a "master control" mechanism that dictates the muscle movements based on the linguistic goal. In the most extreme case, the command system would be oblivious to the state of the articulators at any moment and would administer the muscle commands without regard for the articulator conditions of the moment. The beauty of such a model is the direct access that the motor system has to the language processor. Individual phonemes would be represented by a burst of neural excitation, so that the plan for a /t/ would be expertly executed with faithful precision. This elegantly addresses to a major problem: The articulatory act for any phoneme requires precise activation of an overwhelming number of neurons and muscle fibers, and the activation must be accurate, timely, and result in correct movement. Thus, simply activating a program that your brain knows will produce a /t/ is much simpler than having to micro-manage your articulatory system.

Clearly, feedback from sensors within the articulators and related structures, as well as from the auditory signal itself, had to be accounted for. Without feedback we would be unable to arrive at a production that was accurate and acceptable by our communicative partners. Fairbanks (1954) posed the earliest and most stringent of the **feedback theories**, holding that the brain commands the articulators to achieve a target, and that a mismatch between the feedback and the ideal results in a correction of the output. Modification of articulation is driven by afferent information on an ongoing basis. In this view, the sensory system plays a dominant role in the production of speech.

The downside of these models is that they fail to account for the flexibility of the articulatory system in response to varying environmental conditions. If you pay attention to your tongue as you say the words *beat* and *toot*, you will note that the tongue is in two very different locations as it moves up for the final /t/, yet you are perfectly able to achieve both goals. Central control theories are forced to establish individual articulatory patterns to represent each allophone to accommodate this need—a very weighty proposition. Although the notions of central control remain robust and promising (e.g., MacKay, 1982), clearly there is a need to explain how we are able to articulate with such precision in the face of continuous variability.

Dynamic or Action Theory Models

As theorists worked to explain accurate and variable articulatory ability, the notion of **articulatory goals** evolved. The end product of muscle activity (and central control) was viewed as being a major determinant in execution. Saltzman (1986) viewed goal-related movement as composed of an **effector system**, a portion of which is the **terminal device**. The effector system would include the entire group of articulators involved in a given action, and the terminal device, or **end-effector** (such as the dorsum of the tongue for the articulation of the phoneme /i/), is that portion of the effector system directly related to the articulatory goal. By differentiating these components, one can account for the problem of having to coordinate large numbers of muscle fibers in concert. From this point, one can view the articulatory effector system in a dynamic fashion. The components of the effector system are assigned the goal of articulation but are free to work within the degrees of freedom inherent in the system to accomplish the task. That is, no two acts are ever produced the same way twice, and yet there are definitely commonalities among motor acts. The dynamic models state that the commonality is that the motor act is accurately achieved within the bounds of variability.

The functional units of activation are groups of **coordinative structures**. Coordinative structures are functionally defined muscle groups that, when activated, contribute to achieving the goal at the terminal effector. An important element of this is the concept of motor equivalence. If the goal is, for instance, production of the vowel /i/, there might be many different articulatory solutions to the problem of getting an acoustic production that would be judged as correct. The mandible could be clamped and immobile, which would require a different gesture than that of someone with a slack jaw. Motor equivalence states that a goal can be achieved through various means and systems.

Trajectories, or movement paths, can be seen as targets of movement, and the structures involved in achieving a target are grouped as coordinative structures. If the movement is disturbed during execution, the coordinative structures are capable of altering their degree of activation to compensate for this perturbation without an altered central command. As an example, if you were to pick up a glass of milk, your target would be the accurate movement of the glass rim to your lips. Unknown to you, the glass has a very heavy base. When you lift the glass, you expect it to be lighter than it is, so your muscular effort is less than if you had expected a heavier glass. If you depended on a central program to correct your movement, the glass might not reach your lips, and you would probably pour the milk down your shirt. As it is, your effector system adapts its activities to match the trajectory (table to lips), you add extra force, and your thirst is quenched. This ability to compensate is essential for speech production.

The **dynamic models** take into account the physical properties of the systems involved in articulation. Muscles and connective tissue have elastic properties that result in recoil, and dynamic models account for these variables in the equation. These models have more quickly accommodated the role of afferent information concerning the state of the musculature. According to Kelso and Ding (1993), there are many solutions to achieving any trajectory, and the relationship of the coordinative structures simply defines the solution from a given point of trajectory initiation to the point of termination.

Models of speech production must also somehow account for the fact that speech occurs at an extraordinarily rapid rate and that, somehow, the articulatory system is very resistant to perturbation. We can accommodate a wide range of surprises in speech with no trouble at all. Dynamic models account for the dynamic aspects of

Apraxia

Apraxia refers to a deficit in the programming of musculature for voluntary movement with an absence of any muscular weakness or paralysis. There appear to be many types and subtypes of apraxia. **Limb apraxia** is identified as the inability to perform volitional gestures using the limbs. A patient with limb apraxia might reveal deficits in voluntarily using multiple objects to perform a sequence of acts upon request, such as making a sandwich. The act may be fluent, but the object is used inappropriately. The patient's ability to perform the act through imitation would be much less impaired.

A patient with **oral apraxia** might reveal difficulty using the facial and lingual muscles for non-speech acts. When this individual is asked to blow out a candle, he or she may experience a great deal of effortful groping in an attempt to find the right configuration of his or her lips in coordination with the outward flow of air. Often the oral apractic individual also has a verbal apraxia.

Verbal apraxia refers to a deficit in planning the motor act and programming the articulators for speech sound production. The individual with verbal apraxia will make errors in correct articulation of the sounds of speech, although the errors vary widely from one attempt to another. The individual is aware of the error and will make frequent attempts at production, so that the flow of speech is greatly impeded. This patient will have more difficulty with multisyllabic than monosyllabic words, and semiautomatic speech (such as greetings) may be quite fluent.

By definition, apraxias occur without muscular weakness, although muscular weakness or paralysis may co-occur with the apraxia. Apraxias may arise from lesions to a variety of brain structures. Damage to the left hemisphere premotor region of the cerebral cortex appears to have the greatest probability of producing apraxia. The specific premotor region involved with speech is known as Broca's area, and the insular cortex, which is deep to Broca's area, was identified by Dronkers (1996) and Dronkers, Pinker, and Damasio (2000) as a site involved in verbal apraxia, although others disagree (Hillis et al., 2004).

---

the physical system required to achieve a specific target within the environment. If the articulatory command specifies an output product rather than a specific movement, the system retains the flexibility to adapt to changes in the environment.

These models attempt to account for many difficulties in articulation theory, not the least of which is coarticulation (the overlapping effect of one articulatory gesture on another). During running speech, we will begin movement toward an articulatory posture well in advance of when it is needed *if* that activation does not interfere with the articulations preceding it. For example, pay attention to your lips when you say the words *see* and *sue*. The /s/ in *see* is made with retracted lips, whereas the /s/ in *sue* is produced with rounded lips, both illustrating preparatory articulation. You will *not* see this effect in the word *booty*, however. Try saying that word with your lips retracted for the /I/, and you will hear an unacceptable vowel production.

We are amazingly resilient in our articulatory abilities, and our resistance to **perturbation** (sudden, unexpected force applied to an articulator) supports the notion of functional synergies or coordinative structures. A functionally defined group of muscles and associated articulators are assigned a task, such as "close the lips," but they have many different ways to accomplish the task. A perturbation or bite block reduces the number of ways available to accomplish the task, but as long as there is a solution, the articulators will find it.

The DIVA Model of Speech Production

Models of speech production must necessarily include some forms of feedback about the accuracy of articulation. This feedback may take the form of auditory information (hearing your own production to determine how accurate your attempt at speech was), tactile and kinesthetic feedback (perceiving how accurately your physical target was achieved in articulation), or even feedback from external sources (the frown on someone's face when he or she does not understand what you have said). Guenther, Hampson, and Johnson (1998) and Callan, Kent, Guenther, and Vorperian (2000) proposed the DIVA (directions into velocities of articulation) model, which utilizes auditory feedback and feedforward as the dominant inputs. Guenther et al. (2006) and Guenther and Vladusich (2012) propose that a model of speech production must include both a learning component based upon feedback, and a means of allowing the speech system to produce accurate speech without requiring the same level of monitoring that occurs during the learning process. While this model is designed simply to control the output of a speech synthesizer, Guenther and his colleagues have made a solid connection between the model processes and neural processes, as we will discuss shortly.

You may want to refer to Figure 7-4 as we discuss this model. In simple terms, the model is designed to control output commands that represent muscles of speech. The initial input to the system is the auditory model that the articulatory system is supposed to attempt. For instance, the /i/ phoneme may serve as an input to the system, and the job of the system is to replicate the /i/ by means of regulating the control characteristics of a speech synthesizer. The input signal (/i/) activates "sound map cells" in the modeled premotor cortex, which are themselves modeled after mirror neurons that have been found in the frontal and temporal lobes, and which provide a match-to-model feedback mechanism within the real human brain. Upon activating a sound map cell, an "image" of the sound target is sent to the auditory and somatosensory regions responsible for monitoring accuracy of speech production, representing areas of both the cerebellum and cerebral cortex. Note in Figure 7-4 that both the auditory and somatosensory monitoring regions receive input not only from the cerebral cortex premotor (planning) region but also receive real-world input from the auditory mechanism (hearing) and the somatosensory system (tactile and kinesthetic input related to the state of the articulators at a given moment). This input from the auditory and somatosensory "universe" of your body is a reality check for the system itself: If the command coming from the premotor region results in a distorted acoustic production, the auditory error map

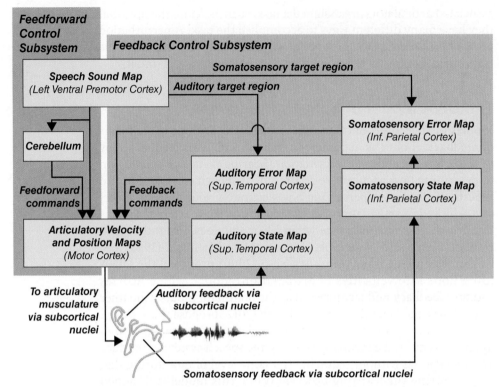

Figure 7-4. DIVA model proposed by Guenther. The speech sound map of the premotor cortex controls the articulator velocity and position maps (lower left) which, in turn, control the muscles of speech. The output of the cortex is fed to somatosensory and auditory error-map regions responsible for monitoring the accuracy of production based on the proposed plan produced at the premotor cortex. The error monitoring systems serve as feedback control, which modifies the output over time during learning stages. Eventually the feedforward control has been modified sufficiently that feedback is no longer critically essential until, of course, a perturbation occurs in the system to require error correction again. Such a perturbation could be as simple as oral anesthesia from dental work to motor disturbance arising from neuromuscular disease.

Source: From Guenther, F. H., Satrajit, S. G., Nieto-Castonon, A., & Tourville, J. A. (2006). A neural model of speech production. In Harrington, J. & Tabain, M. (Eds.) Speech Production: Models, Phonetic Processes, and Techniques. New York: Psychology Press, pp. 27–39, redrawn by permission.

will compare the ideal that the premotor region "desired" with the reality that the motor system produced and cause a change in the articulator velocity and position maps. This change will result in the muscles being activated differently on the next trial. If the change in muscle function results in the acoustic signal being closer to the target, another change in the same direction will be made, and the production tried again. Each successive attempt at that /i/ phoneme will result in its moving closer and closer to the ideal target, until some close acoustical approximation is reached. If a modification of the articulator velocity and position maps results in the action moving farther from the goal, it will be abandoned and a different modification will be tried.

To this point the model relates nicely to what we know about learning in general, and to other models of speech production. We know from our attempts to learn to drive a car that our parents will first take us out to some country road where the variables we have to contend with are limited. Those early attempts to drive the car between the white lines require a great deal of mental effort and the correction of the steering wheel. The visual feedback (watching the road) and tactile feedback (holding the steering wheel, etc.) both provide us with information about how to control the automobile. Every time we oversteer and the car moves too close to the ditch our visual system gives us input that causes a correction in the opposite direction. Eventually we can keep the car between the lines.

Guenther's model is an elegant expression of this speech production process, and if it stopped there it would be an entirely pleasing model. Remarkably, there is much more that the model provides. First of all, learning is predictably accomplished through the feedback system. Guenther's group notes that this motor learning process, in reality, is rather cumbersome as a direct result of the real-time requirements of the neurophysiology underpinning the feedback. It takes between 75 and 150 ms for auditory information to reach the cerebral cortex and for one to act on that information. That is to say, if we use the auditory error map to control speech, we must wait around 100 ms after production in order to tell whether it was correct (Guenther, 2006). This may seem like a small amount of time, but realize that the unstressed monosyllabic word in rapid speech is spoken in less than this duration. This significant time delay explains a lot about the slow rate of speech during the learning process, as well as natural dysfluencies that arise during development. Dysfluency models have long incorporated an auditory feedback component that was either temporarily disruptive (developmental and temporary dysfluency) or permanently disruptive (some basic neurophysiological difference that maintains a feedback disruption). In the DIVA model, motor learning is established through the feedback system of error correction, but significantly, once the target is accurately learned, the feedback system takes the back burner to the feedforward system. That is to say, we no longer use the output of the feedback system to correct our speech continually, but rather we count on our learned accuracy to carry us through the task of talking. We do not stop monitoring our speech, and if we do have some perturbing event (such as oral anesthesia), we can then return to the feedback system to help us correct the errors. Note that when you *do* have anesthesia, your speech is necessarily a bit slower as you try to speak clearly: This is because you must rely on the feedback system, which is slow. Mithen (2008) examined neural function change throughout the process of learning to sing and found a supportive phenomenon: While learning to sing increased responses in the right hemisphere area 45 and in the planum polare of the temporal lobe, activity in regions related to auditory working memory, spatial attention maintenance, and verbal comprehension declined. This reduction in the auditory working memory areas of the cortex would be predicted by DIVA.

Guenther hypothesizes that mirror neurons in the cerebrum may play an important role in the process. Mirror neurons fire when we perform an action, but also fire when we see someone else perform the action. They are, in effect, a sort of environmental monitoring system that could be responsible for a number of phenomena, including empathy and motor learning. Guenther's hypothesis is that these neurons may play a role in the match system between the model and the output of the speaker. Indeed, Prather, Peters, Nowicki, and Mooney (2008) have shown that mirror neurons in the swamp sparrow are responsible for identification of species-specific calls and seem to be critical for "language" learning in sparrows. This adds to a growing list of species (until now, all mammal) with mirror neuron systems.

As if the model's elegance were not enough, Guenther's group has taken three more remarkable steps with it. First, when the model is implemented on a speech synthesizer, dysfluency that is very similar to stuttering can be achieved by disabling the feedforward system and setting a requirement for a more rapid rate of speech output. Essentially, the model demonstrates that one neurophysiological cause of dysfluency may be some inability to disable the feedback systems after speech patterns are learned. This certainly fits with therapies that use slowed rate of speech or highly monitored speech to maintain fluency, as both of these would keep the individual safely within the feedback loop and out of the feedforward system.

A second remarkable achievement by Guenther's group has been to successfully relate the model's input and output systems to neurophysiological systems (Peeva, Guenther, Tourville, Nieto-Castanon, Anton, Nazarian & Alario, 2010). That is to say, the group has identified cortical structures that correspond to elements of the DIVA model. They have then compared the effects of perturbations to the model output to similar perturbations presented to listeners undergoing functional magnetic resonance imaging (fMRI). Remarkably, the model is able to predict the neurophysiological findings of the fMRI, which means that the field may well be on its way to understanding the neurophysiology of speech.

As a result of this groundbreaking development, the group announced that it has begun trials for the therapeutic use of the DIVA model. In collaboration with a neurosurgeon, sensors have been implanted in the model-appropriate regions of the brain of a young man who has "locked-in" syndrome, which resulted from a stroke following traumatic brain injury (Brumberg, Nieto-Castanon, Kennedy & Guenther, 2010). This individual is incapable of any voluntary movement for communication beyond an eye blink. The researchers first identified the area of the brain that was active when the subject imagined himself speaking, since this region would likely be involved in the active production of speech (ventral precentral gyrus) and then implanted a "neural prosthesis" that could read activity within this region. The electrodes within the brain allow the model, implemented on computer, to run a speech synthesizer based on the specific phoneme that the young man is thinking of producing. At this time the model–human combination has successfully and consistently produced three vowels, and the researchers are working to expand the ability of the individual to speak through thought, via machine.

✔ *To summarize:*

- Major theories of motor function approach the task from opposite directions.
- **Central control theories** postulate that a command for muscle movement originates in response to the linguistic needs.
- **Task dynamic theories** posit that the movement arises from the response by coordinated structures to an implicit trajectory.
- **Central control theories** account for the **linguistic dominance** of articulation for speech, while the **dynamic models** account for **variability** and **coarticulatory** effects.
- Both theories account for feedback in speech.

CHAPTER SUMMARY

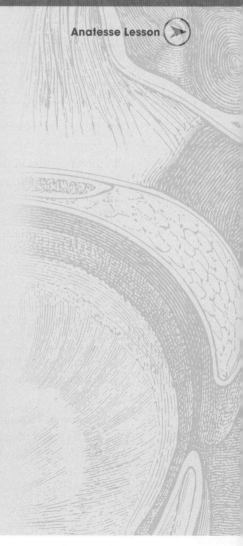

Anatesse Lesson

The lower lip is much faster and stronger than the upper lip and responds reflexively to increases in pressure. Movement of the mandible for speech is slight when compared with its movement for chewing. The mandibular posture for speech is one of sustained dynamic tension between antagonists. The tongue is versatile, with the extrinsic muscles providing the major movement of the body and the intrinsic muscles providing the shaping of the tongue. The velum must be maintained in a reasonably elevated position for most speech sounds, although it is capable of a range of movements.

Development of articulatory function involves gaining control of postural muscles that provide trunk stability and differentiation of muscle group function. Reflexive responses are protective and nurturant, and these primitive patterns gradually develop with voluntary control patterns to facilitate the control of the trunk, neck, and limbs, and finally differentiation for graded oral movement.

Complex speech production requires the control of many parameters simultaneously. We use sensory feedback to learn articulator function in speech and probably use it for error control as well. Central control theories hold that the motor command for an articulation is driven by an articulatory configuration determined through consideration of linguistic elements. The motor command specifies the characteristics of muscle contraction without respect to the speaking environment, but the theories cannot account for articulatory variability or the nearly infinite variety of speaking environments. Dynamic theories hold that coordinative structures interact to accomplish completion of a trajectory, and the theories accommodate the wide variability and flexibility of the articulatory system in speech.

Media Connection

Go to the accompanying online resources at CengageBrain.com and have fun learning! Study with the Anatesse software program, play games, view animations and videos, and take practice tests to help reinforce the key concepts you learned in this chapter.

Study Questions

1. Identify the muscle that best fits the statement. (In some cases there is more than one muscle that fits the bill.)

   a. _____ elevates tongue tip.

   b. _____ depresses tongue tip.

   c. _____ protrudes tongue.

   d. _____ retracts tongue.

   e. _____ elevates posterior tongue.

   f. _____ narrows tongue.

   g. _____ flattens tongue.

   h. _____ depresses velum.

   i. _____ constricts esophageal opening.

   j. _____ constricts upper pharynx.

   k. _____ elevates velum.

2. The _____ (lower lip/upper lip) is faster and stronger than the _____ (lower lip/upper lip).

3. Motor control in the body develops from (head/tail) to _____ (head/tail) and from _____ (proximal/distal) to (proximal/distal).

4. The _____ theory of motor control would require the speaker to learn the sequences of motor acts required for articulation and to link these sequences of motor acts to form an articulatory movement.

5. _____ is the overlapping effect of one articulatory movement on another.

6. _____ theory holds that there is a "master control" mechanism that dictates the muscle movements based up on the linguistic goal.

7. _____ theories generally see articulation as a process of achieving a goal through interaction of coordinative structures. Coordinative structures are muscle groups that, when activated, contribute to achievement of the goal at the terminal effector.

8. Tongue movement depends on the graceful balance of many muscles. Which of the muscles will be involved in elevation of the back of the tongue? As you think of this, ponder the muscles that must work as antagonists to help structures as well.

Study Question Answers

1. Identify the muscle that best fits the statement (In some cases there is more than one muscle that fills the bill.)
   a. **SUPERIOR LONGITUDINAL INTRINSIC** elevates tongue tip.
   b. **INFERIOR LONGITUDINAL INTRINSIC** depresses tongue tip.
   c. **GENIOGLOSSUS, POSTERIOR PORTION** protrudes tongue.
   d. **GENIOGLOSSUS, ANTERIOR PORTION; STYLOGLOSSUS** retracts tongue.
   e. **PALATOGLOSSUS** elevates posterior tongue.
   f. **TRANSVERSE INTRINSIC** narrows tongue.
   g. **VERTICAL INTRINSIC; GENIOGLOSSUS** flattens tongue.
   h. **PALATOGLOSSUS; PALATOPHARYNGEUS** depresses velum.
   i. **CRICOPHARYNGEUS** constricts esophageal opening.
   j. **SUPERIOR PHARYNGEAL CONSTRICTOR** constricts upper pharynx.
   k. **LEVATOR VELI PALATINI** elevates velum.

2. The **LOWER LIP** is faster and stronger than the **UPPER LIP**.

3. Motor control in the body develops from **HEAD** to **TAIL** and from **PROXIMAL** to **DISTAL**.

4. The **ASSOCIATED CHAIN** theory of motor control would require the speaker to learn the sequences of motor acts required for articulation and to link these sequences of motor acts to form an articulatory movement.

5. **COARTICULATION** is the overlapping effect of one articulatory movement on another.

6. **CENTRAL CONTROL** theory holds that there is a "master control" mechanism that dictates the muscle movements based upon the linguistic goal.

7. **TASK DYNAMIC** theories generally see articulation as a process of achieving a goal through interaction of coordinative structures. Coordinative structures are muscle groups that, when activated, contribute to achievement of the goal at the terminal effector.

8. Elevation of the posterior tongue requires active contraction of the palatoglossus, and perhaps the styloglossus, as well as the vertical intrinsic muscle. In addition, realize that the tongue is pulling against the soft palate to achieve elevation, because the palatoglossus is a velar depressor as well. When the palatoglossus contracts to elevate the tongue, the levator veli palatini must contract to keep the soft palate elevated.

Bibliography

Abbs, J. H. (1973). The influence of the gamma motor system on jaw movements during speech: A theoretical framework and some preliminary observations. *Journal of Speech and Hearing Research, 16,* 175–200.

Abbs, J. H., & Cole, K. J. (1991). Consideration of bulbar and suprabulbar afferent influences upon speech motor coordination and programming. In Grillner, S., Lindblom, B., Lubker, J., & Persson, A. (Eds.), *Speech motor control* (pp. 159–186). Oxford: Pergamon Press.

Abrahams, P. H., McMinn, R. M. H., Hutchings, R. T., Sandy, C., & Mark, S. (2003). *McMinn's color atlas of human anatomy* (5th ed.). Philadelphia, PA: Mosby.

Bailey, E. F., Rice, A. D., & Fuglevand, A. J. (2007). Firing pattern of human genioglossus motor units during voluntary tongue movement. *Journal of Neurophysiology, 97,* 933–936.

Baken, R. J., & Orlikoff, R. F. (1999). *Clinical measurement of speech and voice* (2nd ed.). San Diego, CA: Singular Publishing Group.

Barlow, S. M., & Netsell, R. (1986). Differential fine force control of the upper and lower lips. *Journal of Speech and Hearing Research, 29,* 163–169.

Barlow, S. M., & Rath, E. M. (1985). Maximum voluntary closing forces in the upper and lower lips of humans. *Journal of Speech and Hearing Research, 28,* 373–376.

Basmajian, J. V. (1975). *Grant's method of anatomy.* Baltimore, MD: Williams & Wilkins.

Bateman, H. E., & Mason, R. M. (1984). *Applied anatomy and physiology of the speech and hearing mechanism.* Springfield, IL: Charles C. Thomas.

Beck, E. W., Monson, H., & Groer, M. (1982). *Mosby's atlas of functional human anatomy.* St. Louis, MO: C. V. Mosby.

Black, S. M. (2008). Head and neck: External skull. In Strandring, S. (Ed.) *Gray's anatomy: The anatomical and clinical basis of practice* (40th ed., pp. 409–422). London: Churchill Livingstone.

Blair, C. & Muller, E. (1987). Functional identification of the perioral neuromuscular system: A signal flow diagram. *Journal of Speech and Hearing Research, 30,* 60–70.

Bly, L. (1983). *The components of normal movement during the first year of life and abnormal motor movement.* Chicago: Neuro-Developmental Treatment Association.

Bly, L. (1994). *Motor skills acquisition in the first year.* Tucson, AZ: Therapy Skill Builders.

Brumberg, J. S., Nieto-Castanon, A., Kennedy, P. R., & Guenther, F. H. (2010). Brain–computer interface for speech production. *Speech communication, 52,* 367–379.

Bunton, K., & Weismer, G. (1994). Evaluation of a reiterant force-impulse task in the tongue. *Journal of Speech and Hearing Research, 37,* 1020–1031.

Callan, D. E., Kent, R. D., Guenther, F. H., & Vorperian, H. K. (2000). An auditory-feedback-based neural network model of speech production that is robust to developmental changes in the size and shape of the articulatory system. *Journal of Speech, Language, and Hearing Research, 43,* 721–736.

Chusid, J. G. (1985). *Correlative neuroanatomy and functional neurology* (17th ed.). Los Altos, CA: Lange Medical Publications.

DeNil, L. F., & Abbs, J. H. (1991). Influence of speaking rate on the upper lip, lower lip, and jaw peak velocity sequencing during bilabial closing movements. *Journal of the Acoustical Society of America, 89(2),* 845–849.

Dronkers, N. F. (1996). A new brain region for coordinating speech articulation. *Nature, 384(6605),* 159–161.

Dronkers, N. F., Pinker, S. & Damasio, A. (2000). Language and the aphasia. In Kandell, E. R., Schwartz, J. H., & Jessell, T. M. (Eds.), *Principles of neural science* (4th ed., pp. 1169–1186). New York: McGraw-Hill.

Duffy, J. R. (1995). *Motor speech disorders.* St. Louis, MO: C. V. Mosby.

Ettema, S. L., & Kuehn, D. P. (1994). A quantitative histologic study of the normal human adult soft palate. *Journal of Speech and Hearing Research, 37,* 303–313.

Fairbanks, G. (1954). A theory of the speech mechanism as a servosystem. *Journal of Speech and Hearing Disorders, 19,* 133–139.

Flege, J. E. (1988). Anticipatory and carry-over nasal coarticulation in the speech of children and adults. *Journal of Speech and Hearing Research, 31,* 525–536.

Folkins, J. W., & Abbs, J. H. (1975). Lip and jaw motor control during speech: Responses to resistive loading of the jaw. *Journal of Speech and Hearing Research, 18,* 207–220.

Folkins, J. W., & Canty, J. L. (1986). Movements of the upper and lower lip during speech: Interactions of the lips with the jaw fixed at different positions. *Journal of Speech and Hearing Research, 29,* 348–356.

Folkins, J. W., & Larson, C. R. (1978). In search of a tonic vibration reflex in the human lip. *Brain Research, 151,* 409–412.

Folkins, J. W., Linville, R. N., Garrett, J. D., & Brown, C. K. (1988). Interactions in the labial musculature during speech. *Journal of Speech and Hearing Research, 31,* 253–264.

Ganong, W. F. (2003). *Review of medical physiology* (21st ed.). New York: McGraw-Hill/Appleton & Lange.

Garcia-Colera, A., & Semjen, A. (1988). Distributed planning of movement sequences. *Journal of Motor Behavior, 20*(3), 341–367.

Gelb, H. (1985). *Clinical management of head, neck and TMJ pain and dysfunction*. Philadelphia: W. B. Saunders.

Gilroy, A. M., MacPherson, B. R., Ross, L.M. (2012). *Atlas of anatomy* (2th ed.). New York: Thieme.

Goffman, L., & Smith, A. (1994). Motor unit territories in the human perioral musculature. *Journal of Speech and Hearing Research, 37*, 975–984.

Gracco, V. L. (1994). Some organizational characteristics of speech movement control. *Journal of Speech and Hearing Research, 37*, 4–27.

Gracco, V. L. (1988). Timing factors in the coordination of speech movements. *Journal of Neuroscience, 8*(12), 4628–4639.

Gracco, V. L., & Abbs, J. H. (1989). Sensorimotor characteristics of speech motor sequences. *Experimental Brain Research, 75*, 586–598.

Gray, H., Bannister, L. H., Berry, M. M., & Williams, P. L. (Eds.). (1995). *Gray's anatomy*. London: Churchill Livingstone.

Groher, M. E. (1984). *Dysphagia*. Boston: Butterworths.

Guenther, F. H. (2001). Neural modeling of speech production. *Proceedings of the Fourth International Nijmegen Speech Motor Conference*. Nijmegen, The Netherlands, June 13–16.

Guenther, F. H. (2002). Neural control of speech movements. In A. Meyer, & N. Schiller, (Eds.), *Phonetics and phonology in language comprehension and production: Differences and similarities* (pp. 209–240). Berlin: Mouton de Gruyter.

Guenther, F. H. (2006). Cortical interactions underlying the production of speech sounds. *Journal of Communication Disorders, 39*, 360–365.

Guenther, F. H., Nieto-Castanon, A., Tourville, J. A., & Ghosh, S. S. (2001). Effects of categorization training on auditory perception and cortical representations. *Proceedings of the Speech Recognition as Pattern Classification (SPRAAC) Workshop*, Nijmegen, The Netherlands, July 11–13.

Guenther, F. H., Castanon-Nieto, A., Ghosh, S. S., & Tourville, J. A. (2004). Representation of categories in auditory cortical maps. *Journal of speech, Language and Hearing Research, 47*, 46–57.

Guenther, F. H., Ghosh, S. S., & Tourville, J. A. (2006). Neural modeling and imaging of cortical interactions underlying syllable production. *Brain & Language, 96*(3), 280–301.

Guenther, F. H., Hampson, M., & Johnson, D. (1998). A theoretical investigation of reference frames for the planning of speech movements. *Psychological Review, 105*, 611–633.

Guenther, F. H. & Vladusich, T. (2012). A neural theory of speech acquisition and production. *Journal of neurolinguistics, 25*, 408–422.

Hall, P. K., Hardy, J. C., & LaVelle, W. E. (1990). A child with signs of developmental apraxia of speech with whom a palatal lift prosthesis was used to manage palatal dysfunction. *Journal of Speech and Hearing Disorders, 55*, 454–460.

Hellstrand, E. (1981). The neuromuscular system of the tongue. In Grillner, S., Lindblom, B., Lubker, J., & Persson, A. (Eds.), *Speech motor control* (pp. 141–157). Oxford: Pergamon Press.

Hickock, G., & Poerppel, D. (2007). The cortical organization of speech processing. *Nature Reviews Neuroscience, 8*, 393–402.

Hillis, A. E., Work, M., Barker, P.B., Jacobs, M. A., Breeze, E. L., & Maurer, K. (2004). Re-examining the brain regions crucial for orchestrating speech articulation. *Brain, 127*, 1479–1487.

Horak, M. (1992). The utility of connectionism for motor learning: A reinterpretation of contextual interference in movement schemas. *Journal of Motor Behavior, 24*(1), 58–66.

Jordan, M. I. (1990). Motor learning and the degrees of freedom problem. In Jeannerod, M. (Ed.), *Attention and performance XIII: Motor representation and control*. Hillsdale, NJ: Lawrence Erlbaum.

Ostry, D. J., Vatikiotis-Bateson, E., & Gribble, P. L. (1997). An example of the degrees of freedom of human jaw motion in speech and mastication. *Journal of Speech-Language-Hearing Research, 40*, 1341–1351.

Landgren, S., & Olsson, K. A. (1981). Oral mechanoreceptors. In Grillner, S., Lindblom, B., Lubker, J., & Persson, A. (Eds.), *Speech motor control* (pp. 129–139). Oxford: Pergamon Press.

Kandel, E. R., Schwartz, J. H., Jessell, T. M., Siegelbaum, S. A., & Hudspeth, A. J. (2013). *Principles of neural science* (5th ed.). New York: McGraw Hill.

Kaplan, H. M. (1971). *Anatomy and physiology of speech.* New York: McGraw-Hill.

Katz, W. F., Kripke, C., & Tallal, P. (1991). Anticipatory coarticulation in the speech of adults and young children: Acoustic, perceptual, and video data. *Journal of Speech and Hearing Research, 34,* 1222–1249.

Kelso, J. A., & Ding, M. (1993). Fluctuations, intermittency, and controllable chaos in biological coordination. In Newell, K. M., & Corcos, D. M. (Eds.), *Variability and motor control* (pp. 291–316). Champaign, IL: Human Kinetics.

Kelso, J. A. S., Tuller, B., Vatikiotis-Bateson, E., & Fowler, C. A. (1984). Functionally specific articulatory cooperation following jaw perturbations during speech: Evidence for coordinative structures. *Journal of Experimental Psychology: Perception and Performance, 19,* 812–832.

Kent, R. D. (1997). *The speech sciences.* San Diego, CA: Singular Publishing Group.

Kent, R. D., Kent, J. F., & Rosenbek, J. C. (1987). Maximum performance tests of speech production. *Journal of Speech and Hearing Disorders, 52,* 367–387.

Kent, R. D., & Vorperian, H. K. (1995). *Development of the craniofacial-oral-laryngeal anatomy: A review.* San Diego, CA: Singular Publishers.

Kuehn, D. P., Lemme, M. L., & Baumgartner, J. M. (1989). *Neural bases of speech, hearing, and language.* Boston: Little, Brown.

Kuehn, D. P., Templeton, P. J., & Maynard, J. A. (1990). Muscle spindles in the velopharyngeal musculature of humans. *Journal of Speech and Hearing Research, 33,* 488–493.

Landgren, S., & Olsson, K. A. (1981). Oral mechanoreceptors. In Grillner, S., Lindblom, B., Lubker, J., & Persson, A. (Eds.), *Speech motor control* (pp. 129–139). Oxford: Pergamon Press.

Langley, M. B., & Lombardino, L. J. (1991). *Neurodevelopmental strategies for managing communication disorders in children with severe motor dysfunction.* Austin, TX: Pro-Ed.

Lashley, K. S. (1951). The problem of serial order in behavior. In Jerrers, L. A. (Ed.), *Cerebral mechanisms in behavior* (pp. 506–528). New York: John Wiley.

Lieberman, P. (1977). *Speech physiology and acoustic phonetics: An introduction.* New York: Macmillan.

Linvelle, S. E. (2001). *Vocal aging.* San Diego, CA: Singular Publishing Group.

Liss, J. M. (1990). Muscle spindles in the human levator veli palatini and palatoglossus muscles. *Journal of Speech and Hearing Research, 33,* 736–746.

Logemann, J. (1983). *Evaluation and treatment of swallowing disorders.* Boston: College-Hill Press.

Love, R. J., Hagerman, E. L., & Taimi, E. G. (1980). Speech performance, dysphagia, and oral reflexes in cerebral palsy. *Journal of Speech and Hearing Disorders, 45,* 59–75.

McClean, M. (1973). Forward coarticulation of velar movement at marked junctural boundaries. *Journal of Speech and Hearing Research, 16,* 286–296.

MacKay, D. G. (1982). The problem of flexibility, fluency, and speed-accuracy trade-off in skilled behavior. *Psychological Review, 89,* 483–506.

McNeil, M. R., Weismer, G., Adams, S., & Mulligan, M. (1990). Oral structure nonspeech motor control in normal, dysarthric, aphasic, and apraxic speakers: isometric force and static position control. *Journal of Speech and Hearing Research, 33,* 255–268.

Mithen, S. (2008). The diva within. *New Scientist, 197* (2644), 38–39.

Møller, A. R. (2003). *Sensory systems: Anatomy and physiology.* New York: Academic Press.

Moore, C. A. (1993). Symmetry of mandibular muscle activity as an index of coordinative strategy. *Journal of Speech and Hearing Research, 36,* 1145–1157.

Moore, C. A., Smith, A., & Ringel, R. L. (1988). Task-specific organization of activity in human jaw muscles. *Journal of Speech and Hearing Research, 31,* 670–680.

Netsell, R. (1973). Speech physiology. In Minifie, F. D., Hixon, T. J., & Williams, F. (Eds.), *Normal aspects of speech, hearing, and language.* Englewood Cliffs, NJ: Prentice-Hall.

Netter, F. H. (1997). *Atlas of human anatomy.* Los Angeles: Icon Learning Systems.

Peeva, M. G., Guenther, F. H., Tourville, J. A., Nieto-Castanon, A., Anton, J., Nazarian, B., Alario, F. (2010). Distinct representations of phonemes, syllables, and supra-syllabic sequences in the speech production network. *Neuroimage, 50*, 626–638.

Perkell, J. S., Matthies, M. L., Tiede, M., Lane, H., Zandipour, M., Marrone, N., et al. (2004). The distinctness of speaker's /s/-/ʃ/ contrast is related to their auditory discrimination and use of an articulator saturation effect. *Journal of Speech, Language, and Hearing Research, 47*, 1259–1269.

Prather, J. F., Peters, S., Nowicki, S., & Mooney, R. (2008). Precise auditory-vocal mirroring in neurons for learned vocal communication. *Nature, 451*, 305–310.

Raibert, M. H. (1977). Motor control and learning by the state space model. Technical report. MIT Artificial Intelligence Laboratory.

Rohen, J. W., Yokochi, C., Lutjen-Drecoll, E. L., & Romrell, L. J. (2002). *Color atlas of anatomy: A photographic study of the human body* (5th ed.). Philadelphia: Williams & Wilkins.

Rosenbaum, D. A., Kenny, S. B., & Derr, M. A. (1983). Hierarchical control of rapid movement sequences. *Journal of Experimental Psychology: Human Perception and Performance*, 9(1), 86–102.

Rosse, C., Gaddum-Rosse, P., & Rosse, G. (1997). *Hollinshead's textbook of anatomy*. Philadelphia: Lippincott-Raven.

Saltzman, E. (1986). Task dynamic coordination of the speech articulators: A preliminary model. *Experimental brain research* (pp. 129–144). Berlin-Heidelberg: Springer-Verlag.

Schmidt, R. A. (1975). A schema theory of discrete motor skill learning. *Psychological Review, 82*, 225–260.

Schuenke, M., & Ross, L. M., (2010). *Thieme atlas of anatomy*. New York: Thieme.

Seibel, L. M., & Barlow, S. M. (2007). Automatic measurement of nonparticipatory stiffness in the perioral complex. *Journal of Speech, Language and Hearing Research, 50*, 1272–1279.

Shaffer, L. H. (1976). Intention and performance. *Psychological Review, 33*(5), 375–393.

Shriberg, L. D., & Kent, R. D. (2002). *Clinical phonetics* (3rd ed.). New York: Allyn & Bacon.

Small, A. M. (1973). Acoustics. In Minifie, F. D., Hixon, T. J., & Williams, F. (Eds.), *Normal aspects of speech, hearing, and language*. Englewood Cliffs, NJ: Prentice-Hall.

Smith, A., McFarland, D. H., & Weber, C. M. (1986). Interactions between speech and finger movements: An exploration of the dynamic pattern perspective. *Journal of Speech and Hearing Research, 29*, 471–480.

Square-Storer, P., & Roy, E. A. (1989). The apraxias: Commonalities and distinctions. In Square-Storer, P. (Ed.), *Acquired apraxia of speech in aphasic adults: Theoretical and clinical issues*. London: Taylor & Francis.

Standring, S. (2008). *Gray's anatomy: The anatomical and clinical basis of practice* (40th ed.). London: Churchill Livingstone.

Steeve, R. W., & Moore, C. A. (2006). Mandibular motor control during the early development of speech and nonspeech behaviors. *Journal of Speech, Language and Hearing Research, 52*, 1530–1544.

Tasko, S. M., & Greilik, K. (2010). Acoustic and articulatory features of diphthong production: A speech clarity study. *Journal of Speech, Language and Hearing Research, 53*, 84–99.

Ucar, F. I., & Uysal, T. (2011). Orofacial airway dimensions in subjects with Class I malocclusion and different growth patterns. *Angle Orthodontist, 81*(3), 460–468.

Vorparian, H. K., & Kent, R. D. (2005). Vowel acoustic space development in children: A synthesis of acoustic and anatomic data. *Journal of Speech, Language, and Hearing Research, 50*, 1510–1545.

Vorparian, H. K., Kent, R. D., Lindstrom, M. J., Kalina, C. M., Gentry, L. R. & Yandell, B. S. (2005). Development of vocal track length during early childhood: A magnetic resonance imaging study. *Journal of the Acoustical Society of America, 117*(1), 338–350.

Vorperian, H. K., Kent, R. D., Lindstrom, M. J., Kalina, C. M., Gentry, L. R. &Yandell, B. S. (2005). *The Journal of the Acoustical Society of America, 117*, 338.

Vorperian, H. K., Wang, S., Chung, M. K., Schimek, E. M., Durtschi, R. B., Kent, R. D., Ziergert, A. J., & Gentry, L. R. (2009). Anatomic development of the oral and pharyngeal portions of the vocal tract: An imaging study. *Journal of the Acoustical Society of America, 125*(3), 1666–1678.

Vorperian, H. K., Wang, S., Schimek, E. M., Durtschi, R. B., Kent, R. D., Gentry, L. R., & Chung, M. K. (2011). Developmental sexual dimorphism of the oral and pharyngeal portions of the vocal tract: An imaging study. *Journal of Speech, Language and Hearing Research, 54*(4), 995–1010.

Weber, C. M., & Smith, A. (1987). Reflex responses in human jaw, lip, and tongue muscles elicited by mechanical stimulation. *Journal of Speech and Hearing Research, 30*, 70–79.

Westbury, J. R. (1988). Mandible and hyoid bone movements during speech. *Journal of Speech and Hearing Research, 31*, 405–416.

Wickens, J., Hyland, B., & Anson, G. (1994). Cortical cell assemblies: A possible mechanism for motor programs. *Journal of Motor Behavior, 26*(2), 66–82.

Wilson, E. M., Green, J. R., & Weismer, G. (2012). A kinematic description of the temporal characteristics of jaw motion for early chewing: Preliminary findings. *Journal of Speech, Language and Hearing Research, 55*, 626–638.

Wohlert, A. B. (1993). Event-related brain potentials preceding speech and nonspeech oral movements of varying complexity. *Journal of Speech and Hearing Research, 36*, 897–905.

Wohlert, A. B. (1996). Reflex responses in lip muscles in younger and older women. *Journal of Speech and Hearing Research, 39*, 578–589.

Wohlert, A. B., & Goffman, L. (1994). Human perioral muscle activation patterns. *Journal of Speech and Hearing Research, 37*, 1032–1040.

Zemlin, W. R. (1998). *Speech and hearing science: Anatomy and physiology* (4th ed.). Needham Heights, MA: Allyn & Bacon.

Zickefoose, W. (1989). *Techniques of oral myofunctional therapy*. Sacramento, CA: O.M.T. Materials, Inc.

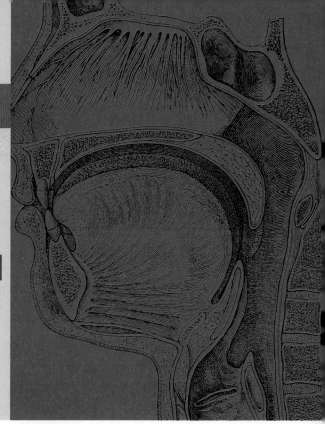

Chapter 8

PHYSIOLOGY OF MASTICATION AND DEGLUTITION

In Chapter 1 we introduced you to the concept of the relationship between the biological and speech function in anatomy and physiology. Humans have done a marvelous job of taking the anatomical structures and their physiology and capitalizing on those functions for speech. In many ways, the physiology of **mastication** (the process of preparing food for swallowing, also known as chewing) and **deglutition** (the processes of swallowing) provides an exquisite view of those integrated systems we use so effortlessly in speech. As we discuss these very basic and fundamental processes, you will see that we must invoke the respiratory, phonatory, articulatory, and nervous systems. Further, keep an eye on the Clinical Notes we provide in boxes to see just how problematic it can be when the anatomy and physiology of *any one of these systems* is disrupted. As practicing speech-language pathologists, you may very likely be deeply involved in these processes, so we hope you will take this information to heart.

mastication: the process of preparing food for swallowing

deglutition: the process of swallowing

MASTICATION AND DEGLUTITION

Mastication refers to the processes associated with grinding and crushing food in preparation for swallowing. *Deglutition* refers to swallowing, which is a complex process of moving the bolus into the pharynx and propelling it into the esophagus. These two biological processes require the integration of lingual, velar, pharyngeal, and facial muscle movement (Chapter 7) with laryngeal adjustments (Chapter 5) and respiratory control (Chapter 2). Consider this:

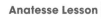 **Anatesse Lesson**

During the adult's mastication and deglutition process, all muscles inserting into the orbicularis oris may be called into action to open, close, purse, and retract the lips as food is received into the oral cavity. All intrinsic and extrinsic muscles of the tongue will be called into action to move the food into position for chewing and preparation of the **bolus** (either liquid or a mass of food) for swallowing. (The term "bolus" comes from the Greek word for "lump." It's that "lump" of food in your mouth that is being prepared for swallowing.) The velar elevators seal off the nasal cavity to prevent regurgitation, and the pharyngeal constrictors must contract in a highly predictable fashion to move the bolus down the pharynx and into the esophagus. With the addition of tongue movement and laryngeal elevation, we have just invoked more than 55 pairs of muscles whose timing and innervation patterns must be coordinated through the accurate activation of cranial and spinal nerves. All this for a snack.

> **bolus:** ball of food or liquid to be swallowed

As you ponder the biological processes associated with deglutition, please do not lose sight of the relationship between feeding and speech. We have long recognized that feeding skills are both preparatory and supportive of the speech act, and inadequate development of feeding reflects directly on speech development. In this chapter, we will first discuss developmental and adult mastication and deglutition patterns as related to the underlying anatomy and physiology, and then we will discuss the neuroanatomical underpinnings of these processes in an attempt to integrate this important function with its control mechanisms.

Instrumentation in Swallowing Function

Because of the complex nature of swallowing, there is a wide array of tools designed to probe swallowing function. Articulator function measures of force are the same as those discussed in Chapter 7, but in this context they may signal the potential for swallowing deficit (e.g., Yoshida, Kikutani, Tsuga, Utanohara, Hayashi, & Akagawa, 2006). For instance, tongue force can be measured pretty simply using the Iowa Oral Pressure Instrument (IOPI) or a similar device, which involves pushing against a flexible ball that measures force. This force measurement may translate directly into a person's ability to move a bolus in the mouth, or to squeeze the tongue onto the roof of the mouth to support movement of the bolus in swallowing. Remember that the articulators have the primary responsibility of mastication, and that speech is a secondary pursuit. Similarly, electromyography (EMG) is widely used in research to measure muscle function during swallowing (e.g., Crary, Carnaby-Mann, & Groher, 2007; McKeown, Torpey, & Ghem, 2002). To examine the complex kinematics of oral and pharyngeal structures, researchers depend on visualization methods that result in three-dimensional representations, such as multislice computer aided tomography (e.g., Fujii, Inamoto, Saitoh, Baba, Okada, Yoshioka, Nakai, Ida, Katada, & Palmer, 2011), and pressure measures such as pharyngeal manometry (e.g., Hoffman, Mielens, Ciucci, Jones, Jiang, & McCulloch, 2012; Mattioli, Lugaresi, Zannoli, Brusori, & d'Ovidio, 2003).

Frequently the tool of choice for testing swallowing function is the modified barium swallow study (MBSS), which involves videoradiographically recording the swallow of an individual who has ingested a bolus of food or liquid that has been mixed with a radio-opaque material (barium). The MBSS allows both lateral and anterior view of the structures active during swallowing and is considered the definitive test for oropharyngeal dysphagia. Another excellent tool for examining swallow function is use of nasoendoscopy, which allows direct visualization of the pharyngeal space during swallowing by means of fiber optic technology. (This is sometimes referred to as fiber endoscopic evaluation of swallowing [FEES]; Langmore, Schatz, & Olson, 1991). It eliminates issues related to radiation exposure, but has some limitations, in that the researcher cannot visualize the oral phase, and portions of the pharyngeal phase are not visible due to movement of the tongue into the pharynx. These limitations are more than made up for by the fact that the clinician or researcher can directly detect aspiration, and more accurately assess pharyngeal residue. Unlike MBSS, endoscopy allows direct visualization of structural changes, such as tumors or other lesions. It also avoids the use of barium, allowing a more natural swallow. Because nasoendoscopy eliminates the dangers of radiation exposure, the clinician can spend much more time assessing structures and function than with MBSS, which means that your knowledge of the structures of the larynx will be very important. A final tool is ultrasound, which also provides a means of observing movement during swallow, although the presence of bone impedes visualization.

Anatomical and Physiological Developmental Issues

As we discussed in Chapter 7, maturation of the infant nervous system provides a stable base of trunk, neck, and head upon which mastication and deglutition are developed. The maturation process of the physical and physiological systems sets an important stage for the adult swallowing function.

Development of swallowing begins well before birth. It has been observed as early as 10 weeks gestational age, and most fetuses display nonnutritive sucking by 15 weeks, and suckling is stimulable at this point in development as well. Tongue movements associated with suckling and swallowing (e.g., tongue cupping, anterior thrusting, suckling movements) have all been seen by ultrasound by 24 months gestational age (reviewed in Delaney & Arvedson, 2008).

At birth, the neonate is restricted to reflexive responses. The infant gains nutrition through the **rooting reflex**, which involves orienting toward the direction of tactile contact with the mouth region (**perioral region**). The full rooting response involves head rotation and mouth opening. Soft tactile contact with the inner margin of the lips will elicit the **sucking reflex**, which involves piston-like tongue protrusion and retraction in preparation for receiving food from the mother's breast. In the first six months of life, this reflex

perioral region: region around the mouth

sucking reflex: reflex involving tongue protrusion and retraction in preparation for receipt of liquid; stimulated by contact to the upper lip is manifest as a suckling pattern, which is the piston-like movement of the tongue. This pattern is replaced by sucking, a more complex process in which the tongue raises and lowers, which, in combination with stronger labial seal, causes a negative pressure that draws liquid into the mouth. This development is dependent on the increased size of the oral cavity, which allows the superior-inferior movement of the tongue. Although both suckling and sucking are supported by mandibular movement, the pattern of the tongue movement and degree of lip occlusion are the primary differences. Nonnutritive suckling experiences are gained by use of pacifiers, which help the infant organize the oral behavior.

Movements at this stage are gross and reflexive. The gross movements of the mandible during suckling and sucking will ultimately give way to refined movement of the mandible during speech in normal development. Tongue protrusion distal to the mouth during suckling will evolve into a sucking gesture that does not require tongue protrusion.

Early postnatal development is a time for organization: The infant must develop the coordination of sucking, swallowing, and breathing. Early on, infants may take up up to three sucks before swallowing, and will have an apneic period between suck–swallow runs (Arvedson & Brodsky, 2002). As the infant develops, the ratio of sucks to swallows moves from 3:1 to 1:1, with respiration occurring after between 10 and 30 suck–swallow sequences (Arvedson & Brodsky, 2002; Lau, Smith, & Schanler, 2003).

Figures 8-1 and 8-2 show the infant oral-pharyngeal structures and those of the adult. If you look closely at these figures, you will realize that there are marked differences between these two systems. The infant's oral cavity is necessarily smaller, but notice also the location of the laryngeal structures and the size of the velum relative to the pharynx. The larynx is markedly elevated at birth but descends over the course of the first four years. The hyoid is elevated and relatively forward as compared with the adult, and there is no dentition in the neonate. The relatively larger velum and elevated larynx play a vital role in respiration and deglutition, as we shall see.

The suckling response is critically important because it is the means by which the infant gets nutrition: Absent or weak suckling reflex will require intervention by a feeding specialist who can help to stimulate it, and alternate forms of nutrient intake may be required until the reflex is established. This reflex is elicited by the tactile stimulation of the lips and perioral space, as well as through the visual presentation of a food source in older infants (Miller, 2002), and involves protrusion of the tongue with sufficient force to initiate the flow of milk from the breast. Repeated forward pumping of the tongue-mandible unit results in milk entering the oral cavity. After a few thrusts of the tongue, a swallow is triggered, with the tongue base lowered to permit the milk bolus to enter the oropharynx during the next forward pumping action of the tongue. This suckling response will evolve into a more mature sucking response that will include tongue elevation and greater lip seal.

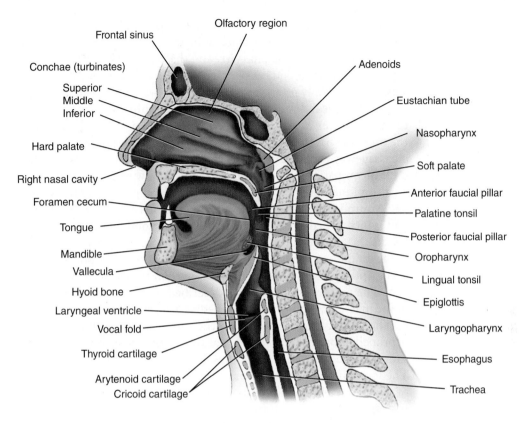

Figure 8-1. Oral, pharyngeal, and laryngeal structure of an adult.
Source: (After Netter, 1976.)

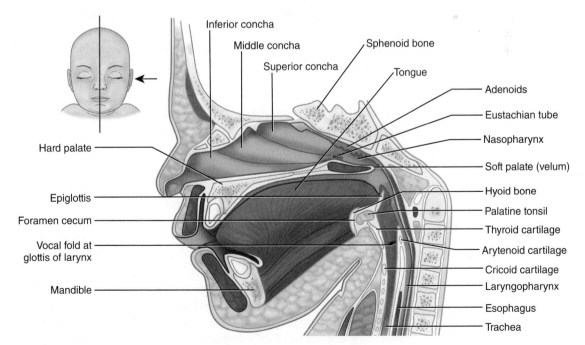

Figure 8-2. The relationship between oral and velar structures in the neonate.
Source: (After Netter, 1976.)

This swallow pattern of the neonate is precisely supported by the anatomy of the infant. Take a look at Figure 8-2 again. You can see that the larynx is high in the pharynx, and the velum of the infant "locks" into the space between the epiglottis and tongue at the location of the valleculae, partially protecting the infant's airway from the liquid bolus.

With typical development, this relationship changes as the oral cavity increases in size and as the hyoid and larynx drop relative to the oropharynx, to their adult positions. The adult pharynx serves as a passageway for both the respiratory and gastrointestinal systems, a clear incompatibility. The adult human swallow pattern compensates for this vulnerability by reflexively closing and protecting the airway.

Around the sixth month, dentition begins erupting, and the infant is introduced to his or her first relatively solid food. The dentition blocks the anterior protrusion of the tongue and supports retraction of the tongue during the swallow. Further, dentition supports chewing and grinding movements, which strengthen the muscles of mastication. The mature swallow (to be described later) requires contraction of the masseter, temporalis, and medial pterygoid muscles to counteract the force of the tongue upon the roof of the mouth as the bolus is propelled backward. The immature swallow does not require this same degree of force to move the liquid bolus into the oropharynx. The force directed onto the palate is critical for proper development of the dental arches and hard palate. If the muscles of mastication are not utilized during the transitional and mature swallow, the maxillary dental arch may collapse medially and a vaulted palate may develop (see Figure 6-28C). A cross-bite may develop, in which the upper dentition does not make proper contact with the lower dentition. This oral configuration may also result in an elongated and narrowed maxilla, giving the impression of a long and narrow face, classically referred to as the "mouth breather **facies**," because it is often associated with nasal obstruction that prohibits proper nasal respiration.

ORGANIZATIONAL PATTERNS OF MASTICATION AND DEGLUTITION

Mastication and deglutition in the adult consist of a sequence of three extremely well-orchestrated events or stages. These stages are the oral stage, pharyngeal stage (pharyngeal swallow), and esophageal stage (esophageal transit). The oral stage can be further subdivided into the oral preparatory stage (mastication) and the oral transport stage (movement of the bolus through the oral cavity), and we will discuss them this way for the purposes of functional clarity. Although the oral preparatory stage is traditionally considered to be voluntary in nature (i.e., under volitional control), it is strongly dependent upon the centrally generated patterns of mastication and tongue movements. We are very adept at using these reflexes to complete tasks, thereby requiring little voluntary activity until called upon by some unexpected change. (Can you remember the last time you encountered something surprising in your food, such as a piece of hull in handful of chopped almonds?

The snack immediately got your full attention, which may have been previously focused somewhere else.) The beauty of these centrally generated patterns of the oral mechanism is that we can control them when we want to, or let them run more-or-less automatically (Matsuo & Palmer, 2013). The pharyngeal and esophageal stages are considered to be reflexively controlled (Ertekin & Aydoglu, 2003). The oral transport stage (moving the bolus into the oropharynx) can be either voluntary or involuntary, but the pattern of movement is the same in either case (Lang, 2009). Transport of the bolus from mouth to stomach (oral transport, pharyngeal, and esophageal stages) is governed by pools of neurons that provide the ordered, sequential motor activity associated with swallowing (e.g., Lang, 2009). As Lang notes, if you initiate the oral phase of swallowing experimentally, the pharyngeal and esophageal phases will occur in sequence (it is worth noting that "failed" swallows, such as dry swallows that don't involve a bolus will not result in an esophageal stage). If you stimulate the pharyngeal stage, the esophageal stage will follow, but you will never see the oral transport stage occur. The pools of neurons controlling each stage are separate, but clearly connected, as demonstrated by their sequential activation. We'll return to this issue of transport later. You may want to refer to the timeline of the swallow in Figure 8-3 that has been outlined by Dodds, Stewart, and Logemann (1990) as we discuss the stages of swallowing.

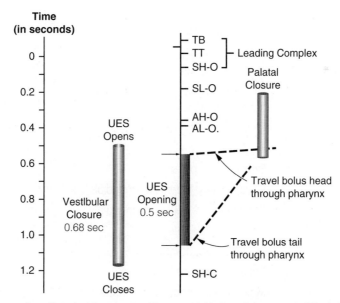

Figure 8-3. Timeline of the swallow. Note that time starts with zero at initiation of movement of the bolus. Tongue Base movement (TB), governed by suprahyoid muscles, is initiated prior to movement of the bolus, and is indicated by electromyographic activity measured in the submental region (SM-O). Tongue Tip (TT) elevates, followed quickly by movement of the hyoid superiorly (SH-O). As part of this set of "leading components" of swallow, the vocal folds close by around .1 second. The larynx begins elevation (SL-O), and palatal closure closely follows as the bolus enters the oropharynx. Around .4 seconds (400 ms post initiation) the hyoid moves forward (AH-O), followed quickly by forward movement of the larynx (AL-O). The upper esophageal sphincter (UES) opens as the head of the bolus reaches it, at about .5 seconds post-initiation. Notice that the laryngeal vestibule is closed as long as the bolus is in the pharynx.

Source: From Dodds, W. J., Stewart, E. T., & Logemann, J. A. (1990). Physiology and radiology of the normal and pharyngeal phases of swallowing. *American Journal of Roentgenology, 154,* 953-963.

Oral Stage: Oral Preparation

In this stage, food is prepared for swallowing. To complete this task, a number of processes must occur at virtually the same time (Table 8-1). It should be emphasized that although this may be a voluntary process, it can be performed automatically without conscious effort.

First, we anticipate the food. This is an important part of the oral stage because the view and smell of food provide us with a motivation to ingest it, which helps us maintain nutrition. The food is introduced into the mouth and kept there by occluding the lips (referred to as the preparatory phase). This lip seal requires breathing through the nose, so the tongue bunches up in the back and the soft palate is pulled down to keep the food in the oral cavity.

Table 8-1 **Muscles of the oral preparation stage**

Muscle	Function	Innervation (Cranial Nerve)
Facial Muscles		
Orbicularis oris	Maintains oral seal	VII
Mentalis	Elevates lower lip	VII
Buccinator	Flattens cheeks	VII
Risorius	Flattens cheeks	VII
Mandibular Muscles		
Masseter	Elevates mandible	V
Temporalis	Elevates mandible; retracts and protrudes mandible	V
Medial pterygoid	Elevates mandible; moves mandible grinds mandible laterally;	V
Lateral pterygoid	Protrudes and grinds mandible	V
Tongue Muscles		
Mylohyoid	Elevates floor of mouth	V
Geniohyoid	Elevates hyoid; depresses mandible	XII
Digastric	Elevates hyoid; depresses mandible	V, VII
Superior longitudinal	Elevates tip; deviates tip	XII
Inferior longitudinal	Depresses tip; deviates tip	XII
Vertical	Cups and grooves tongue	XII
Genioglossus	Moves tongue body; cups tongue	XII
Styloglossus	Elevates posterior tongue	XII
Palatoglossus	Elevates posterior tongue	IX, X, XI
Soft Palate Muscles		
Palatoglossus	Depresses velum	IX, X, XI
Palatopharyngeus	Depresses velum	X, XI

The tongue cups in preparation for the input food. A food bolus must be ground up (the reduction phase) so that it can easily pass through the esophagus for digestion, and this is performed by the coordinated activity of the muscles of mastication as well as the lingual muscles. The tongue is in charge of keeping the food in the oral cavity, and it does so by creating a seal along the alveolar ridge. As it holds the food in place, it may compress it against the hard palate, partially crushing it in preparation for the teeth. The tongue then begins moving the food onto the grinding surfaces of the teeth, pulling the food back into the oral cavity to be mixed with saliva, and then moving it back to the teeth for more of a work-up. The salivary glands (parotid, submandibular, and sublingual glands) secrete saliva into the oral cavity to help form the mass of food into a bolus for swallowing. The facial muscles of the buccal wall (risorius and buccinator) contract to keep the food from entering the lateral sulcus (between the gums and cheek wall). The cheeks are critical players in mastication: When they are experimentally inhibited from functioning the bolus is poorly mixed and poorly formed (Mazari, Heath, & Prinz, 2007).

This is quite a feat of coordination. To prove this to yourself, take a bite of a cracker and attend to the process. If you count the number of times you chew on the cracker, you will realize that you grind it between 15 and 30 times before you swallow any of it. As you introduce the cracker into your mouth, your tongue may push it up against the anterior hard palate to begin breaking it down. Your tongue then performs the dance of mastication, flicking in between the molars as your mandible lowers, then quickly moving out of the way before the jaw closes forcefully to continue grinding. Your tongue organizes the ground food onto its dorsum, mixes the food with saliva, and moves it back out to the teeth if the bolus does not meet your specification for "ready to swallow." We are quite adept at creating the "ideal" bolus for swallowing, which is amazingly similar in consistency among individuals (Hoebler et al., 1998; Mishellany, Woda, Labas, & Peyron, 2006; Peyron, Mishellany, & Woda, 2004; Printz & Lucas, 1995). That is to say, humans have a common perception of how dense, large, masticated and moist a bolus should be, and unconsciously strive to create such a bolus before swallowing. This person-to-person consistency of bolus may reflect an important organizing principle: We do not have to worry about *how* we create the bolus (i.e., how many times we chew, or how often we have to mix saliva with the particles), but we are very aware of the outcome (Mishellany et al., 2006). To create this ideal bolus may require a degree of grinding and manipulation, but the product is the same: When we achieve the physical qualities of the ideal bolus the swallow is initiated.

The sensory receptors in your oral cavity monitor the bolus continually as it is being prepared (Ertekin & Aydogdu, 2003). Mechanoceptors in the tongue and hard and soft palates provide input to the nervous system concerning the physical characteristics of the bolus, including the particle size, texture, ductility (ability to be pulled apart) and malleability (ability to be compressed), and degree of cohesion. Chemoreceptors (receptors that differentially respond to chemical composition) play an important role in the taste component

Deficits of the Oral Preparatory Stage

Numerous problems arise when the neuromuscular control of mastication is compromised. Loss of sensation and awareness, coupled with weak buccal musculature, can lead to pocketing of food in the lateral or anterior sulci. Weak muscles of mastication can cause inadequately chewed food; weak lingual muscles may result in poor mixing of saliva with the food, inadequate bolus production, poor lip seal and posterior tongue elevation to impound the bolus, and difficulty compressing the bolus onto the hard palate. If the muscles of the soft palate are compromised, the velum may not be fully elevated and the tongue may not be elevated in the back, permitting food to escape into the pharynx before initiation of the pharyngeal reflexes. This is life-threatening because food entering the pharynx in the absence of the reflexive response may well reach the open airway. Aspiration pneumonia (pneumonia secondary to aspirated matter) is a constant concern for individuals with dysphagia (a disorder of swallowing).

of foods, but also have an important place in stimulation of the pharyngeal swallow, as we will discuss. Thermoreceptors provide sensation concerning the temperature of the bolus, which is also important for both taste and stimulation of the pharyngeal swallow.

If you still question the grace of this process, try to remember the last time you bit your tongue, lip, or cheek. A snack of 10 crackers may invoke at least 600 oscillations of the mastication musculature, and a full meal clearly requires thousands of grinding gestures. Despite this, you can scarcely remember the last painful time your tongue and mandible failed the coordination test.

Oral Stage: Transport

When the bolus of food is finally ready to swallow, the **transport stage** of swallowing begins (see Table 8-2). Interestingly, oral transport can be either voluntary or involuntary (automatic might be a better term). We can voluntarily and willfully move the bolus into the oropharynx as part of the oral preparatory stage, or it may arise as part of the involuntary, automatic sequence that leads to the pharyngeal and esophageal stages of swallowing. In either case, the motor sequence is the same.

In the oral transport stage, several processes must occur sequentially. The tongue base is elevated at the posterior during mastication, but now it drops down and pulls posteriorly. Mastication stops, and the anterior tongue elevates to the hard palate as the vocal folds close to terminate respiration at about 0.1 second after initiation. The tongue tip and dorsum move to squeeze the bolus back toward the faucial pillars. Importantly, the tongue movement is characterized as a front-to-back squeezing motion. Tongue tip function shows a lot of variability among people (Dodds, Stewart, & Logemann, 1990) refer to "tippers" and "dippers" as individuals who elevate the tip or depress the tip during swallow, but the dorsum and posterior tongue are easier to characterize. X-ray microbeam studies of swallowing using water verify the anterior-to-posterior movement of the tongue during swallowing of liquid (Tasko, Kent & Westbury, 2002). Notably, the mandible elevates to counteract the pressure of the tongue on the roof of the mouth, although the extent and degree of movement are quite variable as well.

Contact with the faucial pillars, soft palate, or posterior tongue base has been proposed as the stimulus that triggers the reflexes of the pharyngeal stage (Ertekin, Kiylioglu, Tarlaci, Truman, Secil, & Aydogdu, 2011), but Lang (2009) states that the physical presence of adequate bolus in the oropharynx is the prerequisite for the patterned pharyngeal swallow to occur. Indeed, the pharyngeal swallow does not occur with every completed transport event that occurs, but only after there is adequate mass of bolus in the oropharynx.

> **oral transit time:** time required to move the bolus through the oral cavity to the point of initiation of the pharyngeal stage of swallowing

Table 8-2 Muscles of the oral stage required to propel the bolus into the oropharynx

Muscle	Function	Innervation (Cranial Nerve)
Mandibular Muscles		
Masseter	Elevates mandible	V
Temporalis	Elevates mandible	V
Internal pterygoid	Elevates mandible	V
Tongue Muscles		
Mylohyoid	Elevates tongue and floor of mouth	V
Superior longitudinal	Elevates tongue tip	XII
Vertical	Cups and grooves tongue	XII
Genioglossus	Moves tongue body; cups tongue	XII
Styloglossus	Elevates posterior tongue	XII
Palatoglossus	Elevates posterior tongue	IX, X, XI

© Cengage Learning®.

Deficits of the Oral Transit Stage

Deficits of the oral stage center around sensory and motor dysfunction. Weakened movements cause reduced **oral transit time** of the bolus toward the pharynx. With greater motor involvement, food may remain on the tongue or hard palate following transit.

In patients with oral-phase involvement, there is a tendency for the epiglottis to fail to invert over the laryngeal opening and to have limited elevation of the hyoid. Perlman, Grayhack, and Booth (1992) found that individuals with such a deficit showed increased pooling of food or liquid within the valleculae.

Difficulty initiating a reflexive swallow may be the result of sensory deficit. Application of a cold stimulus to the anterior faucial pillars coupled with instructions to attempt to swallow is a time-honored method to assist these individuals in initiating a swallow, although ongoing clinical research is needed to determine its efficacy (Rosenbek, Robbins, Fishback, & Levine, 1991).

pharyngeal stage: the stage
of swallow in which the bolus
is from the oral cavity, through
the pharynx, and to the
entryway to the esophagus;
involves numerous
physiological protective
responses

Pharyngeal Stage

The **pharyngeal stage** consists of a complex sequence of reflexively controlled events (see Table 8-3 and Figure 8-4). As the bolus reaches the region of the faucial pillars (or, alternatively, farther back at the posterior base of the tongue near the valleculae in older individuals; for examinations of the effects of age on pharyngeal stage initiation, see Martin-Harris., Brodsky, Michel, Lee, and Walters [2007] and Stephens, Taves, Smith, & Martin [2005]. For age effects on transit time see Mendell & Logemann, [2007]), the pharyngeal swallow stage begins. Events happen fast during the pharyngeal stage, which is a highly coordinated and well-orchestrated sequence of patterned motor operations. It's important to realize that, although the pharyngeal stage is classically referred to as "reflexive" in nature, it is considerably more complex than that, as will be discussed. The pharyngeal stage is a programmed stage of transit, such that the sequence of events that we conveniently label as the pharyngeal stage really reflects a component of oropharyngeal transit. Assemblies of neurons called central pattern generator (CPG) circuits create the control mechanism for highly organized and yet involuntary movements, such as those that control swallowing from tongue tip to lower esophageal sphincter. (We should mention here that we are only talking about single swallows: If a person takes multiple swallows or if the bolus is large the pharyngeal stage may not be initiated until the bolus is in the valleculae: Stephens, Taves, Smith, and Martin [2005]).

CPGs are neural circuits that, when initiated, will produce the same sequence of events unless modified by influences from the cerebral cortex. They are similar to reflexes (which are simple patterned responses to an environmental stimulus), but consist of a complex sequence of motor responses. Here is a contrast between reflexes and central pattern generators. If you hold your mandible in a relaxed state and pull rapidly down on your chin with your thumb, your mouth may snap closed. The stretch receptors in the masseter and temporalis are stimulated by your movement of the mandible, and cause the muscles to contract. That's the bite reflex. On the other hand, when you take a bite of cookie, you automatically start chewing it (unless you consciously decide not to), and the movement is a complex interaction among the masseter, temporalis, internal and external pterygoid muscles, and muscles of the tongue. To grind a hard bolus we must alternate contraction of the muscles of mastication side-to-side, all the while controlling where our tongue is. This is the product of a central pattern generator. If you think of the very complex process of the pharyngeal stage of swallowing, which will use many muscles in a highly orchestrated manner to protect the airway and transfer the bolus from the mouth to the esophagus, you will quickly recognize how elegant this CPG is.

Because of the complexity of the pharyngeal stage (see Figure 8-3), we will characterize the activities as separate functional operations, including hyolaryngeal elevation, pharyngeal timing, pharyngeal

Table 8-3 **Muscles of the pharyngeal stage required to propel the bolus toward the esophagus, elevate the larynx, and close the airway**

Muscle	Function	Innervation (Cranial Nerve)
Tongue Muscles		
Mylohyoid	Elevates hyoid and tongue	V
Geniohyoid	Elevates hyoid and larynx; depresses mandible	XII
Digastricus	Elevates hyoid and larynx	V, VII
Genioglossus	Retracts tongue	XII
Styloglossus	Elevates posterior tongue	XII
Palatoglossus	Narrows fauces; elevates posterior tongue	IX, X, XI
Stylohyoid	Elevates hyoid and larynx	VII
Hyoglossus	Elevates hyoid	XII
Thyrohyoid	Elevates hyoid	XII
Superior longitudinal	Elevates tongue	XII
Inferior longitudinal	Depresses tongue	XII
Transverse	Narrows tongue	XII
Vertical	Flattens tongue	XII
Soft Palate Muscles		
Levator veli palatini	Elevates soft palate	X, XI
Tensor veli palatini	Dilates Eustachian tube	V
Musculus uvulae	Shortens soft palate	X, XI
Pharyngeal Muscles		
Palatopharyngeus	Constricts oropharynx to channel bolus	X, XI
Salpingopharyngeus	Elevates pharynx	XI
Stylopharyngeus	Raises larynx	IX
Cricopharyngeus	Relaxes esophageal orifice	X, XI
Middle constrictor	Narrows pharynx	X, XI
Inferior constrictor	Narrows pharynx	X, XI
Laryngeal Muscles		
Lateral cricoarytenoid	Adducts vocal folds	X
Transverse arytenoid	Adducts vocal folds	X
Oblique arytenoid	Adducts vocal folds	X
Aryepiglotticus	Retracts epiglottis; constricts aditus	X
Thyroepiglotticus	Dilates airway following swallow	X

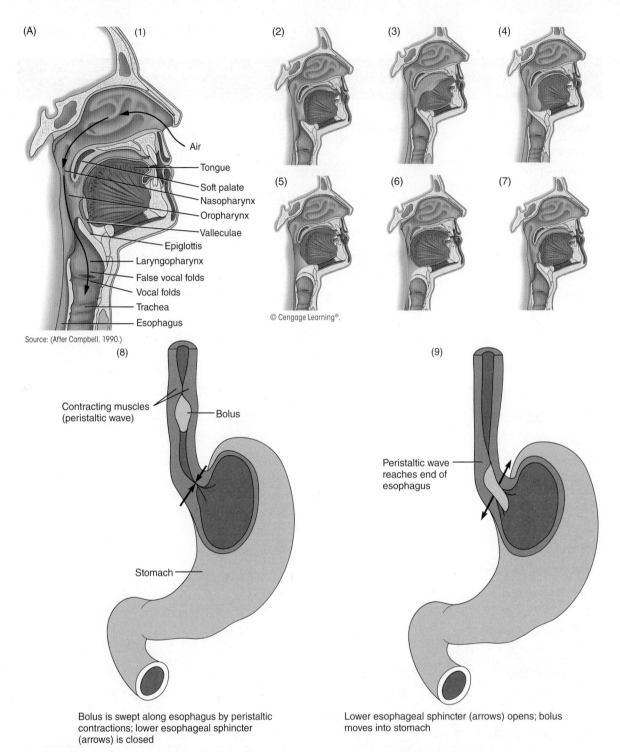

Figure 8-4. (A) (1) Tongue is at rest and respiration occurs. No bolus is present. (2) Bolus rests on tongue after having been prepared for swallowing. (3) Anterior tongue elevates to hard palate, and hyoid elevates. (4) Posterior tongue elevates, which propels the bolus into the oropharynx. At the same time the larynx moves up and forward, and the velum elevates. The upper esophageal sphincter opens as the larynx elevates. Vocal folds adduct. (5) The epiglottis inverts, closing off the vestibule. The bolus passes over inverted epiglottis, divides into 2 portions, and enters the pyriform sinuses of the hypophyarnx. (6) Tongue moves posteriorly to contact posterior pharyngeal wall, increasing pharyngeal pressure. The divided boluses recombine at the esophageal opening, and bolus passes through upper esophageal sphincter into esophagus. (7) Bolus has cleared the hypopharynx, epiglottis elevates, hyoid and larynx descend, velum depresses, and respiration (typically expiration) is initiated. (8) Bolus is swept along esophagus by peristaltic contractions; lower esophageal sphincter (arrows) is closed. (9) Lower esohageal phincter (arrows) opens; bolus moves into stomach. (continues).

Source: (After Campbell, 1990.)

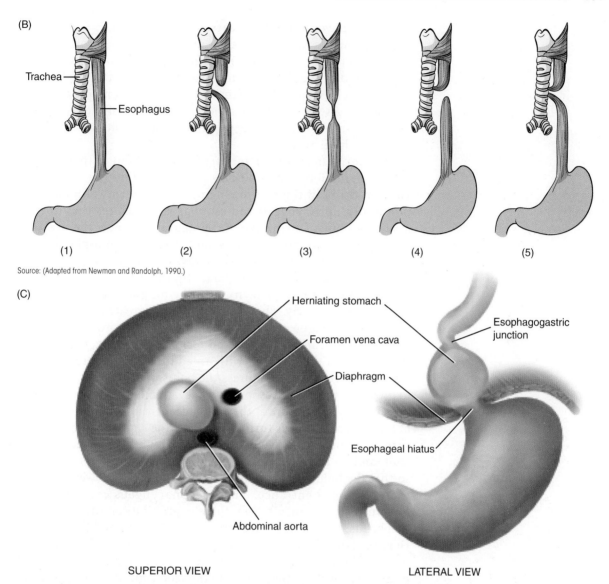

(B)

Trachea

Esophagus

(1) (2) (3) (4) (5)

Source: (Adapted from Newman and Randolph, 1990.)

(C)

Herniating stomach

Foramen vena cava

Esophagogastric junction

Diaphragm

Esophageal hiatus

Abdominal aorta

SUPERIOR VIEW

LATERAL VIEW

Figure 8-4 continued. (B) Developmental malformations of the esophagus. (B-1) Normal esophagus. (B-2) Esophagus anastomosing with trachea. (B-3) Esophageal stenosis. (B-4) Esophageal discontinuity with tracheal porting. (B-5) Esophageal fusing with trachea, resulting in esophageal porting. (C) Herniation of stomach through esophageal hiatus of diaphragm. *Left*: View from above the diaphragm, showing herniation of stomach. *Right*: Lateral view. Note the position of the lower esophageal sphincter (esophagastric junction).

Source: (After Healey and Seybold, 1969, and Payne and Ellis, 1984.)

pressurization, airway protection, and upper esophageal sphincter (UES) action. (You will remember discussion of the cricopharyngeus muscle in Chapter 7: It makes up the bulk of the upper esophageal sphincter, which is responsible for keeping the esophagus closed until a bolus is ready to enter the esophagus.) Realize this is simply a way to organize discussion of the movements, but these are not isolated events during the pharyngeal stage of the swallow.

Hyolaryngeal elevation: Movement of the hyolaryngeal complex (hyoid and larynx) begins with anterior movement of the tongue base and tongue tip at the initiation of the swallow. Nearly simultaneously the hyoid and larynx elevate as a result of contraction of the suprahyoid muscles (Pearson, Langmore, Uy, & Zumwalt, 2012), followed quickly by anterior movement of the hyoid and larynx. All of these movements make mechanical sense. The upward movement of the larynx also supports inversion of the epiglottis by virtue of its mechanical attachment to the larynx and proximity to the tongue. As we will discuss shortly, elevation of the larynx is a key player in relaxation of the upper esophageal sphincter and protection of the airway.

Pressurization of the Pharynx: Pressurization of the pharynx is the driving force behind bolus propulsion into the esophagus. You can think of the swallowing process in terms of manipulation of oral, pharyngeal, and esophageal pressures that in turn move the bolus. During the oral preparatory stage, the oral and pharyngeal cavity pressures are equalized with atmospheric pressure, because of the open nasal airway. When entering the transit stage of the swallow, the soft palate tightly closes, separating the oropharynx and nasopharynx, and the tongue begins squeezing the bolus posteriorly. The positive pressure created by the movements of the tongue propels the bolus toward the oropharynx. The tongue makes contact with the posterior oropharynx, transferring the bolus into the pharynx with an additional pressure gradient. The pharyngeal walls compress the bolus, increasing the pressure to prompt it toward the esophagus. Elevation of the larynx creates a relatively lower pressure at the esophageal entryway, and relaxation of the cricopharyngeus further increases the superior-inferior pressure gradient. The laryngeal entryway is tightly clamped to avoid confounding the pressures of deglutition with those of respiration so that the bolus is naturally drawn to the area of lower pressure, the esophageal entrance. The cricopharyngeus contracts most forcefully during inspiration, thereby prohibiting inflation of the esophagus. Peristaltic contraction of the superior, middle, and inferior constrictor muscles will help to clear the pharynx of residue to protect the airway, but the pressures generated are the primary means of propelling the bolus into the esophagus (Gumbley, Huckabee, Doeltgen, Witte, & Moran, 2008).

Airway protection: The airway must be protected. To accomplish the protective function, the vocal folds tightly adduct at the initial stage of the swallow, as part of what Dodd et al. (1990) refer to as the "leading complex" of actions (Figure 8-3). As the larynx elevates, the false folds close (in most people), and the epiglottis inverts to cover the laryngeal aditus. If you reflect back on Figure 8-3, you'll see that the laryngeal vestibule is completely sealed off as long as the bolus is in the pharynx.

Pharyngeal timing: Doty and Bosma (1956) performed the seminal research that defined the muscular sequence of the pharyngeal swallow, and since that time researchers have acknowledged that the highly complex neuromuscular activity arises from a centrally generated

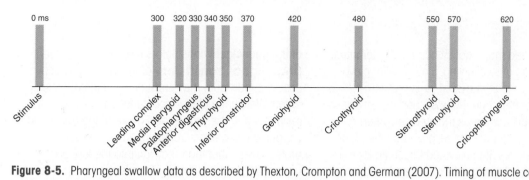

Figure 8-5. Pharyngeal swallow data as described by Thexton, Crompton and German (2007). Timing of muscle contraction during pharyngeal stage of swallow. Stimulus presentation was a milk bolus delivered orally to decerebrate pigs. EMG recordings were verified through videoradiograph recordings. Note that the leading complex included the hyoglossus, stylohyoid, mylohyoid, middle pharyngeal constrictor and styloglossus muscles. The following are implied muscular functions and timings: 300 ms Leading complex, including hyoglossus (hyoid elevation), Stylohyoid (hyoid elevation), mylohyoid (hyoid elevation), Middle pharyngeal constrictor (pharyngeal constriction), and Styloglossus (tongue retraction); 320 ms Medial pterygoid (mandible elevation); 330 ms Palatopharyngeus (pharyngeal elevation and constriction), Omohyoid (hyoid depression or fixation); 340 ms Anterior digastricus (forward hyoid movement); 350 ms Thyrohyoid (elevation of larynx); 370 ms Inferior constrictor (narrowing of hypopharynx); 420 ms Geniohyoid (hyoid elevation); 480 ms Cricothyroid (anterior rocking of thyroid); 550 ms Sternothyroid (fixation of larynx); 570 ms Sternohyoid (fixation of hyoid); 620 ms Cricopharyngeus (UES activation).

Source: From data of Thexton, A. J., Crompton, A. W. & German, R. Z. (2007). Electromyographic activity during the reflex pharyngeal swallow in the pig: Doty and Bosma (1956) revisited. Journal of Applied Physiology, 102, 587-600.

neuromuscular pattern. Thexton, Crompton, and German (2007) have elaborated the sequence of events in the pharyngeal swallow, as you can see from Figure 8-5. Although this study was performed on nonhumans, it should be noted that the swallow across mammals is extraordinarily similar in both sequence and timing (Jean, 2001). In Figure 8-5, the term "leading complex" refers to the first set of muscles that are activated in the patterned response. As you can see, those muscles are the hyoglossus, stylohyoid, mylohyoid, middle pharyngeal constrictor, and styloglossus: They contract about 300 ms (about 1/3 second) after the liquid bolus is introduced orally. This coincides with the timeline identified by Dodds et al. (1990; Figure 8-3), with three of these muscles causing hyoid elevation and one (styloglossus) involved in tongue retraction (the Dodds et al. timeline is relative to the first muscle activation rather than introduction of the bolus, which is how we have drawn Figure 8-5). An important thing to remember is that the act of swallowing is the product of a central pattern within the brain stem that orchestrates the series of movements illustrated here. Once initiated, this patterned activity will continue to its conclusion. This motor sequence is built into the functioning mammal (Ertekin & Aydogdu, 2003).

Upper esophageal sphincter action: The UES consists of the cricopharyngeus muscle of the inferior constrictor, which is tonically

Deficits of the Pharyngeal Stage

Sensory and motor deficit can be dangerous at this stage of swallowing. Slowed velar elevation may result in **nasal regurgitation** (loss of food or liquid through the nose, and loss of pharyngeal pressure), whereas reduced sensation at the fauces, posterior tongue, pharyngeal wall, or soft palate may result in elevated threshold for the trigger of the swallowing reflex. Reduced function of the pharyngeal constrictors may result in slowed **pharyngeal transit time** of the bolus, in which case the individual may prematurely reinitiate respiration. Weakened pharyngeal function may result in residue left in the valleculae. Failure of the hyoid and thyroid to elevate may result in the loss of airway protection, so that food may fall into the larynx and be aspirated on reinflation of the lungs.

nasal regurgitation: loss of food or liquid through the nose

pharyngeal transit time: The time from initiation of the pharyngeal stage of swallowing (clinically identified as elevation of the larynx) to the passage of the bolus through the esophageal entrance (clinically identified as the depression of the larynx).

esophageal reflux: esophageal regurgitation into the hypopharynx

esophageal stage: the stage of swallow in which food is transported from the upper esophageal region to the stomach

peristaltic: wavelike

contracted during respiration, but during the swallow the UES relaxes and opens up as the larynx and hyoid move up and forward. This relaxation is produced by the inhibition of the portion of the recurrent laryngeal nerve of the vagus that innervates the cricopharyngeus. During respiration (i.e., when a person is not swallowing), the UES is continually (tonically) contracted, which keeps gastric contents from escaping into the laryngopharynx (**esophageal reflux**). Relaxing this muscle gives the bolus a place to go.

Esophageal Stage

During the pharyngeal stage, the bolus passed over the epiglottis, was divided into two roughly equal masses, and passed into the pyriform sinuses on either side of the larynx. The bolus recombines at the esophageal entrance.

The **esophageal stage** is purely reflexive and is not within voluntary control. This stage begins when the bolus enters the esophagus, and appears to be triggered by distension of the upper 2 cm of the esophagus by the bolus (Lang, 2009). The bolus is transported through the esophagus to the lower esophageal sphincter (LES) by means of segmental and inferiorly directed **peristaltic** contraction and gravity, arriving at the stomach for the process of digestion after 10 to 20 seconds of transit time. When the bolus passes the UES into the esophagus for transit to the stomach, the cricopharyngeus will again contract, the laryngeal valves open, the soft palate will be depressed, and respiration will begin again.

In the normal swallow, respiration is stopped for only about a second. Reinitiation of respiration increases pressure in the laryngopharynx, and food at the laryngeal entryway will typically be blown clear and propelled to the pharynx as most individuals exhale after swallowing.

The esophageal stage is similar to the pharyngeal stage in terms of motor control. Jean (2001) characterizes the sequential contraction of the esophageal musculature as being governed by a brain stem pattern generator, although the esophageal pattern is simpler.

The UES is composed of three muscle components (the inferior pharyngeal constrictor, upper esophageal muscle, and the cricopharyngeus), with the cricopharyngeus being the dominant muscle. Of these, only the cricopharyngeus is functional in all states of the swallow. The pharyngeal plexus innervates the cricopharyngeus. The superior laryngeal nerve of the X vagus forms the primary innervation of the cricopharyngeus, although muscle is also innervated by the recurrent laryngeal nerve, the pharyngoesophageal nerve, the glossopharyngeal nerve, and the cervical sympathetic system (Lang & Shaker, 1997). If the superior laryngeal nerve (SLN) is stimulated electrically, it will cause the entire transport sequence of swallow, including esophageal peristalsis, to occur (Goyal, Padmanabhan, & Sang, 2001), and it is likely that the SLN provides significant sensory input to the swallowing circuit generally (Lang et al., 1997). The tonic contraction of the cricopharyngeus is likely the product of interaction with other muscular systems (e.g., the thyropharyngeus), rather than a circuit designed to maintain the tone. For instance, either increased esophageal pressure or increased pharyngeal stimulation near the UES will cause increases in tone (Lang et al., 1997).

Deficits of the Esophageal Stage

Although the disorders of the esophageal stage are not directly treated by an SLP, a working knowledge of problems associated with this stage is certainly important to the speech-language pathologist. Gastroesophageal reflux disease (GERD) is significant and potentially life threatening. You may have experienced "heartburn" at one time or another, but that burning feeling may have been the acids from your stomach (i.e., gastric region) being refluxed into your esophagus or pharynx. In some individuals the lower esophageal sphincter relaxes, allowing gastric juices to enter the esophagus. If the upper sphincter is likewise weakened or flaccid, these acids may "reflow" (reflux) into the pyriform sinus, assaulting the delicate pharyngeal tissue. If this occurs during the night when you are supine, the acid may flow into the airway, resulting in aspiration. (We know of

one client with oral, pharyngeal, and esophageal dysphagia secondary to irradiation for cancer. Her pharyngeal dysphagia was being well controlled through treatment directed toward improving pharyngeal responses, and her esophageal reflux had been controlled surgically. The surgical procedure to prevent reflux failed and she was hospitalized with aspiration pneumonia.)

The stomach can herniate through the esophageal hiatus (see Figure 8-4C), a condition termed a *hiatal hernia*. When this occurs, the lower esophageal sphincter may malfunction, allowing reflux into the esophagus. More rarely, a congenital malformation of the esophagus, such as stenosis (see Figure 8-4B), may cause a severe, life-threatening loss of nutrition in a newborn. Rare maldevelopment of the esophagus may even result in the esophageal contents directly entering the trachea.

oral preparatory stage:
the stage in which food is
prepared for swallow

oral transport stage: the
stage of swallow in which the
bolus is transmitted to the
pharynx

✔ *To summarize:*

- Mastication and deglutition involve a complex set of motor acts that are strongly governed by the sensory environment.
- The oral stage can be subdivided into the oral preparatory and transport stages. In the **oral preparatory stage**, food is introduced into the oral cavity, moved onto the molars for chewing, and mixed with saliva to form a concise bolus between the tongue and the hard palate. In the **oral transport stage**, the bolus is moved back toward the oropharynx by the tongue.
- The **pharyngeal stage** begins when the bolus reaches the faucial pillars. The soft palate and larynx have begun elevation during the transport stage, and contact of the tongue with the posterior pharyngeal wall pressurizes the pharynx, propelling the bolus to the upper esophageal sphincter, which has relaxed to receive the material. The epiglottis has dropped to partially cover the laryngeal opening, whereas the intrinsic musculature of the larynx has effected a tight seal to protect the airway. Food passes over the epiglottis and through the pyriform sinuses to the esophagus.
- The final, **esophageal stage** involves the peristaltic movement of the bolus through the esophagus.
- **Central pattern generators (CPGs)** govern the complex, hierarchical movement of muscles in oral, pharyngeal and esophageal stages. Although each stage is independently controlled, the control systems are linked, providing efficiently controlled deglutition. The oral preparatory stage is considered to be a voluntary stage.

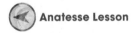

Anatesse Lesson

NEUROPHYSIOLOGICAL UNDERPINNINGS OF MASTICATION AND DEGLUTITION

It is critically important for the experience of eating to be pleasant and behaviorally reinforcing. Natural drives related to hunger bring you to the process of acquiring nutrition, but the food must be palatable for it to be consumed in sufficient quantities to properly nourish you. Further, there must be an adequate neuroanatomical substrate that supports the stages of swallowing. Let us discuss these substrates in turn, and then see how they integrate into the acts of mastication and deglutition.

There are three primary brainstem elements that govern swallowing: the sensory (afferent) component, the cranial motor nuclei, and the network that organizes these two elements into "the program" for swallowing, or the swallowing CPG (Broussard & Altschuler, 2000; Ertekin & Aydogdu, 2003; Jean, 2001). Let us look at each of these elements.

Sensation Associated with Mastication and Deglutition

Numerous types of stimulus receptors are critical for completion of the chewing, sucking, and swallowing (CSS) elements associated with mastication and deglutition. (For a thorough review of sensory systems, see Møller, 2003, and Kandel, Schwartz, Jessell, Siegelbaum, & Hudspeth, 2013). Among these are the gustatory (taste), tactile (touch), temperature (thermal), and pressure senses, as well as pain sensation (nociception). Each plays a critical role in successful completion of the CSS routines. We will go into considerable detail in our discussion of these senses, but some of the material may become clear to you only upon studying the underlying neuroanatomy (Chapters 11 and 12).

Gustation

Gustation (taste) is a complex and critical component of CSS. Taste drives the desire to continue eating, which fulfills the nutritional requirements of the body. Taste receptors (**taste buds**, or **taste cells**) consist of a class of sensors known as **chemoreceptors**, in that they respond when specific chemicals come in contact with them. Taste receptors are found interspersed in the epithelia of the tongue within **papillae**, or prominences (see Figure 8-6). An opening in the epithelium called the **taste pore** permits the isolation of a sample of the tasted substance, which is held in place by **microvilli** (small hair-like fibers projecting

taste buds (taste cells): chemoreceptors for gestation

chemoreceptors: neural receptors that respond to specific chemical compositions

papillae: prominences

taste pore: opening in the lingual epithelium that houses taste cells

microvilli: small, hairlike fibers projecting from the taste cell into the taste pore

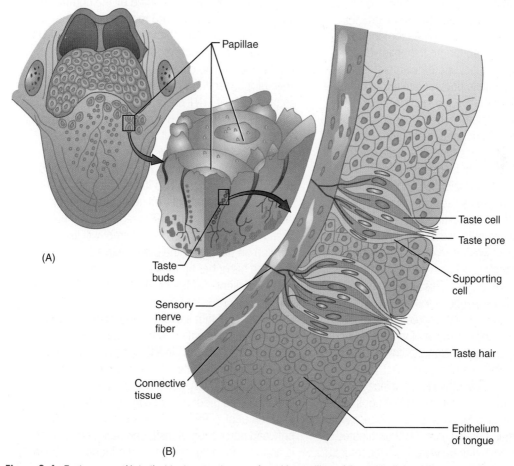

(A)

Papillae

Taste buds

Sensory nerve fiber

Connective tissue

(B)

Taste cell

Taste pore

Supporting cell

Taste hair

Epithelium of tongue

Figure 8-6. Taste sensor. Note that taste receptors are found in papillae of the epithelium of the tongue, within taste pores.

Source: (Adapted from Buck, 2000.)

from the taste cell into the taste pore). There are five basic tastes: sweet, salty, sour, bitter, and umami. We are familiar with the first four terms, but you may have never run across *umami*, though you most certainly have tasted it. Umami is the taste of monosodium glutamate, which tastes "meaty," or protein-like. For over a century, we believed that taste receptors were restricted to zones of the tongue, with sweet tastes being sensed at the tip, salty at the sides in front, and sour at the sides in the back. Bitterness was thought to be sensed on the posterior tongue. The reality is that all the tastes can be sensed all over the tongue.

If you examine Figure 8-6 (see Figure 6-36), you can see that the tongue is richly invested with papillae of various forms. The filiform papillae are the dominant papillary formation of the tongue. They appear

What Did They Do with the Tongue Map?

Hoffman (1875) was the first to state that the basic tastes of sweet, sour, salty, and bitter were represented in zones of the tongue, so that sweet taste was mediated by the tongue tip, bitter taste was sensed by the posterior tongue, and so on. His work arose from both the observation that there was differential anatomy among taste receptors (circumvallate papillae are found in the posterior middle of the tongue, and foliate papillae are in the posterior lateral aspect; fungiform papillae are found on the anterior and lateral surfaces of the tongue) and that humans tended to taste the four basic tastants in different locations. His work and that of many perceptual scientists who followed him defined the tongue tip as sensitive to sweet taste, the anterior and antero-lateral surface as responsive to salty, with sour taste being sensed at the mid-lateral regions. Bitter taste was reserved for the posterior dorsum of the tongue, just above the junction of the hard and soft palates. This view began to blur, however, as knowledge of taste receptors improved. Hoon et al. (1999) showed that taste receptors were actually a subset of what is termed G protein coupled receptor signal pathways (GPCR). Two specific GPCRs were identified: T1R1 (found predominantly in the circumvallate papillae) and T1R2 (found in abundance in the foliate papillae). What the authors also found was that the receptors were mixed, rather than isolated: T1R2 dominated the foliate papillae, but there were T1R1 receptors there as well. Eventually, two more receptors were

found (T1R3 and T12Rs) and added to the mix. Perception studies revealed that, in humans, the sense of sweetness is mediated by the combined activation of T1R2 and T1R3 receptors (Nelson, Hoon, Chandrashekar, Zhang, Ryba, & Zuker, 2001), and bitter sense is activated by the T2Rs receptors. The taste of amino acids (such as umami, the taste of monosodium glutamate) is mediated by a combination of T1R1 and T1R3 sensors. A receptor for sour taste (PK2DL1: Huang, et al., 2006) left salt as the only outlier without a receptor. Salty taste evidently is mediated by direct sodium migration into the cell (Oka, Butnaru, von Buchholtz, Ryba, & Zuker, 2013). The taste bud itself, which is not neural tissue, can be genetically altered in lab animals so that, for instance, a bitter TRC feeds a sweet neural fiber. When this is done, a lab animal will likely develop an affinity for the bitter taste, ostensibly because his or her brain perceives sweet when bitter taste is presented (Mueller, Hoon, Erlenbach, Zuker, & Ryba, 2005).

Where did that leave our historical taste map? Although it is appealing to think that specific regions of the tongue are sensitive to specific tastes, this view gets blurred quite a bit by the reality of the receptor distribution. Each taste bud has many TRCs, and there is a great deal of overlap of TRC fields. As Hoon et al. (1999) state, there is a "correlation" between perception of taste and receptors, but there is no room for a rigidly demarcated tongue map in current physiology.

as small threads on the surface of the tongue, are pink or gray in color, and make the dorsum of the tongue look rough. They include not only taste sensors but also mechanoreceptors to provide a fine tactile sensory ability to the tongue, permitting fine discrimination of the bolus characteristics (discussed later). Fungiform papillae are bright red and are found interspersed with filiform papillae on the tip and sides of the tongue. Vallate papillae are the large V-shaped formation of circles seen in the posterior dorsum of the tongue. There are typically a dozen or so on a tongue, and each has a "moat" surrounding it. Foliate papillae are sparsely present on the lateral margins of the tongue.

Taste is mediated by means of four cranial nerves. The VII facial nerve mediates the sense of taste from the anterior two-thirds of the tongue, specifically involving sweet, salty, and sour sensations (Segerstad & Hellekant, 1989: see Figure 8-7), whereas the IX glossopharyngeal nerve transmits information from the posterior one-third of the tongue (Geran & Travers, 2011; Ninomaya, Imoto, & Sugimura, 1999). Taste receptors of the palate are innervated by the VII facial nerve. Although not shown in Figure 8-7, taste receptors of the epiglottis and esophagus are innervated by the X vagus nerve. The V trigeminal is responsible for the mediation of chemesthetic sense, as we will discuss below.

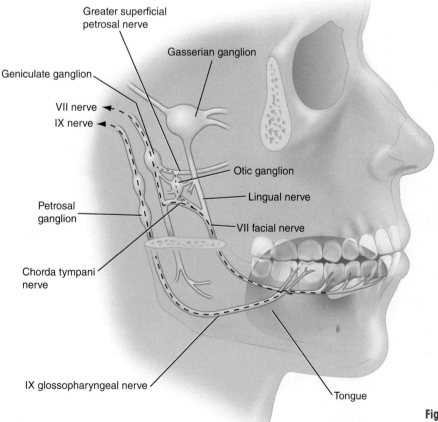

Figure 8-7. Innervation schematic for anterior and posterior tongue.
Source: (Adapted from Mountcastle, 1974.)

Taste stimulus to the VII facial nerve is relayed through the geniculate ganglion to the solitary tract within the medulla, to terminate at the rostral and lateral aspects of the solitary tract nucleus in the gustatory region of the brainstem. Taste sensation from the IX glossopharyngeal nerve is mediated via the petrosal ganglion, and fibers also terminate in the solitary tract nucleus. Epiglottal and esophageal taste senses are transmitted via the X vagus nerve through the nodose ganglion, likewise to the solitary tract nucleus. This taste information is then relayed to the ventral posterior medial nucleus (VPMN) of the thalamus, which subsequently relays this information ipsilaterally to the anterior portion of the insula of the cerebral cortex. Figure 8-8 illustrates the taste pathways in humans.

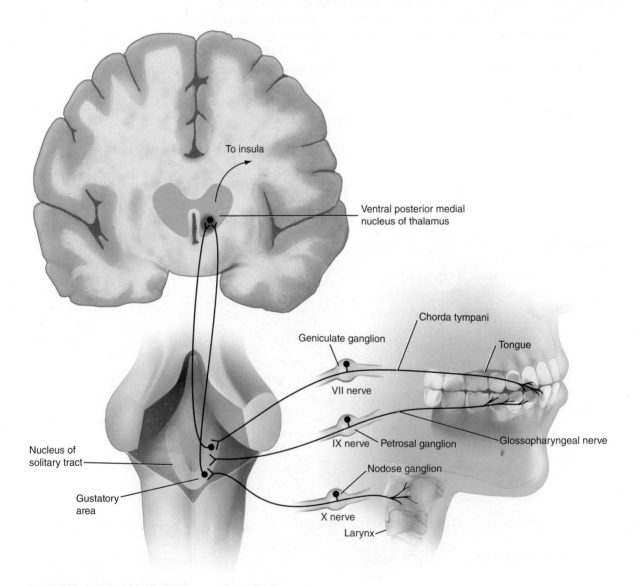

Figure 8-8. Pathways mediating the sensations of taste.
Source: (After Buck, 2000.)

Now examine Figure 8-9, which illustrates the relative contribution of each nerve to taste perception. First, notice the relative magnitude of tastes mediated by each of the nerves (VII, IX, and X) in relation to their locations and distribution. This information converges on the rostral nucleus of the solitary tract (rNST) and is then sent to the ventral posterior nucleus (VPN) of the thalamus. The sensation is subsequently transmitted to the primary sensory cortex (located in the postcentral gyrus of the cerebrum) and to the insular cortex of the frontal lobe (located in a fold of the cerebral cortex underlying the operculum), as well as the operculum overlying the insula. Taste and smell are probably integrated at the insula (Møller, 2003). Fibers from the insula project into the limbic system and the motor regions of the brain stem.

The NST also projects into the motor cortex, specifically the region serving the tongue. This is important. Our nutritional needs govern our selection of sweet and umami tastes, as these indicate the presence of carbohydrates (sweet) and protein (umami). Salt is also a necessary mineral, so we "crave" that taste as well. These tastes may elicit salivation, as well as ingestive responses, including tongue protrusion to receive the food, release of insulin, mastication, and

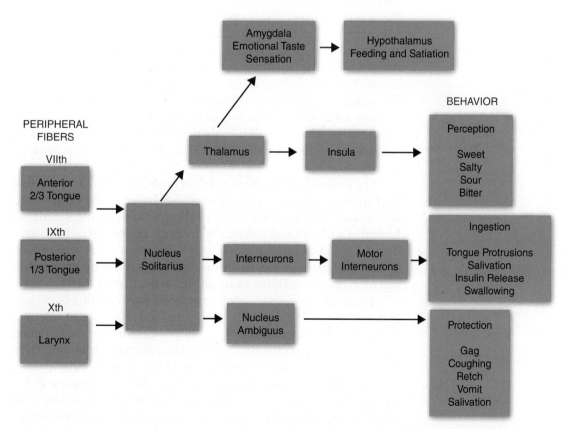

Figure 8-9. Schematic illustration of routing and response to taste within the nervous system.

Source: Modified, after S. A. Simon & S. D. Roper [1993]. Mechanisms of taste transduction. Boca Raton, FL: CRC Press.

deglutition. In contrast, bitter and sour tastes typify poisons, and they will often elicit protective responses that include gagging, coughing, apnea, and salivation (salivation in this case encapsulates the material and protects the oral cavity). The receptors sensitive to bitter taste are even found in the cilia of the airway, and presence of bitter materials increases the beating of those cilia, apparently as a means of eliminating a potentially toxic material from the airway (Shah, Ben-Shahar, Moninger, Kline, & Welsh, 2009). Admittedly, we *do* eat sour and bitter foods, but notice next time you encounter a particularly bitter taste how you find it difficult to swallow, or at least become wary of it. This underscores a critically important point. Tastes can elicit motor responses that may or may not be under volitional (or even conscious) control. The gag response is a complex motor act involving elevation of the larynx and clamping of the vocal folds, elevation of the velum, and protrusion of the tongue. Coughing entails tightly closing the vocal folds, compressing the abdomen and thorax and forcefully blowing the vocal folds apart. Now recognize that each of these responses has components of the swallow embedded within it, and you can see that deglutition is made up of a complex set of motor responses dictated by stimuli in the oral and pharyngeal spaces.

Some foods are capable of activating nontaste sensors, which can have both positive and negative effects on swallowing. Oral chemesthesis is the process of detection of chemical stimuli by thermal and pain receptors within the mouth (Green, 2011). Obviously, pain is an aversive stimulus that typically causes a person to stop whatever activity induced the pain (think of the last time you burned your finger). In contrast, thermal stimuli (heat and cold) mediate qualities of the bolus that are important, although there are extremes there as well. A warm drink is very satisfying in winter, but if it is too hot the sense of pain takes over. We will talk about pain and thermal sense shortly, but first let us consider the interaction of these protective senses in gustation.

The study of oral chemesthesis has provided insight into swallowing behavior. Some chemesthetic stimuli enhance swallowing function by lowering the threshold of the swallow, although others signal the body that a foreign and potentially dangerous material has been introduced. Oral chemesthesis can tell your body that it has been invaded by bacteria that have caused chemical changes in the oral mucosa, for instance, causing sneezing or nasal rhinorrhea (Green, 2012).

These "chemosensor" components are only one side of chemesthesis, however. We regularly indulge in foods that trigger responses from pain and thermal sensors. Chili powder, for instance, contains capacin that triggers pain and thermal receptors in the mouth, giving the burning sensation and, some would say, sense of pain from the chili (Cometto-Muniz, Cain, & Abraham, 2004). (There are at least two words for "hot" in Spanish: *picante* and *caliente*, with *picante* referring to the heat associated with capacin and *caliente* referring to the heat associated with cooking.) Researchers are examining the possibility that clinicians can utilize oral chemesthesis to their advantage in therapy. There are several examples of the cross-modality function of chemesthesis. For example, carbonation triggers a painful sensation, and gingerol in very strong ginger ale stimulates thermal receptors. The conversion of CO_2 to carbonic acid in carbonated water, a reaction catalyzed by the salivary enzyme carbonic anhydrase, activates lingual nociceptors, which causes trigeminal neurons to signal oral irritation to higher centers (Cowart 1998; Dessirier, Simons, Carstens, O'Mahony, & Carstens, 2000). Carbonated water, with and without the addition of the thermal irritant ginger (in strong ginger ale) (Krival & Bates, 2011), as well as high concentrations of sucrose, salt, and citric acid (Pelletier & Dhanaraj, 2006) all increased lingua-palatal pressure in people with normal swallow function. In adults with dysphagia, high levels of citric acid and carbonation have each been shown to reduce the latency of swallow initiation as well as to reduce the occurrence of aspiration in experimental MBSS studies (Bülow, Olsson, & Ekberg, 2003; Logemann, 1995; Pelletier & Lawless, 2003; Sdravou, Walshe, & Dagdilelis, 2012). Although to date no studies have examined the effectiveness of these chemesthetic stimuli on swallowing over time, the fact that immediate changes in swallowing occur suggests that capitalizing on the oral chemesthetic sense has promise for increasing lingual force and pharyngeal swallowing in people with dysphagia. A caution though: in many of these studies the effect on swallowing was achieved only when the bolus was so strongly irritating that it was deemed unpalatable by the research participants (Logemann, 1995; Pelletier & Dhanaraj, 2006).

Olfaction

Olfaction (the sense of smell) plays a vital role in appetite and taste. Molecules arising from food pass over olfactory chemoreceptors to increase the magnitude of the taste perception, a fact to which you can relate if you remember how "flat" your favorite food tasted when you had nasal congestion. In fact, if you tightly occlude your nares and blindly take a bite of apple and then a bite of onion, you will likely not be able to taste the difference.

Olfactory sensors arise from the olfactory bulb and have the distinction of a short life and continual replacement. They last only about 60 days before being replaced by new sensors. Olfactory sensors are found within the epithelial lining of the upper posterior nasal cavity (see Figure 8-10). There are small cilia protruding from the olfactory sensor, similar to the microvilli of the taste cell. These cilia are highly specialized, in that they transduce the molecular stimulant into the perception of smell that is transmitted to the olfactory bulb located within the cranial space. Recent research has revealed that although the basic structure of the odor receptors on the cilia is similar for all olfactory sensors, the specific structure of the receptor varies slightly, so that more than 1,000 different odors are decoded by the olfactory system.

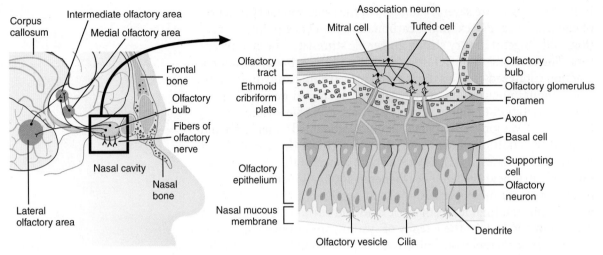

Figure 8-10. Detail of olfactory bulb.
© Cengage Learning®.

After an odorant stimulates a specific receptor, information that the receptor has been activated is transmitted to the olfactory bulb, which resides within the braincase. More than 1,000 axons of sensory cells converge on each olfactory interneuron (termed a **glomerulus**) in the olfactory bulb. This information is transmitted by means of the olfactory tract to the olfactory region of the cortex, which includes the amygdala, the anterior olfactory nucleus, the piriform cortex, the olfactory tubercle, and a portion of the entorhinal cortex. Information from some of these brain centers is routed through the thalamus and subsequently relayed to the frontal lobe of the cerebral cortex, orbital region. Olfactory information from the amygdala is transmitted to the hypothalamus, whereas olfactory information from the entorhinal area terminates in the hippocampus within the temporal lobe. The functional implications are that olfaction arrives at the cerebral cortex through multiple pathways, including the thalamus and that the information serves as a stimulus to emotion and motivation (amygdala), physiological responses (hypothalamus), and memory encoding (hippocampus). The information reaching the orbitofrontal region of the cerebral cortex appears to be involved in olfactory discrimination (i.e., conscious, discriminative processing of smell). Again, recognize that motor responses are readily mediated by reception of olfactory stimulation. Salivation may result from pleasant food odors, whereas gagging or even vomiting can be triggered by unpleasant odors.

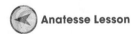
Anatesse Lesson

mechanoreceptors: neural receptors designed to sense mechanical forces

glabrous: hairless

Tactile Sense

The sense of touch is mediated by a number of **mechanoreceptors**, which are sensors that are sensitive to physical contact. Generally, sensors differ based on whether the epithelium contains hair or is hairless (**glabrous** skin). Glabrous skin of the hands contains "fingerprints" that are, in reality, the overlay for dense collections of mechanoreceptors. Touch receptors are broadly distributed about the body and are differentiated based on the type of stimulus that causes them to respond (see Figure 8-11). Hairy skin receptors are less critical to our discussion of swallowing, as the epithelial linings of the oral and pharyngeal cavities are hairless.

Glabrous (hairless) skin contains **Meissner's corpuscles** and **Merkel disk receptors**. Meissner's corpuscles are physically coupled to the papilla in which they reside (similar to taste receptors) and respond to minute mechanical movement. Merkel disk receptors transmit the sense of pressure. Meissner's corpuscles adapt quickly to stimulation (i.e., they stop responding after a brief period of sustained stimulation), whereas Merkel disk receptors respond for longer periods of time to sustained stimulation. Both of these receptors are found within the superficial layer of the lingual epithelium. Both Meissner's corpuscles and Merkel disk receptors are found at the end of the papillary ridge. Deep cutaneous tissues contain **Pacinian corpuscles** and cells with the **Ruffini ending**. The Pacinian corpuscle is similar to the Meissner's corpuscle and responds to rapid deep pressure to the

Meissner's corpuscles: superficial cutaneous mechanoreceptors for minute movement

Merkel disk receptors: superficial cutaneous mechanoreceptors for light pressure

Pacinian corpuscles: deep cutaneous mechanoreceptors for deep pressure

Ruffini endings: deep cutaneous mechanoreceptors for tissue stretch

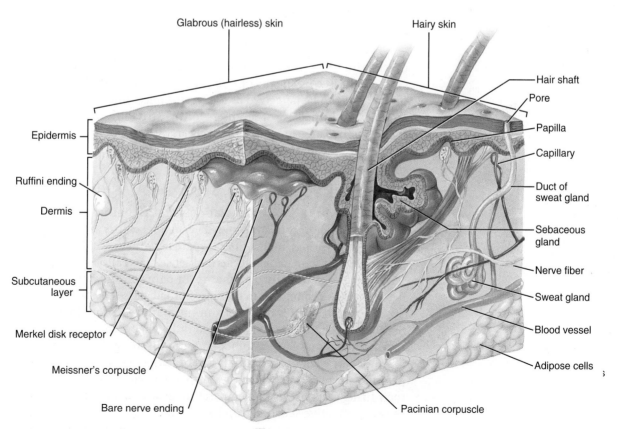

Figure 8-11. Detail of mechanoreceptors.
© Cengage Learning®.

outer epithelium. Ruffini endings sense stretch within the deep tissues and are critical to our perception of the shape of objects perceived by touch. It is important to note that Meissner's corpuscles and Merkel disk receptors have small receptor fields, which means that their effective sensory area is more limited than those of the deeply embedded Ruffini endings and Pacinian corpuscles, which have larger receptive fields. Deep pressure has the potential to stimulate a larger field and greater array of sensors than light pressure, an issue that is important in the treatment of dysphagia.

Vibration sense is a subclass of tactile sense. Vibration may be considered as either deep or superficial pressure, depending on the amplitude of the vibration. In both cases, vibration is sensed as individual deformation of tactile sensors. Pacinian corpuscles (deep pressure sensors) respond most efficiently to stimulation between 70 and 500 Hz (best frequency is 280 Hz), whereas Meissner's corpuscles respond best to stimulation between 10 and 100 Hz, with a shallow best frequency of 50 Hz. (**Best frequency** refers to the frequency of vibration at which a sensor responds most effectively.) Though both of these receptors are rapidly adapting sensors, Pacinian corpuscles (deep receptors) have a markedly lower threshold to vibration than Meissner's corpuscles (superficial receptors). Rapidly adapting sensors have lower thresholds of stimulation than slowly adapting receptors, meaning that Meissner's and Pacinian corpuscles will respond to lower levels of stimulation than Ruffini endings and Merkel disk receptors.

The classic test for spatial density of receptors is of two-point discrimination, wherein an individual is provided a pressure of calibrated force by means of two probes. The distance between the probes that can be perceived as two versus one stimulus is considered an index of the density of receptors for the structure. That is to say, if the two points are close enough together, they will both stimulate the same single receptor, giving the perception of a single contact point.

Thermal Receptors

Four classes of thermal stimulation are differentiated by human senses: warm, hot, cool, and cold. Thermal receptors are actually the same as pain sensors, in that they are bare nerve endings. Although it is convenient to group pain and thermal sense, the reality is that thermal sensors are functionally different from pain sensors, with different nerve endings responding to these two broad classes of stimulation.

Thermal receptors differ from mechanoreceptors in a critical manner: Mechanoreceptors respond only when stimulated, whereas thermal receptors have a tonic, ongoing discharge. The individual receptors for each of the four classes of temperature have "best temperature" responses to which they respond. Cold sensors will increase their firing response as the temperature of stimulation drops, even as the cool-sensitive sensors drop back to their basal firing rate. Thermal receptors, apparently, are most effective at identifying thermal stimulation that differs markedly from the ambient temperature of

Sensory Examination

The clinical or bedside evaluation tests both motor and sensory functions of swallowing. Logemann (1993) provides an excellent discussion of both sensory and motor examinations. In brief, the sensory examination is designed to assess the tactile sense (2-point discrimination), thermal sense (cold, hot), and taste sense (sweet, sour, bitter, salty, and umami). As you examine these elements, you must remove visual cues to the stimulus and must remember to test multiple locations within the oral cavity. One way to test the gustatory element is to dip cotton-tipped applicators in water and then into the dry compound (salt, sugar or sugar-free sweetener, bitters, lemon, umami) and then touch a location in the oral cavity, asking what the person tastes.

the skin. Thus, a slow increase or decrease in stimulus temperature will be more difficult to detect than a rapid change in temperature. At high temperatures, heat sensors cease firing and pain sensors fire instead. Thermal sense requires longer duration of stimulation for the perception of sensation, but the sensation is retained for longer periods of time.

Pain Sense (Nociception)

Pain sense is included in this discussion because of its importance in the development of structural disorders of swallowing. As an example, structural defects such as oral or pharyngeal lesions (e.g., cold sores) can cause pain that can interfere with swallowing responses.

Nociceptors (pain sensors) respond directly to a noxious stimulus (e.g., chemical burn), to molecules released by injured tissue (such as positive potassium ions, serotonin, and acetylcholine), to acidity caused by injury, or to direct contact with a traumatic source. Some nociceptors respond to mechanical trauma, whereas others respond to thermal stimulation. Most nociceptors respond to general destruction of tissue rather than to the specific quality of a stimulus, and the perception arising from the stimulation of these receptors (termed *polymodal nociceptors*) is a burning sensation.

nociceptors: pain sensors

Nociceptors

Nociceptors produce the perception of pain when they are traumatized, such as in burning. The direct trauma to a nerve ending relays this information to higher centers so that you can withdraw from the painful stimulus. If the nerve ending is destroyed entirely, there will be no perception of pain; this is one indication of the third-degree burn.

Muscle Stretch and Tension Sense

Muscle stretch is sensed by muscle spindle fibers, which consist of nuclear chain fibers and nuclear bag fibers within muscle tissue itself. Stretch receptors are found predominantly in larger muscles, such as the antigravity muscles of the legs, but are also found within oral musculature. The mandibular elevators (masseter, temporalis, and lateral and medial pterygoid muscles) are richly endowed with stretch receptors, as are the deep tongue fibers of the genioglossus and the palatoglossus muscles. Facial muscles are notably deficient in stretch receptors.

Muscle spindle fibers return a muscle to its original position following passive stretching. As an example, if you were to pull sharply down on your relaxed mandible, the mandible would quickly elevate thereafter, to the point that your teeth might make contact (depending on how relaxed you are and how low your threshold of stimulation is). This sensor system is designed to maintain a muscle at a preset length, so that the monitored muscle group contracts in response to passive stretching. The spindle function is normally inhibited during active contraction, although damage to the upper motor neuron can cause hyperactive stretch reflexes and spasticity (to be discussed in Chapters 11 and 12).

Muscle tension is sensed by Golgi tendon organs (GTOs), found within the tendons and fascia. These organs respond to the active contraction of muscles and serve to inhibit the muscle spindle fibers.

Muscle tone is regulated partially through the interaction of muscle spindles and GTOs. **Muscle tone** refers to the perception of resistance to the passive movement of stretching. A high tone of spasticity results from an inadequately inhibited response from muscle spindle sensors,

Mouth Breathing

Chronic mouth breathing is more than an unpleasant habit; it is at the root of facial malformation and the cause of hearing loss. Mouth breathing is often, attributed to hypertrophy of the tonsilar ring, prohibiting adequate nasal respiration. In children with this condition, the adenoids are frequently enlarged, blocking the nasal choanae and also the orifice of the Eustachian tube. Inadequate ventilation of the middle ear cavity may result in otitis media (inflammation of the middle ear cavity). Chronic otitis media is often associated with fluid in the middle ear (serous otitis media), a condition resulting in conductive hearing impairment.

The hypertrophy also makes mouth breathing mandatory. During normal nasal respiration, the tongue maintains fairly constant contact with the upper alveolar ridge and hard palate, but with the mouth open constantly for respiration, the tongue can exert little pressure there. Without that pressure, the dental arch may narrow and the palate may bulge upward to an extreme vault as the facial bones develop. With narrow dental arches, the permanent teeth may not have adequate space, so they become crowded and prone to caries (decay of bone or tooth). The narrowed maxillae may cause the upper lip to pull up, exposing the upper front teeth. The nasal cavity may become narrow, increasing the probability of later nasal obstruction. The look of "adenoid facies" includes an open mouth, narrow mandible, and dental crowding. When coupled with persistent conductive hearing loss, mouth breathing presents a sizable (yet, generally preventable) deficit to the developing child.

whereas low tone results from inadequate tonic stimulation, either from lower motor neuron disease or cerebellar lesion. Muscular rigidity arises from a basal ganglia lesion and occurs because of the co-contraction of agonists and antagonists. Reflexes may be normally elicited despite abnormally high muscle tone. High muscle tone resulting from muscle spindle disinhibition may result in a clasp-knife response to passive stretching. This disinhibition likely arises from GTOs (Brown, 1994). In this response, there is an initial resistance to a stretch that is released, apparently because of input from cutaneous sensors and nociceptors. Thus, it is possible that cutaneous, thermal, and pain sensors may be used to reduce or inhibit spastic responses in pathological conditions.

Mechanical deformation (touch and pressure), thermal sense, pain sense, and joint and tendon sense of the face and oral cavity are primarily mediated by the V trigeminal nerve, although the IX glossopharyngeal and X vagus also have pathways associated with these sensations (Møller, 2003).

Salivation Response

Related to taste, smell, and noxious stimulation is the salivation response. **Salivation** (the production and release of saliva into the oral cavity) is not a sensory system, but rather a motor response. It is an essential and often overlooked component of mastication and deglutition and deserves attention in this discussion of normal function. When saliva mixes with tasteless starch, the combination produces sugars that taste sweet and thus make the food more desirable.

Salivation is the product of three major glands: the parotid, submandibular, and sublingual. In addition, mucus-secreting accessory salivary glands are present throughout the oral cavity, embedded within the mucosa. These glands are activated by the stimulation of taste receptors (the anterior two-thirds of the tongue), mediated by the VII facial nerve via the nucleus solitarius of the dorsal pons (sublingual and submandibular glands) and IX glossopharyngeal nerve (parotid gland). This nucleus projects into the inferior and superior salivatory nuclei of the pons, which excites the salivary glands to secrete saliva.

The submandibular gland is found behind the free margin of the mylohyoid muscle, between the mylohyoid muscle and the submandibular fossa of the inner mandible. It extends as far posteriorly as the second molar and extends forward as the submandibular duct (see Figure 8-12). The duct courses anteriorly and medially, opening into the oral cavity just lateral to the lingual frenulum.

The sublingual gland is above the mylohyoid muscle and medially placed. It is an elongated mass located in the floor of the mouth, with the right and left glands meeting in the front of the oral cavity. The visual manifestation of the gland is a ridge seen to follow the base of the tongue along the floor of the mouth, upon elevation of the tongue. The sublingual gland empties into the mouth through ducts within the sublingual fold. The parotid gland is located posterior to the mandibular ramus and superior to the sternocleidomastoid muscle, and secretions from it empty into the pharynx.

salivation: production and release of saliva into the oral cavity

Disorders of Salivation

Disorders of salivation can occur for numerous reasons. If an individual has the reduced sensation of salivary output, it is termed **xerostomia**, or "dry mouth." This can have numerous causes, but the most frequent cause is one of hundreds of medications, such as diuretics, antihypertensive medications, and of course antihistamines. It is also frequently caused by the irradiation of face and neck for cancer treatment, or by chemotherapy agents. Sjogren's disease is an autoimmune disorder wherein the salivary glands and tear ducts are disabled. Finally, peripheral and central nerve damage can result in the loss of salivary function.

If the submandibular and sublingual glands are affected, the person may have difficulty with bolus formation, as these two glands help to make the bolus cohesive. If the parotid gland is affected, the pharyngeal stage swallow may be affected, as the type of saliva secreted is much thinner, facilitating movement of the bolus through the pharynx.

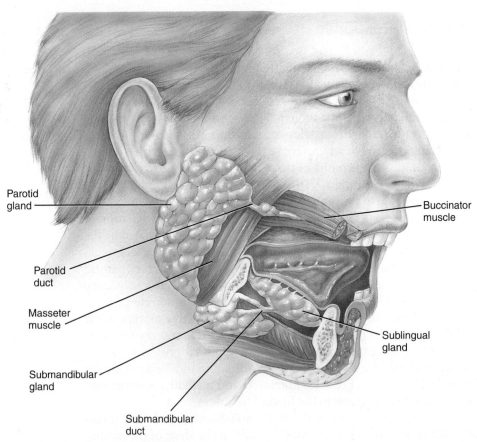

Figure 8-12. Salivary glands and ducts.
© Cengage Learning®.

mucus: thick, high-viscosity saliva

Each of these glands has distinctly different secretions. The sublingual gland produces **mucus**, a high-viscosity (thick), protein-rich secretion that helps in the formation of the bolus of food. Its ropey quality helps encapsulate food particles, permitting tongue action to prepare the food for propulsion to the pharynx.

The submandibular gland produces both **serous** and mucus secretions. Serous saliva has markedly lower viscosity (i.e., it is thinner in consistency) and serves as a lubricant to the bolus. The posteriorly placed parotid gland produces only serous saliva, which is instrumental in the active and rapid propulsion of the bolus into and through the pharynx.

Salivary flow is stimulated behaviorally by the sight, smell, and taste of food. The salivary glands produce as much as 1.2 liters of saliva per day, although the production is reduced to minute quantities during sleep.

serous: thin, low-viscosity saliva

✔ *To summarize:*

- **Gustation** (taste) is mediated by **chemoreceptors** that transmit information to the brain via the IX glossopharyngeal, X vagus, and VII facial nerves. Taste sensors are specialized for sweet, sour, salty, bitter, and umami sense.
- Taste sense determines whether a **bolus** is ingested or ejected from the oral cavity.
- **Olfaction** (the sense of smell) is mediated by chemoreceptors within the nasal mucosa.
- The sense of touch (**tactile** sense) is mediated by means of **mechanoreceptors** that respond to deep or shallow touch.
- Four classes of **thermal stimulation** are differentiated by human senses: warm, hot, cool, and cold.
- Pain sense (**nociception**) is a response to a noxious stimulus.
- Muscle **stretch** is sensed by muscle spindle fibers, and muscle **tension** is sensed by Golgi tendon organs (GTOs), found within tendons and fascia.
- Tactile sense, thermal sense, pain sense, and joint and tendon sense of the face and oral cavity are mediated by the V trigeminal, IX glossopharyngeal, and X vagus nerves.
- **Salivation** occurs because of the stimulation of salivary glands.
- The type of saliva varies between glands. The **sublingual gland** produces thick **mucus** secretions, the **submandibular gland** produces both thin **serous** and mucus secretions, and the **parotid gland** secretes only serous saliva.

REFLEXIVE CIRCUITS OF MASTICATION AND DEGLUTITION

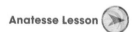 Anatesse Lesson

The individual reflex circuits associated with mastication and deglutition are the building blocks for the normal processes associated with the intake of food and drink. Recognize that these reflexes are mediated at the level of the brain stem and do not require cortical involvement. This does not imply that there is no cortical activity associated with CSS, but rather that the cortex is not essential. We have included **expulsive reflexes** here as well (gag, retch) because of their close association with the systems of mastication and deglutition. Most of the reflexes that we will discuss are controlled by circuitry within the phylogenetically old reticular formation of the posterior brainstem (see Figure 8-13).

(A)

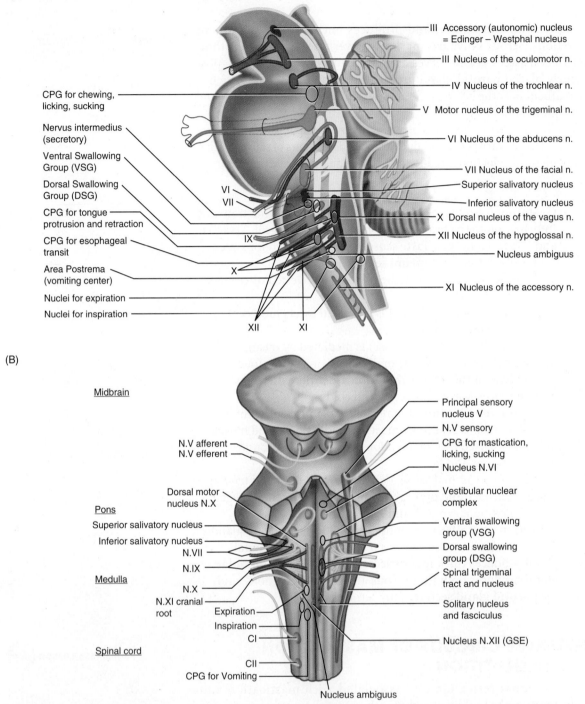

III Accessory (autonomic) nucleus
= Edinger – Westphal nucleus

III Nucleus of the oculomotor n.

IV Nucleus of the trochlear n.

CPG for chewing,
licking, sucking

V Motor nucleus of the trigeminal n.

Nervus intermedius
(secretory)

VI Nucleus of the abducens n.

Ventral Swallowing
Group (VSG)

VII Nucleus of the facial n.

Dorsal Swallowing
Group (DSG)

Superior salivatory nucleus

Inferior salivatory nucleus

CPG for tongue
protrusion and retraction

X Dorsal nucleus of the vagus n.

XII Nucleus of the hypoglossal n.

CPG for esophageal
transit

Nucleus ambiguus

Area Postrema
(vomiting center)

XI Nucleus of the accessory n.

Nuclei for expiration

Nuclei for inspiration

VI
VII

IX

X

XII   XI

(B)

Midbrain

Principal sensory
nucleus V

N.V sensory

N.V afferent
N.V efferent

CPG for mastication,
licking, sucking

Nucleus N.VI

Dorsal motor
nucleus N.X

Vestibular nuclear
complex

Pons

Ventral swallowing
group (VSG)

Superior salivatory nucleus

Inferior salivatory nucleus

Dorsal swallowing
group (DSG)

N.VII

N.IX

Spinal trigeminal
tract and nucleus

Medulla

N.X

N.XI cranial
root

Solitary nucleus
and fasciculus

Expiration

Inspiration

CI

Nucleus N.XII (GSE)

Spinal cord

CII

CPG for Vomiting

Nucleus ambiguus

Figure 8-13. Locations of centers for swallowing, mastication/sucking, vomiting, and respiration. (A) Lateral view of brainstem. Central Pattern Generator (CPG) for planning (Dorsal Swallowing Group DSG) is located within the Solitary Tract Nucleus and reticular formation, whereas the CPG for execution (Ventral Swallowing Group VSG) is located above the Nucleus Ambiguus (Ertekin & Aydogdu, 2003; Jean, 2001). Motor cranial nerve nuclei involved in oropharyngeal swallowing include those of the V, VII (mastication and sucking) and XII (mastication, sucking, transport, including tongue retraction and protrusion), the nucleus ambiguus (IX and X: rostral for esophagus, pharynx, larynx; intermediate for pharynx and velum; caudal for larynx), and the dorsal motor nucleus of vagus (Jean, 2001). The CPG for inspiration is located in the reticular formation below the motor nucleus for vagus, and the CPG for expiration is located between the nucleus for vagus and the nucleus for the hypoglossal nerve (Duus, 2005). The vomiting center is located in the Area Postrema (dorsal reticular formation) below the hypoglossal nerve nucleus (Duus, 2005). The center for mastication, sucking and licking is located in the pons, above the nuclei of the facial (VII) and trigeminal (V) nerves (Lund & Kolta, 2006). (B) Posterior view of brainstem, with centers located.

Chewing Reflex

Chewing is a complex reflex that can be triggered by deep pressure on the roof of the mouth, as when you bite a cracker. It involves alternating left-side and right-side contraction of the muscles of mandibular elevation (masseter and medial pterygoid muscles), such that a rotatory motion of the mandible is produced. The alternating contraction of these mandibular elevators is interspersed with the depression of the mandible, which allows the lingual musculature to move the bolus onto and off the molars. The chewing center complex is made up of a CPG for the rhythmic mandibular movement (located above the motor nuclei for the V trigeminal and VII facial nerves in the pons), as well as the nucleus pontis caudalis in the caudal reticular formation (Lund & Kolta, 2006). Hardness of food is sensed by the pressure on the teeth (periodontal afferents), which is fed into the central program generator and which increases the force exerted by the muscles of mastication. This center is also involved in the reflexive movements of the tongue for sucking and licking (Baehr & Frotscher, 2012; Lund & Kolta, 2006).

Orienting, Rooting and Suckling/Sucking Reflexes

The **rooting** and sucking reflexes—very functional for neonates and infants—rely on tactile stimulation of the perioral region. The suckling response is considered to be an earlier developmental stage of the sucking reflex. Lightly stroking the lips or cheek on one side will cause the infant's mouth to open and its head to turn toward the stimulus; this is termed the rooting reflex. Light contact within the inner margin of the lips will initiate a sucking response, which involves generating a labial seal (contraction of the upper and lower orbicularis oris), and alternatively protruding and retracting the tongue. Tactile stimulation of the perioral region is mediated by the V trigeminal nerve, and central mediation of sucking is within the midbrain reticular formation. If the side of the newborn's tongue is touched, the infant's tongue will move in the direction of the stimulus, and this is called the **orienting reflex**. The rooting and sucking reflexes are actually composites of more basic reflexive responses (Miller, 2003).

> **rooting reflex:** reflexive response of infant to tactile stimulation of the cheek or lips; causes the infant to turn toward the stimulus and open his or her mouth

Uvular (Palatal) Reflex

Uvular elevation occurs in response to the excitation of IX glossopharyngeal general visceral afferent (GVA) component (see Appendix G) by irritation. It appears to be mediated in a manner similar to the gag reflex (see next section), involving the palatal muscles innervated by the X vagus.

Gag (Pharyngeal) Reflex

The **gag reflex** is elicited by tactile stimulation of the faucial pillars, posterior pharyngeal wall, or posterior tongue near the lingual tonsils (Miller, 2003). Tactile stimulation (light or deep touch) of this region is mediated by the IX glossopharyngeal nerve GVA component.

Desensitizing the Gag Reflex

A hyperactive gag reflex can be quite problematic. Although the gag reflex for most of us is stimulated by contacting the posterior tongue, or lateral and posterior pharyngeal walls, some people experience a hyperactive gag reflex. In our clinic, we have seen children with gag reflexes that are so sensitive that simply touching the lips triggers a gag response. You may have experienced a little twinge when trying to brush your tongue when brushing your teeth, so you have a notion of how sensitive the gag can be. This points out how important it is to desensitize the gag reflex, as well, because children with hyperactive gag reflex do not enjoy brushing their teeth.

Desensitizing the gag reflex involves slowly and systematically stimulating the oral and perioral regions, so that you never actually trigger the response itself. It is a slow work that requires a lot of trust by the client, but the benefits are great for the client, the parents, and you, the clinician.

Dendrites convey sensation through the petrosal (inferior) and superior ganglia of the IX glossopharyngeal to the solitary nucleus and solitary fasciculus of the medulla oblongata in the brain stem. Connection with the X vagus nerve via interneurons activates the muscles of general visceral efferent (GVE) lineage, including abdominal muscles and muscles of the velum and pharynx, causing the soft palate to elevate and the pharynx to elevate and constrict. Note that, as mentioned earlier, the gag reflex can be elicited by taste, specifically mediated by the IX glossopharyngeal nerve, special visceral afferent (SVA) component.

Retch and Vomit Reflex

Retching is an involuntary attempt at vomiting. **Vomiting** (emesis) refers to the oral expulsion of gastrointestinal contents. The retching reflex is a complex response mediated by noxious smells (I olfactory), tastes (IX glossopharyngeal), gastrointestinal distress (X vagus), vestibular dysfunction (VIII vestibulocochlear), or even a distressing visual or mental stimulation. Stimulation by one or more of these sensory systems activates a retching center located near the swallow center in the reticular formation of the medulla oblongata, near the motor nuclei associated with the complex of responses associated with vomiting. The vomit response includes multiple simultaneous or synchronous reflexes, including occlusion of the airway by vocal fold adduction, extreme contraction of abdominal muscles, relaxation of the upper and lower esophageal sphincters, elevation of the larynx and velum, depression of the epiglottis, elevation of the pharynx, and tongue protrusion (Miller, 2003).

Cough Reflex

The **cough** reflex is typically initiated by noxious stimulation of the pharynx, larynx, or bronchial passageway. The GVA component of the vagus nerve transmits information concerning this stimulation to the nucleus solitarius of the medulla. Interneurons activate the expiration center of the medullary reticular formation, which causes the abdominal muscles to contract. The nucleus ambiguus, the motor nucleus of the X vagus, causes laryngeal adduction before exhalation, permitting sufficient subglottal pressure to be generated to dislodge the irritating substance from the airway.

Pain Reflex

Although not technically a reflex associated with mastication or deglutition, the **pain withdrawal reflex** can have an effect on mastication and swallowing. You may remember the unpleasant sensation of having a lesion on your tongue or oral mucosa. When you masticate, you become very aware of the area and tend to avoid it if possible. This response represents a conscious version of the withdrawal response, a natural response to noxious stimuli. The classic withdrawal reflex involves rapid, total removal of a limb from a noxious stimulus, such as a hot stove. Oral and pharyngeal pain responses include the removal of noxious bolus (spicy or excessively hot food), either by expectoration or by swallowing.

Apneic Reflex

The apneic reflex is a protective response that is active during swallowing. It can be elicited through stimulation of the oral cavity, pharynx or larynx, which results in adduction of the vocal folds, elevation of the larynx, and inversion of the epiglottis, as well as cessation of respiration (Miller, 2003).

Respiration Reflexes

Respiration occurs reflexively but can be voluntarily controlled to a degree. A sensor system near the carotid sinus (the **carotid body**) responds to the quantity of oxygen and carbon dioxide in the blood, as well as to blood acidity. When oxygen levels decline below a specific criterion level, or when carbon dioxide or acidity increases beyond a specific level, a signal mediated by the IX glossopharyngeal nerve via the nucleus solitarius is relayed to the respiratory center, which increases the respiration rate. There are individual inspiratory and expiratory centers: excitation of inspiration inhibits expiratory musculature, and vice versa. The two respiratory centers are located in the lower medulla (the inspiratory and expiratory controls are separate). Mechanical stimulation of the nasopharynx can cause reflexive inhalation (known as the sniff reflex or aspiration reflex), and stimulation of the pharynx can cause forced expiration. Obstructing or restricting the nasal passageway will result in oral respiration (Miller, 2003).

✔ *To summarize:*

- **Chewing, sucking**, and **swallowing** are the products of numerous individual reflex patterns executed in a synchronous sequence.
- The **chewing reflex** involves rotatory movement of the mandible, coordinated with movement of the bolus by the tongue.
- The **rooting reflex** involves orientation to light tactile stimulation of the cheek area, which causes the infant's head to turn toward the stimulus.
- The **sucking reflex** is elicited by soft contact with the inner margin of the lips, causing protrusion and retraction of the tongue, as well as closing of the lips.
- **Uvular elevation** occurs in response to the tactile stimulation of faucial pillars, lingual tonsils, or upper pharynx.
- The **gag reflex** is elicited by the tactile stimulation of faucial pillars, posterior faucial wall, or posterior tongue near the lingual tonsils. It results in the termination of respiration and elevation of the larynx.
- The **retching** and **vomiting reflexes** are complex responses that are similar to the gag.
- The **cough reflex** involves laryngeal adduction, abdominal contraction to develop increased subglottal pressure, and forceful exhalation.
- The **pain withdrawal reflex** causes withdrawal from a noxious stimulus.
- **Respiration** occurs because of inadequate oxygenation of or excessive carbon dioxide in the blood or blood acidity.

REEXAMINATION OF THE PATTERNS FOR MASTICATION AND DEGLUTITION: A COMPLEX INTEGRATION OF REFLEXES AND VOLUNTARY ACTION

The patterns associated with mastication and deglutition are governed by unconscious, automatic sensorimotor systems. Again, this does not mean that the processes will not reach consciousness or that they cannot be controlled voluntarily (i.e., cortically), but rather that they spring from basic protective and nutritive reflexes and, more importantly, a superordinate CPG. Let us examine the processes of mastication and deglutition from a brain stem control perspective.

Receipt of food by the tongue appears to have evolved from the basic tongue posture of the neonate. The infant suckling gesture involves three to four piston-like pumps followed by a protrusive swallow. During the suck cycles, the liquid is pooled on the tongue in preparation for swallowing, a gesture not unlike the tongue dishing that occurs as adults and infants receive food into the mouth. In the mature mastication pattern, food is moved from the tongue to the molars for chewing, processes that are governed by the chewing response of the midbrain, and is mixed with saliva, production of which is triggered by taste primarily on the anterior two-thirds of the tongue. Tactile sensation within the oral cavity provides feedback concerning the consistency, size, and shape of the bolus. The bolus is retained within the oral cavity with the aid of the buccal musculature and orbicularis oris, as well as the depressed velum and elevation of the posterior tongue.

When the consistency of the bolus is sensed to be adequate, the mature swallow is initiated. The palatal reflex is stimulated by the contact of an object with the fauces or pharynx and causes the velum to elevate. The pharyngeal reflex is initiated by similar contact with the fauces, posterior tongue base, or valleculae by the bolus. In reality, the determination of whether these two reflexes result in ingestion or expulsion of the bolus depends on the nature of the stimulus (see Figure 8-13). Both noxious and benevolent stimuli result in the elevation of the larynx and opening of the cricopharyngeus, but only noxious stimuli elicit abdominal contraction related to vomiting or retching. When the bolus is propelled posteriorly, the orbicularis oris, buccinator, risorius, masseter, temporalis, medial pterygoid, and superior constrictor all contract, which in turn pulls the superior constrictor forward by virtue of its attachment. If the bolus is "palatable," the middle and inferior constrictors will assist in ingestion, whereas an unpalatable bolus would stimulate an opposite response.

The process of bolus transport through the oral cavity, transport through the pharynx, and movement through the esophagus, is tightly orchestrated at the brain stem level by the CPG for swallowing (Jean, 2001; Ertekin & Aydogdu, 2003). There is no doubt that reflexes play an important role in swallowing, but it is the highly ordered activity involving those reflexes that results in swallowing.

The CPG for swallowing is a complex set of neural structures that work in a coordinated fashion to orchestrate the act of swallowing. If you have ever played with dominoes by standing them on end so that you can see them fall sequentially, you will have a fairly good analogy for the swallowing CPG. You can push the first domino in the sequence and watch them fall one at a time. You can also pick a domino in the middle of the sequence and push it over, watching the sequence play out from that point. There is evidence that the swallowing CPG will move toward its end point, even if the CPG is triggered in the middle of the sequence. If you trigger the CPG at the pharyngeal elevation, for instance, you would not get the early "dominoes" to fall (e.g., velar elevation), but you will get the rest of the sequence to faithfully occur. The swallowing CPG is frankly amazing, so let's take a look at the neural components.

The swallowing CPG is actually made up of two networks of autonomous excitatory and inhibitory premotor interneurons that generate rhythmic outputs without requiring sensory input (Pearson & Gordon, 2013): The dorsal swallowing group (DSG) and ventral swallowing group (VSG), both within the medulla oblongata. (Before going too far into this discussion, we must note that, while sensory input is not *required* for the rhythmic output to occur, the CPG for swallowing is sensitive to environmental variables that modify the output, such as bolus size and texture.) The DSG is located in the medulla oblongata near the solitary tract nucleus, but the VSG is near the nucleus ambiguus. The DSG is responsible for generation of the swallowing pattern, whereas the VSG is responsible for activation of the nuclei that will actually elicit the motor response (Ertekin & Aydogdu, 2003). There are swallowing CPG circuits on both left and right sides of the medulla, and the VSG on one side activates the DSG on the contralateral side (Jean, 2001).

The VSG receives its sensory input from the maxillary branch of the V trigeminal nerve, the IX glossopharyngeal nerve, and the SLN of the X vagus (Jean, 2001), which convey sensory information to the solitary tract nucleus from the tongue dorsum, epiglottis, fauces, and posterior pharyngeal wall. Electrical stimulation of either the solitary tract nucleus or superior laryngeal nerve is like pushing the "start button:" it will invariably elicit a complete swallow sequence.

It is important to recognize that the swallowing CPG interacts with the respiratory CPG. Respiration is the product of pools of neurons that create rhythmic motor responses, but obviously the apneic period of swallowing must be coordinated with the transport period. This obligatory coordination occurs as a result of shared neuron pool components (Broussard & Altschuler, 2000).

We speak of swallowing as a strictly involuntary (albeit highly patterned) phenomenon, but we must also acknowledge the ability to initiate the swallow voluntarily under cortical control. It appears that the cortex can activate the medullary circuitry for swallowing, and a cortical lesion (for instance, from cerebrovascular accident) can disrupt swallowing despite leaving an intact brainstem physiology. In addition, we should acknowledge the fact that the structures governed by the reflexive and patterned neuronal systems can be voluntarily moved, which is very good news for the clinician. Procedures such as the Mendelsohn maneuver and the supraglottic swallow (e.g., Logemann, 1998) capitalize on a client's ability to voluntarily protect the airway, even if reflexive systems are deficient. Indeed, pleasant tastes evoke stronger pharyngeal motor responses than bitter tastes when subjects were stimulated transcranially (Mistry, Rothwell, Thompson, & Hamdy, 2006), which supports the therapeutic use of gustation in clients with oropharyngeal dysphagia.

We think of mastication and deglutition as common and every day, and we perform these acts easily and seamlessly. Nonetheless, these actions are comprised of motor elements that have their roots in basic reflexive responses to specific types of stimulation. This understanding is critical for those speech-language pathologists who work with all children (whether they have swallowing disorders or not) and adults who may have acquired swallowing disorders. This knowledge will allow you, as a speech-language pathologist, to approach the diagnosis and treatment of the disordered swallow stages with a better understanding of the systems you are attempting to evaluate, remediate, and provide compensation for.

CHAPTER SUMMARY

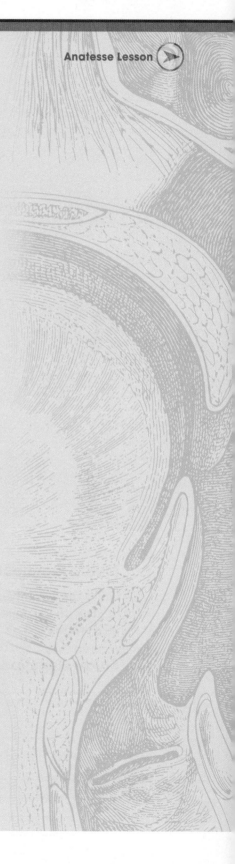

Anatesse Lesson

Mastication and deglutition can be viewed behaviorally or as a system of reflexive responses. The behavioral stages of mastication and deglutition include the oral (oral preparatory and oral transport), pharyngeal, and esophageal stages. In the oral preparatory stage, food is introduced into the oral cavity, moved onto the molars for chewing, and mixed with saliva to form a concise bolus between the tongue and the hard palate. In the oral transport stage, the bolus is moved back toward the oropharynx by the tongue. The pharyngeal stage begins when the bolus reaches the faucial pillars. The soft palate and larynx elevate, and the bolus is propelled through the pharynx to the upper esophageal sphincter, which has relaxed to receive the material. The tongue contacts the posterior pharyngeal wall, increasing pharyngeal pressure and driving the bolus into the open, awaiting esophagus. The epiglottis has dropped to partially cover the laryngeal opening, whereas the intrinsic musculature of the larynx has effected a tight seal to protect the airway. The final, esophageal stage involves the peristaltic movement of the bolus through the esophagus. Sensory elements of mastication and deglutition are critical for the elicitation of the muscular components of chewing and swallowing, as well as the maintenance of the various qualities of these processes. Gustation (taste) is mediated by chemoreceptors that transmit information to the brain via the IX glossopharyngeal and VII facial nerves. Taste sensors are specialized for sweet, sour, salty, bitter, and umami taste senses. Taste sense determines whether a bolus is ingested or removed from the oral cavity. Oral chemesthesis refers to detection of chemicals by means of pain and thermal sensors within the oral cavity, and stimuli eliciting these responses may be used to facilitate swallowing responses.

Olfaction (the sense of smell) is mediated by chemoreceptors within the nasal mucosa. The tactile sense (sense of touch) is mediated by mechanoreceptors that respond to deep or shallow touch. Four classes of thermal stimulation are differentiated by human senses: warm, hot, cool, and cold. Pain sense (nociception) is a response to a noxious stimulus, and acts as a protective response against the inappropriate entry of foreign objects into the gastrointestinal system. Muscle stretch is sensed by muscle spindle fibers, and muscle tension is sensed by Golgi tendon organs, found within tendons and fascia. Tactile sense, thermal sense, pain sense, and joint and tendon sense of the face and oral cavity are mediated by the V trigeminal, IX glossopharyngeal, and X vagus nerves. Oral chemesthesis is mediated by the V trigeminal nerve. Salivation occurs because of the stimulation of salivary glands. The type of saliva produced varies by gland: the sublingual gland produces thick mucus secretions, the submandibular gland produces both thin serous and mucus secretions, and the parotid gland secretes only serous saliva.

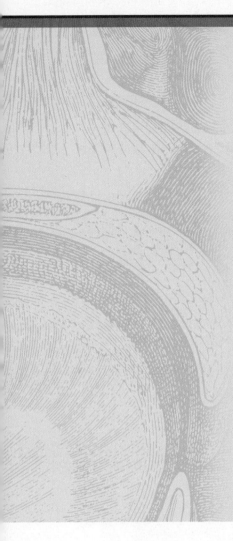

A neurophysiological view of CSS patterns reveals that chewing, sucking, and swallowing are the products of numerous individual reflex patterns executed in a synchronous sequence. The chewing reflex involves rotatory movement of the mandible, coordinated with the movement of bolus by the tongue. The rooting reflex is oriented to light tactile stimulation of the cheek area, which causes the infant's head to turn toward the stimulus. The sucking reflex, which supports the developmentally earlier suckling response, is elicited by soft contact with the inner margin of the lips and causes protrusion and retraction of the tongue, as well as closing of the lips. The uvular elevation of the palatal reflex occurs in response to the tactile stimulation of the faucial pillars, lingual tonsils, or upper pharynx. The gag reflex is elicited by the tactile stimulation of the faucial pillars, posterior faucial wall, or posterior tongue near the lingual tonsils. It results in the termination of respiration and the elevation of the larynx. The retching and vomiting reflexes are complex responses similar to the gag. The cough reflex involves laryngeal adduction, abdominal contraction to develop increased subglottal pressure, and forceful exhalation. The pain withdrawal reflex causes withdrawal from a noxious stimulus. Respiration occurs because of inadequate oxygenation of or excessive carbon dioxide in the blood or blood acidity. The oral transport, pharyngeal, and esophageal stages are a seamless series of highly orchestrated actions that are the actions of many reflexes under control of the central pattern generators (CPGs) for swallowing. The dorsal swallowing generator (DSG) is responsible for planning the pharyngeal swallow, whereas the ventral swallowing generator (VSG) is responsible for the execution of the plan. There are likewise CPGs for respiration and mastication, sucking and licking.

Media Connection

Go to the accompanying online resources at CengageBrain.com and have fun learning! Study with the Anatesse software program, play games, view animations and videos, and take practice tests to help reinforce the key concepts you learned in this chapter.

Study Questions

1. _____ refers to the process of preparing food for swallowing.

2. _____ refers to the process of swallowing.

3. _____ refers to a "ball" of food or drink.

4. List five of the elements of the oral preparatory stage of mastication and deglutition.

   a. _____

   b. _____

   c. _____

   d. _____

   e. _____

5. List three of the elements of the oral transport stage of deglutition.

    a. _____

    b. _____

    c. _____

6. List seven of the critical elements of the pharyngeal stage of deglutition.

    a. _____

    b. _____

    c. _____

    d. _____

    e. _____

    f. _____

    g. _____

7. The _____ reflex involves orienting toward the direction of tactile stimulation to the cheek.

8. _____ refers to "mouth region."

9. The _____ reflex is elicited by soft contact with the lower lip and results in tongue protrusion and retraction.

10. List two essential differences between the oral-pharyngeal anatomy and physiology of an infant and that of an adult.

    a. _____

    b. _____

11. The _____ stage is the stage in which food is prepared for a swallow.

12. The _____ stage is the stage of swallow involving the oral transit of the bolus to the pharynx.

13. The _____ stage is the stage of swallow involving the transit of the bolus to the esophagus and includes numerous physiological protective responses.

14. The _____ stage is the stage of swallow in which food is transported from the upper esophageal region to the stomach.

15. _____ refers to wavelike action.

16. List three critical elements related to the pressures of deglutition.

    a. _____

    b. _____

    c. _____

17. _____ refers to the sense of taste.

18. _____ is the class of receptors that respond to chemical stimulation.

19. _____ refers to the detection of chemicals that stimulate pain and thermal sense within the oral cavity.

20. Taste from the anterior two-thirds of the tongue is mediated by the _____ cranial nerve (name and number).

21. Taste from the posterior one-third of the tongue is mediated by the _____ cranial nerve (name and number).

22. Taste from the epiglottis and esophagus is mediated by the _____ cranial nerve (name and number).

23. The taste of bitterness is predominantly transmitted by the _____ cranial nerve (name and number).

24. The taste of sweetness is predominantly mediated by the _____ cranial nerve (name and number).

25. The tastes of sourness and saltiness are predominantly mediated by the _____ cranial nerve (name and number).

26. Oral chemesthetic sensations are mediated by the _____ cranial (nerve and number).

27. _____ refers to the sense of smell.

28. _____ corpuscles respond to minute mechanical movements in the superficial epithelia.

29. _____ receptors transmit the sense of pressure within the superficial epithelia.

30. _____ respond to rapid deep pressure.

31. Cells with _____ endings sense stretch within the deep layers of the epithelium.

32. List the four classes of thermal receptors that mediate thermal events.

    a. _____
    b. _____
    c. _____
    d. _____

33. T/F Thermal sensors and pain sensors share the same morphology.

34. _____ refers to the sense of pain.

35. Muscle stretch is sensed by _____.

36. T/F Facial muscles have muscle spindles.

37. _____ sense muscle tension.

38. _____ refers to the production and release of saliva into the oral cavity.

39. The parotid glands release _____ (type of saliva) into the posterior oral cavity and pharynx.

40. The sublingual glands release _____ (type of saliva) into the anterior oral cavity.

41. The _____ reflex involves rotary motion of the muscles of mastication.

42. The _____ reflex involves elevation of the soft palate.

43. The _____ reflex involves evacuation of the contents of the stomach.

44. The _____ reflex involves contracting the muscles of adduction and forcefully blowing them open to expel foreign matter from the respiratory passageway.

Study Question Answers

1. **MASTICATION** refers to the process of preparing food for swallowing.

2. **DEGLUTITION** refers to the process of swallowing.

3. **BOLUS** refers to a "ball" of food or drink.

4. List five of the elements of the oral preparatory stage of mastication and deglutition.

    a. Food is received in mouth, and food is impounded in mouth by lip sealing, tongue dorsum elevating and velum depressing

    b. Food is moved onto molars by tongue

    c. Food is mixed with saliva

    d. Food is formed into bolus

    e. Food is removed from buccal cavity by tongue action

5. List three of the elements of the oral transport stage of deglutition.

    a. Tongue tip elevates to alveolar ridge

    b. Bolus is propelled posteriorly by squeezing action

    c. Bolus makes contact with faucial pillars and velum

6. List seven of the critical elements of the pharyngeal stage of deglutition. Answer could include any of the following:

- Bolus enters oropharynx
- Velum elevates
- Larynx elevates
- Vocal folds adduct
- Epiglottis inverts to protect airway
- Tongue contacts posterior pharyngeal wall
- Upper esophageal sphincter opens
- Pharynx contracts with peristaltic action

7. The **ROOTING** reflex involves orienting toward the direction of tactile stimulation to the cheek.

8. **PERIORAL** refers to "mouth region."

9. The **SUCKING** reflex is elicited by soft contact with the lower lip, and results in tongue protrusion and retraction.

10. List two essential differences between the oral-pharyngeal anatomy and physiology of an infant and that of an adult.

    a. **LARYNX IS ELEVATED IN INFANT**

    b. **TONGUE FILLS GREATER PROPORTION OF ORAL CAVITY**

11. The **ORAL PREPARATORY** stage is the stage in which food is prepared for a swallow.

12. The **ORAL** stage is the stage of swallow involving the oral transit of the bolus to the pharynx.

13. The **PHARYNGEAL** stage is the stage of swallow involving the transit of the bolus to the esophagus, and includes numerous physiological protective responses.

14. The **ESOPHAGEAL** stage is the stage of swallow in which food is transported from the upper esophageal region to the stomach.

15. **PERISTALSIS** refers to wavelike action.

16. List three critical elements related to the pressures of deglutition.

    a. **VELUM ELEVATES**

    b. **TONGUE AND LIPS FORM ORAL SEAL**

    c. **CRICOPHARYNGEUS OPENS AS LARYNX ELEVATES**

17. **GUSTATION** refers to the sense of taste.

18. **CHEMORECEPTOR** is the class of receptors that respond to chemical stimulation.

19. **ORAL CHEMESTHESIS** refers to the detection of chemicals that stimulate pain and thermal sense within the oral cavity.

20. Taste from the anterior two-thirds of the tongue is mediated by the **VII FACIAL** cranial nerve (name and number).

21. Taste from the posterior one-third of the tongue is mediated by the **IX GLOSSOPHARYNGEAL** cranial nerve (name and number).

22. Taste from the epiglottis and esophagus is mediated by the **X VAGUS** cranial nerve (name and number).

23. The taste of bitterness is predominantly transmitted by the **IX GLOSSOPHARYNGEAL** cranial nerve (name and number).

24. The taste of sweetness is predominantly mediated by the **VII FACIAL** cranial nerve (name and number).

25. The tastes of sourness and saltiness are predominantly mediated by the **VII FACIAL** cranial nerve (name and number).

26. Oral chemesthetic sensations are mediated by the **V TRIGEMINAL** cranial nerve (name and number).

27. **OLFACTION** refers to the sense of smell.

28. **MEISSNER'S** corpuscles respond to minute mechanical movements in the superficial epithelia.

29. **MERKEL DISK** receptors transmit the sense of pressure within the superficial epithelia.

30. **PACINIAN CORPUSCLES** respond to rapid deep pressure.

31. Cells with **RUFFINI** endings sense stretch within the deep layers of the epithelium.

32. List the four classes of thermal receptors that mediate thermal events.
    a. **COOL**
    b. **COLD**
    c. **WARM**
    d. **HOT**

33. **T** Thermal sensors and pain sensors share the same morphology.

34. **NOCICEPTION** refers to the sense of pain.

35. Muscle stretch is sensed by **MUSCLE SPINDLES**.

36. **FACIAL** muscles have muscle spindles.

37. **GOLGI TENDON ORGANS** sense muscle tension.

38. **SALIVATION** refers to the production and release of saliva into the oral cavity.

39. The parotid glands release **SEROUS** (type of saliva) into the posterior oral cavity and pharynx.

40. The sublingual glands release **MUCUS** (type of saliva) into the anterior oral cavity.

41. The **CHEWING** reflex involves rotary motion of the muscles of mastication.

42. The **UVULAR (PALATAL)** reflex involves elevation of the soft palate.

43. The **VOMIT** reflex involves evacuation of the contents of the stomach.

44. The **COUGH** reflex involves contracting the muscles of adduction and forcefully blowing them open to expel foreign matter from the respiratory passageway.

Bibliography

Arvedson, J. C., & Brodsky, L. (2002). *Pediatric swallowing and feeding: Assessment and management* (2nd ed.). Clifton Park, NY: Delmar Publishers.

Baehr, M., & Frotscher, M. (2012). *Topical diagnosis in neurology.* New York: Thieme.

Bateman, H. E., & Mason, R. M. (1984). *Applied anatomy and physiology of the speech and hearing mechanism.* Springfield, IL: Charles C. Thomas.

Beck, E. W., Monson, H., & Groer, M. (1982). *Mosby's atlas of functional human anatomy.* St. Louis, MO: C. V. Mosby.

Bhatnagar, S. C. (2007). *Neuroscience for the study of communicative disorders* (3rd ed.). Philadelphia, PA: Lippincott, Williams & Wilkins.

Bly, L. (1983). *The components of normal movement during the first year of life and abnormal motor movement.* Chicago: Neuro-Developmental Treatment Association.

Bly, L. (1994). *Motor skills acquisition in the first year.* Tucson, AZ: Therapy Skill Builders.

Bowman, J. P. (1971). *The muscle spindle and neural control of the tongue.* Springfield, IL: Charles C. Thomas.

Broussard, D. L., & Altschuler, S. M. (2000). Brainstem viscerotopic organization of afferents and efferents involved in the control of swallowing. *American Journal of Medicine, 108*(4A), 79S–86S.

Brown, P. (1994). Pathophysiology of spasticity. *Journal of neurology neurosurgery and psychiatry, 57,* 773–777.

Buck, L. B. (2000). Smell and taste: The chemical senses. In E. R. Kandel, J. H. Schwartz, & T. M. Jessell (Eds.), *Principles of neural science* (4th ed.). New York: McGraw-Hill.

Bülow, M., Olsson, R., & Ekberg, O. (2003). Videoradiographic analysis of how carbonated thin liquids and thickened liquids affect the physiology of swallowing in subjects with aspiration on thin liquids. *Acta Radiologica, 44*(4), 366–372.

Burbank, E., Seikel, J., & Burke, R. (2006). The perception of umami in non-pathological individuals. Poster presented at the Annual Convention of the American Speech-language Hearing Association.

Campbell, N. A. (1990). *Biology.* Redwood City, CA: Benjamin/Cummings.

Carpenter, M. B. (1991). *Core text of neuroanatomy* (4th ed.). Baltimore: Williams & Wilkins.

Chusid, J. G. (1985). *Correlative neuroanatomy and functional neurology* (17th ed.). Los Altos, CA: Lange Medical Publications.

Commetto-Muñiz, J. E., Cain, W. S., & Abraham, M. H. (2004). Chemosensory additivity in trigeminal chemoreception as reflected by detection of mixtures. *Experimental brain research, 158,* 196–206.

Corbin-Lewis, K., Liss, J. M., & Sciortino, K. L. (2005). *Clinical anatomy & physiology of the swallow mechanism.* Clifton Park, NJ: Thomson Delmar Learning.

Cotman, C. W., & McGaugh, J. L. (1980). *Behavioral neuroscience.* New York: Academic Press.

Cowart, B. J. (1998). The addition of CO_2 to traditional taste solutions alters taste quality. *Chemical senses, 23*(4), 397–402.

Crary, M. A., Carnaby-Mann, G. D., & Groher, M. E. (2006). Identification of swallowing events from sEMG signals obtained from healthy adults. *Dysphagia, 22,* 94–99.

Delaney, A. L., & Arvedson, J. C. (2008). Development of swallowing and feeding: Prenatal through first year of life. *Developmental disabilities research reviews, 14,* 105–117.

Dodds, W. J., Stewart, E. T., & Logemann, J. A. (1990). Physiology and radiology of the normal and pharyngeal phases of swallowing. *American Journal of Roentgenology, 154,* 953–963.

Doty, R. W., & Bosma, J. F. (1956). An electromyographic analysis of reflex deglutition. *Journal of neurophysiology, 19,* 44–60.

Dessirier, J. M., Simons, C. T., Carstens, M. I., O'Mahony, M., & Carstens, E. (2000). Psychophysical and neurobiological evidence that the oral sensation elicited by carbonated water is of chemogenic origin. *Chemical senses, 25*(3), 277–284.

Ertekin, C. & Aydogdu, I (2003). Nerophysiology of swallowing. *Clinical Neurophysiology, 114,* 2226–2244.

Ertekin, C., Kiylioglu, N., Tarlaci, S., Truman, A. B., Secil, Y. & Aydogdu, I. (2011). Voluntary and reflex influences on the initiation of swallowing reflex in man. *Dysphagia, 16,* 40–47.

Fujii, N., Inamoto, Y., Saitoh, E., Baba, M., Okada, S., Yoshioka, S., Nakai, T., Ida, Y., Katada, K., & Palmer, K. (2011). Evaluation of swallowing using 320-detector-row multislice CT. Part I. Single- and Multiphase volume scanning for three-dimensional morphological and kinematic analysis. *Dysphagia, 27,* 99–107.

Ganong, W. F. (2005). *Review of medical physiology* (22nd ed.). New York: McGraw-Hill/Appleton & Lange.

Geran, L. C. & Travers, S. P. (2011). Glossopharyngeal nerve transection impairs unconditioned avoidance of diverse bitter stimuli in rats. *Behavioral Neuroscience, 125*(4), 519–528.

Gilroy, A. M., MacPherson, B. R., & Ross, L. M. (2012). *Atlas of anatomy* (2nd ed.). New York: Thieme.

Gosling, J. A., Harris, P. F., Humpherson, J. R., Whitmore, I., & Willan, P. L. T. (1985). *Atlas of human anatomy*. Philadelphia: J. B. Lippincott.

Goyal, R. K., Padmanabhan, R., & Sang, Q. (2001). Neural circuits in swallowing and abdominal vagal afferent-mediated lower esophageal sphincter relaxation. *The American Journal of Medicine, 111*(8A), 1–11.

Gray, H., Bannister, L. H., Berry, M. M., & Williams, P. L. (1995). *Gray's anatomy*. London: Churchill Livingstone.

Green, B. G. (2012). Chemesthesis and the chemical senses as components of a "chemofensor complex." *Chemical senses, 37*, 201–206.

Grobler, N. J. (1977). *Textbook of clinical anatomy* (Vol. 1). Amsterdam: Elsevier Scientific.

Groher, M. E. (1997). *Dysphagia* (3rd ed.). St. Louis, MO: Butterworth-Heinemann.

Healey, J. E., & Seybold, W. D. (1969). *A synopsis of clinical anatomy*. Philadelphia: W. B. Saunders.

Gumbley, F., Huckabee, M. L., Doeltgen, S. H., Witte, U., & Moran, C. (2008). Effects of bolus volume on pharyngeal contact pressure during normal swallowing. *Dysphagia, 23*, 280–285.

Hoebler, C., Karinthi, A., Devaux, M. F., Guillon, F., Gallant, D.J.G., Bouchet, B., Melegari, M., & Barry, J. L. (1998). Physical and chemical transformations of cereal food during oral digestion in human subjects. *British Journal of Nutrition, 80*, 429–436.

Hoffman, M. R., Mielens, J. D., Ciucci, M. R., Jones, C. A., Jiang, J. J., & McCulloch, T. M. (2012). High-resolution manometry of pharyngeal swallow pressure events associated with effortful swallow and the Mendelsohn maneuver. *Dysphagia, 27*, 418–426.

Hoon, M. A., Adler, E., Lindemeier, J., Battey, J. F., Ryba, N. J. P., & Zuker, C. S. (1999). Putative mammalian taste receptors: A class of taste-specific GPCRs with distinct topographic selectivity. *Cell, 96*, 541–551.

Huang, A. L., Chen, X., Hoon, M. A., Chandrashekar, J., Guo, W., Trankner, D., Ryba, N. J. P., & Zuker, C. S. (2006). The cells and logic for mammalian sour taste detection. *Nature, 442*, 934–938.

Jean, A. (2001). Brain stem control of swallowing: Neuronal network and cellular mechanisms. *Physiological reviews, 81*(2), 929–969.

Kahane, J. C., & Folkins, J. F. (1984). *Atlas of speech and hearing anatomy*. Columbus, OH: Charles E. Merrill.

Kandel, E. R., Schwartz, J. H., Jessell, T. M., Siegelbaum, S. A., & Hudspeth, A. J. (2013). *Principles of neural science* (5th ed.). New York: McGraw Hill.

Kliegman, R. M., Behrman, R. E., Jenson, H. B., & Stanton, B. F. (2007). *Nelson textbook of pediatrics*. Philadelphia, PA: Saunders.

Krival, K., & Bates C. (2012). Effects of club soda and ginger brew on linguapalatal pressures in healthy swallowing. *Dysphagia, 27*(2), 228–239.

Krival, K., & Bates, C. (2012). Effects of club soda and ginger brew on linguapalatal pressures in healthy swallowing. *Dysphagia, 27*, 228–239.

Kuehn, D. P., Lemme, M. L., & Baumgartner, J. M. (1991). *Neural bases of speech, hearing, and language*. Boston: Little, Brown.

Kuehn, D. P., Templeton, P. J., & Maynard, J. A. (1990). Muscle spindles in the velopharyngeal musculature of humans. *Journal of Speech and Hearing Research, 33*, 488–493.

Landgren, S., & Olsson, K. A. (1981). Oral mechanoreceptors. In S. Grillner, B. Lindblom, J. Lubker, & A. Persson (Eds.), *Speech motor control* (pp. 129–139). Oxford: Pergamon Press.

Lang, I. M. (2009). Brain stem control of the phases of swallowing. *Dysphagia, 24*, 333–348.

Lang, I. M., & Shaker, R. (1997). Anatomy and physiology of the upper esophageal sphincter. *The American journal of medicine. 103*(5A), 50s–55s.

Langley, M. B., & Lombardino, L. J. (1991). *Neurodevelopmental strategies for managing communication disorders in children with severe motor dysfunction*. Austin, TX: Pro-Ed.

Langmore, S. E., Schatz, K. & Olson, N. (1991). Endoscopic and videofluorsoscopic examination of swallowing and aspiration. *Annals of Otology, Rhinology and Laryngology, 100*(8), 678–681.

Lau, C., Smith, E. O., & Schanler, R. J. (2003). Coordination of suck-swallow and swallow respiration in preterm infants. *Acta Paediatrica, 92*(6), 721–727.

Liss, J. M. (1990). Muscle spindles in the human levator veli palatini and palatoglossus muscles. *Journal of Speech and Hearing Research, 33*, 736–746.

Logan, B. M., Hutchings, R. T., & Reynolds, P. (2003). *McMinn's color atlas of head and neck anatomy* (3rd ed.). Edinburgh, NY: Mosby.

Logemann, J. A. (1995). Dysphagia: evaluation and treatment. *Folia phoniatrica et logopedica, 47*(3), 140–164.

Logemann, J. (1998). *Evaluation and treatment of swallowing disorders* (2nd ed.). Austin, TX: Pro-Ed.

Lund, J. P., & Kolta, A. (2006). Generation of the central masticatory pattern and its modification by sensory feedback. *Dysphagia, 21*, 167–174.

Mackay, D. G. (1982). The problems of flexibility, fluency, and speed-accuracy trade-off in skilled behaviors. *Psychological Review, 89*, 483–506.

Martin-Harris, B., Brodsky, M. B., Michel, Y, Lee, F-S., & Walters, B. (2007). Delayed initiation of the pharyngeal swallow: Normal variability in adults swallows. *Journal of speech-language-hearing research, 50*, 585–594.

Mendell, D. A., & Logemann, J. A. (2007). Temporal sequences of swallowing events during the oropharyngeal swallow. *Journal of Speech-Language-Hearing Research, 50*, 1256–1271.

Matsuo, K., & Palmer, J. B. (2013). Oral phase prepration and propulsion: Anatomy, physiology, rheology, mastication, and transport. In Shaker, R., Belafsky, P. Co., & Postma, G. N. (Eds.), *Principles of deglutition: A multidisciplinary text for swallowing and its disorders* (pp. 117–132). New York: Springer.

Mattioli, S., Lugaresi, M., Zannoli, R., Brusori, S., & d'Ovidio, F. (2003). Ballon sensors for the manometric recording of the pharyngoesophageal tract: An experimental study. *Dysphagia, 18*, 249–254.

Mazari, A., Heath, M. R., & Prinz, J. F. (2007). Contribution of the cheeks to the intraoral manipulation of food. *Dysphagia, 22*, 117–121.

McKeown, M. J., Torpey, D. A., & Gehm, W. C. (2002). Non-invasive monitoring of distinctive muscle activations during swallowing. *Clinical Neurophysiology, 113*, 354–366.

Miller, A. (2002). Oral and pharyngeal reflexes in the mammalian nervous system: Their diverse range in complexity and the pivotal role of the tongue. *Critical Reviews in Oral Biology and Medicine, 13*, 409–425.

Mishellany, A., Woda, A., Labas, R., & Peyron, M.A. (2006). The challenge of mastication: Preparing a bolus suitable for deglutition. *Dysphagia, 21*, 87–94.

Mistry, S., Rothwell, J. C., Thompson, D. G., & Hamdy, S. (2006). Modulation of human cortical motor pathways after pleasant and aversive taste stimuli. *American Journal of Physiology: Gastrointestinal and Liver Physiology, 291*, G666–G671.

Møller, A. R. (2003). *Sensory systems: Anatomy and physiology.* New York: Academic Press.

Mountcastle, V. B. (1974). *Medical physiology.* St. Louis, MO: Mosby.

Mueller, K. L., Hoon, M. A., Erlenbach, I., Zuker, C. S., & Ryba, N. J., (2005). The receptors and coding logic for bitter taste. *Nature, 434*(7030), 225–229.

Nelson, G., Hoon, M. A., Chandrashekar, J., Zhang, Y., Ryba, N. J. P., & Zuker, C. S. (2001). Mammalian sweet taste receptors. *Cell, 106*, 381–390.

Netter, F. (1976). *Clinical symposia: Development of the upper respiratory system.* Summit, NJ: CIBA Pharmaceutical Company.

Netter, F. H. (1983). *The CIBA collection of medical illustrations. Vol. 1. Nervous system. Part I. Anatomy and physiology.* West Caldwell, NJ: CIBA Pharmaceutical Company.

Netter, F. H. (1997). *Atlas of human anatomy.* Los Angeles: Icon Learning Systems.

Newman, K. D., & Randolph, J. (1990). Surgical problems of the esophagus in infants and children. In D. C. Sabiston & F. C. Spencer (Eds.), *Surgery of the chest* (5th ed., pp. 815–839). Philadelphia: W. B. Saunders.

Ninomaya, Y., Imoto, T., & Sugimura, T. (1999). Sweet taste responses of mouse chorda tympani neurons: Existence of Gurmarin-sensitive and insensitive receptor components. *Journal of Neurophysiology, 81*(6), 3087–3091.

Nolte, J. (2002). *The human brain* (5th ed.). St. Louis, MO: Mosby.

Oka, Y., Butnaru, M., von Buchholtz, L., Ryba, N. J. P., & Zuker, C. S. (2013). High salt recruits aversive taste pathways. *Nature, 494*, 472–475.

Payne, W. S., & Ellis, F. H., Jr. (1984). Esophagus and ciaphragmatic hernias. In S. I. Schwartz, G. T. Shires, F. C. Spencer, & E. H. Storer (Eds.), *Principles of surgery* (4th ed., pp. 1063–1112). New York: McGraw-Hill.

Pearson, K. G., & Gordon, J. E. (2013). Locomotion. In Kandel, E. R., Schwartz, J. H., Jessell, T. M., Siegelbaum, S. A. & Hudspeth, A. J. (Eds.). *Principles of neural science* (5th ed.). New York: McGraw Hill, 812–834.

Pearson, W. G., Langmore, S. E., Uy, L. B., & Zumwalt, A. C. (2012). Structural analysis of muscles elevating the hyolaryngeal complex. *Dysphagia, 27*, 445–451.

Pelletier, C. A., & Dhanaraj, G. E. (2006). The effect of taste and palatability on lingual swallowing pressure. *Dysphagia, 11*, 121–128.

Pelletier, C. A., & Lawless, H. T. (2003). Effect of citric acid and citric acid-sucrose mixture on swallowing in neurogenic oropharyngeal dysphagia. *Dysphagia, 18*(4), 231–241.

Perlman, A. L., Grayhack, J. P., & Booth, B. M. (1992). The relationship of vallecular residue to oral involvement, reduced hyoid elevation, and epiglottic function. *Journal of Speech and Hearing Research, 35*, 734–741.

Perlman, A. L., Luschei, E. S., & Du Mond, C. E. (1989). Electrical activity from the superior pharyngeal constrictor during reflexive and nonreflexive tasks. *Journal of Speech and Hearing Research, 32*, 749–754.

Perlman, A. L., & Schulze-Delrieu, K. (1997). *Deglutition and its disorders.* San Diego, CA: Singular Publishing Group.

Peyron, M. A., Mishellany, A., & Woda, A. (2004). Particle size distribution of food boluses after mastication of six natural foods. *Journal of Dental Research, 83*, 573–582.

Printz, J. F., & Lucas, P. W. (1995). Swallow thresholds in human mastication. *Archives of Oral Biology, 40*(5), 401–403.

Rademaker, A. W., Pauloski, B. R., Logemann, J. A., & Shanahan, T. K. (1994). Oropharyngeal swallow efficiency as a representative measure of swallowing function. *Journal of Speech and Hearing Research, 37*, 314–325.

Reid, J. A., King, P. L., & Kilpatrick, N. M. (2000). Desensitization of the gag reflex in an adult with cerebral palsy: a case report. *Special Care in Dentistry, 20*(2), 56–60.

Rohen, J. W., Yokochi, C., & Lutjen-Drecoll, E. (2006). *Color atlas of anatomy* (6th ed.). Philadelphia: Williams & Wilkins.

Rosenbek, J. C., Robbins, J., Fishback, B., & Levine, R. L. (1991). Effects of thermal application on dysphagia after stroke. *Journal of Speech and Hearing Research, 34*, 1257–1268.

Rosse, C., Gaddum-Rosse, P., & Rosse, G. (1997). *Hollinshead's textbook of anatomy.* Philadelphia: Lippincott-Raven.

Schuenke, M., & Ross, L. M., (2010). *Thieme atlas of anatomy.* New York: Thieme.

Sdravou, K., Walshe, M., & Dagdilelis, L. (2012). Effects of carbonated liquids on oropharyngeal swallowing measures in people with neurogenic dysphagia. *Dysphagia, 27*(2), 240–250.

Segerstad, C. H., & Hellekant, G. (1989). The sweet taste in the calf. I. Chorda tympani proper nerve response to taste stimulation of the tongue. *Physiology and Behavior, 45*(3), 633–638.

Shah, A. S., Ben-Shahar, Y., Moninger, T. O., Kline, J. N., & Welsh, M. J. (2009). Motile cilia or human airway epithelia are chemosensory. *Science, 325*(5944), 1131–1134.

Sonies, B. C. (1997). *Dysphagia. A continuum of care.* Gaithersburg, MD: Aspen.

Standring, S. (2008). *Gray's anatomy: The anatomical and clinical basis of practice* (40th ed.). London: Churchill Livingstone.

Stephens, J. R., Taves, D. H., Smith, R. C., & Margin, R. E. (2005). Bolus location at the initiation of the pharyngeal stage of swallowing in healthy older adults. *Dysphagia, 20*, 266–272.

Tasko, S. M., Kent, R. D., & Westbury, J. R. (2002). Variability in tongue movement kinematics during normal liquid swallowing. *Dysphagia, 17*, 126–138.

Thexton, A. J., Crompton, A. W., & German, R. Z. (2007). Electromyographic activity during the reflex pharyngeal swallow in the pig: Doty and Bosma (1956) revisited. *Journal of Applied Physiology, 102*, 587–600.

Weber, C. M., & Smith, A. (1987). Reflex responses in human jaw, lip, and tongue muscles elicited by mechanical stimulation. *Journal of Speech and Hearing Research, 30*, 70–79.

Wickens, J., Hyland, B., & Anson, G. (1994). Cortical cell assemblies: A possible mechanism for motor programs. *Journal of Motor Behavior, 26*(2), 66–82.

Winans, S. S., Gilman, S., Manter, J. T., & Gatz, A. J. (2002). *Manter and Gatz's essentials of clinical neuroanatomy and neurophysiology* (10th ed.). Philadelphia: F. A. Davis.

Wohlert, A. B., & Goffman, L. (1994). Human perioral muscle activation patterns. *Journal of Speech and Hearing Research, 37*, 1032–1040.

Yoshida, M., Kikutani, T., Tsuga, K., Utanohara, Y., Hayashi, R., & Akagawa, Y. (2006). Decreased tongue pressure reflects symptoms of dysphagia. *Dysphagia, 21*, 61–65.

Zemlin, W. R. (1998). *Speech and hearing science: Anatomy and physiology* (4th ed.). Needham Heights, MA: Allyn & Bacon.

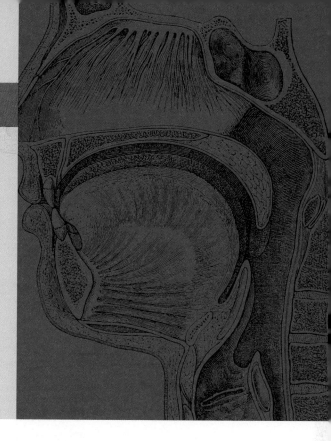

Chapter 9

ANATOMY OF HEARING

I t is a recurring theme that communication ability is superimposed on a physical system clearly designed for another function. The auditory system is the only system that has no other function besides communication. One might argue that our distant ancestors were more interested in the sounds that supported survival than those that arose from society, but nonetheless **audition** (the process associated with hearing) is an essential element of verbal communication.

The mechanisms of hearing are extraordinary in scope and complexity. In this chapter we will discuss the structures of hearing. Chapter 10 will be devoted to the reasons these structures exist: the physiology of hearing.

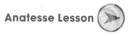

Anatesse Lesson

THE STRUCTURES OF HEARING

The physical structures of the ear are deceptively simple, especially in light of their exquisite function. The ear is an energy **transducer**, which means that it converts acoustic energy into electrochemical energy. The details of these structures will set the stage for the discussion of the transduction process in Chapter 10.

We will talk about the ear in terms of the basic elements involved: the outer ear, the middle ear, the inner ear, and, in Chapter 10, the auditory pathways (see Figure 9-1).

transducer: L., trans, across + ducer, to lead

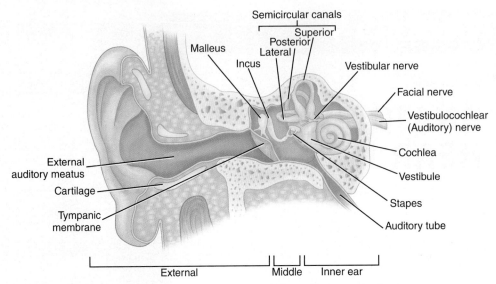

Figure 9-1. Schematic of frontal section revealing outer, middle, and inner ear structures.
© Cengage Learning®.

OUTER EAR

The outer ear is composed of two basic components with which you are quite familiar (Table 9-1). The **pinna** (or auricle) is the prominence we colloquially refer to as the ear, although it serves primarily as a collector of sound to be processed at deeper levels (e.g., the middle ear and the cochlea). The structure of the pinna is provided by a cartilagenous framework.

The pinna has several important functions, including aiding the localization of sound in space and "capturing" sound energy. Landmarks of the pinna are important for a number of reasons, not the least of which is their diagnostic significance for some genetic conditions (see Figure 9-2). The **helix** forms the curled margin of the pinna, marking its most distal borders. The superior-posterior bulge on the helix is known as the **auricular tubercle** (or **Darwin's tubercle**). Immediately anterior to the helix is the **antihelix**, a similar fold of tissue marking the entrance to the concha. Between the helix and antihelix is the **scaphoid fossa**. The antihelix bifurcates superiorly, producing the **crura anthelicis**, and the space between them forms the **triangular fossa (fossa triangularis)**. The **cymba conchae** is the anterior extension of the helix marking the anterior entrance to the concha, and the **cavum conchae** is the deep portion of the concha. The **concha** (or **concha auriculae**) is the entrance to the ear canal, known as the **external auditory meatus** (abbreviated [EAM]; alternately **meatus acousticus externus**). A flap of epithelium-covered cartilage known as the **tragus** looks as if it could cover the entrance to the meatus (and probably did in an earlier version of the auditory mechanism). Superior to the tragus is the **tuberculum supratragicum**. Posterior and inferior to the tragus is the **antitragus** (the region between tragus and antitragus is termed the **intertragic incisure** or **incisura intertragica**), and below the antitragus is the **lobule** or **lobe**.

pinna: L., feather

helix: Gr., coil

concha: Gr., konche, shell

tragus: Gr., tragos, goat

Table 9-1 **Landmarks of the outer ear**
Auricle (Pinna)
Helix
Auricular tubercle (Darwin's tubercle)
Antihelix
Crura
Crura anthelicis
Triangular fossa
Scaphoid fossa
Concha
Cymba conchae
Cavum conchae
Tragus
Intertragic incisure
Antitragus
Lobule
External Auditory Meatus
Cartilagenous meatus
Osseous meatus
Isthmus
Tympanic membrane

© Cengage Learning®.

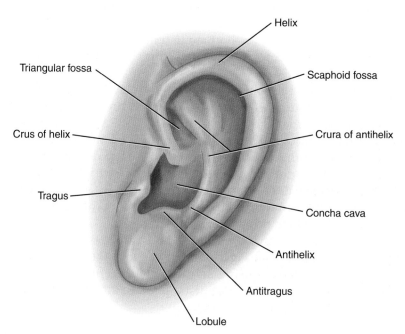

Figure 9-2. Landmarks of the auricle or pinna.
© Cengage Learning®.

Anatesse Lesson

speculum: L., mirror

If you palpate these structures on yourself, you will realize that the lobule is one of the few structures devoid of cartilage. The **auricular cartilage** is a unitary structure closely following the landmarks we have just described and is covered with a layer of epithelial tissue invested with fine hairs that are useful for keeping insects and dirt out of the ear canal.

The **external auditory meatus** is approximately 7 mm in diameter and 2.5 cm long when measured from the depth of the concha, but you would add another 1.5 cm to its length if you chose to measure it from the tragus. This is, in reality, not a trivial matter: The EAM and conchae are resonating cavities that both contribute to hearing and are a major determinant of the resonant frequency, as we shall see in Chapter 10.

The lateral third of the canal is comprised of cartilage and is about 8 mm long; the medial two-thirds is the bony meatus of the temporal bone. The EAM is S-shaped: If you were a fly walking toward the **eardrum (tympanic membrane [TM])**, you would start out hiking generally medially, forward, and up. At the juncture of the osseous and cartilaginous EAM, you would take a turn down as you made your approach. During your hike you would see two constrictions: The first marks the end of the cartilaginous portion and the beginning of the osseous EAM. The second constriction, termed the **isthmus**, is about 0.5 cm from the TM itself. At the end of your hike, you would run into the TM, a thin trilaminar sheet of tissue that sits at an oblique angle in the EAM. The epithelial cover of the pinna continues into the EAM and serves as the outer layer of the tympanic membrane, to be discussed.

Because the adult ear canal takes a turn downward, you cannot see the medial end of the canal without some effort. If you were to look into the ear canal (you will have to manipulate the pinna and use a **speculum**, a device used to view cavities of the body), you would see that the outer third of the EAM is lined with hairs, and has **cerumen**, or "ear wax." These are both quite functional additions to the canal, as they trap insects and dirt, protecting the medial-most point of the outer ear, the TM.

The TM marks the boundary between the outer and middle ear. It completely separates the two spaces, being an extremely thin three-layered sheet of tissue. The epithelial lining of the EAM continues as the external layer of the TM, while the lining of the middle ear provides the inner layer. Sandwiched between these two delicate epithelial linings is a layer of fibrous tissue that provides structure for the TM. This intermediate layer really consists of two layers of fibers. The radial and circular fibroelastic connective tissues provide optimal strength and tension to this intermediate layer.

The TM is approximately 55 mm^2 in area and has a number of important landmarks (see Figure 9-3). If you take the time to view one of your friend's TM using an otoscope (carefully), you will see the **umbo**, which is the most distal point of attachment of the inner TM to one of the bones of the middle ear, the malleus. The TM is particularly taut at this point, and the location inferior and anterior to this is referred to as the **cone of light** because it reflects the light of the audiologist's otoscope. You may be able to see the handle (or manubrium) of the malleus behind the TM, appearing as a streak on the membrane; if you are looking at the left TM, the handle of the malleus will look like the hand of a clock pointing to the 11.

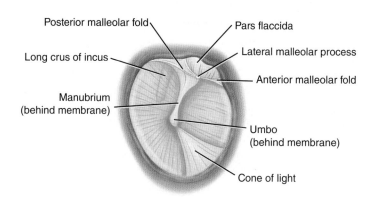

Posterior malleolar fold

Pars flaccida

Long crus of incus

Lateral malleolar process

Anterior malleolar fold

Manubrium
(behind membrane)

Umbo
(behind membrane)

Cone of light

Figure 9-3. Right ear tympanic membrane, as viewed from the external auditory meatus.
© Cengage Learning®.

Otitis Externa and Cerumen

The epithelial lining of the auricle and EAM is tightly bound to the cartilage and bone of these structures, and this binding accounts for the pain involved in any swelling of the tissue. **Otitis externa** refers to inflammation of the skin of the external ear. When tissue is inflamed, it responds with **edema** (swelling). If the epithelium is tightly bound to its underlying structure, as it is in the EAM and pinna, the swelling increases the tension on the epithelium, making it quite painful.

Otitis externa may result from bacterial infection following trauma or abrasion. Failure to clean probe tips and specula could result in the transmission of the infection between clients. Otitis externa may also result from viral infection, including infection with herpes zoster virus. This painful infection may lead to facial paralysis or hearing loss if the facial or vestibulocochlear nerves are involved.

The EAM is invested with cilia and ceruminous glands, largely restricted to the cartilaginous portion of the canal. Cerumen (ear wax) is secreted by the glands into the ear canal, trapping insects and dirt that would otherwise threaten the TM. Individuals with overly active ceruminous glands may find that the EAM becomes occluded, and removal of the cerumen may be required. Attempts to remove the cerumen by the individual using cotton swabs often result in cerumen and dirt being packed against the inferior boundary of the TM, as the oblique angle forms a perfect "pocket" to catch the matter.

The interested student and budding audiologist would be well advised to read the descriptions of these and other conditions provided by Martin and Clark (1995, 2006).

Malformations of the Pinna and EAM

As many as 8.3 out of 10,000 live births include anomalies of the outer ear. **Auricular malformations** arise from issues in embryological development, while **deformations** arise from the effects of physical forces on the prenatal structures (Porter & Tan, 2005). The auricle develops between the fifth and ninth prenatal week, and malformations likely arise from the compounded effects of multiple genes, as well as introduction of teratogens (e.g., Wei, Makori, Peterson, Hummler, & Henrickx, 1999). Failure of cartilage to develop (failure of **chondrogenesis**) can result in auricular or **meatal atresia** (absence of the external auditory meatus), or less severely in **microtia** (small auricle). Parts of the auricle can become duplicated, referred to as **polyotia**. In this case, for instance, a person may develop a second tragus, which may occur in hemifacial microsomia (Lam & Dohil, 2007). **Pre-auricular tags** are prominences that form prenatally anterior to the pinna, while **cryptotia** is congenital atresia (absence) or maldevelopment of the upper portion of the ear. **Anotia** refers to complete absence of the pinna, and **Stahl's ear** refers to pointy, elfin-shaped ears.

A number of genetic syndromes manifest in auricle anomalies. Children affected by branchio-oto-renal syndrome will often have cupped ears or microtia, in conjunction with stapes disconnection and conductive or sensorineural hearing loss. A high proportion of individuals with Down syndrome (Trisomy 21) will show microtia, often have small earlobes and helix malformation, and occasionally show stenosis of the ear canal.

Many deformities require surgical intervention, although some may be treated by molding techniques postnatally (applying continued force in specific directions). The cartilage of the auricle is more malleable in the first three months, making molding a more attractive treatment than surgery, when applicable. Deformities of the auricle and external auditory meatus affect a person's ability to hear, but have a significant impact on appearance as well.

If the pinna is subjected to trauma, as in that inflicted during the sport of boxing, the result can be permanent deformation of its structure. Trauma can cause hemorrhaging between the epithelium and cartilage, and, if left untreated, the resulting swelling may cause a permanent distortion.

The TM is slightly concave when viewed from the EAM, and the umbo is the most depressed portion of this concavity. Although most of the TM is invested with fibrous tissue, the **pars flaccida** is not, and this "flaccid part" may be seen in the superior quadrant of the TM. On either side of the pars flaccida is a recess, consisting of the **anterior** and **posterior malleolar folds**. These folds and the region at the cone of light are the result of the malleus pushing distally on the membrane, much as if you were to stretch an unfilled balloon and push it from behind. This tight binding between membrane and malleus permits ready transmission of acoustic energy from the TM to the ossicular chain. If the TM is particularly transparent, you may also be able to see the long process of the incus parallel to the lateral process of the malleus. In addition, the chorda tympani may sometimes be seen through the superior tympanic membrane.

✔ *To summarize:*

- The outer ear is composed of the pinna, the structure that serves primarily as a sound collector, and the **external auditory meatus (EAM)** or ear canal.
- Landmarks of the pinna include the margin of the **auricle**, called the **helix**, and the **auricular tubercle** on the helix.
- The **cymba conchae** is the anterior extension of the helix and is the anterior entrance of the concha.
- The EAM has both osseous and cartilaginous parts.
- The distal, cartilaginous portion makes up one-third of the ear canal; the other two-thirds are housed in bone.
- At the terminus of the EAM is the **tympanic membrane (TM)**, the structure separating the outer and middle ear.

MIDDLE EAR

Anatesse Lesson

The middle ear is a small but extremely important space occupied by three of the smallest bones of the body. By birth, the middle ear is adult size, and the ossicles and tympanic membrane are almost as large as they will ever be (Gleeson, 2008). First, let us examine these bones and their attachments, and then discuss the landmarks of the cavity itself (Table 9-2).

Ossicles

The bones of the ear, known as the **ossicles**, include the malleus, incus, and stapes (see Figure 9-4 through Figure 9-6). This **ossicular chain** of three articulated bones provides the means for transmission of acoustic energy impinging on the TM to the inner ear.

Structure of the Tympanic Membrane

The tympanic membrane is a roughly oval structure, approximately 10 mm in diameter in the superior-inferior dimension. The anterior-posterior dimension is slightly smaller (about 9 mm in diameter), and the entire membrane is placed within the canal at a 55° angle with the floor. The circumference of the membrane is a fibrocartilaginous ring that fits into the **tympanic sulcus**, a groove in the temporal bone. The sulcus is incomplete in the superior aspect, accommodating the anterior and posterior malleolar folds.

The TM is made up of three layers of tissue: the outer, intermediate, and inner layers. The **outer (cuticular) layer** is a continuation of the epithelial lining of the EAM and pinna. The **intermediate (fibrous) layer** is made up of two parts: The superficial layer is composed of fibers that radiate out from the handle of the malleus to the periphery. The deep layer is made up of circular fibers that are found mostly in the periphery of the membrane. The **inner (mucous) layer** is continuous with the mucosa of the middle ear.

Table 9-2 **Landmarks of the middle ear**

Ossicles

Malleus

    Manubrium (handle)

    Head (caput)

    Lateral process

    Anterior process

    Facet for incus

    Ligaments

        Superior ligament

        Lateral ligament

        Anterior ligament

Incus

    Short process (crus breve)

    Long process (crus longum)

    Lenticular process

    Facet for malleus

    Superior ligament of incus

    Posterior ligament of incus

Stapes

    Head (caput)

    Neck

    Posterior crus (crus posterius)

    Anterior crus (crus anterius)

    Base (footplate)

Muscles

Stapedius muscle

Tensor tympani muscle

Medial Wall

Promontory

    Oval window

    Round window

    Prominence of facial nerve

Prominence of lateral semicircular canal

Canal of tensor tympani

Anterior Wall

Entrance of auditory tube

Posterior Wall

Prominence of stapedial pyramid

Origin of prominence of facial nerve

Aditus to mastoid antrum

Floor

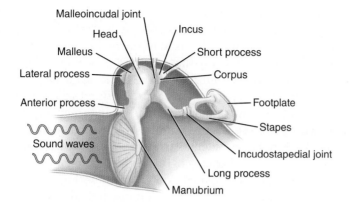

Figure 9-4. Articulated ossicular chain of the right ear in medial view.

Source: Clark/Ohlemiller. (2008). Anatomy and Physiology of Hearing for Audiologists.

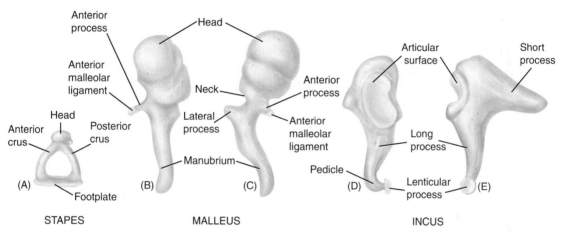

Figure 9-5. Ossicles of the middle ear and their landmarks. (A) Stapes landmarks. (B) Posteromedial view of malleus. (C) Anteromedial view of malleus. (D) Anteromedial view of incus. (E) Posteromedial view of incus.
© Cengage Learning®.

The **malleus** is the largest of the ossicles, providing the point of attachment with the TM.

As you can see in Figure 9-5, the handle or **manubrium** of the malleus is a long process, separated from the **head** by a thin neck. The **anterior** and **lateral processes** provide points of attachment for ligaments, to be discussed. The manubrium attaches to the TM along its length, terminating with the **lateral process**. This attachment of the lateral process with the TM forms the anterior and posterior malleolar folds and the pars flaccida.

Examination of the malleus will reveal that the bulk of the bone is in the head (or **caput**)—not coincidentally the point of articulation with the incus. The head of the malleus protrudes into the epitympanic recess of the middle ear, to be discussed. Although the malleus is the largest of the ossicles, it is only 9 mm long and it weighs a mere 25 mg.

malleus: L., hammer

manubrium: L., handle

incus: L., anvil

lenticular process: the process of the incus with which the stapes articulates

stapes: L., stirrup

The **incus** (fancied to be shaped like an anvil) provides the intermediate communicating link of the ossicular chain. The **body** of the incus articulates with the head of the malleus by means of the **malleolar facet** in such a way that the **long process** of the incus is nearly parallel with the manubrium of the malleus; the body is nearly entirely within the epitympanic recess. The **short process** projects posteriorly, while the end of the long process bends medially, forming the **lenticular process** with which the stapes will articulate. Needless to say, this is not an accidental arrangement of nature, but we will reserve discussion of the benefits of this configuration for Chapter 10.

The incus weighs approximately 30 mg, and its longest process is approximately 7 mm. The malleus and incus articulate by means of a saddle joint, although it appears that the movement at the joint is quite limited. Rather, the malleus and incus appear to move as a unit upon movement of the TM.

The **stapes**, or "stirrup," is the third bone of this chain. The head (caput) of the stapes articulates with the lenticular process of the incus, and the neck of the stapes bifurcates to become the crura. The arch formed by the **anterior** and **posterior crura** converges on the **footplate** or **base** of the stapes. The footplate of the stapes rests in the oval window of the temporal bone, held in place by the **annular ligament**. This is the smallest of the ossicles, weighing approximately 4 mg, with the area of the stapes being only about 3.5 mm². The articulation of the incus and the stapes (the **incudostapedial joint**) is of the ball-and-socket type.

The ossicular chain is held in place by a series of strategically placed ligaments that suspend the ossicles from the walls of the middle ear cavity. The **superior ligament of the malleus** holds the head of the malleus within the epitympanic recess. An **anterior ligament of the malleus** binds the neck of the malleus to the anterior wall of the middle ear, and the **lateral ligament of the malleus** attaches the head of the malleus to the lateral wall. The **posterior ligament of the incus**

Otitis Media with Effusion

Serous (secretory) otitis media refers to any condition in which fluid accumulates in the middle ear cavity. The typical sequence is as follows: The auditory tube stops functioning properly, allowing the middle ear space to become anaerobic as tissue within the space absorbs the available oxygen. Parallel to this, the poorly functioning auditory tube may not allow equalization of pressure between the middle ear space and the environment.

In either condition, a relatively negative pressure may build in the middle ear space, pulling serous fluid from the blood of the middle ear tissues (termed **transudation**). The negative air pressure may also stimulate secretion of mucus from the middle ear tissue. This state, termed **middle ear effusion**, creates a barrier to sound transmission, in that the movement of the tympanic membrane is greatly inhibited.

suspends the incus by means of its short process, while a poorly formed **superior ligament of the incus** may be seen to bind the incus to the epitympanic recess.

Tympanic Muscles

- **Stapedius**
- **Tensor tympani**

Two important muscles of the middle ear are attached to the ossicles. These are the smallest muscles of the human body, appropriately so considering their attachment to the smallest bones (see Figure 9-5).

Stapedius

The **stapedius** muscle, approximately 6 mm long and 5 mm^2 in cross-sectional area, is embedded in the bone of the posterior wall of the middle ear, with only its tendon emerging from the **pyramidal eminence** in the middle ear space. The muscle inserts into the posterior neck of the stapes, so that when it contracts, the stapes is rotated posteriorly. Muscle spindles have been found in the stapedius muscle. Innervation of the stapedius is by means of the stapedial branch of the VII facial nerve.

Tensor Tympani

The **tensor tympani** is approximately 25 mm in length and nearly 6 mm^2 in cross-sectional area, arising from the anterior wall of the middle ear space, superior to the orifice of the auditory tube (also known as the Eustachian tube or pharyngotympanic tube). As with the stapedius, only the tendon of the tensor tympani is found in the middle ear space; the muscle itself is housed in bone. The muscle originates from the cartilaginous part of the auditory tube, as well as from the greater wing of the sphenoid, coursing through the **canal for the tensor tympani** in the anterior wall of the middle ear. The tendon for the tensor tympani emerges from the canal, courses around a bony outcropping called the **trochleariform process** (alternately **cochleariform process**), and inserts into the upper manubrium malli. Contraction of this muscle pulls the malleus anteromedially, thereby reducing the range of movement of the TM by placing indirect tension on it. Indeed, both the tensor tympani and the stapedius muscles stiffen the middle ear transmission system, thereby reducing transmission of acoustical information in the lower frequencies. That is, contraction of these muscles reduces the strength of the signal reaching the cochlea, potentially protecting it from damage due to high signal intensity. Unfortunately, the protective function is compromised, in that the stiffening of the ossicular chain provides little barrier to transmission of the high-frequency sound so dominant in modern industrial societies. Innervation of the tensor tympani is by the V trigeminal nerve via the otic ganglion.

Muscle:	Stapedius
Origin:	Posterior wall of middle ear space of temporal bone
Course:	Anteriorly
Insertion:	Posterior crus of stapes
Innervation:	VII facial nerve
Function:	Rotates footplate of stapes posteriorly, thereby stiffening ossicular chain

Muscle:	Tensor tympani
Origin:	Cartilaginous portion of auditory tube and greater wing of sphenoid
Course:	Posteriorly through canal for tensor tympani and around trochleariform process
Insertion:	Manubrium malli
Innervation:	V trigeminal nerve via the otic ganglion
Function:	Pulls malleus anteromedially and stiffens ossicular chain

Acoustic Reflex

The **acoustic reflex** (also known as the **stapedial reflex**) is a staple of the audiologist's diagnostic toolkit. The stapedius muscle applies a force on the footplate of the stapes that reduces the amplitude of excursion of the footplate, thereby reducing the sound pressure level reaching the cochlea. It is thought that this is a basic protective mechanism for the cochlea, as it is triggered by loud sounds, typically greater than 85 dB SPL. The acoustic reflex may also include response by the tensor tympani muscle.

The neural circuit for the acoustic reflex is such that stimulation of either ear results in response by both ears, although attenuation of the signal by the ipsilateral ear is stronger than the attenuation in the contralateral ear. As outlined by Møller (2006), a stimulus entering the right ear is transduced by the right cochlea, right ventral cochlear nucleus, and right medial superior olive, consecutively. The right medial superior olive communicates with both the right- and left-side nuclei of the VII facial and V trigeminal nerves, so that the appropriate stimulus triggers a response in stapedius muscles on both left and right sides.

The arrangement of these ligament and muscle attachments is critical to the function of the middle ear. As we shall see in Chapter 10, the attachments of the ossicles provide the precise "tuning" necessary to support vibration while prohibiting continued oscillation.

Landmarks of the Middle Ear

The middle ear space is invested with numerous landmarks of importance in the study of auditory function. Figure 9-6 is a drawing of the right middle ear, to help our discussion.

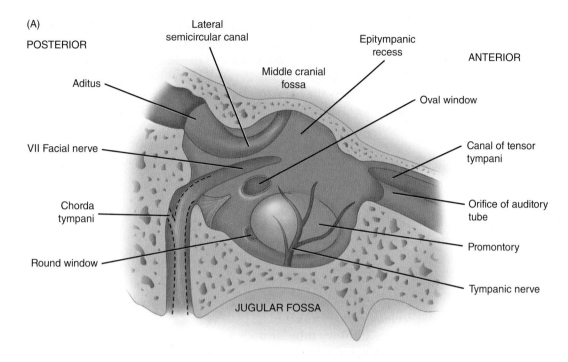

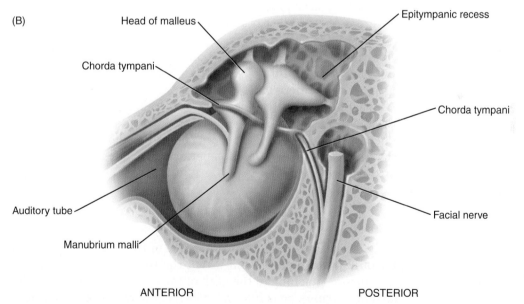

Figure 9-6. (A) Schematic representation of the middle ear cavity of the right ear, as viewed from the external auditory meatus with tympanic membrane and ossicles removed. (B) View of medial surface of tympanic membrane in situ, showing the course of the chorda tympani nerve.

© Cengage Learning®.

Medial Wall

Four landmarks related to the cochlea and the vestibular system lie immediately medial to the space. The **oval window (fenestra vestibuli; fenestra ovalis)**, in which the footplate of the stapes is embedded, lies in the superior-posterior aspect, and below that point is the **round window (fenestra cochlea; fenestra rotunda)**, an opening sealed by the **secondary tympanic membrane** and marking the entrance into the scala tympani of the cochlea. Between these two is the **promontory**, a bulge created by the basal turn of the cochlea. Immediately above the oval window is the prominence of the **lateral semicircular canal** of the vestibular mechanism, to be discussed. In addition to these landmarks, you can see a portion of the canal within which the tensor tympani is housed, and from which its tendon emerges, as well as the **prominence of the facial nerve**.

Anterior Wall

Examination of the anterior wall reveals the **entrance to the auditory tube**, and within that wall the internal carotid artery courses. The canal for the tensor tympani arises from the medialmost aspect of this wall, marked by the trochleariform process, as mentioned previously (see Figure 9-6).

The **auditory tube** (also known as the **pharyngotympanic tube**) was discussed previously in Chapter 6. This important structure provides the sole means for bringing oxygen to the middle ear space (**aeration**), a crucial process for maintaining equilibrium between the pressure in the middle ear and atmospheric pressure. The auditory tube is about 36 mm in length, coursing anteriorly and medially on its way to the nasopharynx. The bony portion of the auditory tube (approximately 12 mm in length) terminates at the juncture of the petrous and squamous parts of the temporal bone. The cartilaginous auditory tube is twice as long as the bony tube and in cross-section is seen to be incomplete along the entire inferior aspect. That is, the auditory tube is capable of expanding by pulling the inferior margins away from each other, a function performed by the tensor veli palatini, discussed in Chapter 6.

Posterior Wall and Floor

On the posterior wall is the **prominence of the stapedial pyramid (pyramidal eminence)** from which the tendon of the stapedius arises before attaching to the neck of the stapes. The **aditus to the mastoid antrum** opens into the epitympanic recess of the mastoid antrum. Within the posterior wall courses the chorda tympani, and the VII facial nerve prominence may be seen to continue on the medial wall.

Beneath the floor of the middle ear cavity lies the jugular bulb. **Mastoid air cells** comprising much of the mastoid process may extend to the floor of the middle ear cavity. Infection of the middle ear space may result in subsequent infection of the mastoid air cells, sometimes requiring mastoidectomy.

Mastoiditis

Mastoiditis refers to inflammation ("itis") of the mastoid bone. This is a serious condition that can result in unilateral deafness, and even infection of the brain and death. The typical means of infection of the mastoid air cells is by means of the auditory (Eustachian) tube. Bacteria enter the auditory tube, migrate to the middle ear, and enter the *aditus ad antrum* and subsequently the air cells of the mastoid. The infection can then spread to the dura mater lining of the brain within the middle cranial fossa, causing bacterial meningitis, which is life threatening. Infection within the mastoid bone may include the area behind the auricle (post-auricular abscess or Bezold's abscess), or the anterior portion of the mastoid process where the posterior digastricus and sternocleidomastoid attach. If the anterior portion is infected, turning the head will be painful (Gleeson, 2008). Mastoiditis is typically related to chronic otitis media, which is infection of the middle ear space. Treatment of mastoiditis involves antibiotics, but persistent and resistant mastoiditis may require a surgical procedure (mastoidectomy) to remove the infected bony tissue.

Mastoiditis can cause infection of the cochlea and vestibular mechanism (labyrinthitis), and may result from permanent sensorineural hearing loss, vestibular dysfunction, and tinnitus (ringing of the ears).

✔ *To summarize:*

- The middle ear cavity houses the important middle ear ossicles and has a number of important landmarks.
- The **malleus** is the largest of the ossicles, providing the point of attachment with the tympanic membrane.
- The **incus** provides the intermediate communicating link for the ossicular chain, and the **stapes** is the third bone of this chain.
- The ossicular chain is held in place by a series of important ligaments: the **superior, anterior,** and **lateral ligaments of the malleus**; and the **posterior** and **superior ligaments of the incus**.
- The **stapedius muscle** inserts into the posterior neck of the stapes and pulls the stapes posteriorly.
- The **tensor tympani** muscle inserts into the upper manubrium malli and pulls the malleus anteromedially.
- Landmarks of the medial wall of the middle ear cavity include the **oval window**, the **round window**, the **promontory** of the cochlea, and the **prominence of the facial nerve**.
- The anterior wall houses the entrance to the **auditory tube**, and the posterior wall houses the **prominence of the stapedial pyramid**.

INNER EAR

The inner ear houses the sensors for balance (the vestibular system) and hearing (the cochlea) (see Table 9-3). The entryway to the cochlea is termed the **vestibule**.

Anatesse Lesson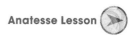

Table 9-3 **Landmarks of the inner ear**

Vestibule
- Saccule
- Utricle
- Macula
- Otolithic membrane
- Stereocilia
- Kinocilium
- Ductus reunien
- Endolymphatic duct

Semicircular canals
- Lateral semicircular canal
- Anterior vertical semicircular canal
- Posterior vertical semicircular canal
- Ampulla
- Crista ampularis
- Stereocilia
- Kinocilium

Cochlea
- Scala vestibuli
- Scala tympani
- Scala media (cochlear duct)
  - Reissner's membrane
  - Basilar membrane
  - Spiral ligament
  - Stria vascularis
  - Organ of Corti
    - Inner and outer hair cells with stereocilia
    - Deiter's cells
    - Tunnel of Corti
    - Spiral limbus
    - Inner spiral sulcus
    - Tectorial membrane
    - Reticular lamina
    - Hensen's cells
    - Cells of Claudius
    - Rods of Corti

Osseous spiral lamina
- Habenula perforate

Helicotrema

Examination of Figure 9-7 will help in this preliminary discussion of the inner ear. Depicted in this figure is the **osseous** or **bony labyrinth**, representing the cavities (tunnels) within which the inner ear structures (the **membranous labyrinth**) are housed. The bony labyrinth is embedded within the petrous portion of the temporal bone, which is the densest bone in the body. The epithelial lining of

(A)

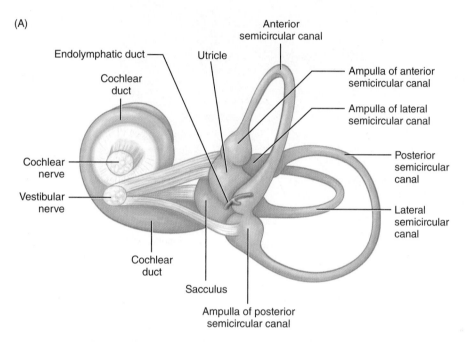

(B)

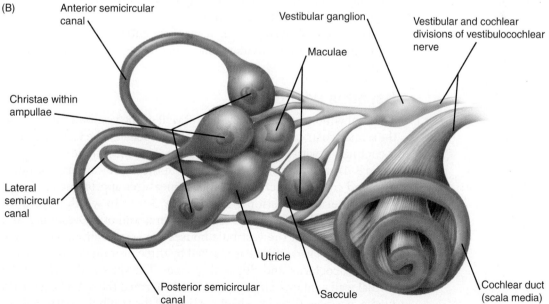

Figure 9-7. (A) Schematic of relationship of semicircular canals, and cochlea. (B) The membranous labyrinth, revealing components of the inner ear. Note that the vestibule is not shown because it is external to the membranous vestibular duct and is filled with perilymph. (continues).

(C)

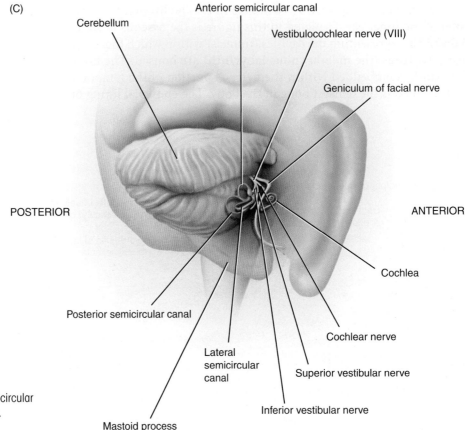

Cerebellum

Anterior semicircular canal

Vestibulocochlear nerve (VIII)

Geniculum of facial nerve

POSTERIOR

ANTERIOR

Cochlea

Posterior semicircular canal

Cochlear nerve

Lateral semicircular canal

Superior vestibular nerve

Inferior vestibular nerve

Mastoid process

Figure 9-7 continued.
(C) Orientation of the semicircular canals in the erect human.
© Cengage Learning®.

the bony labyrinth secretes perilymph, the fluid that is found in the superficial cavities of the labyrinth.

The osseous labyrinth is made up of the entryway to the labyrinth, the vestibule, the semicircular canals, and the osseous cochlear canal.

Osseous Vestibule

The oval window is within the lateral wall of the vestibule, anterior to the semicircular canals and posterior to the cochlea. The vestibule space is continuous with both the vestibular mechanism and the cochlea (see Table 9-4), although it is separated from the membranous vestibular duct and cochlear duct. The vestibule measures approximately 5 mm in the anterior-posterior dimension by 3 mm in width (Hackney, 2008). The oval window resides in the lateral wall of the vestibule, and the medial wall of the vestibule houses the vestibular aqueduct (see Figure 9-7a). The vestibule is marked by three prominent recesses, the spherical, cochlear, and elliptical recesses. The **spherical recess** of the medial wall contains minute perforations termed the **macula cribrosa media**, passages through which portions of the vestibular nerve pass to the saccule of the membranous labyrinth. The **cochlear recess** provides a similar communication between the vestibule and the basal end of the cochlear duct. The **elliptical recess** is similarly perforated, providing

Table 9-4 **Critical values of the labyrinthine spaces. Volumes and lengths of vestibular and cochlear spaces, as indicated by source**

Structure or Space	Dimension	Source
Volume of inner ear	208.26 µL	Buckingham and Valvassori (2001); Igarashi, Ohashi, and Oshii (1986); Melhem et al. (1998)
Volume of cochlear endolymph	7.7 µL	Igarashi, Ohashi, and Oshii (1986)
Volume of perilymph (vestibular and cochlear)	162.45 µL	Buckingham and Valvassori (2001); Igarashi, Ohashi, and Oshii (1986)
Volume of scala tympani	44.3 µL	Igarashi, Ohashi, and Oshii (1986)
Length of scala tympani	28.46	Thorne et al. (1999);
Volume of scala vestibuli	31.5 µL	Igarashi, Ohashi, and Oshii (1986)
Area of round window	2.22 mm^2	Okuno and Sando (1988)
Length of cochlear aqueduct	6–12 mm	Gopen et al. (1997)
Diameter of cochlear aqueduct	138 µm	Gopen (1997)

Source: Derived from data compiled by A. Salt, Ph.D. of the Cochlear Fluids Research Lab of Washington University.

communication between the utricle it houses and the ampullae of the superior and lateral semicircular canals, to be discussed.

Osseous Semicircular Canals

The osseous semicircular canals house the sense organs for the movement of the body in space. These consist of the **anterior** (anterior vertical; superior), **posterior** (posterior vertical), and **lateral** (horizontal) **semicircular canals**, the names describing the orientation of each canal. You can envision the canals as a series of three rings attached to a ball (the vestibule) and lying behind and above that ball. Each ring is in a plane at right angles to other rings, so that the interaction of the three permits the brain to code three-dimensional space. The semicircular canals all open onto the vestibular space by means of apertures, although the vertical canals (anterior and posterior semicircular canals) share an aperture, the **crus commune**. Near the opening to the vestibule in each canal is an enlargement that houses the ampulla, to be discussed.

The anterior vertical canal is vertical in orientation, so that it senses movement in a plane roughly perpendicular to the long axis of the temporal bone. The anterior end of the canal houses the ampulla; the other end combines with the non-ampulated end of the posterior vertical canal at the crus commune.

The posterior vertical semicircular canal is vertically oriented as well, but is in the plane roughly parallel to the long axis of the temporal bone. Its ampulla is housed in the lower crus, entering the vestibule below the oval window.

The horizontal (lateral) semicircular canal senses movement roughly in the transverse plane of the body. Its ampulated end enters the vestibule near that of the anterior semicircular canal, above the level of the oval window.

Binaural orientation of the two semicircular canals is such that the anterior semicircular canal of one ear is parallel to the posterior canal of the other. The horizontal canals lie in the same plane, but the ampullae are in mirror-image locations. This horizontal orientation of the canal helps your brain differentiate rotatory movement toward the left versus right. The anterior semicircular canals sense movements of your head as it moves toward your shoulder, while the posterior semicircular canals sense movement if you move your head to nod "yes." Shaking your head "no" is sensed by the lateral semicircular canals. The utricle and saccule are responsible for mediating the sense of acceleration of your head in space, such as in sudden movement or falling.

Osseous Cochlear Labyrinth

The osseous labyrinth has the appearance of a coiled snail shell ("cochlea" comes from the Greek word *cochlos*, meaning "snail"). It coils out from its base near the vestibule, wrapping around itself 2-5/8 times before reaching its **apex**. The core of the osseous labyrinth, the **modiolus**, is a finely perforated bone: Fibers of the VIII vestibulocochlear nerve pass through these perforations en route to ganglion cells within the modiolus (the modiolus is actually the combination of the core space, known as Rosenthal's canal, and the spiral ganglion nerve fibers: Coleman et al., 2006). The core of the modiolus is continuous with the **internal auditory meatus** of the temporal bone, through which the vestibulocochlear nerve passes.

The labyrinth is divided into two incomplete chambers, the **scala vestibuli** and the **scala tympani**, by an incomplete bony shelf protruding from the modiolus, the **osseous spiral lamina**. This very important structure forms the point of attachment for the scala media, which houses the sensory organ for hearing. The osseous spiral lamina becomes progressively smaller approaching the apex, such that the space between it and the opposite wall of the labyrinth increases. At the apex the two chambers formed by the incomplete lamina become hooklike (hence the name **hamulus**), forming the **helicotrema**, the region through which the scala tympani and scala vestibuli will communicate.

The osseous labyrinth has three prominent openings. The round window (foramen rotundum; fenestra rotundrum) provides communication between the scala tympani and the middle ear. The oval window, upon which the stapes is placed, permits communication between the scala vestibuli and the middle ear space. The **cochlear canaliculus** or **cochlear aqueduct** is a minute opening between the scala tympani in the region of the round window and the subarachnoid space of the cranial cavity. It is hypothesized that **perilymph**, the fluid that fills the

modiolus: L., hub

scala vestibuli and scala tympani, passes through this duct, although this has not been demonstrated. There is about 204 μL of fluid in the entire labyrinth, with only 38 μL of endolymph and about 166 μL of perilymph. The vestibule has only about 7 μL of fluid in it. To get a notion of scale, 1 mL is 1/1000 of a liter, and 1 μL is 1/1,000,000 of a liter.

✔ *To summarize:*

- The inner ear houses the sensors for balance (the vestibular system) and hearing (the cochlea).
- The entryway to these structures is termed the **vestibule**.
- The **osseous labyrinth** is made up of the entryway to the labyrinth, the vestibule, the semicircular canals, and the osseous cochlear canal.
- The osseous labyrinth has the appearance of a coiled snail shell.
- The labyrinth is divided into two incomplete chambers, the **scala vestibuli** and the **scala tympani**, by the **osseous spiral lamina**, an incomplete bony shelf protruding from the modiolus.
- The **round window** provides communication between the scala tympani and the middle ear space.
- The **oval window** permits communication between the scala vestibuli and the middle ear space.
- The **cochlear aqueduct** connects the upper duct and the subarachnoid space.

Membranous Labyrinth

Anatesse Lesson ➤

The structure of the membranous labyrinth parallels that of the bony labyrinth. First, orient yourself to the oval window, recognizing its link to the stapes of the middle ear. Beneath it, but not quite visible, is the round window. The vestibule or entryway to the inner ear is a space shared by the sense organ of hearing, the cochlea, and the sense organs of balance, the semicircular canals. The same fluid flows through all of the membranous labyrinth, making balance and hearing intimately related in both function and pathology. Let us examine the sensory components of the inner ear (see Figure 9-8).

Vestibular System

The membranous labyrinth can be thought of as a fluid-filled sac that rests within the cavity of the osseous labyrinth. This sac does not completely fill the labyrinth but rather forms an additional space within the already fluid-filled region. The cochlear duct forms only a small portion of the membranous labyrinth and contains fluid of a slightly different composition from that of the region surrounding the duct. This fluid in the cochlear duct is termed **endolymph**.

In the vestibular system, the membranous labyrinth houses the vestibular organ. As you will recall, the **ampulla** is the expanded region of the semicircular canals near one opening to the vestibule. Each ampulla houses a **crista ampularis**, over which a gelatinous

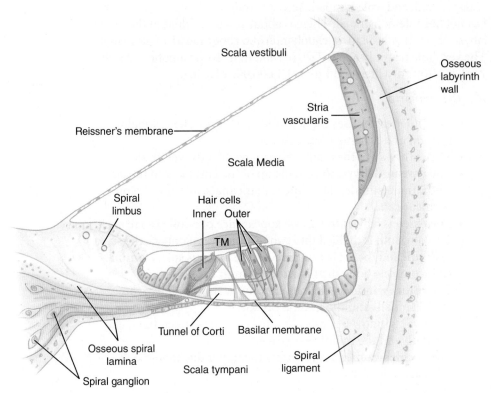

Figure 9-8. Cross-section of the cochlea, revealing scala vestibule; scala media; scala tympani; and TM, tectorial membrane.

© Cengage Learning®.

crista: receptor organ for movement within vestibular mechanism

cupola lies. The **crista** is the receptor organ for movement, being made up of ciliated receptor cells and a supporting membrane. From each of the 6,000 receptor cells protrude approximately 50 **stereocilia**, minute hairs that sense movement in fluid, and one **kinocilium**. A **cupola** overlays the crista ampularis such that the cilia are embedded within the cupola.

Within the vestibule lie the **utricle** and the **saccule**, housing for the otolithic organs of the vestibular system. The utricular **macula** is the sensory organ, which is endowed with hair cells and cilia. It is covered by the **otolithic membrane**, which is invested with crystals (**otoliths**). The saccule lies near the scala vestibuli in the vestibule and is similarly endowed with macula and otolithic membrane. The saccule and utricle communicate by means of the **endolymphatic duct**, which is embedded in the dura mater. The saccule communicates with the cochlea by means of the minute **ductus reuniens**.

Cochlear Duct

The membranous labyrinth of the cochlea, the **cochlear duct**, resides between the scala vestibuli and scala tympani, making up the intermediate **scala media**. This structure houses the sensory apparatus for hearing.

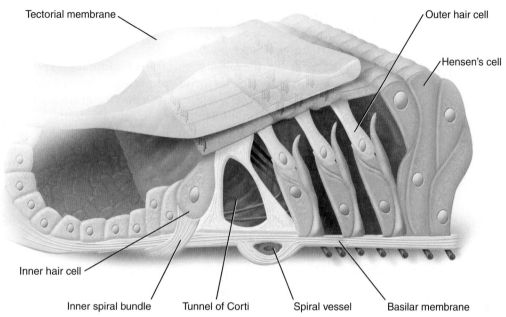

Tectorial membrane

Outer hair cell

Hensen's cell

Inner hair cell

Inner spiral bundle

Tunnel of Corti

Spiral vessel

Basilar membrane

Figure 9-9. Landmarks and structures of the organ of Corti.
© Cengage Learning®.

A cross-section through the region of the scala media reveals its extraordinary structure, as shown in Figure 9-9. Note first the osseous spiral lamina, discussed previously. This shelf courses the extent of the osseous labyrinth, forming the major point of attachment for the cochlear duct. Again, looking at Figure 9-8, you can see **Reissner's membrane**, an extremely thin separation between the perilymph of the scala vestibuli and the endolymph of the scala media. One end is continuous with the **stria vascularis**, highly vascularized tissue that is firmly attached to the **spiral ligament**, and which is responsible for the potassium used by the hair cells. Disruption of the blood supply to the cochlea, such as can occur during surgery for a cerebellar tumor, results in immediate hearing loss, arising from reduced potassium output into the endolymph of the scala media (Mom, Chazal, Gabrillargues, Gilian, & Avan, 2005).

The **basilar membrane** forms the "floor" of the scala media, separating the scala media and scala tympani. It is on this membrane that the organ of hearing is found. The basilar membrane is extremely thin, because of its role in supporting the traveling wave (to be discussed).

The **organ of Corti** is grossly similar to the design of the vestibular organs. There are four rows of hair cells resting on a bed of Deiters' cells for support. The outer three rows of hair cells, known as **outer hair cells**, are separated from the single row of **inner hair cells** by the **tunnel of Corti**, the product of **pillar cells of Corti**. The superior surface of the outer hair cells and the phalangeal processes of Deiters' cells form a matrix termed the *reticular lamina*, through which the cilia protrude. The vascular supply for the organ of Corti arises from the labyrinthine artery (which itself arises from the basilar artery, to be discussed in Chapter 11). The cochlear branch of the labyrinthine artery divides into between 12 and 14 "twigs" that serve the spiral lamina, basilar membrane, stria vascularis, and other cochlear structures (Hackney, 2008).

On the modiolar side of the cochlear duct is found the **spiral limbus**, from which arises the **tectorial membrane**. The tectorial membrane overlays the hair cells and has functional significance in the processing of acoustic stimuli. The outer hair cells are clearly embedded in this membrane, but the inner hair cells do not make physical contact with the tectorial membrane, although its proximity to the hair cells is an important contributor to hair cell excitation, as will be discussed.

Inner and outer hair cells differ markedly in number. The hair cells on the modiolar side of the tunnel of Corti are termed the inner hair cells (see Figure 9-10). The 3,500 inner hair cells form a single

(A)

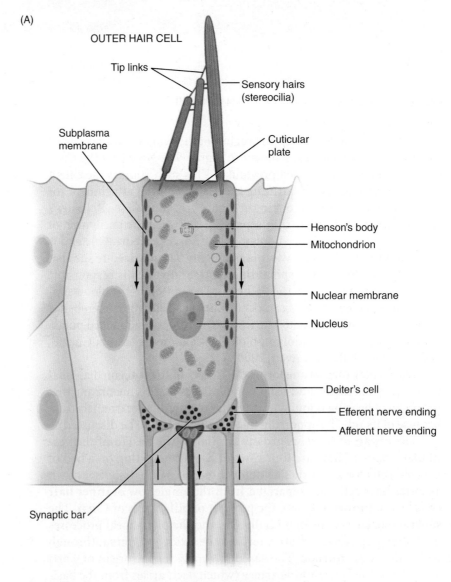

Figure 9-10. Details of hair cells. (A) Outer hair cell. (continues).
© Cengage Learning®.

(B)

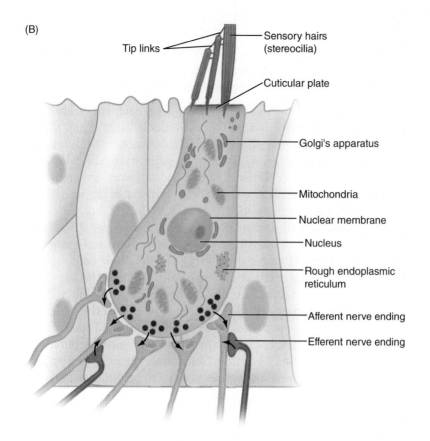

Tip links

Sensory hairs (stereocilia)

Cuticular plate

Golgi's apparatus

Mitochondria

Nuclear membrane

Nucleus

Rough endoplasmic reticulum

Afferent nerve ending

Efferent nerve ending

Figure 9-10 continued.
(B) Inner hair cell. Note presence of both afferent and efferent fibers innervating both types of sensory cells.

Source: From Stach. (2009). Clinical Audiology: An Introduction, 2nd ed. Clifton Park, NY: Delmar Cengage Learning. Reprinted with permission.

row stretching from the base to apex. The upper surface of each hair cell is graced with a series of approximately 50 **stereocilia** forming a slight "U" pattern opened toward the modiolar side. There are three rows of outer hair cells, broadening to four rows in the apical end, numbering approximately 12,000. As with the inner cells, the stereocilia protrude from the surface of each outer hair cell, but with a "W" or "V" pattern formed by approximately 150 stereocilia. In both the inner and outer hair cells, the stereocilia for a given cell are graduated in length, so that the longer cilia are distal to the modiolar side. The cilia of a hair cell are all connected by thin, filamentous links. Shorter cilia are connected to the taller cilia by "tip links," and cilia are also linked laterally, thus ensuring that movement of one cilia involves disturbance of adjacent cilia on a hair cell. Stereocilia found in the apex are longer than those found in the base.

The morphology between inner and outer hair cells differs markedly. The inner hair cells are teardrop or gourd shaped, with a broad base and narrowed neck. The outer hair cells, in contrast, are shaped like a test tube. Inner hair cells are embedded in a matrix of inner phalangeal cells for support, while outer hair cells are nested in outer phalangeal cells of Deiters'. Phalangeal processes apparently replace hair cells lost through acoustic trauma, thereby maintaining the delicate cuticular plate.

Innervation Pattern of the Organ of Corti

The hair cells of the cochlea receive both afferent and efferent innervation, as discussed in Chapter 12. The pattern of innervation is strikingly different between outer and inner hair cells.

Afferent Innervation. As shown in Figure 9-11, each inner hair cell is connected to as many as 10 VIII vestibulocochlear nerve fibers, referred to as *many-to-one* innervation. In contrast, each outer hair cell shares its innervation with 10 other outer hair cells, all being innervated by the same VIII nerve fiber ("one-to-many" innervation).

VIII vestibulocochlear nerve fibers consist of Type I fibers (large, myelinated fibers) and Type II fibers (small, both myelinated and unmyelinated fibers). Type I fibers, making up 95 percent of the VIII nerve, apparently innervate the inner hair cells, whereas unmyelinated Type II fibers innervate the outer hair cells. Type I fibers innervating hair cells course medially through the habenula perforata, after which point myelin will be found on the fiber. Most of the Type II outer hair cell fibers course medially to the habenula perforata as the inner radial bundle. A small portion of Type II fibers courses within the tunnel of Corti apically to join with the outer spiral bundle. The outer spiral bundle fibers innervating the outer hair cells contain both afferent and efferent fibers, to be discussed.

Efferent Innervation. As will be discussed in Chapter 11, the efferent innervation of the outer hair cells is inhibitory, reducing the afferent output caused by hair cell stimulation. The pathway and circuitry involved is termed the olivocochlear bundle because it arises from

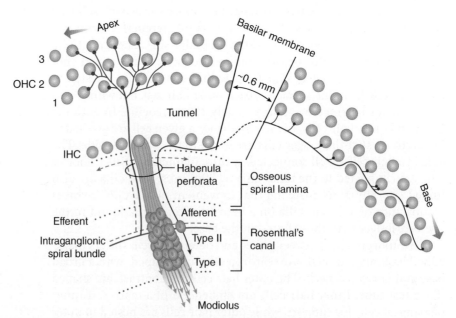

Figure 9-11. Innervation scheme of organ of Corti. Note that many nerve fibers innervate each inner hair cell, while many outer hair cells are innervated by one nerve fiber.

Source: From Primary neurons and synapses, by H. H. Spoendlin, Ultrastructural atlas of the inner ear, by I. Friedmann and J. Ballantyne, 1984, London: Buttersworth, 133–164.

the region of the olivary complex of the brainstem auditory pathway. This bundle of fibers consists of about 1,600 neurons and is divided into crossed and uncrossed pathways. The crossed olivocochlear bundle (COCB) arises from a region near the medial superior olive of the olivary complex, and descends to the fourth ventricle, where the majority of the fibers decussate and proceed to innervate the outer hair cells. The uncrossed olivocochlear bundle (UCOB) originates near the lateral superior olive of the olivary complex and courses primarily ipsilaterally to the inner hair cells of the cochlea. Activation of the olivocochlear bundle appears to be controllable through cortical activity and assists in the detection of signal within a background of noise.

✔ *To summarize:*

- The **membranous labyrinth** can be thought of as a fluid-filled sac that rests within the cavity of the osseous labyrinth and is filled with **endolymph**.
- In the vestibular system, the membranous labyrinth houses the vestibular organ.
- The **ampulla** is the expanded region of the semicircular canals containing the **crista ampularis**. Within the vestibule lie the **utricle** and the **saccule**.
- The membranous labyrinth of the cochlea resides between the scala vestibuli and scala tympani, making up the intermediate **scala media**.
- **Reissner's membrane** forms the upper boundary of the scala media, and the basilar membrane forms the floor.
- The **organ of Corti** has four rows of hair cells resting on a bed of Deiters' cells for support.
- The **outer hair cells** are separated from the **inner hair cell** row by the **tunnel of Corti**.
- The upper surface of each hair cell is graced with a series of **stereocilia** connected by tip links.
- Each inner hair cell is connected with as many as 10 VIII vestibulocochlear nerve fibers, and each outer hair cell shares its innervation with 10 other outer hair cells, all being innervated by the same VIII nerve fiber.

CHAPTER SUMMARY

Anatesse Lesson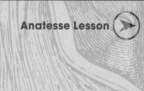

The outer ear is composed of the pinna and the external auditory meatus. Landmarks of the pinna include the margin of the auricle, the helix, and the auricular tubercle on the helix. The EAM has both osseous and cartilaginous parts: The cartilaginous portion makes up one-third of the ear canal, while the other two-thirds are housed in bone. At the terminus of the external auditory meatus is the tympanic membrane, the structure separating the outer and middle ear.

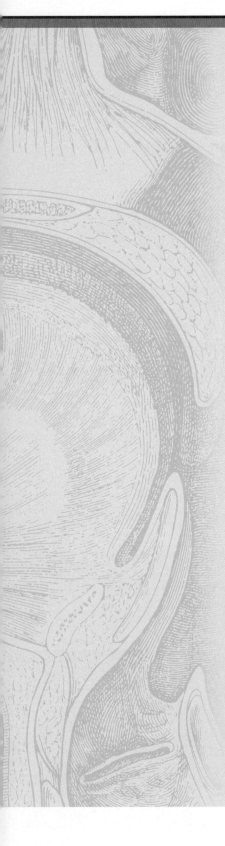

The middle ear cavity houses the middle ear ossicles. The malleus is the largest of the ossicles, providing the point of attachment with the TM. The incus provides the intermediate communicating link of the ossicular chain, and the stapes is the third bone of this chain. The ossicular chain is held in place by a series of important ligaments. The stapedius muscle inserts into the posterior neck of the stapes and pulls the stapes posteriorly; the tensor tympani muscle inserts into the upper manubrium malli, pulling the malleus antero-medially. Landmarks of the medial wall of the middle ear cavity include the oval window, the round window, the promontory of the cochlea, and the prominence of the facial nerve. The anterior wall houses the entrance to the auditory tube, and the posterior wall houses the prominence of the stapedial pyramid.

The inner ear houses the sense mechanism for balance (the vestibular system) and hearing (the cochlea). The entryway to these structures is termed the vestibule. The osseous labyrinth is made up of the entryway to the labyrinth, the vestibule, the semicircular canals, and the osseous cochlear canal. It has the appearance of a coiled snail shell and is divided into two incomplete chambers, the scala vestibuli and the scala tympani, by the osseous spiral lamina, an incomplete bony shelf protruding from the modiolus. The round window provides communication between the scala tympani and the middle ear space. The oval window permits communication between the scala vestibuli and the middle ear space. The cochlear aqueduct connects the upper duct and the subarachnoid space.

The membranous labyrinth can be thought of as a fluid-filled sac that rests within the cavity of the osseous labyrinth and is filled with endolymph. In the vestibular system, the membranous labyrinth houses the vestibular organ. The ampulla is the expanded region of the semicircular canals containing the crista ampularis. Within the vestibule lie the utricle and saccule. The membranous labyrinth of the cochlea resides between the scala vestibuli and the scala tympani, making up the intermediate scala media. Reissner's membrane forms the distal boundary of the scala media, and the basilar membrane forms the proximal boundary. The organ of Corti has four rows of hair cells resting on a bed of Deiters' cells for support. The outer hair cells are separated from the row of inner hair cells by the tunnel of Corti. The upper surface of each hair cell is graced with a series of stereocilia. Each inner hair cell is innervated by as many as 10 VIII nerve fibers, while each outer hair cell shares its innervation with 10 other outer hair cells, all being innervated by the same VIII nerve fiber.

Media Connection

Go to the accompanying online resources at CengageBrain.com and have fun learning! Study with the Anatesse software program, play games, view animations and videos, and take practice tests to help reinforce the key concepts you learned in this chapter.

Study Questions

1. The ear is a _____, in that it converts acoustical energy into electrochemical energy.

2. The _____ serves the function of sound collection.

3. The _____ meatus is a conduit for sound reaching the tympanic membrane.

4. The _____ meatus is a conduit for the VIII nerve fibers coursing to the brain stem.

5. The tympanic membrane (or eardrum) is made up of _____ layers of tissue.

6. The outer layer of the tympanic membrane is continuous with the _____.

7. The _____ layer of the tympanic membrane is made up primarily of radiating fibers.

8. The _____ is a landmark produced by the most distal part of the manubrium malli.

9. The _____ is the bone of the middle ear directly attached to the tympanic membrane.

10. The _____ is the bone of the middle ear directly communicating with the oval window.

11. The _____ of the malleus attaches to the tympanic membrane.

12. The _____ of the stapes articulates with the oval window.

13. The _____ muscle pulls the stapes posteriorly.

14. The _____ muscle pulls the malleus anteromedially.

15. The entryway to the cochlea and vestibular system is via the space known as the _____.

16. The _____ is the system of cavities within bone that houses the membranous labyrinth.

17. The scala _____ and scala _____ are incomplete spaces within the osseous labyrinth.

18. The _____ window provides communication between the scala tympani and the middle ear.

19. The _____ window permits communication between the scala vestibuli and the middle ear space.

20. The _____ is a fluid-filled sac attached to the walls of the osseous labyrinth and is filled with endolymph.

21. _____ membrane separates the scala vestibuli and the scala media; the _____ membrane separates the scala media from the scala tympani.

22. There is are _____ row(s) of outer hair cells and row(s) of inner hair cells.

23. The _____ separates the outer and inner hair cells.

24. The hair cells are innervated by the _____ nerve.

25. Microsurgery procedures have advanced rapidly in recent years, permitting rearticulation of ossicles that have become disarticulated. Considering how well protected the ossicles are, what could cause them to become disarticulated?

Study Question Answers

1. The ear is a **TRANSDUCER**, in that it converts acoustical energy into electrochemical energy.

2. The **OUTER EAR** serves the function of sound collection.

3. The **EXTERNAL AUDITORY** meatus is a conduit for sound reaching the tympanic membrane.

4. The **INTERNAL AUDITORY** meatus is a conduit for the **VIII** nerve fibers coursing to the brain stem.

5. The tympanic membrane (or eardrum) is made up of **THREE** layers of tissue.

6. The outer layer of the tympanic membrane is continuous with the **EPITHELIUM OF THE EXTERNAL AUDITORY MEATUS**.

7. The **INTERMEDIATE** layer of the tympanic membrane is made up primarily of radiating fibers.

8. The **UMBO** is a landmark produced by the most distal part of the manubrium malli.

9. The **MALLEUS** is the bone of the middle ear directly attached to the tympanic membrane.

10. The **STAPES** is the bone of the middle ear directly communicating with the oval window.

11. The **MANUBRIUM** of the malleus attaches to the tympanic membrane.

12. The **FOOTPLATE** of the stapes articulates with the oval window.

13. The **STAPEDIUS** muscle pulls the stapes posteriorly.

14. The **TENSOR TYMPANI** muscle pulls the malleus anteromedially.

15. The entryway to the cochlea and vestibular system is via the space known as the **VESTIBULE**.

16. The **OSSEOUS LABYRINTH** is the system of cavities within bone that houses the membranous labyrinth.

17. The scala **VESTIBULI** and scala **TYMPANI** are incomplete spaces within the osseous labyrinth.

18. The **ROUND** window provides communication between the scala tympani and the middle ear.

19. The **OVAL** window permits communication between the scala vestibuli and the middle ear space.

20. The **MEMBRANOUS LABYRINTH** is a fluid-filled sac attached to the walls of the osseous labyrinth and is filled with endolymph.

21. **REISSNER'S** membrane separates the scala vestibuli and the scala media; the **BASILAR** membrane separates the scala media from the scala tympani.

22. There are **THREE** rows of outer hair cells and **ONE** row of inner hair cells.

23. The **TUNNEL OF CORTI** separates the outer and inner hair cells.

24. The hair cells are innervated by the **VIII VESTIBULOCOCHLEAR** nerve.

25. As with any other body structure, the ossicles are subject to trauma. A frequent cause of disarticulation of the ossicles is head trauma that involves the temporal bone (this may also cause a perilymph fistula, which is a tear in the basilar or Reissner's membrane that allows perilymph and endolymph to mingle). Another cause of disarticulation is noise or high-pressure trauma: The high-pressure forces associated with explosions can easily cause disarticulation.

Bibliography

Altschuler, R. A., Bobbin, R. P., & Hoffman, D. W. (1986). *Neurology of hearing: The cochlea.* New York: Raven Press.

Anson, B. J., & Donaldson, J. R. (1973). *Surgical anatomy of the temporal bone and ear.* Philadelphia, PA: W. B. Saunders.

Beck, E. W., Monson, H., & Groer, M. (1982). *Mosby's atlas of functional human anatomy.* St. Louis, MO: C. V. Mosby.

Black, S. M. (2008). Head and neck: External skull. In Strandring, S. (Ed.) *Gray's anatomy: The anatomical and clinical basis of practice* (40th ed., pp. 409–422). London: Churchill Livingstone.

Buckingham, R. A., & Valvassori, G. E. (2001). Inner ear fluid volumes and the resolving power of magnetic resonance imaging: Can it differentiate endolymphatic structures? *Annals of Otology, Rhinology, and Laryngology, 110*(2), 113–117.

Carpenter, M. B. (1991). *Core text of neuroanatomy* (4th ed.). Baltimore, MD: Williams & Wilkins.

Cazals, Y., Demany, L., & Horner, K. (1991). *Auditory physiology and perception.* Oxford: Pergamon Press.

Chusid, J. G. (1985). *Correlative neuroanatomy and functional neurology* (17th ed.). Los Altos, CA: Lange Medical Publications.

Coleman, B., Hardman, J., Coco, A., Epp, S., de Silva, M., Crook, J., & Shepherd, R. (2006). Fate of embryonic stem cell migration in the deafened mammalian cochlea. *Cell transplantation, 15*(5), 369–380.

Clark, W. W., & Ohlemiller, K. K. (2008). *Anatomy and physiology of hearing for audiologists.* Thomson- Delmar.

Dallos, P. (1973). *The auditory periphery.* New York: Academic Press.

Duifhuis, H., Horst, J. W., van Dijk, P., & van Netten, S. M. (1993). *Biophysics of hair cell sensory systems.* Singapore: World Scientific.

Durrant, J. D., & Lovrinic, J. H. (1995). *Bases of hearing science* (3rd ed.). Baltimore, MD: Williams & Wilkins.

Engstrom, H., Ades, H. W., & Andersson, A. (1966). *Structural pattern of the organ of Corti.* Baltimore, MD: Williams & Wilkins.

Gardner, E., Gray, D. J., & O'Rahilly, R. (1986). *Anatomy: A regional study of human structure* (5th ed.). Philadelphia, PA: W. B. Saunders.

Gelfand, S. A. (2001). *Hearing.* New York: Thiene Medical Publishers.

Gilroy, A. M., MacPherson, B. R., & Ross, L.M. (2012). *Atlas of anatomy* (2nd ed.). New York: Thieme.

Gopen, Q., Rosowski, J. J., & Merchant, S. N. (1997). Anatomy of the normal human cochlear aqueduct with functional implications. *Hearing Research, 107*(1–2), 9–22.

Gray, H., Bannister, L. H., Berry, M. M., & Williams, P. L. (Eds.). (1995). *Gray's anatomy.* London: Churchill Livingstone.

Green, D. (1976). *An introduction to hearing.* Hillsdale, NJ: Lawrence Erlbaum Associates.

Gulick, W. L. (1971). *Hearing physiology and psychophysics.* New York: Oxford University Press.

Hackney, C. M. (2008). Inner ear. In S. Standring (Ed .), *Gray's anatomy: The anatomical and clinical basis of practice* (40th ed., pp. 633–650). London: Churchill Livingstone.

Henson, O. W. (1974). Comparative anatomy of the middle ear. In H. Autrum, R. Jung, W. R. Loewenstein, D. M. MacKay, & H. L. Teuber (Eds.), *Handbook of sensory physiology* (pp. 40–110). New York: Springer-Verlag.

Igarashi, M., Ohashi, K., & Oshii, M. (1986). Morphometric comparison of endolymphatic and perilymphatic spaces in human temporal bones. *Acta Otolaryngolica, 101*(3–4), 161–164.

Kandel, E. R., Schwartz, J. H., Jessell, T. M., Siegelbaum, S. A., & Hudspeth, A. J. (2013). *Principles of neural science* (5th ed.). New York: McGraw Hill.

Kiang, N. Y. S. (1965). *Discharge patterns of single fibers in the cat's auditory nerve.* Cambridge, MA: The MIT Press.

Kuehn, D. P., Lemme, M. L., & Baumgartner, J. M. (1991). *Neural bases of speech, hearing, and language.* Boston: Little, Brown.

Lam, J., & Dohil, M. (2007). Multiple accessory tragi and hemifacial microsomia. *Pediatric Dermatology, 24*(6), 657–658.

Lewis, E. R., Leverenz, E. L., & Bialek, W. S. (1985). *The vertebrate inner ear.* Boca Raton, FL: CRC Press.

Lim, D. J. (1980). Cochlear anatomy related to cochlear micromechanics: A review. *Journal of the Acoustical Society of America, 67*(5), 1686–1695.

Lim, D. J. (1986). Effects of noise and ototoxic drugs at the cellular level in the cochlea. *American Journal of Otolaryngology, 7,* 73–99.

Martin, F., & Clark, J. G. (1995). *Hearing care for children.* Boston, MA: Allyn & Bacon.

Martin, F., & Clark, J. G. (2006). *Elements of audiology: A learning aid with cases.* Boston, MA: Allyn & Bacon.

Martin, F. N. (1981). *Medical audiology.* Englewood Cliffs, NJ: Prentice-Hall.

Melhem, E. R., Shakir, H., Bakthavachalam, S., MacDonald, C. B., Gira, J., Caruthers, S. D., et al. (1998). Inner ear volumetric measurements using high-resolution 3D T2-weighted fast spin-echo MR imaging: Initial experience in healthy subjects. *American Journal of Neuroradiology, 19*(10), 1807–1808.

Minifie, F. D., Hixon, T. J., & Williams, F. (Eds.). (1992). *Normal aspects of speech, hearing, and language.* Englewood Cliffs, NJ: Prentice-Hall.

Møller, A. R. (1973). *Basic mechanisms of hearing.* New York: Academic Press.

Møller, A. R. (1983). *Auditory physiology.* New York: Academic Press.

Møller, A. R. (2003). *Sensory systems: Anatomy and physiology.* New York: Academic Press.

Møller, A. (2006). *Neural plasticity and disorders of the nervous system.* Boston, MA: Cambridge University Press.

Mom, T., Chazal, J., Gabrillargues, J., Gilian, L., & Avan, P. (2005). Cochlear blood supply: An update on anatomy and function. *French Oto-rhino-laryngology, 88,* 81–88.

Netter, F. H. (1997). *Atlas of human anatomy.* Los Angeles: Icon Learning Systems.

Okuno, H., & Sando, I. (1988). Anatomy of the round window. A histopathological study with a graphic reconstruction method. *Acta Otolaryngologica. 106*(1–2), 55–63.

Gleeson, M. (2008). The external and middle ear. In S. Standring (2008). *Gray's anatomy: The anatomical and clinical basis of practice* (40th ed., pp. 614–632). London: Churchill Livingstone.

Pickles, J. O. (1988). *An introduction to the physiology of hearing* (2nd ed.). London: Academic Press.

Porter, C. J. W., & Tan, S. T. (2005). Congenital auricular anomalies: Topographic anatomy, embryology, classification and treatment strategies. *Plastic and Reconstructive Surgery, 115*(6), 1701–1712.

Rohen, J. W., Yokochi, C., Lutjen-Drecoll, E., & Romrell, L. J. (2002). *Color atlas of anatomy* (5th ed.). Philadelphia, PA: Williams & Wilkins.

Rosse, C., & Gaddum-Rosse, P. (1997). *Hollinshead's textbook of anatomy* (5th ed.). Philadelphia, PA: Lippincott-Raven.

Rossing, T. D. (1990). *The science of sound.* Reading, MA: Addison-Wesley.

Schuenke, M., & Ross, L. M., (2010). *Thieme atlas of anatomy.* New York: Thieme.

Standring, S. (2008). *Gray's anatomy: The anatomical and clinical basis of practice* (40th ed.). London: Churchill Livingstone.

Spoendlin, H. (1978). The afferent innervation of the cochlea. In R. F. Naunton & C. Fernandez (Eds.), *Evoked electrical activity in the auditory nervous system.* New York: Academic Press.

Syka, J., & Masterton, R. B. (1988). *Auditory pathway structure and function.* New York: Plenum Press.

Thorne, M., Salt, A. N., DeMott, J. E., Henson, M. M., Henson, O. W. Jr., Gewalt, S. L., et al. (1999). Cochlear fluid space dimensions for six species derived from reconstructions of three-dimensional magnetic resonance images. *Laryngoscope, 109*(10), 1661–1668.

Tobias, J. V., & Schubert, E. D. (1983). *Hearing research and theory* (Vol. 2). New York: Academic Press.

von Békésy, G. (1960). *Experiments in hearing.* New York: McGraw-Hill.

Wei, X., Makori, N., Peterson, P. E., Hummler, H., & Hendrickx, A. G. (1999). Pathogenesis of retinoic acid-induced ear malformations in primate model. *Teratology, 60*(2), 83–92.

Williams, P. L., Bannister, L. H., Berry, M. M., Collins, P., Dyson, M., Dussek, J. E., et al. (1995). *Gray's anatomy* (38th ed.). New York: Churchill Livingstone.

Wilson, J. P., & Kemp, D. T. (1989). *Cochlear mechanisms: Structure, function, and models.* New York: Plenum Press.

Yost, W. A. (2000). *Fundamentals of hearing: An introduction* (4th ed.). New York: Academic Press.

Zemlin, W. R. (1998). *Speech and hearing science: Anatomy and physiology* (4th ed.). Needham Heights, MA: Allyn & Bacon.

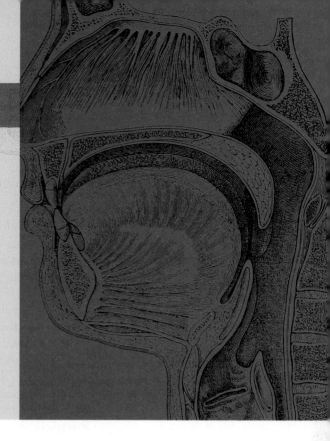

Chapter 10

AUDITORY PHYSIOLOGY

The auditory mechanism is responsible for processing the acoustic signal of speech. Auditory stimuli can arrive at the tympanic membrane in an amazingly wide range of sound pressures, from the whisper of a leaf blowing in the breeze to the pressures associated with painfully loud sound. Likewise, the human auditory mechanism has a frequency range of approximately 10 octaves, spanning 20 to 20,000 Hz. Within these broad requirements of transducing sounds in a range of frequencies are much finer tasks, including differentiating small increments in frequency and intensity. Even beyond these tasks are the everyday requirements of listening to a signal embedded in a background of noise and listening to extremely rapid sequences of sounds. The beauty of the auditory system is that it performs all of these tasks and more with breathtaking ease. This chapter cannot provide a thorough examination of all aspects of auditory physiology, but we hope it will show you why audiologists are so excited by their field.

The field of audiology owes a great deal to the extraordinary scientist Georg von Békésy, whose work earned him a Nobel Prize in 1961 (Evans, 2003). Von Békésy (1960) performed exceedingly intricate measurements on the auditory mechanism, and was at times forced to create tools where none existed. We will refer frequently to his work, which defined the basic function of the middle and inner ear, as we discuss the basic physiological principles involved in the translation of an acoustic stimulus into a form that is interpretable by the brain. The organizing principle to keep in mind is this: The outer ear collects sound and "shapes" its frequency components somewhat; the middle ear matches the airborne acoustic signal with

An octave is a doubling in frequency.

See Chapter 4 for a discussion of frequency and periodicity.

Anatesse Lesson

the fluid medium of the cochlea; the inner ear performs temporal and spectral analyses on the ongoing acoustical signal; the auditory pathway conveys and further processes that signal. The cerebral cortex interprets the signal.

INSTRUMENTATION IN HEARING RESEARCH

There are a number of tools available for the study of hearing. Of critical importance is knowledge of the temporal and spectral characteristics of a signal being transduced by the listener, so spectral and temporal acoustic analysis tools (discussed in Chapters 5 and 7) serve that purpose. Impedance of the middle ear is measured by tympanometry, and recent developments in wideband acoustic reflectance measures have become important tools for elaborating middle ear function (e.g., Sanford & Feeney, 2008). The cochlea provides significant challenges for study due to its extremely small size, and the fact that it is embedded within the densest bone in the body. While it can be visualized through high-resolution functional magnetic resonance imaging for purposes of identifying malformations, the physical study of the cochlea relies on postmortem micrographic imaging and histological techniques. Researchers have been able to identify neural receptors and functional proteins within the cochlea (e.g., Spicer & Schulte, 1996, to be discussed) using ultrastructural visualizing methods.

Questions about the function of the cochlea have resulted in the development of instruments that ultimately entered the clinical realm for diagnostic purposes. You have likely been exposed to the clinical audiometer, which is a means of behaviorally assessing the hearing threshold of individuals. Otoacoustic emissions testing involves introducing tones into the ear and recording the reflection from the cochlea as a means of determining the viability of the outer hair cells. This important assessment tool began as a research instrument (e.g., Norton & Neely, 1987) and has evolved into a critically important clinical tool (e.g., Seixas, Kujawa, Norton, Sheppard, Neitzel & Slee, 2004).

Electrophysiological methods provide a window to the neurophysiology of the auditory mechanism. Research on nonhuman animals often involves direct, single-cell measurement of the auditory pathway, which gives a great deal of insight into the detail of auditory transmission (there have been a few direct measurements in humans as well). The acoustic reflex permits examination of the integrity of the early stages of the auditory pathway. For years auditory brain stem evoked responses (ABR) and electrocochleography (EcOG) have allowed researchers and clinicians to examine the integrity of the auditory pathway, and cortical auditory functioning (and even cognitive processes) can be illuminated through numerous late cortical responses to acoustic stimuli (e.g., P300, P400, contingent negative variation). Functional magnetic resonance imaging (fMRI) provides a unique window to auditory cortical functioning (although the extraordinarily high sound pressure levels of the instrument provide a particularly daunting challenge to the researcher trying to present auditory stimuli to a subject).

Instrumentation in hearing science began with the pioneering work of von Békésy and Helmholtz before him, and continues to develop as technology of acoustical, physical, and physiological measurement becomes more refined.

OUTER EAR

The outer ear can be seen primarily as a collector of sound. The **pinna**, with its ridges, grooves, and dished-out regions, is an excellent funnel for sound directed toward the head from the front or side, although less effective for sound arising from behind the head.

Indeed, the crevices and crannies of the pinna are functional. If you have blown across the lip of a soda bottle and produced a tone, you know that cavities have characteristics that make them particularly responsive to specific frequencies. When a tube or bottle is excited by an input stimulus, it will tend to select energy at its resonant frequency, while tending to reject energy at frequencies other than the resonant frequency. The result is **selective enhancement** of certain frequencies (see Figure 10-1).

Because the outer ear has no active (moveable) elements, it can have only a passive effect on the input stimulus. The pinna acts as a "sound funnel," focusing acoustic energy into the external auditory meatus (EAM), and the EAM funnels sound to the TM. Both of these

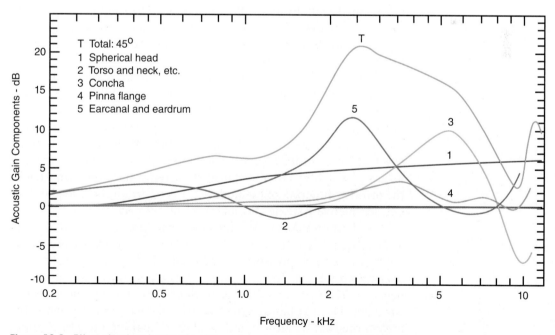

Figure 10-1. Effect of various landmarks of the outer ear upon the input acoustic signal.

Source: Reprinted by permission from the External Ear by E. A. G. Shaw, 1974, p. 95. In W. D. Keidel & W. D. Neff, Eds., *Handbook of Sensory Physiology*. Copyright 1974 by Springer-Verlag, Inc. New York: Springer-Verlag.

structures, however, have shapes that boost the relative strength of the signal through resonance, with the result being relatively enhanced signal intensity between 1,500 and 8,000 Hz.

As can be seen in Figure 10-1, the components of the pinna contribute a relatively small amount to the overall gain as compared with that of the EAM. Nonetheless, the contribution of the entire system results in a net gain reaching 20 dB at approximately 2,100 Hz. Kruger (1989) showed that the resonant frequency of the outer ear changes from birth until about 3 years: The neonate has a peak resonance that is closer to 6,000 Hz, but that resonance shifts down steadily as the auricle and EAM grow, reaching 2,500 Hz at 37 months.

MIDDLE EAR FUNCTION

As you remember, the primary structures of the middle ear are the TM, the ossicles, and the entry to the cochlea, the oval window. These are the players in one of the most important evolutionary dramas of the auditory mechanism.

If you can recall a dreamy summer day at a swimming pool, you may also remember that it would have been almost impossible to communicate vocally with someone in that pool if the person was submerged. When you tried to yell at your friend from above the water, nearly all of the sound energy of your speech would have reflected off the surface of the water.

The cochlea is a fluid-filled cavity, and were it not for the presence of the middle ear mechanism, talking to each other would be like trying to talk to someone under water: The sound energy would reflect off the oval window because of the vast differences in the liquid and gaseous media of perilymph and air. Somewhere in our evolution a mechanism arose to improve our plight.

The middle ear mechanism is designed to increase the pressure approaching the cochlea, thereby overcoming the resistance to flow of energy, termed **impedance**. You will recall from Chapter 2 that **pressure = force/area**. That is, to increase pressure, you must either increase the force or decrease the area over which the force is being exerted. The middle ear mechanism uses the latter as the primary means of matching the impedance of the outer and inner ear. That is, the primary function of the middle ear is to match the impedance of two conductive systems, the outer ear and the cochlea.

The first mechanism of impedance matching is achieved through addressing the area parameter of the TM and the oval window. As mentioned earlier, pressure can be increased by decreasing the area over which force is distributed: A lightweight individual in a spike heel can do much more damage to floor tiles than a piano mover in sneakers. The TM has an effective area of about 55 mm², while the area of the oval window is about 3.2 mm², making the TM 17 times larger, depending on species size. Sound energy reaching the TM is "funneled" to the much smaller area of the oval window, so there is a gain of 17:1, which translates to an increase of about 25 dB.

The second impedance-matching function is achieved by a lever difference. The length of the manubrium is approximately 9 mm, while that of the long process of the stapes is about 7 mm, giving an overall gain of about 1.2. The lever effect arising from this gain is nearly 2 dB.

A third effect arises from the buckling of the TM. As it moves in response to sound, the TM buckles somewhat, such that the arm of the malleus moves a shorter distance than the surface of the TM. This results in a reduction in velocity of displacement of the malleus, with a resulting increase of force that provides a 4–6 dB increase in effective signal.

Combined, the area, lever, and buckling effects result in a signal gain of about 31 dB, from the TM to cochlea, depending on the stimulus frequency. Again, were the middle ear removed, a signal entering the EAM would have to be 31 dB more intense to be heard. This middle ear transformer action is very important to audition, and any process that reduces the effectiveness of this function (such as otitis media, otosclerosis, or glomus tumors) can have a serious impact on the conduction of sound to the inner ear.

✔ *To summarize:*

- The outer and middle ears serve as funneling and impedance-matching devices.
- The **pinna** funnels acoustical information to the **external auditory meatus** and aids in the **localization** of sound in space.
- The **resonant frequencies** of the pinna and the external auditory meatus are those of the important components of the speech signal, between 1,500 and 8,000 Hz.
- Resistance to the flow of energy is termed **impedance**.
- The middle ear mechanism is an **impedance-matching device**, increasing the pressure of a signal arriving at the cochlea.
- The **area ratio** between the tympanic membrane and the oval window provides a 25 dB gain.
- The **lever advantage** of the ossicles provides a 2 dB gain.
- The buckling effect provides a 4–6 dB gain.

INNER EAR FUNCTION
Vestibular Mechanism

Anatesse Lesson ⊳

The semicircular canals are uniquely designed to respond to rotatory movements of the body. By virtue of their orientation, each canal is at approximate right angles to the other canals, so that all movements of the head can be mapped by combinations of outputs of the sensory components, the cristae ampulares. Activation of the sensory element arises from inertia: As your head rotates, the fluid in the semicircular canals tends to lag behind. The result of this is that the cilia are stimulated by relative movement of the fluid during rotation. The utricle and saccule sense acceleration of the head rather than rotation, during body or head tilting. When you are standing erect, the macula of the utricle is roughly horizontal to the plane of movement, so straight-line acceleration in a forward or backward movement will be sensed there. The saccule, in contrast, is oriented more vertically. You can thank the macula of the utricle for the sensation associated with rapid acceleration during take-off of a jet. In contrast, the saccule can be blamed for that sinking feeling when you hit turbulence that causes the plane to drop suddenly, and the semicircular canals can take care of the other movements. Taken together, the vestibular mechanisms provide the major input to the proprioceptive system serving the sense of one's body in space. This information is integrated with joint sense, muscle spindle afferents, and visual input to form the perception of body position.

Auditory Mechanism: Mechanical Events

One simply must be awed by the cochlea. This structure would neatly fit on the eraser of a pencil, and the fluid within it would be but a drop on your tabletop. The structures are astoundingly small and delicate, and yet this mechanism, given some reasonable care, can serve a lifetime of hearing without appreciable degeneration. Admittedly, the high-impact noise of modern society takes a rapid toll on such a delicate mechanism, but that is another story. Let us examine what is arguably the most amazing sensory system of the human body, the cochlea.

Clinical Manipulation of the Vestibular Mechanism

Audiologists are involved in working with assessment and treatment of disorders of the auditory mechanism, as you know. Among those disorders are *vestibular disorders*. Disorders that cause a sense of vertigo (perception of spinning or rotation) or dizziness (lightheadedness), loss of balance, and visual disturbances arising from difficulty in integrating body sense with the visual input. Benign paroxysmal positional vertigo (BPPV) is quite common, providing the patient with a spinning perception (vertigo) that occurs suddenly (paroxysmal), relative to body position (Hackney, 2008). The "benign" part is good news, because that means it is not associated with a degenerative or organic disease condition. Nystagmus (ratcheting oscillation of the eyes) typically occurs, resulting from the brain's perception that it needs to adjust to head movement (which is perceived, but not real). It is thought that BBPV arises because the calcium carbonate crystals of the otoliths in the semicircular canals drop into the ampulla of the posterior semicircular canal. This is where the audiologist (and physical therapist) come in.

Audiologists and physical therapists will often team up to perform the Epley maneuver. In this treatment, the client is placed in a series of positions that cause the crystals to move out of the ampulla and into the vestibule, where they no longer cause vestibular mischief. This maneuver is highly successful in alleviating the dizziness, vertigo, and cognitive distress that comes with BBPV, and all of this without requiring surgery!

As we mentioned in the introduction to this chapter, the inner ear is responsible for performing spectral and temporal acoustic analyses of the incoming acoustical signal. By **spectral analysis**, we refer to the process of extracting or defining the various frequency components of a given signal. You will recall from our discussion in Chapter 5 that frequency and intensity of vibration define the psychological correlates of "pitch" and "loudness." The cochlea is specifically designed to sort out the frequency components of an incoming signal, determine their amplitude, and even identify basic temporal aspects of that signal. These processes make up the first level of auditory processing of an acoustic signal. Subsequent processing occurs as the signal works its way rapidly along the auditory pathway, ultimately to the brain. To get a notion of how this happens, we need to consider the input to the cochlea.

As you remember, sound is a disturbance in air. The airborne disturbance causes the TM to move, and that movement is translated to the oval window. When the TM moves inward, the stapes footplate in the oval window also moves in; and when the TM moves out, so does the footplate. This movement is a direct analog to the compressions and rarefactions of sound, so that, for the most part, the complexities of sound are directly translated to the cochlear fluid medial to the stapes footplate.

When the stapes compresses the perilymph of the scala vestibuli, Reissner's membrane is distended toward the scala media, and the basilar membrane is distended toward the scala tympani. That is, a compression in the fluid of the scala vestibuli is translated directly to the basilar membrane. You will remember that the frequency of a sound is determined by the number of oscillations or vibrations per second. In this case, it is the number of oscillations of the TM-ossicle-footplate combination: A 100 Hz signal results in the footplate moving inward and outward 100 times per second, and that periodic vibration is translated to the basilar membrane, where it initiates a wave action known as the **traveling wave**.

Georg von Békésy discovered that the basilar membrane is particularly well designed to support wave action that directly corresponds to the frequency of vibration of the input sound. Specifically, when high-frequency sounds impinge on the inner ear, they cause vibration of the basilar membrane closer to the vestibule, the basal end of the cochlea. Low-frequency sounds result in a long traveling wave that reaches toward the apex, covering a greater distance along the basilar membrane. In this way, the traveling wave separates out the frequency components of complex sounds, because high-frequency sounds are processed in basal regions, whereas low-frequency sounds are processed nearer the apex. When a sound has both high- and low-frequency components, those components are separated out and processed at their respective portions of the basilar membrane.

If you have experienced an ocean beach, you will be familiar with wave action. Waves roll in from the ocean and swell to a large amplitude as they break on the beach. Although the analogy is not perfect, it may help you to recognize the driving force behind differentiating frequency components: The point of maximum amplitude excursion of the traveling wave on the basilar membrane is the primary point of neural excitation of the hair cells within the organ of Corti. Said another way, the traveling wave moves along the basilar membrane, growing and swelling as it travels, until it reaches a point of maximum growth. The wave very quickly damps down after that point, so there is only one truly *strong* point of disturbance from the traveling wave. In this manner, the low-frequency sound discussed earlier will cause the traveling wave to "break" closer to the apex, and that place of maximum disturbance determines the frequency information that is transmitted to the brain.

Our understanding of the mechanism that determines *where* the point of maximum amplitude excursion occurs is another of von Békésy's legacies. He fashioned instruments from exotic materials such as pig bristles to measure the stiffness of the basilar membrane. As stiffness increases, the natural frequency of vibration of a body increases. (See the software auditory physiology lessons to test the effects of stiffness on the traveling wave.) Von Békésy's pig bristle experiments revealed that the basal end of the basilar membrane is stiffer than the apical end, and that the stiffness decreases in a graded fashion from base to apex. (In fact, the cochlear duct is flaccid at its most apical end, where it is not connected to the bony labyrinth, to form the helicotrema.) In addition, we know that as mass of a structure increases, its resonant frequency decreases. The basilar membrane becomes increasingly massive, from base to apex. Finally, the basilar membrane becomes progressively wider from base to apex. These three components—graded stiffness, graded mass, graded width—combine to make the basilar membrane an excellent frequency analyzer. Verification of the importance of these resonance characteristics is provided by the fact that the traveling wave can be stimulated in the absence of the middle ear mechanism (as in bone conduction testing of an individual without middle ear ossicles). No matter how the traveling wave is initiated, it *always* travels from base to apex, because of the impedance gradient of the basilar membrane.

Excitation of the hair cells occurs as the result of several interacting variables. First, the cilia of the outer hair cells are embedded within the tectorial membrane (see Figure 10-2). As the traveling wave moves along the basilar membrane, the hair cells are displaced relative to the tectorial membrane. This produces a **shearing action** that is, of course, greatest at the point of maximum perturbation of the basilar membrane.

Tonndorf (1958) and later Møller (1973) and Dallos (1973) described another mechanism that helps to explain how the inner hair cells are excited. Recall that the inner hair cells are not embedded in the tectorial membrane, so they are not subjected to the same forces as the outer hair cells. Further, their placement closer to the osseous spiral lamina gives them reduced opportunity to capitalize on shear. Rather, it appears that the inner hair cells depend on fluid movement of the

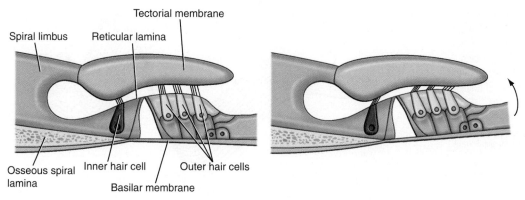

Figure 10-2. Schematic representation of shearing action of basilar membrane-tectorial membrane relationship.
© Cengage Learning®.

endolymph to excite them. As the traveling wave moves along the basilar membrane, it effectively slides past the fluid molecules. Put another way, the fluid moves relative to the hair cell. The cilia are displaced by the fluid movement, just as grass in a riverbed is drawn by the fluid flow. If you invoke the Bernoulli principle studied in Chapter 5, you will see the final stage of excitation. At the point of maximum excursion, the basilar membrane is "humped" up, essentially protruding into the fluid stream. The Bernoulli principle states that at the constriction, velocity of fluid flow will increase. This disturbance at the point of maximum excitation causes a turbulence, which produces eddies or swirls of fluid molecules. In this way, the fluid is more turbulent at the point of maximum excitation, meaning that the hair cells are more likely to be excited at that point than at other, less turbulent locations.

Stimulation of the hair cell presents a paradox, however. A hair cell is stimulated when the cilia are bent in a direction away from the modiolus, but the traveling wave produces a disturbance that is apically directed along the length of the basilar membrane, at right angles to the pattern that excites the hair cell. This dilemma is easy to resolve, however. Remember that the basilar membrane is anchored to the spiral lamina. When the traveling wave perturbs the basilar membrane, the shearing action on the cilia is produced in the medial-proximal dimension because of the hinge-like function of the lamina. Because of the nature of the traveling wave, the primary shear at the peak of the traveling wave is radial, as described, whereas the shear apical to the maximum of the wave is longitudinal, a direction that does not stimulate the hair cell (see Figure 10-3).

The hinge-like arrangement of the basilar membrane and spiral limbus place the outer hair cells in a position to be activated by a lower-level stimulus than the inner hair cells. Thus, it appears that, at least for intensities less than 40 dB SPL, the outer hair cells are an important mechanism for coding intensity, although the inner hair cells are essential for frequency coding. Loss of outer hair cells does not result in complete loss of hearing, but rather elevation of the threshold of audition.

Figure 10-3. Traveling wave patterns. (A) Pattern of oscillation in absence of lateral restraints. (B) Pattern of vibration arising from stimulation, but accounting for lateral attachment of basilar membrane.

Source: Reprinted with permission from "Shearing Motion in Scala Media of Cochlear Models," by J. Tonndorf, 1960, *Journal of the Acoustical Society of America*, 32(2), p. 241. Copyright 1960 by American Institute of Physics.

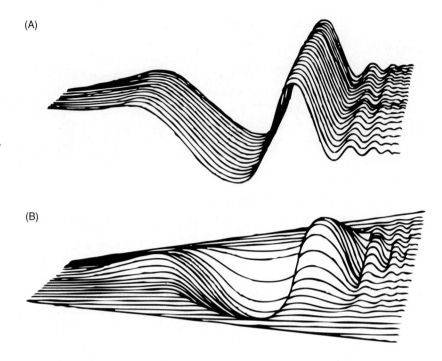

(A)

(B)

Hair Cell Regeneration

Gene therapy is being developed to regenerate hair cells. We have known for a few years that avian hair cells regenerate, but only recently have researchers identified a means for regenerating hair cells in mammals. Izumikawa et al. (2005) genetically modified a cold virus and injected it into guinea pigs. Not only did new hair cells grow, but when the guinea pigs were tested using auditory brainstem responses, it was clear that the hair cells were working. The first clinical trial for hair cell regeneration in humans has been initiated by a research group at the University of Kansas Medical School. In 2013, Kraft, Hsu, Brough, and Staecker inserted *Atoh1* genes into mice with cochleas that had been damaged using ototoxic drugs and found that the hearing improved 20 dB as a result of the therapy. The researchers have initiated a clinical trial on 45 humans with severe sensorineural hearing loss arising from ototoxic drugs. The research community is anxiously awaiting the results of this clinical trial. If the expanded trial proves successful it could mean return to hearing for over 7 million people in the United States alone.

✔ *To summarize:*

- The inner ear is responsible for performing **spectral** (frequency) and **temporal acoustic analyses** of the incoming acoustical signal.
- Movement of the tympanic membrane is translated into an analogous movement of the stapes footplate and the fluid in the scala vestibuli.

- Compression of the fluid of the scala vestibuli is translated directly to the basilar membrane, and the disturbance at the basilar membrane initiates the **traveling wave**.
- The cochlea has a **tonotopic arrangement**, with high-frequency sounds resolved at the base and low-frequency sounds processed at the apex.
- The point of **maximum excursion** of the basilar membrane determines the frequency information transmitted to the brain.
- The traveling wave quickly **damps** after reaching its point of maximum excursion.
- The frequency analysis ability of the basilar membrane is determined by its graded **stiffness**, **thickness**, and **width**. The basilar membrane is stiffer, thinner, and narrower at the base than at the apex.
- Excitation of the **outer hair cells** occurs primarily as a result of the **shearing effect** on the cilia.
- Excitation of the **inner hair cells** is produced by the effect of **fluid flow** and **turbulence** of the endolymph.

Superior Semicircular Canal Dehiscence

We know that movement of the ossicles causes the traveling wave of the cochlea: When you hear a sound, it moves the ossicles and causes displacement of the footplate of the stapes, which translates into a pulsatile action at the vestibule. The traveling wave is generated in the cochlea, and the point of maximum perturbation of the basilar membrane is identified as the major frequency component of the sound. So far, so good. If you look at Figure 9-7 again, however, you'll see that the vestibular mechanism and the cochlear duct (scala media) are connected: they share endolymph, and therefore they share perturbations that occur in the endolymph. If you think about it a minute, it seems that the perturbation that occurs when the stapes footplate moves in response to sound ought to cause a disturbance in both the cochlea and the vestibular mechanism. Said another way, what stops sound from activating the semicircular canals?

The answer to this is in hydraulics. Remember that the cochlea is designed with two windows (oval window and round window), and that the impulse creating the traveling wave (arising from that movement of the stapes) translates directly from the scala vestibuli to the scala media and then to the scala tympani. The micropressure is relieved by the round window. In contrast, you cannot pressurize one end of a semicircular canal without also pressurizing the other end, since both ends open onto the vestibule.

This answer also reveals a pathology. Superior semicircular canal dehiscence is a condition that arises when the bone overlying the superior semicircular canal erodes, allowing the membranous sac within which the canal resides to be continuous with the brain space (e.g., Banerjee & Nikkar-Esfahani, 2011). In other words, a hole develops in the bone that is the equivalent of another round window, within the vestibular mechanism. In this case, a disturbance at the vestibule caused by movement of the stapes in response to sound will cause a disturbance in the superior semicircular canal. The result is sound-induced vertigo, or Tullio phenomenon (Watson, Halmagyi, & Colbach, 2000), as well as hyperacusis (hypersensitivity to sound) and autophony (unusually loud perception of one's own voice or heartbeat).

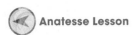 **Anatesse Lesson**

Electrical Events

The cochlea is both a spectrum analyzer and a transducer. The mechanical properties of the components of the organ of Corti provide spectral analysis, and the stimulation of hair cells permits the mechanical energy arriving at the cochlea in the form of movement of the stapes footplate to be converted into electrochemical energy. As with any other neural component of the nervous system, the hair cells are designed to transmit information. When the basilar membrane is displaced toward the scala vestibuli, the hair cells are activated, whereas when the basilar membrane is displaced toward the scala tympani, electrical activity of the hair cell is inhibited. Stimulation of the hair cells results in four electrical potentials.

So how is it that an electrical event is initiated? The mechanism for initiating a response in the cochlea hinges, quite literally, on the sterocilia. You will recall from Chapter 9 that each hair cell is endowed with stereocilia. These cilia are linked together by means of molecules of fibrin, which provides a rigid connection between cilia. The core of each sterocilia is coated with a plasma membrane, and each cilia tapers down from top to bottom. That is to say, the cilia are markedly thinner near the hair cell, which gives them an ideal mechanism for pivoting. Each hair cell has a rudimentary kinocilium, which is a type of cilia.

In the resting state, about 15 percent of the ion channels are open at any time. When the cilia are pivoted toward the tallest stereocilia (the kinocilium), the hair cell depolarizes; when it is tilted away from the kinoclium, the hair cell is hyperpolarized (cannot fire). This depolarization produces a graded receptor potential that increases as the amplitude of the stimulus increases. Realize that this involves a rather small movement, in reality, because movement of 100 nm provides 90 percent of its dynamic range, while 0.3 nm worth of deflection is the threshold of hearing. A nanometer is 1 billionth of a meter (the hair on your head is about 10 μm wide, which is 10 millionths of

Noise Pollution

Psychologically, auditory noise is anything that gets in the way of what we want to hear, the signal. Noise is more than a psychological phenomenon, however. Haralabidis et al. (2008) examined the effects of nighttime noise on individuals living near airports in Europe. When a subject heard noise at or above 35 dB HL the systolic blood pressure increased by 6.2 mmHg and diastolic pressure increased by 6.4 mmHg. The authors found that every 10 dB increase in noise during the night raised the likelihood of a person developing high blood pressure (hypertension) by 14 percent. The authors note that it is not just airplane noise, but even a loudly snoring partner can have the same effect. Considering that hypertension is one of the most significant predictors of stroke, it would do well to sleep in the quiet.

a meter), so virtually the entire range of a hair cell involves movement that is 1/10,000 of the width of a human hair. The scale of function in the cochlea is astounding.

Each hair cell has around 100 channels for ion transduction (approximately 1 per cilia): When the cilia are mechanically deflected toward the highest stereocilia, the channels are drawn open. The tip links on the cilia act like tiny springs that cause the ion channels to open rapidly. At the base of the hair cell is the active zone: The neurotransmitter glutamate (which is the most prevalent neurotransmitter in the nervous system: von Bohlen und Halbach & Dermietzel, 2006), is released here as a result of depolarization of the hair cell, and this is used as a signal to the VIII nerve fiber. You will remember discussion of the stria vascularis from Chapter 9 and its critical role in maintaining ion balance within the scala media. Potassium enters the hair cell when the cilia are deflected through disturbance of the basilar membrane and, remarkably, passes through the basilar membrane into the perilymph within the scala tympani. From there it is taken up by the stria vascularis and recycled into the endolymph. In this manner, the K^+ rich environment of the endolymph is maintained (Spicer & Schulte, 1996). The ions move as a result of a cross-membrane ion gradient through the superficial stria vascularis and ion pumps for Na^+, Cl^- and K^+. Enriching the endolymph with potassium is not a trivial matter: The superficial cells of the stria vascularis have K^+ ion channels that allow osmotic movement into the endolymph, and when mice are genetically engineered without the ability to move potassium via the superficial cells they have a demonstrable hearing loss (Casimiro et al., 2001). It is precisely the establishment of the ion gradient between the intermediate cells of the stria vascularis and the endolymph that create the +80 mV potential difference that drives hearing function (Wangemann, 2006). The hair cell, in contrast, has a negative potential of –70 mV, which produces a powerful 150 mV differential between the endolymph and the hair cell, as we will discuss shortly.

Depolarizing the inner hair cells causes excitation of the VIII nerve as a result of glutamate release, while depolarizing the outer hair cells causes a "motor" response that actually moves the basilar membrane. The IHC transmit information about the site of excitation and the OHC amplify the signal by moving the basilar membrane at the site of activation, a phenomenon recorded by the audiologist as otoacoustic emissions (Musiek & Baran, 2006).

Resting Potentials

The **resting** or **standing potentials** are those voltage potential differences that can be measured from the cochlea at rest. Ions do not travel between the endolymphatic region (scala media) and those of the perilymph (scala tympani and scala vestibuli), and there are cochlear potential differences among those spaces. The scala vestibuli is slightly more positive than the scala tympani (about +5 mV), but the scala media is considerably more positive (about +80 mV). That is, the scala media has a constant positive potential (the **endocochlear potential**) relative to the scala tympani and scala vestibuli. The strong positive potential arises from passive osmosis and active ion pumping by the stria vascularis. Another resting potential, the **intracellular resting potential**, is found within the hair cells. The potential difference between the endolymph and the intercellular potential of the hair cell is –70 mV relative to the endolymph, giving a very large 150 mV difference between the hair cells and the surrounding fluid.

Potentials Arising from Stimulation

Stimulation of the hair cells results in the generation of a number of potentials, although not all of them are thought to be important in auditory processing. The **cochlear microphonic** was once thought to be the "prime mover" of cochlear activity, and for good reason. Wever and Bray (1930) found that the cochlear microphonic recorded from a living cat's cochlea directly followed the speech signal (see Figure 10-4). It was felt that the potential was "microphonic" (like a microphone), directly responding to the input signal. They were correct at first blush: The potential *does* directly follow the movement of the basilar membrane, and it appears to be generated by the outer hair cells or current changes at the reticular lamina in the vicinity of the outer hair cells. Although microelectrode recording of inner hair cell intracellular potentials shows an alternating current (AC) potential, the potential is not large enough to account for the microphonic. In any case, the cochlear microphonic is an AC potential that follows the movement of the input signal as it impinges upon the basilar membrane.

The **summating potential** is a sustained, direct current (DC) shift in the endocochlear potential that occurs upon stimulation of

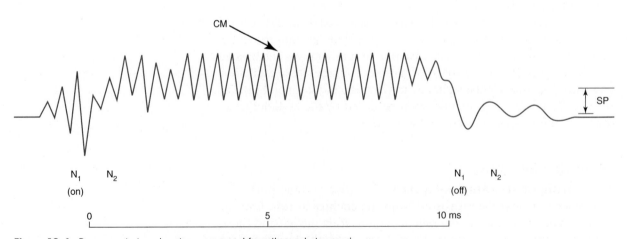

Figure 10-4. Response to tone burst, as measured from the scala tympani.

Source: Pickles, J. O. (2012). An introduction to the physiology of hearing (Vol. 4). Emerald Group Publishing Limited, figure 3.25.

the organ of Corti by sound (see Figure 10-4). The inner hair cells are depolarized when stimulated by sound, and that results in reduced intracellular potential (a less negative potential). This potential difference between the hair cell and the endolymph may produce the summating potential. It is seen as a DC shift in electrical output that is maintained as long as an auditory stimulus is presented to the ear.

The **whole-nerve action potential** (also known as the **compound action potential**), abbreviated AP, arises directly from stimulation of a large number of hair cells simultaneously, eliciting nearly simultaneous individual action potentials in the VIII nerve, as discussed in Chapter 9. Measured extracochlearly, the whole-nerve action potential represents the sum of action potentials generated by stimulation of the hair cells. It is best elicited using clicks with broad spectral content rather than tones, although tones certainly can be used. The AP has two major negative components, N_1 (occurring around 1 ms post-stimulus onset) and N_2 (around 2 ms post-stimulus onset) and the amplitude of the AP increases as the sound stimulus intensity increases (Musiek & Baran, 2006). The whole-nerve action potential is first detected at between 10 and 20 dB above a person's behavioral threshold (Eggermont & Odenthal, 1974), and this potential can be measured by means of the auditory brainstem response (ABR) or through ECoG. The individual action potential arising from stimulation of an individual VIII nerve fiber tells a very important story at the microscopic level. Looking at single-unit (single VIII nerve fiber) responses reveals that the cochlear mechanism has an extraordinarily fine ability to differentiate frequency components (frequency specificity), and by processing data from a large number of individual fibers we can learn a great deal about the coding of simple and complex stimuli by the auditory nervous system.

✔ *To summarize:*

- When the basilar membrane is displaced toward the scala vestibuli, the hair cells are activated, resulting in **electrical potentials**.
- **Resting** or **standing potentials** are those voltage potential differences that can be measured from the cochlea at rest.
- The scala vestibuli is 5 mV more positive than the scala tympani, but the scala media is 80 mV more positive.
- The **intracellular resting potential** within the hair cell reveals a potential difference between the endolymph and the hair cell of –70 mV, giving a 150 mV difference between the hair cells and the surrounding fluid.
- Stimulus-related potentials include the alternating current **cochlear microphonic** generated by the outer hair cells; the **summating potential**, a direct current shift in the endocochlear potential; and the **whole-nerve action potential**, arising directly from stimulation of a large number of hair cells simultaneously.

Neural Responses

There are two basic types of VIII nerve neurons: **low spontaneous rate** (high-threshold) and **high spontaneous rate** (low-threshold) fibers. High-threshold neurons require a higher level of stimulation to fire, respond to the higher end of our auditory range of signal intensity, and have little or no random background firing noise. Low-threshold fibers, in contrast, respond at very low signal intensities and display random firing even when no stimulus is present. Thus, it appears that the low-threshold neurons may be a mechanism for hearing sound at near-threshold levels, whereas high-threshold fibers may pick up where the low-threshold fibers stop, as the signal increases.

The background "chatter" of random firing poses some problems for examining neuron response, however. The task of neurophysiologists is to identify neuron responses related to a specific stimulus and to separate them from the background noise of random firing. Two basic techniques have evolved to manage that problem, and both have provided important clues to neural function. Let us look at these techniques and the results of their application.

Post-Stimulus Time Histograms

Histograms are a convenient method of looking at data that occur over time. When you are taking an anatomy exam, you know that the whole class does not finish at the same time. Rather, the first person may finish after 40 minutes, the next one at 43 minutes, then a couple more at 44 minutes, and so on. If you were interested in the *modal* finishing time for an exam, you could plot the elapsed test-taking time for each person in the form of a bar graph (**histogram**) and identify the point at which the greatest number of people left at the same time. You can also look at the response time of neurons the same way. Auditory physiologists record bursts of electrical activity of single neurons and plot their response. Because they know when the stimulus was presented (just as your instructor knows when the test started), the researcher can plot the responses relative to the onset of the stimulus—hence, post-stimulus time (PST) histogram.

Because neurons are all-or-none devices, every unit response is equal to the next in intensity and duration. Thus, the only way neurons can provide differential response is by having different rates of firing. Single-unit neural information is conveyed in the timing of its response. If you were to record the spike-rate activity of a neuron that is firing randomly, in the absence of a stimulus, there would be no real dominant mode of activity; rather, the neural response would be spread fairly evenly over the entire recording period. If you were to record that activity in response to a tonal stimulus, you would get a response more like that of Figure 10-5. When an VIII nerve fiber responds to tonal stimulation, there is an initial burst of strong activity, followed by a decline to a plateau of discharge over the duration of the tone. When the tone is terminated, the response of the fiber drops to below baseline levels, rising up to the baseline "noise" level after recovery.

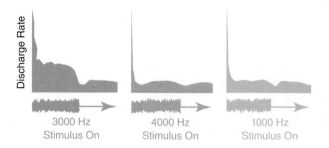

Figure 10-5. Schematic representation of post-stimulus time histogram for 3000 Hz, 4000 Hz, and 1000 Hz tones, as recorded from a nerve fiber with a characteristic frequency of 3000 Hz.
© Cengage Learning®.

This fairly straightforward PST histogram has provided us with very important verification of the **frequency specificity**, the ability of the cochlea to differentiate different spectral components of a signal. Figure 10-5 displays a hypothetical array of spike rate PST histograms generated for the same neuron under different stimulus conditions. In this case, we have placed an electrode on a fiber serving the area of the cochlea in which 3,000 Hz signals are processed. Look at the responses. When we deliver a 3,000 Hz signal, the fiber has a strong response shortly after onset, with the characteristic plateau until the tone ends. Now see what happens when we present a 4,000 Hz signal. The response is *much* weaker to that stimulation than it is to the 1,000 Hz signal. As you know from the traveling wave theory, signals above 3,000 Hz will not cause much disturbance on the basilar membrane at the 3,000 Hz point. Likewise, the traveling wave must necessarily pass through the region of our electrode on its way to the 1,000 Hz point (toward the apex, or low-frequency region), but the traveling wave has not gained much amplitude at that point so there is not much excitation. In other words, if we record the firing rate of a neuron, we can get a fair estimate of its **characteristic** or **best frequency**. The characteristic frequency (CF) of a neuron is the frequency to which it responds best. In the case shown in Figure 10-5, the CF of the neuron we were recording was 3000 Hz.

One goal of auditory physiology is to explain humans' extraordinary ability to discriminate signals in the frequency domain. Researchers who study auditory perceptual abilities as they relate to the physical mechanism (**psychoacousticians**) have found that, in general, humans can discriminate change in frequency of signals of about 1 percent. (Recognize that this gross generalization ignores differences in signal intensity, variations based on different stimulus frequency, signal duration, etc.) That is, if a 100 Hz tone is presented, you can hear the difference between it and a 102 Hz tone, an increase of 2 percent. The challenge to physiologists was to identify how the cochlea could produce such fine discriminations.

Figure 10-6 shows a "tuning curve" for a single-unit recording. A tuning curve is basically a composite of the responses of a single fiber at each frequency of presentation. To demonstrate this, researchers placed an electrode on a neuron and presented different frequencies of stimulation. They then recorded the stimulus intensity at which the neuron began to fire in response to the stimulus

Figure 10-6. Schematic representation of tuning curve for VIII nerve fiber with characteristic frequency of 10000 Hz.

© Cengage Learning®.

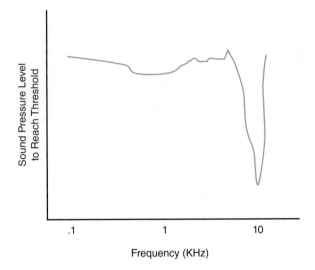

(its threshold) and plotted that intensity. In Figure 10-6, you can see that the fiber was most sensitive to the 10,000 Hz signal. As the signal frequency decreased to 8,000 Hz, the signal had to be of greater intensity to cause the neuron to fire. The signal at 5,000 Hz had to be 60 dB stronger than that at the CF for that neuron, 10,000 Hz.

This tuning curve is a measure of neural specificity in one sense, but probably as much a measure of basilar membrane response. The electrode is, in effect, measuring the activity at one point on the basilar membrane (10,000 Hz, near the base), and the activity farther up the cochlea toward the apex has less and less effect on the neuron we are recording. The sharper the tuning curve, the greater the frequency specificity of the basilar membrane. Indeed, when Khanna and Leonard (1982) compared the tuning curves of the basilar membrane and the auditory nerve, they found that the two curves were quite similar. That is, the basilar membrane is a very finely tuned filter capable of fine differentiation.

What happens when the stimulation to the cochlea is more complex than a simple sinusoid curve? For instance, if a tone complex including 500, 1,000, 1,500, and 2,000 Hz were presented to the ear, how would the cochlea and VIII nerve respond? Essentially, the nerve fibers with characteristic frequencies of the stimulus components (500 Hz, 1,000 Hz, etc.) will respond, whereas those fibers with other CFs (i.e., 510 Hz, 511 Hz, 512 Hz, etc.) outside the range of direct stimulation will take much more stimulation to fire. You will notice that we judiciously avoided 505 Hz in our list of off-stimulus CF, because that difference is probably not discriminable. That is, the cochlea generally cannot differentiate a difference smaller than that, so the fibers at 502 Hz would respond the same as those at 500 Hz. To the brain, those two frequencies are indiscriminable.

The PST histogram provides excellent support for the **place theory of hearing**, stating that the frequency resolution of the cochlea occurs as a result of place of stimulation by the traveling wave. The tonotopic array of the cochlea is clearly relayed to the auditory nervous system in the form of individual nerve fiber activation.

Firing rate is also used to encode intensity of the stimulation (see Figure 10-7). As the intensity of stimulation increases, the rate of firing increases, up to a point. Because neurons are limited by the refractory period, they typically cannot fire more than once per millisecond. The dynamic range for intensity that can be encoded in rate of firing is in the order of 30 to 40 dB, far too small for encoding

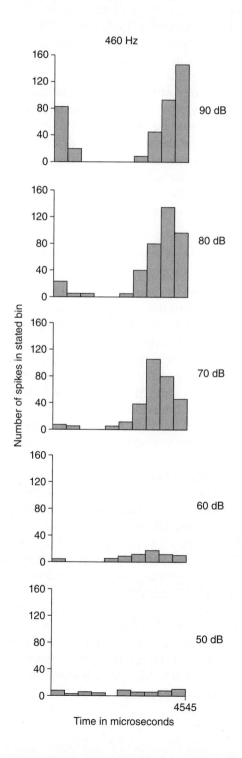

Figure 10-7. Effect of signal intensity on firing rate for a single neuron. From Anderson, D. J., Rose, J. E., Hind, J. E. & Brugge, J. F (1980). Temporal position of discharges in single auditory nerve fibers within the cycle of a sine-wave stimulus: frequency and intensity effects. *Journal of the Acoustical Society of America*, 49, 1131-11-38.

Source: *Journal of the Acoustical Society of America*, 49, 1131-11-38.

of intensity. We are capable of differentiating a much greater range of intensities than this. Recall that different neurons have different thresholds of response (low- and high-threshold neurons). Apparently intensity is coded by using both types of neurons: Low-threshold neurons can process low-intensity signals, while high-threshold neurons carry the load of higher intensity sound. Taken together, they account for the dynamic range of hearing for intensity. Evidence from Kiang, Liberman, Sewell, and Guinan (1986) reveals that outer hair cells (OHCs) augment the function of the inner hair cells in frequency discrimination, as evidenced by a marked loss of tuning curve sharpness when the OHCs are traumatized.

The efferent system of the auditory mechanism has the effect of reducing neural response. When the crossed-olivocochlear and uncrossed-olivocochlear bundles are stimulated, the firing rate of neurons innervated by them is reduced dramatically (Winslow & Sachs, 1988). This has the effect of reducing response to unwanted information, perhaps permitting the nervous system to "focus" on a desired signal while damping the response to noise. The efferent system also appears to have a role in frequency discrimination.

Interspike Interval and Period Histograms

Although rate histograms reveal a great deal about how the cochlea and VIII nerve respond to sound, **interspike interval** (ISI) histograms provide details of the temporal structure of the VIII nerve response. With ISI histograms, the interval between successive firings of a neuron is measured and recorded. Figures 10-8 and 10-9 show "phase-locking" of a neuron to stimulation. The stimulus is an 812 Hz tone, and the period of vibration associated with an 812 Hz tone is approximately 1.2 ms. If you look closely at the response, you will recognize that the interval between the spikes of the histogram is 1.2 ms, the period of the tone. **Phase-locking** refers to the quality of a neuron wherein it responds to the period of the stimulus, in this case 1.2 ms. Because a neuron requires 1 ms to recover from depolarization, we should not expect to see phase-locking to signals above 1000 Hz (period = 1 ms), but we do see it. Phase-locking is seen in signals up to 5,000 Hz, although this does not mean that the basic physiology of neural excitation should be redefined. The VIII nerve fiber responds to the phase of the signal, but not necessarily to *every* cycle of vibration. As you can see in Figure 10-9, a fiber will respond when it is capable of responding, and it will respond at whole-number multiples of the period of excitation.

One can reorganize the interval histogram data by examining a period histogram. A **period histogram** displays the point in the cycle of vibration at which firing occurs (Figure 10-8). In this manner, the degree of phase-locking is represented in the major peak of the figure. As the signal increases, the histogram becomes more peaked, representing a greater degree of phase-locking.

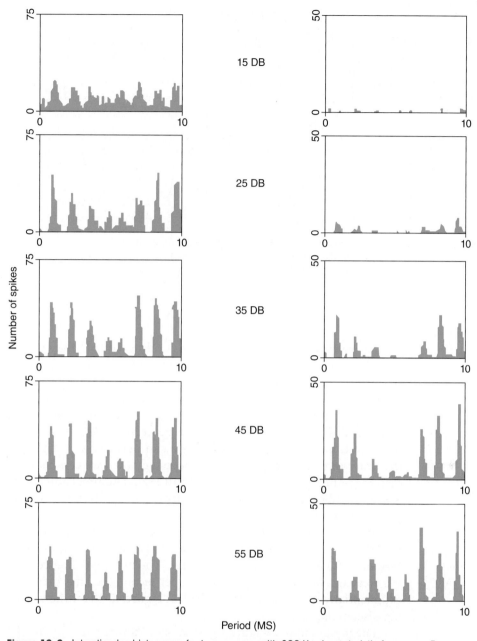

Figure 10-8. Interstimulus histograms for two neurons with 800 Hz characteristic frequency. From Javel, E. (1980). Coding of AM tones in the chinchilla auditory nerve: Implications for the pitch of complex tones.

Source: *Journal of the Acoustical Society of America*, 68(1), 133-146.

It is clear from the interval and period histograms that temporal information of the waveform is preserved and potentially transmitted to the brain by the auditory nervous system. It appears that both place and temporal information are used in the coding of acoustical information, extracting important redundancy of information from the acoustical signal.

Response from single neuron

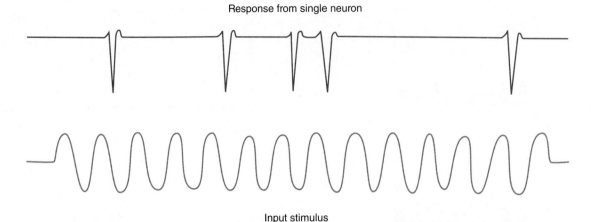

Input stimulus

Figure 10-9. Relationship between neuron response (lower trace) and signal phase (upper trace).

Source: Reprinted with permission from Fundamentals of Hearing: An Introduction (5th ed.), by W. A. Yost, 2007, New York: Elsevier Academic Press. Reprinted with permission.

Frequency Selectivity

Earlier we talked about tuning curves and noted that they reflect specificity of response in the auditory system. The concept is this: If a tuning curve is sufficiently sharp, it will represent a great deal of selectivity on the basilar membrane. Think of a tuning curve as a very sharp pencil making a very thin line. That sharp, precise line is necessary for humans to be able to perceive minute differences between tones. As a matter of fact, we can perceive something in the order of a 1 percent change in frequency (i.e., we can hear the difference between 1,000 Hz and 1,010 Hz). The precision of the basilar membrane in frequency selectivity is reflected in the sharpness of the tuning curve.

Perception is actually a logarithm-based phenomenon: we can hear a 1 Hz difference at 100 Hz (1%) or a 10 Hz difference at 1,000 Hz (1%) or a 100 Hz difference at 10,000 Hz. The differential perception is a constant, but the number of cycles per second (Hz) has increased exponentially up the scale. Take a look at Figure 10-10 for the following discussion.

The top portion of Figure 10-10 shows a tuning curve of an VIII nerve fiber from an area of the basilar membrane that is centered at 11,000 Hz. Next to it is a tuning curve that is centered at 1,100 Hz. The 11,000 Hz plot *looks* sharper than the bottom one, right? Looking at them you would hypothesize that the 11,000 Hz plot has greater specificity. In order to actually compare these two, however, we must calculate a value known as Q_{10}, which is the ratio of the center frequency divided by the bandwidth $Q_{10} = cf/bw_{10db}$. Basically, we measure up 10 dB from the tip, and identify how wide the tuning curve is (bandwidth, in Hz). Then, we divide the bandwidth by the center frequency, in Hz. A higher number indicates sharper tuning. Now look at the derivation of Q_{10} for these same plots.

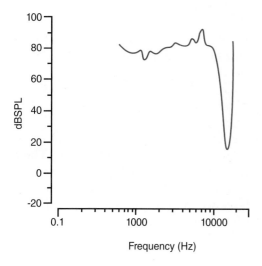

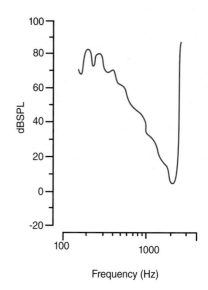

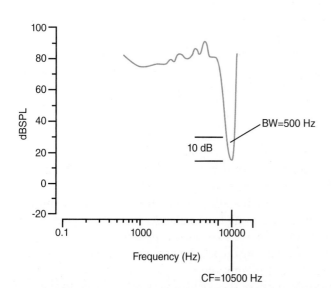

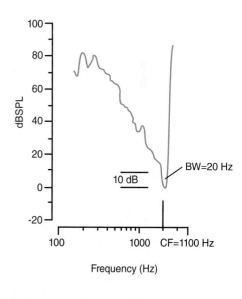

Figure 10-10. Plot of tuning curves from two different VIII nerve fibers, representing characteristic frequencies of 10500 Hz (left) and 1000 Hz (right). Note that the tuning curve on the left looks sharper. Calculation of Q_{10} (lower plots) reveals that the low-frequency fiber is, in reality, markedly more specific (sharper) than the high-frequency fiber, as indicated by the greater Q_{10} value.

Source: Derived from data of "Acoustic Trauma in Cats," by M. C. Liberman and N. Y. S. Kiang, 1978, Otolaryngica, Supplement 358, pp. 1–63. Reprinted with permission.

Calculation for the Q_{10} for the 11,000 Hz fiber is as follows:

Q_{10} = cf/bw
Q_{10} = 10,500/500
Q_{10} = 21

Calculation of Q_{10} for the 1,100 Hz fiber is as follows:

Q_{10} = cf/bw
Q_{10} = 1,100/20
Q_{10} = 55

Clearly, the lower-frequency fiber is sharper than the high-frequency fiber, when you compare its precision using the Q_{10}. There is critical benefit to performing this "normalizing" process when examining tuning curves of fibers or the basilar membrane. Q_{10} allows us to put all tuning curves on common footing and to compare their sharpness relative to their response region.

✔ *To summarize:*

- There are two basic types of VIII nerve neurons, and specific techniques have been developed for assessing their function.
- **High-threshold neurons** require a higher intensity and encompass the higher end of our auditory range of signal intensity.
- **Low-threshold fibers** respond at very low signal levels and display random firing even when no stimulus is present.
- **Low-threshold neurons** may process near-threshold sounds, whereas high-threshold fibers process higher level sounds.
- **Frequency specificity** is the ability of the cochlea to differentiate the spectral components of a signal. It is reflected in the sharpness of the tuning curve. Humans can perceive a change in frequency of approximately 1 percent.
- **Post-stimulus time histograms** are plots of neural response relative to the onset of a stimulus.
- The **characteristic** or **best frequency** of a neuron is the frequency to which it responds best.
- A **tuning curve** is a composite of the responses of a single fiber at each frequency of presentation.
- Q_{10} is a derived ratio that allows comparison of the sharpness of tuning curves all along the basilar membrane. Higher numbers for Q_{10} indicate sharper tuning curves.
- The sharper the tuning curve, the greater the frequency specificity of the basilar membrane.
- The **tonotopic array** of the cochlea is clearly relayed to the auditory nervous system in the form of individual nerve fiber activation.
- As the intensity of stimulation increases, **rate of firing** increases.
- When the **crossed-olivocochlear** and **uncrossed-olivocochlear bundles** are stimulated, the firing rate of neurons innervated by them is reduced dramatically.

- **Interspike interval histograms** record the interval between successive firings of a neuron, revealing phase-locking of neurons to stimulus period.

Auditory Pathway Responses

The cochlea and VIII nerve represent only the first stage of information extraction of an auditory signal. Temporal and tonotopically arrayed information is passed to progressively higher centers for further extraction of information (see Figure 10-11).

Cochlear Nucleus

At the first way station in the auditory pathway, the cochlear nucleus (CN), tonotopic representation is readily observable in tuning curves. There is evidence that significant signal processing occurs at this level of the brain stem.

Pfeiffer (1966) demonstrated at least six different neural responses to auditory stimulation, in contrast to the single-unit response seen at the VIII nerve level (see Figure 10-12). **Primary-like responses** are the firing patterns that most resemble VIII nerve responses. These responses appear to arise from bushy cells in the CN and will have identical rate functions, intensity responses, spontaneous activity, and Q_{10} values as the VIII nerve fibers they reflect. Some neurons exhibit **onset responses**, in which there is an initial response to onset of a stimulus, followed by silence. These responses will have a sharp peak at the onset of a stimulus, and then simply stop firing. They are found throughout the CN and appear to arise from octopus cells. They have a smaller Q_{10} than other responses in the cochlear nucleus (wider tuning curves), and this may represent some sort of summative function. Remember, a wider tuning curve reflects <u>less</u> specificity, and in this case that could mean that the fiber being measured is responding to multiple areas of the basilar membrane. **Chopper responses** do not seem to be related to stimulus frequency, but appear to have a periodic, chopped temporal pattern as long as a tone is present. Chopper response is marked by repeated firing when stimulated by a tone. These responses are strongest in the posteroventral cochlear nucleus (PVCN) and dorsal cochlear nucleus (DCN), although they can be found throughout the CN. They do not seem to be related to any particular cell type, and their firing rate is not really related to the period of the stimulus. It would appear that these chopper cells most likely have numerous inputs and simply move through a "fire–shutdown–fire" cycle as long as they are stimulated. **Pausers**, found in the dorsal cochlear nucleus, take a little longer to respond than other neurons: If the signal is of higher intensity, the pauser has an initial on-response, is quiet, and then responds with a low-level firing rate throughout stimulation. Pausers are found mostly in the DCN and appear to arise from fusiform cells. They respond to complex

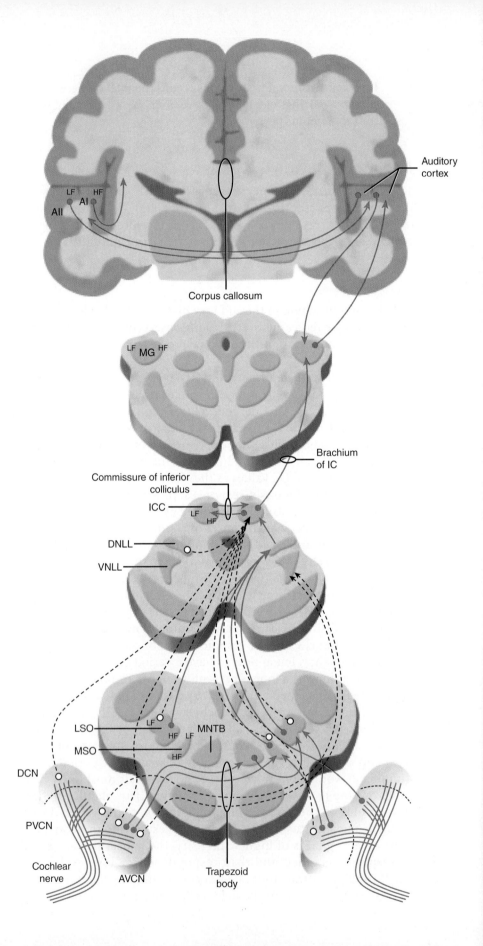

Auditory cortex

Corpus callosum

Brachium of IC

Commissure of inferior colliculus

ICC

DNLL

VNLL

LSO

MSO

MNTB

DCN

PVCN

Cochlear nerve

AVCN

Trapezoid body

Figure 10-11. Schematic representation of auditory pathway in humans. [After Møller, 2003.] Note the following: DCN = dorsal cochlear nucleus; AVCN = anteroventral cochlear nucleus; PVCN = posteroventral cochlear nucleus; LSO = lateral superior olive; and MSO = medial superior olive.
© Cengage Learning®.

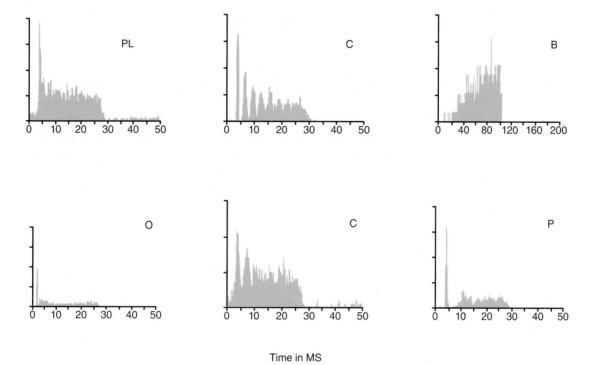

Time in MS

Figure 10-12. Peristimulus time histograms showing response characteristics of cochlear nucleus. Note that PL = Primary Like; O = Onset type; C = Chopper type; B = Buildup type; P = Pauser type.

Source: From "The Use of Intracellular Techniques in the Study of the Cochlear Nucleus," by W. S. Rhode, 1985, by *Journal of the Acoustic Society of America*, 78(1), p. 321. Copyright 1985 by Acoustical Society of America. Reprinted with permission.

stimuli and most likely represent some form of processing of complex acoustic features. **Buildup** neurons slowly increase their firing rate through the initial stages of firing.

These complex responses reflect not only different cell types within the CN but also interactions among neurons. Although all these responses may be seen in different neurons in response to the same tonal stimulus, it would be unwise to assume that they are *simply* responses to stimulation. They are most certainly the result of complex interaction and neural processing.

Complex Interaction within the Cochlear Nucleus. The basic neuron response types that we have just discussed have another layer of complexity we should mention. There are at least four basic types of inhibition found within the CN, which is absent in the VIII nerve that feeds it (remember that the VIII nerve does not have inhibition).

In Type II and III inhibitory patterns, one sees a rather standard tuning curve configuration in response to stimulation, but there are also inhibitory sidebands above and below the characteristic frequency. Response to a signal presented at CF is greatly sharpened if there is stimulation in the sideband, apparently by damping the off-frequency information. These fibers typically do not have spontaneous activity, so they are strictly stimulus bound.

Type IV and V fibers are almost completely inhibitory, arising from the DCN. That is to say, if they receive stimulation, they terminate output. Generally, there is less inhibition in the AVCN, and the most inhibition is found in the DCN. Indeed, it appears that fibers in the AVCN inhibit responses from the DCN. The anteroventral cochlear nucleus (AVCN) and PVCN provide an exact, unadulterated copy of the VIII nerve response to the olivary complex (to be discussed) for the purpose of localization of sound in space, and it appears that the DCN is responsible for performing complex acoustic analysis and forwarding that information to higher brain stem and cortical centers.

There are some other atypical responses found at the level of the CN. Pausers and buildup neurons show a specifically different response to signals that sweep up in frequency versus those sweeping down. That is to say, frequency modulation is a specific feature detected by these neurons: Some will be highly specific to up-sweep and "blind" to down-sweep, while others are specific to down-sweep and do not respond to up-sweep. This response corresponds quite well to characteristics found in the speech signal in transitions from consonants to vowels.

Similarly, some neurons are responsive to minute changes in intensity (as in pulsing intensity), producing very large responses to small changes. Møller (2003) posits that this sensitivity to pulsatile changes reflects a means of identifying the envelope of a signal, which is critical for the identification of syllable boundaries.

Superior Olivary Complex

The superior olivary complex (SOC) is the first site of binaural interaction, receiving information from the cochlear nuclei of both ears, and is specialized for localization of sound in space. There are three outputs from the CN and two of these pathways go to the olivary complex. The dorsal stria arises from the DCN and bypasses the olivary complex. The ventral stria is made up of responses from the AVCN and PVCN, and the intermediate stria arises from the PVCN, and both of these are shunted directly to the olivary complex.

The lateral superior olive (LSO) receives high-frequency information from the ipsilateral cochlear nucleus, and the medial superior olive (MSO) receives low-frequency information. When the LSO is provided with ipsilateral (same side) stimulation, the response is entirely excitatory. The tuning curves look like VIII nerve fibers, with thresholds in the 10–20 dB SPL range. When the neurons are stimulated by contralateral (other side) signals, the response is entirely inhibitory, and these fibers are referred to as E–I (excitatory–inhibitory). In this way, the LSO responds to differences in intensity between the two ears. A difference in intensity between the two ears is heard when one sound has to pass around the head to reach the other ear. When the signals are high in frequency (above about 1,500 Hz), there is a "head shadow" because the wavelength is too short to effectively bend around the head. The result is that a signal presented to the left ear will be louder than that presented to the right ear, and your LSO will process that difference as "location in space."

In sharp contrast to the LSO, the medial superior olive (MSO) receives input from the AVCN for both ears. It is worth remembering that the MSO receives a very "clean" copy of the auditory signal from the AVCN, and that copy arrives quickly since there are not any way stations between the CN and the MSO. The MSO responds to low-frequency sounds (below about 1,500 Hz), being particularly tuned to timing differences in the waveforms presented to each ear. A difference in timing at low frequencies results in a phase difference between signals from the two ears. Essentially, the cells of the MSO are sensitive to the interaural delay time, which is the time difference between the two ears. That time lag is mapped by the MSO as point in space and allows us to localize sounds quite accurately. In fact, the cells of the MSO have a "characteristic delay," similar to the characteristic frequency seen in other cells. This means that each cell is tuned to a specific time delay between the two ears. Most of the cells of the MSO are excited by signals from either ear (EE, excitatory–excitatory). All cells of the MSO are binaural in nature, meaning they respond to sound from either ear. Therefore, it can be seen that two basic responses occur within the SOC. **Contralateral stimulation** (stimulation of the ear opposite the side of the SOC being studied) by high-frequency information results in excitation of the **lateral superior olive** (LSO, or S-segment) that is directly related to stimulus intensity. These so-called **E–E** (excitatory–excitatory) responses provide a means of comparing the intensity of a signal on one side of the head with that on the other side. In the MSO, when low-frequency tones are presented, an **E–I** (excitatory–inhibitory) response occurs, wherein contralateral input excites neurons and **ipsilateral stimulation** causes inhibition of neurons. Said another way, a low-frequency signal arriving at the left ear causes excitation of the right-side MSO, while inhibiting the left-side

Echolocation

Animal sonar systems have been examined extensively for over 40 years, including those in dolphins, whales, and bats. Over 800 species of bats have evolved a means of producing high-frequency (as high as 120 kHz) sounds that bounce off of objects. The reflected sound is received as an auditory echo that is processed by the superior olivary complex (SOC) to determine the spatial location of the object from which the echo was derived. When bats are flying toward an object that is getting closer, the frequency of the reflected sound will shift up (Doppler shift), resulting in a higher-frequency signal being received. This tells the bat that the object of its affection (perhaps a moth) is getting closer and may be available soon for a snack. If the object is moving away from the bat at a faster speed than the bat is flying, the frequency will shift down. Of course, moths and other insects have developed countermeasures. Moths that are preyed upon by bats have developed auditory neurons specifically tuned to the frequency of the bat's sonar, so that when they are "pinged" by a bat's echolocation system they will go into a free fall that foils the bat's predictions. Other moths will flutter their wings chaotically or fly upward in a spiral to defeat the sonar.

MSO. In addition, some cells in the MSO respond to a **characteristic delay** in arrival time, so that the MSO detects minute changes in arrival time of a sound between the two ears. This **interaural phase (time) difference** is the primary mechanism for localization of low-frequency sounds in space; the **interaural intensity** difference is the primary means of localization of high-frequency sound in space. The neurons responding to specific characteristics or features of the stimulus are termed **feature detectors**. That is, they respond to specific features of the stimulus (e.g., interaural phase differences), extract that information from the signal, and convey the results of analysis to the cerebral cortex. In this way the complex acoustic signal can be broken into some subset of characteristics. Indeed, the different responses at the CN (e.g., pauser and onset-response) most likely represent the second level of feature extraction, the first level being at the cochlea.

Inferior Colliculus

The inferior colliculus (IC) receives bilateral innervation from the LSO, as well as indirect input from the CN via the lateral lemniscus. A wide range of responses is apparent at the IC, including those of neurons with sharp frequency tuning curves, inhibitory responses, onset and pauser responses, and intensity-sensitive units. Some neurons are sensitive to interaural time and intensity differences, apparently used for a localization function similar to the SOC. It appears that the IC may be the site at which frequency information from the CN discarded through localization processing at the SOC can be recombined with phase and intensity information.

Responses within the IC are wide-ranging. Cells of the IC have characteristic frequencies with tuning curves, but the range of sharpness (Q_{10}) of the tuning curves is dramatic, being between 25 and 40, among the best in the auditory nervous system. There are also broad tuning curves with very wide bandwidths.

Rate responses are also widely varied in the IC. About half of the cells of the IC show a monotonic rate-intensity response, which means that as intensity increases, rate increases in proportion. The other half are nonmonotonic, which is to say that the response is not a linear function of the stimulus. In fact, as intensity increases many of the neurons change from primary-type response to pauser responses, and even to onset responses, ultimately ending in chopper responses. Some of these neurons are also highly responsive to signals sweeping either up in frequency or down in frequency (but not both), similar to those signals found in the frequency transitions of speech. Neurons of the IC are generally responsive to contralateral stimulation and appear to map auditory information based on interaural timing difference, similar to the MSO, but there are also neurons sensitive to intensity differences, similar to the LSO. This implicates the MSO strongly as a mechanism for localization, but it also serves as an area of intersensory interaction.

Medial Geniculate Body

The medial geniculate body (MGB) is a relay point to the thalamus, the final sensory way station of the brain stem. The ventral portion of the MGB projects information directly to the primary auditory reception area of the temporal lobe, the medial portion projects to other regions of the temporal lobe, and the dorsal portion projects information to association regions of the cerebrum. Although a distinct tonotopic arrangement is apparent even at this level, a complex interaction of response types is also apparent. Surprisingly, these include neurons responsive to minute interaural intensity differences, much like the SOC and IC.

The MGB shows sharp tuning curves similar to those of the VIII nerve fibers. Responses of the MGB neurons include onset responses, as well as sustained excitatory responses. Most neurons within the MGB respond to stimuli from both ears and have nonmonotonic rate-intensity functions. Some of the neurons of the MGB respond to intensity differences much as the LSO does, and, in fact, some neurons are so sensitive to interaural intensity difference that they reach 80 percent of their response rate with as little as 2 dB difference between the ears.

Cerebral Cortex

The cerebral cortex receives input primarily from the contralateral ear via the ipsilateral MGB. A full tonotopic map is found at the primary reception area of the temporal lobe, Heschl's gyrus. In addition, the auditory reception area is organized in columns, with each column having similar CFs, but different tuning curve widths. Further, different neurons within the columns respond to different stimulus parameters, such as frequency up-glides, down-glides, intensity up-glides and intensity down-glides, and so on. It is clear that the neurons of the cerebral cortex use the ipsilateral and contralateral temporal and spectral information extracted at earlier processing stages for identification of the features of speech. For example, neurons that are sensitive to frequency up-glides would be very useful in encoding information concerning formant frequency transitions, whereas the vocal fundamental frequency would be readily coded from the temporal information arising from the phase-locking at the cochlear level and presented, intact, to the cortex.

The brain stem is clearly responsible for initial coding of the neural signal representing the auditory stimulus, but there remain significant challenges to understanding the true mechanism involved in that coding. Work by Gollisch and Meister (2008) with the visual system revealed that the initial spike latencies of the retinal ganglion cells provided very clear spatial coding, despite the rapidly changing nature of the visual system as a result of saccadic eye movements. This unexpected coding mechanism from bipolar cells, in a system that has the benefit of longer sensory memory (i.e., afterimage), may provide a fruitful research path for the auditory system.

While quite complex and daunting, the auditory pathway is simple when compared with the cerebral cortex. Take a look at Figure 10-13. This is an elaborated illustration of the auditory pathway from

Kaas and Hackett (2000), taking into consideration the known direct pathways for audition (we have not mentioned the indirect pathways yet). The area to focus on in this diagram is the top four or so layers. The lower areas, from the cochlea up through the thalamus, are quite familiar to you by now. The representation of Heschl's gyrus may be new to you, so let us discuss that a bit before we talk about physiology.

Typically, we state that Heschl's gyrus is located in the superior aspect of the temporal lobe, at the Sylvian fissure. Brodmann actually described the superior temporal gyrus (STG) as consisting of four distinct regions, based on cell type: areas 22 (most of the lateral surface of the STG), 41 (typically considered to be Heschl's gyrus), 42 (lateral to Heschl's gyrus, being a higher processing region), and area 52 on the medial, and, typically, hidden surface of the STG. If one pulls the temporal lobe out and rotates it out a bit, areas 41, 42, and 52 are revealed in more detail. With the medial surface of the temporal lobe revealed you would see the planum temporale, which is posterior to Heschl's gyrus. The planum polare (also known as the temporal pole) is anterior to Heschl's gyrus.

Kaas and Hackett (2000) have laid to rest the notion that the auditory cortex consists of a simple receptive zone and an adjacent higher-order processing area. Instead, the auditory cortex is seen as consisting of a medially placed core, a more distal belt, and a surrounding parabelt (see Figure 10-13). A great deal of research has elaborated its function in primates, and some research has elucidated its function in humans.

First, look at the elaboration of the receptive region (Figure 10-13B). This receptive region consists of the core, belt, and parabelt.

Core. The core in this figure is represented by areas A1, R, and RT, and makes up most of Heschl's gyrus in humans. The classical notion of auditory reception is represented by A1. The tonotopic relationship that we have been observing throughout the auditory pathway is retained. Low frequency processed on A1 is in the distal or rostral end of the area, while high frequencies are processed more medially (closer to Wernicke's area). To the left of A1 is the rostral portion of the core (R): The tonotopic array is reversed for this portion of the core, so that the high frequencies are processed closer to the temporal pole (anterior aspect). Finally, the rostrotemporal (RT) portion of the core appears to have the tonotopic relationship seen in A1. Essentially then, auditory information arises at this core region in one or more of these three locations. All three of them appear to receive input from the MGB.

Belt. The belt is a 2- to 3-mm region consisting of eight areas surrounding the core. The names simply represent the location of the region. Neurons in the caudomedial (CM) region have some identifiable CFs, but do not really respond well to tones. Note that it also displays a tonotopic processing scheme but is reversed relative to its neighbor, A1. Neurons in the CM respond not only to auditory information but also to somatosensory stimulation of the neck and head. The caudolateral (CL, labeled CC in the figure) region has the

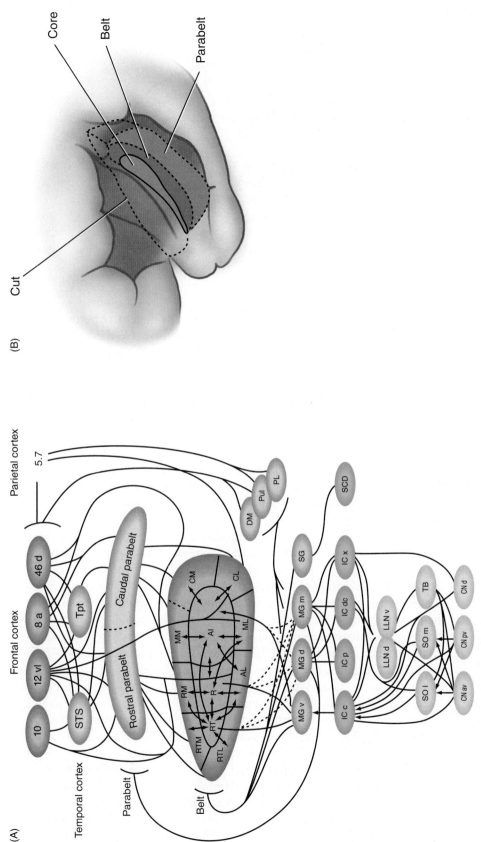

Figure 10-13. (A) Primate auditory pathway, based upon physiological studies. (B) Elaboration of auditory reception area as core, belt, and parabelt. Key: AVCN = anteroventral cochlear nucleus, PVCN = posteroventral cochlear nucleus, DCN = dorsal cochlear nucleus, LSO = lateral superior olive, MSO = medial superior olive, MNTB = medial nucleus of trapezoid body, DNLL = dorsal nucleus of lateral lemniscus, VNLL = ventral nucleus of lateral lemniscus, ICc = Central nucleus of inferior colliculus, ICp = pericentral nucleus of inferior colliculus, ICX = external nucleus of inferior colliculus, MGv = ventral medial geniculate body (thalamus), MGd = dorsal medial geniculate body (thalamus), MGm = magnocellular nucleus of medial geniculate body, Sg = suprageniculate nucleus of medial thalamus, Lim = limitans nucleus of thalamus, PM = medial pulvinar of thalamus, A1 = auditory core of cortex, R = Rostral portion of core, cortex, RT = rostrotemporal aspect of core, CL = caudolateral area of belt, cortex, CM = caudomedial area of belt, cortex, ML = middle lateral area of belt, cortex, MM = middle medial area of belt, cortex, RM = rostromedial area of belt, cortex, AL = anterolateral area of belt, cortex, RTL = rostrotemporal area of belt, cortex, RTM = rostrotemporal area of belt, cortex, CPB = caudal parabelt, RPB = rostral parabelt, Tpt = temporoparietal area of temporal lobe, STS = superior temporal sulcus of temporal lobe, STG = superior temporal gyrus, temporal lobe, 8 = Brodmann area 8a (frontal eye field), 46 = Brodmann area 46d (working memory area), 12vl = Brodmann area 12, prefrontal cortex, 10 = Brodmann area 10, frontal pole, orb = orbitofrontal cortex.

Source: "Kaas, J. A. & Hackett, T. A. (2000). Subdivisions of auditory cortex and processing streams in primates. Proceedings of the National Academy of Science of USA, 97 (22), 11794. Copyright 2000 National Academy of Sciences, U.S.A.

Figure 10-14. Brodmann areas for auditory reception, including areas 41, 42, 52.

© Cengage Learning®.

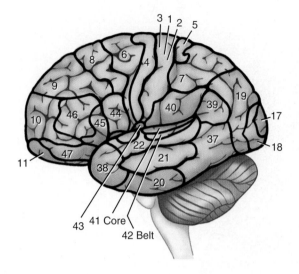

same tonotopic array as the CM, but responds generally better to high-frequency information. It appears to be sensitive to the location of sound in space. The mediolateral (ML) region is also tonotopically arrayed, but parallel to A1. The ML is strongly linked with A1, but only weakly linked with the rostral core (R). The ML projects its output to the area 46 of the frontal lobe, an area involved in visual processing. It receives its input from the MGB, importantly from the pulvinar nucleus, which is involved in language processing. It also receives input from the supergeniculate limitans nucleus of the thalamus. The middle medial (MM) region is not really well defined but appears to represent the A1 portion of the core. Output of the MM is to the rostral parabelt and then to the frontal eye region (8) of the cortex, just as with the ML.

The anterior lateral (AL) region (indicated as RL in this figure) has broadly tuned neurons that respond to tones and has a general tonotopicity. The AL region has a special function: It is responsive to tones, but it is more responsive to complex signals. In fact, it is specifically responsive to species-specific calls. For the macaque monkey, it would be most responsive to macaque calling. For the human, it is most responsive to human speech. Significantly, it is not particularly involved in the location of the calls, but their nature. In fact, Petkov et al. (2008) found that this area in macaque monkeys can differentiate different macaque voices. The AL region is densely connected with the R of the core, and less so with A1. The input of this region is from the posteromedial portion of the thalamus, including the nucleus limitans, medial portion of the MGB, and dorsal portion of the MGB. It projects to the visual region (46) and polysensory region (12) of the frontal lobe.

The rostromedial portion of the belt (RM) appears to be important for both identification and localization of a sound. It communicates with the AL and ML of the belt and has a stronger connection with the R of the core than with A1. The RM region also projects to the parabelt region (to be discussed). The rostromedial (RTM) and lateral rostrotemporal regions (LRT) both project to the rostral parabelt (RPB) of the parabelt.

Parabelt. The parabelt region is lateral to the belt and makes up the third level of processing of the input auditory signal at the reception area. The parabelt is closely linked to the belt. It appears that the RPB is most closely interconnected with the rostral belt, and the caudal parabelt (CPB) is most closely connected with the caudal portion of the belt. The parabelt appears to receive its input from disparate regions of the thalamus, including the dorsal and medial portions of the MGB, suprageniculate nucleus, nucleus limitans, and the posteromedial nucleus. The parabelt projects to area 8 of the frontal lobe, responsible for some high-level visual processing, and may assist in directing vision toward an auditory stimulus. It also projects to area 46 of the frontal lobe, which appears to be an important region for visual-spatial memory processing. The RPB also connects with area 10, which is part of the orbital portion of the cortex. This area appears to be important for the integration of visual and auditory information. The RPB is also responsive to species-specific vocalization (i.e., in humans it is responsive to the human voice), so this region may be involved in identifying the nature of sounds, perhaps helping to define them as linguistic in nature.

It is important to realize that all of the core, belt, and parabelt project to other regions of the temporal lobe. If you once again look at the pathways of Figure 10-13, you will see rich connections running from the core, belt, and parabelt to the rest of the superior temporal gyrus, the superior temporal sulcus, and the temporoparietal region.

Highest-Level Processing. The highest level of auditory processing occurs throughout the rest of the superior temporal gyrus (STG) and the superior temporal sulcus (STS), as well as the temporo-parieto-occipital association area (the area that includes Wernicke's area in humans). Auditory processing is also performed in the prefrontal and orbital regions of the brain, as well as in the temporal pole (anterior temporal lobe). The middle temporal gyrus, just inferior to the STG, is activated more by the recognition of a stimulus than by its location. In nonhumans, the left auditory cortex is necessary for discriminating species-specific vocalizations.

It appears that A1 and the lateral belt region of humans are sensitive to human voices. Physiological studies reveal that the largest responses to human vocalizations are in the superior temporal sulcus, and the responses are strongest when the speech is true as opposed to scrambled. This implies that it is not simply the acoustic elements that are triggering a response, but rather the acoustic elements of a meaningful stimulus. In macaque monkeys this function is lateralized to the left hemisphere, just as it is in humans. The left hemisphere response to speech by humans is very robust in the left planum temporale, medial to the core.

There are other, noncortical processing sites as well for auditory stimuli. The cerebellum has been implicated as a contributor to the millisecond level timing required for speech processing. We have already discussed the role of the SOC and IC of the brain stem for localization of sound in space, but it appears that an intact cortex is a requirement for adequate localization function. Unilateral lesion of the cerebral cortex will cause severe localization deficit. We already know that the superior colliculus has a very well-defined map of the external visual space it processes, and that map is integrated with auditory information so that an auditory-visual map is developed. Is there such a map in the cerebrum for auditory stimuli? That remains to be seen. It does appear that there are two paths taken by stimuli relative to localization and identification. One stream of information courses from the thalamus to A1, and it seems specialized for identification of a stimulus. A posterior stream appears to process the localization information.

A dual stream model of speech processing posits that auditory information arises bilaterally at the STS and STG, where spectral and temporal information are defined. This information is delivered to the phonological processing center in the middle and posterior STS. At that point the information is sent to the dorsal and ventral streams. The dorsal stream information, which is strongly left-hemisphere dominated, is translated to the left parietal-temporal junction at the Sylvian fissure (corresponding to Wernicke's area of the temporal lobe and the supramarginal gyrus of the parietal lobe), and subsequently to the area around (and including) Broca's area and the anterior insula. This dorsal stream also projects information to the supplementary motor area. Conceptually, this dorsal stream dominates the motor patterning associated with articulatory production. The ventral stream similarly arises from the STG and STS (and perhaps the middle temporal gyrus) and is also projected bilaterally to the middle and posterior STS. The ventral stream is much more bilateral, projecting to the middle temporal gyrus and anterior portion of the inferior temporal sulcus to lexical processing areas. This allows phonological information to combine with areas related to word meaning bilaterally, and appears to be essential for processing speech (Hickok & Poeppel, 2007). As you can see from Figure 10-15, the strongly left-hemisphere dorsal stream is involved in translating the speech acoustics into spatial articulatory representations within the frontal lobe, and is involved in a type of auditory-to-motor transformation. Hickok and Poeppel posit that speech perception is processed by the dorsal stream, but speech recognition involves the ventral system. The dorsal stream (speech perception) is a left-hemisphere function, but the ventral stream is bilaterally represented (speech recognition).

According to this dual-stream model, the auditory cortex first performs a spectral or temporal analysis bilaterally, by means of the core, belt, and parabelt. The middle and posterior aspects of the bilateral superior temporal sulcus is involved in phonological processing and phonological representation. From there the dorsal stream converts the phonological and sensory information into linguistically meaningful units (lexicon). The dorsal stream may or may not be involved in spatial processing of speech information but certainly appears to be important for mapping linguistic information to the motor system.

In summary, the cortical processing of stimuli is complex but becoming more apparent. There are at least three locations that receive direct input from the thalamus, and projections from these regions reach frontal, temporal, and parietal lobes of the cerebrum. The core consists

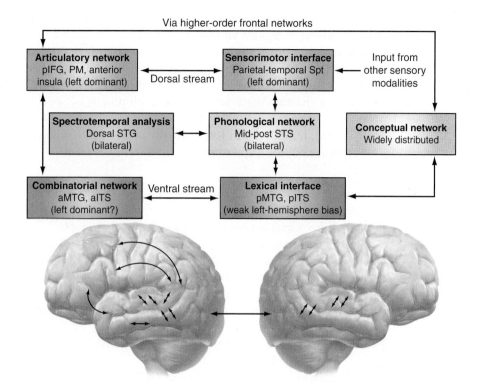

Figure 10-15. Graphic illustration of the proposed pathways of the dual stream model of auditory processing. Hickock and Poeppel propose stages of speech processing as follows. Speech information arises at area 41 (bilateral Heschl's gyrus, superior temporal sulcus, green) where spectral and temporal analysis occurs in both hemispheres. Bilateral phonological processing (yellow, probably dominated by left-hemisphere function) occurs in the superior temporal sulcus (middle and posterior). The flow of processing divides into ventral (pink) and dorsal (blue) streams. The left-hemisphere dorsal stream maps the phonological representations to articulatory processing regions (peri-Broca's region and supplementary motor area, left hemisphere). The ventral pathway maps phonological representations to linguistic or lexical processing regions (region around Spt, the parietal-temporal boundary of the Sylvian fissure, particularly adjacent to and including Wernicke's area and inferior temporal lobes). This area synthesizes sensory and motor information related to language. Based on figure, data, and description of Hickock and Poeppel (2007). Redrawn by permission. Note: STS = superior temporal sulcus, STG = superior temporal gyrus, aITS = anterior inferior temporal sulcus, aMTG = anterior middle temporal gyrus, pIFG = posterior inferior frontal gyrus, PM = premotor region, Spt = sylvian fissure at parietal-temporal lobe boundary (near Wernicke's area).

of three regions with their own tonotopic maps. The belt is made up of at least eight regions, all of which have unique response characteristics. The parabelt region is the highest-input processing region, projecting to other levels of the cortex. The belt and parabelt appear to be critical for recognition of species-specific calls, as well as for localization of sound in space. They also appear to be important for the identification of the nature of a sound, and perhaps the identification of a sound as speech versus nonspeech. Information is projected to an area of the STS that processes phonological information. A dorsal stream projects to motor planning areas and is involved in speech perception, while a ventral stream projects to lexical regions for speech recognition.

The auditory nervous system is a complex processor of sound that defies simplistic description. The audiologist and speech-language pathologist must recognize that this most astounding of the sensory systems provides the raw material for the development of speech and language.

To summarize, temporal and tonotopically arrayed information is passed to progressively higher centers for further extraction of information.

- At the **cochlear nucleus**, tonotopic representation is readily observable in **tuning curves**.
- **Primary-like** responses are the firing patterns that most resemble VIII nerve responses.
- **Onset** responses are those in which there is an initial response to the onset of a stimulus followed by silence.
- **Chopper** responses do not appear related to stimulus frequency but have a periodic, chopped temporal pattern as long as a tone is present.
- **Pausers** take longer to respond than other neurons, having an initial on-response for strong stimuli.
- Q_{10} of neurons in the inferior colliculus (IC) are the highest of the auditory nervous system.
- Rate–intensity functions show both linear and nonlinear responses in the IC.
- Neurons show a wide range of responses to auditory stimuli, including chopper and onset, and some neurons are sensitive to either up-sweep or down-sweep of signals.
- Neurons of the IC are sensitive to interaural intensity and timing differences.
- Neurons in the medial geniculate body (MGB) are responsive to input from both ears, and some are very sensitive to minute differences in interaural intensity.
- **Buildup responses** slowly increase in firing rate through the initial stages of depolarization.
- The superior olivary complex is the primary site of **localization** of sound in space.
- **Contralateral stimulation** of the SOC by high-frequency information results in excitation related to stimulus intensity.
- **Low-frequency stimuli** presented binaurally to the SOC are processed in interaural time difference detection.
- A wide array of responses is seen at the **inferior colliculus**, including inhibitory responses, onset and pauser responses, intensity-sensitive units, and interaural time-sensitive and intensity-sensitive responses.
- The **medial geniculate body** is a relay point to the thalamus.
- The **cerebral cortex** receives input primarily from the contralateral ear via the ipsilateral MGB.
- A full **tonotopic map** on the cortex may be seen at the primary reception area, Heschl's gyrus.

- The **auditory reception area** is organized in columns, with each column having a similar CF.
- Different neurons within the columns respond to different stimulus parameters, such as frequency up-glides, down-glides, intensity up- and down-glides, and so on.
- The Brodmann map of the superior temporal gyrus includes elaboration of the areas known as Heschl's gyrus.
- The auditory pathway is an elaborate set of connections that allows multiple inputs to the auditory reception area of the cerebral cortex.
- The auditory reception area consists of a three-part core, eight-part belt region, and a two-part parabelt. These areas are richly interconnected and provide the initial cortical level auditory processing.
- The parabelt region projects specifically to other areas of the cerebral cortex, particularly the temporal, frontal, and parietal lobes.

CHAPTER SUMMARY

Anatesse Lesson

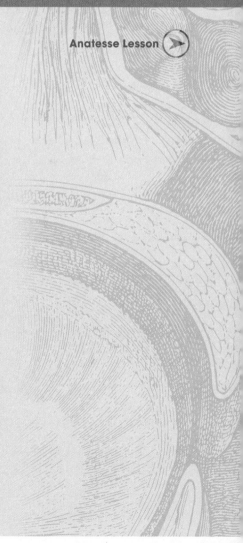

The outer and middle ears serve as funneling and impedance-matching devices. The pinna funnels acoustical information to the external auditory meatus and aids in localization of sound in space. Resistance to the flow of energy is termed impedance. The middle ear plays the role of an impedance-matching device, increasing the pressure of a signal arriving at the cochlea. The area ratio between the tympanic membrane and the oval window provides a significant gain of 25 dB in output over input, and the lever advantage of the ossicles provides a smaller gain of 2dB. The buckling effect grants another 4–6 dB gain.

The inner ear is responsible for performing spectral (frequency) and temporal acoustic analyses of the incoming acoustical signal. Movement of the tympanic membrane is translated into parallel movement of the stapes footplate and the fluid in the scala vestibuli. Movement of the fluid of the scala vestibuli is translated directly to the basilar membrane, and the disturbance at the basilar membrane causes the initiation of the traveling wave. The cochlea has a tonotopic arrangement, with high-frequency sounds resolved at the base and low-frequency sounds processed toward the apex. The point of maximum displacement of the basilar membrane determines the frequency information transmitted to the brain. The traveling wave quickly damps after reaching its point of maximum displacement. The frequency analysis ability of the basilar membrane is determined by graded stiffness, thickness, and width. The basilar membrane is stiffer, thinner, and narrower at the base than at the apex. Excitation of the outer hair cells occurs primarily as a result of a shearing effect on the cilia. Excitation of the inner hair cells is caused by the effect of fluid flow and turbulence of endolymph.

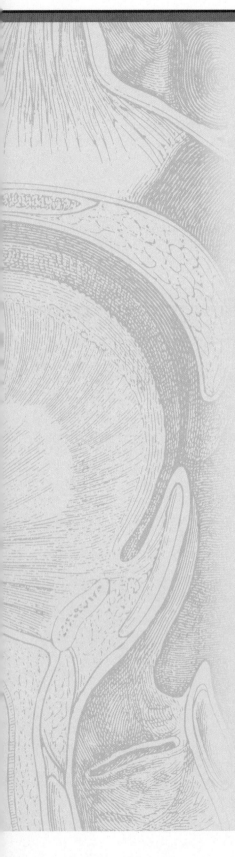

When the basilar membrane is displaced upward, the hair cells are activated, resulting in electrical potentials. Resting or standing potentials are those voltage potential differences that can be measured from the cochlea at rest. The scala vestibuli is 5 mV more positive than the scala tympani, but the scala media is 80 mV more positive. The intracellular resting potential in the hair cells reveals a negative potential difference between the endolymph and the hair cell of 70 mV, giving a 150 mV difference between the hair cells and the surrounding fluid. Stimulus-related potentials include the alternating current cochlear microphonic, generated by the outer hair cells; the summating potential, a direct current shift in the endocochlear potential; and the whole-nerve action potential, arising directly from stimulation of a large number of hair cells simultaneously.

There are two basic types of VIII nerve neurons, and specific techniques have been developed for assessing their function. High-threshold neurons require a higher intensity for response and encompass the higher end of our auditory range of signal intensity. Low-threshold fibers respond at very low signal levels and display random firing even when no stimulus is present. Low-threshold neurons may process near-threshold sounds, whereas high-threshold fibers process higher-level sounds. Frequency specificity is the ability of the cochlea to differentiate the various spectral components of a signal. Post-stimulus time histograms are plots of neural response relative to the onset of a stimulus. The characteristic or best frequency of a neuron is the frequency to which it responds best. A tuning curve is a composite of the responses of a single fiber at each frequency of presentation. The sharper the tuning curve, the greater the frequency specificity of the basilar membrane. The tonotopic array of the cochlea is clearly maintained within the auditory nervous system in the form of individual nerve fiber activation. As the intensity of stimulation increases, the rate of firing increases. When the crossed-olivocochlear and uncrossed-olivocochlear bundles are stimulated, the firing rate of neurons innervated by them is reduced dramatically. Interspike interval histograms record the interval between successive firings of a neuron, revealing phase-locking of neurons to stimulus period.

Temporal and tonotopically arrayed information progresses to higher centers for further extraction of information. The cochlear nucleus reveals tonotopic representation, with a wide variety of neuron responses. Primary-like responses most resemble VIII nerve firing, onset responses show an initial response to the onset of a stimulus followed by silence, and chopper responses show a periodic, chopped temporal pattern as long as a tone is present. Pauser responses take longer to respond than other neurons. Buildup responses slowly increase in firing rate through the initial stages of firing.

The superior olivary complex (SOC) is the primary site of localization of sound in space. Contralateral stimulation of the

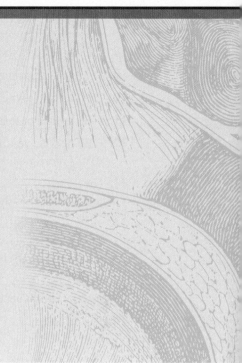

SOC by high-frequency information results in excitation related to stimulus intensity. Low-frequency stimuli presented binaurally to the SOC result in interaural time difference detection. A wide array of responses is seen at the inferior colliculus, including neuron inhibitory responses, onset and pauser responses, intensity-sensitive units, and interaural time- and intensity-sensitive responses. The medial geniculate body is a relay of the thalamus. The cerebral cortex receives input primarily from the contralateral ear via the ipsilateral medial geniculate body (MGB). A full tonotopic map on the cortex may be seen at the primary reception area. The auditory reception area is organized in columns, with each column having a similar characteristic frequency. Different neurons within the columns respond to different stimulus parameters, such as frequency up-glides, down-glides, intensity up-glides and down-glides, and so on. Hickok and Poeppel (2007) propose stages of speech processing that are differentiated based on the level of complexity of the stimulus. Sublexical information appears to be bicortically processed in the superior temporal gyrus by a ventral stream, whereas lexical information is processed by a left-hemisphere dorsal stream.

Media Connection

Go to the accompanying online resources at CengageBrain.com and have fun learning! Study with the Anatesse software program, play games, view animations and videos, and take practice tests to help reinforce the key concepts you learned in this chapter.

Study Questions

1. The _____ of the outer ear is important for the localization of sound in space.

2. Resistance to the flow of energy is termed _____.

3. The area ratio between the tympanic membrane and the oval window provides a _____ dB gain, and the lever advantage gives a _____ dB gain.

4. The cochlea performs both _____ analysis and _____ analysis.

5. Compression of the fluid of the scala vestibuli is translated directly to the basilar membrane, and the disturbance at the basilar membrane causes the initiation of a _____ wave.

6. High-frequency sounds are resolved at the base of the cochlea, with progressively lower-frequency sounds processed at progressively higher positions on the cochlea. This array is termed _____.

7. The frequency analysis ability of the basilar membrane is determined by graded _____ and _____.

8. T/F At the apex, the basilar membrane is thicker than at the base.

9. T/F At the apex, the basilar membrane is narrower than at the base.

10. T/F The cilia of the outer hair cells are embedded in the tectorial membrane.

11. T/F The cilia of the inner hair cells are embedded in the tectorial membrane.

12. T/F The scala vestibuli is 5 mV more positive than the scala tympani, but the scala media is 80 mV more positive the scala vestibuli.

13. The _____ arises directly from the stimulation of a large number of hair cells simultaneously.

14. _____ neurons require a higher intensity and encompass the higher end of our auditory range of signal intensity, whereas _____ neurons respond at very low signal levels and display random firing even when no stimulus is present.

15. _____ refers to the ability of the cochlea to differentiate the various spectral components of a signal.

16. The _____ frequency of a neuron is the frequency to which it responds best.

17. The tuning curves are composites of the responses of a single fiber at each frequency of presentation. The sharper the tuning curve, the greater the _____ of the basilar membrane.

18. The rate of firing of neurons increases as the _____ increases.

19. Stimulation of the _____ bundle and the _____ bundle reduces the firing rate of neurons innervated by them.

20. _____ are those firing patterns that most resemble VIII nerve responses.

21. The _____ is the primary site of localization of sound in space.

22. Comparative anatomy provides insights into function. What changes in the cochlea would you predict when comparing the cochlea of a human with that of a mammal that used ultra-high-frequency sound to echolocate, such as a fruit bat? What changes would you predict that you would find when comparing an elephant's cochlea with that of a human?

23. The _____ is the primary brain stem location for localization of sound in space.

24. The _____ of the brain stem is involved in both localization and intersensory interaction.

25. The _____ of the auditory cortex is responsible for primary reception of the auditory signal and is divided into three portions.

26. The Planum _____ is posterior to Heschl's gyrus.

27. The Planum _____ is anterior to Heschl's gyrus.

28. The _____ region of the auditory cortex surrounds the core area for auditory reception.

29. The _____ of the thalamus is the primary source of input to the core of the auditory cortex.

Study Question Answers

1. The **PINNA** of the outer ear is important for the localization of sound in space.

2. Resistance to the flow of energy is termed **IMPEDANCE**.

3. The area ratio between the tympanic membrane and the oval window provides a **25** dB gain, and the lever advantage gives a **2** dB gain.

4. The cochlea performs both **SPECTRAL** analysis and **TEMPORAL** analysis.

5. Compression of the fluid of the scala vestibuli is translated directly to the basilar membrane, and the disturbance at the basilar membrane causes the initiation of a **TRAVELING** wave.

6. High-frequency sounds are resolved at the base of the cochlea, with progressively lower frequency sounds processed at progressively higher positions on the cochlea. This array is termed **TONOTOPIC**.

7. The frequency analysis ability of the basilar membrane is determined by graded **WIDTH**, **STIFFNESS**, and **THICKNESS**.

8. **T** At the apex, the basilar membrane is **THICKER** than at the base.

9. **F** At the apex, the basilar membrane is **WIDER** than at the base.

10. **T** The cilia of the outer hair cells are embedded in the tectorial membrane.

11. **F** The cilia of the inner hair cells are embedded in the tectorial membrane.

12. **T** The scala vestibuli is 5 mV more positive than the scala tympani, but the scala media is 80 mV more positive than the scala vestibuli.

13. The **WHOLE-NERVE ACTION POTENTIAL** arises directly from the stimulation of a large number of hair cells simultaneously.

14. **HIGH-THRESHOLD** neurons require a higher intensity and encompass the higher end of our auditory range of signal intensity, whereas **LOW-THRESHOLD** neurons respond at very low signal levels and display random firing even when no stimulus is present.

15. **FREQUENCY SPECIFICITY** refers to the ability of the cochlea to differentiate the various spectral components of a signal.

16. The **CHARACTERISTIC** frequency of a neuron is the frequency to which it responds best.

17. The tuning curves are composites of the responses of a single fiber at each frequency of presentation. The sharper the tuning curve, the greater the **FREQUENCY SPECIFICITY** of the basilar membrane.

18. The rate of firing of neurons increases as the **INTENSITY** increases.

19. Stimulation of the **CROSSED-OLIVOCOCHLEAR** bundle and the **UNCROSSED-OLIVOCOCHLEAR** bundle reduces the firing rate of neurons innervated by them.

20. **PRIMARY-LIKE** are those firing patterns that most resemble VIII nerve responses.

21. The **SUPERIOR OLIVARY COMPLEX** is the primary site of localization of sound in space.

22. The fruit bat cochlea is, naturally enough, smaller than that of the human. In addition, the cochlea of the bat is extremely sensitive to ultra-high frequencies (above human range of hearing), because high-frequency sounds are more efficient for echolocation. Elephants, in contrast, have larger cochleas than humans. They process sounds that are lower than those we can hear.

23. The **SUPERIOR OLIVARY COMPLEX** is the primary brain stem location for localization of sound in space.

24. The **INFERIOR COLLICULUS** of the brain stem is involved in both localization and intersensory interaction.

25. The **CORE** of the auditory cortex is responsible for primary reception of the auditory signal and is divided into three portions.

26. The Planum **TEMPORALE** is posterior to Heschl's gyrus.

27. The Planum **POLARE** is anterior to Heschl's gyrus.

28. The **BELT** region of the auditory cortex surrounds the core area for auditory reception.

29. The **MEDIAL GENICULATE BODY** of the thalamus is the primary source of input to the core of the auditory cortex.

Bibliography

Altschuler, R. A., Bobbin, R. P., & Hoffman, D. W. (1986). *Neurobiology of hearing: The cochlea.* New York: Raven Press.

Anson, B. J., & Donaldson, J. R. (1973). *Surgical anatomy of the temporal bone and ear.* Philadelphia, PA: W. B. Saunders.

Banerjee, A., & Nikkar-Esfahani, A. (2011). Occlusion of the round window: A novel way to treat hyperacusis symptoms in superior canal dehiscence syndrome. *Otolaryngology-Head and Neck Surgery, 145*(2 suppl), P89–P99.

Belin, P., & Zatorre, R. J. (2005). Voice processing in human auditory cortex. In R. Konig, P. Heil, E. Budinger, & H. Scheich (Eds.). *The auditory cortex* (pp. 163–180). Mahwah, NJ: Lawrence Erlbaum.

Bhatnagar, S. C., & Andy, O. J. (2002). *Neuroscience for the study of communicative disorders* (2nd ed.). Baltimore, MD: Williams & Wilkins.

Budinger, E. (2005). Introduction: Auditory cortical fields and their functions. In R. Konig, P. Heil, E. Budinger, & H. Scheich (Eds.). *The auditory cortex* (pp. 3–6). Mahwah, NJ: Lawrence Erlbaum.

Carpenter, M. B. (1991). *Core text of neuroanatomy* (4th ed.). Baltimore, MD: Williams & Wilkins.

Casimiro, C. C., Knollmann, B. C., Ebert, S. N., Vary, J. C., Greene, A. E., Franz, M. R., Grinberg, A., Huang, S. P., & Pfeifer, K. (2001). Targeted disruption of the Kcnq1 gene produces a mouse model of Jervell and Lange-Nielsen Syndrome. *Proceedings of the National Academy of Sciences USA, 98*(5), 2526–2531.

Cazals, Y., Demany, L., & Horner, K. (1991). *Auditory physiology and perception.* Oxford: Pergamon Press.

Chusid, J. G. (1985). *Correlative neuroanatomy and functional neurology* (17th ed.). Los Altos, CA: Lange Medical Publications.

Clarke, S., Adriani, M., & Tardif, E. (2005). "What" and "Where" in human audition: Evidence from anatomical, activation, and lesion studies. In R. Konig, P. Heil, E. Budinger, & H. Scheich (Eds.). *The auditory cortex* (pp. 77–94). Mahwah, NJ: Lawrence Erlbaum.

Dallos, P. (1973). *The auditory periphery.* New York: Academic Press.

Dallos, P., Billone, M. C., Durrant, J. D., Wang, C.Y., & Raynor, S. (1972). Cochlear inner and outer hair cells: Functional differences. *Science, 177,* 356–358.

Davis, H. (1958). Transmission and transduction in the cochlea. *Laryngoscope, 68,* 359–382.

Duifhuis, H., Horst, J. W., van Dijk, P., & van Netten, S. M. (1993). *Biophysics of hair cell sensory systems.* Singapore: World Scientific.

Durrant, J. D., & Lovrinic, J. H. (1995). *Bases of hearing science* (3rd ed.). Baltimore, MD: Williams & Wilkins.

Eggermont, J. J., & Odenthal, D. W. (1974). Electrophysiological investigation of the human cochlea: Recruitment, masking and adaptation. *Audiology, 13*(1), 1–22.

Engstrom, H., Ades, H. W., & Andersson, A. (1966). *Structural pattern of the organ of Corti.* Baltimore, MD: Williams & Wilkins.

Evans, R. B. (2003). Georg von Bekesy: Visualization of hearing. *American Psychologist, 58*(9), 742–746.

Gelfand, S. A. (1990). *Hearing.* New York: Marcel Dekker.

Gelfand, S. A. (2001). *Essentials of audiology* (2nd ed.). New York: Thieme Medical Publishers.

Gollisch, T., & Meister, M. (2008). Rapid neural coding in the retina with relative spike latencies. *Science, 319,* 1108–1111.

Gray, H., Bannister, L. H., Berry, M. M., & Williams, P. L. (Eds.). (1995). *Gray's anatomy.* London: Churchill Livingstone.

Green, D. (1976). *An introduction to hearing.* Hillsdale, NJ: Lawrence Erlbaum.

Gulick, W. L. (1971). *Hearing physiology and psychophysics.* New York: Oxford University Press.

Hackney, C. M. (2008). Inner ear. In Standring, S. (2008). *Gray's anatomy: The anatomical and clinical basis of practice* (40th ed., pp. 633–650). London: Churchill Livingstone.

Haralabidis, A. G., Dimakopoulou, K., Vigna-Taglianti, F., Giampaolo, M., Borgini, A., Dudley, M-L., et al. (2008). Acute effects of night-time noise exposure on blood pressure in populations living near airports. *European Heart Journal, 29*(5), 658–664.

Hickok, G., & Poeppel, D. (2007). The cortical organization of speech processing. *Nature Reviews of Neuroscience, 8,* 393–402.

Izumikawa, M., Minoda, R., Kawamoto, K., Abrashkin, K. A., Swiderski, D. L., Dolan, D. F., Brough, D. E., & Raphael, Y. (2005). Auditory hair cell replacement and hearing improvement by Atoh1 gene therapy in deaf mammals. *Nature Medicine, 11,* 271–276.

Javel, E. (1986). Basic response properties of auditory nerve fibers. In R. A. Altschuler, R. P. Bobbin, & D. W. Hoffman (Eds.), *Neurobiology of hearing: The cochlea* (pp. 213–245). New York: Raven Press.

Kaas, J. H., & Hackett, T. A. (2000). Subdivisions of auditory cortex and processing streams in primates. *Proceedings of the National Academy of Sciences USA, 97*(22), 11793–11799.

Kaas, J. H., & Hackett, T. A. (2005). Subdivisions and connections of the auditory cortex in primates: A working model. In R. Konig, P. Heil, E. Budinger, & H. Scheich (Eds.). *The auditory cortex* (pp. 7–26). Mahwah, NJ: Lawrence Erlbaum.

Kandel, E. R., Schwartz, J. H., & Jessell, T. M. (2000). *Principles of neural science* (4th ed.). New York: McGraw-Hill.

Khanna, S. M., & Leonard, D. G. B. (1982). Basilar membrane tuning in the cochlea. *Science, 215,* 305–306.

Kiang, N. Y-S. (1965). *Discharge patterns of single fibers in the cat's auditory nerve.* Cambridge, MA: The MIT Press.

Kiang, N., Y-S., Liberman, M. C., Sewell, W. F., & Guinan, J. J. (1986). Single unit clues to cochlear mechanisms. *Hearing Research, 22,* 171–182.

Konig, R., Heil, P., Budinger, E., & Scheich, H. (2005). *The auditory cortex.* Mahwah, NJ: Lawrence Erlbaum.

Kraft, S., Hsu, C., Brough, D. E., & Staecker, H. (2013). Atoh1 induces hair cell recovery in mice with ototoxic injury. *Laryngoscope, 123*(4), 992–999.

Kruger, B. (1989). An update on external ear resonance in infants and young children. *Ear and Hearing, 8*(6), 333–336.

Kuehn, D. P., Lemme, M. L., & Baumgartner, J. M. (1991). *Neural bases of speech, hearing, and language.* Boston: Little, Brown.

Lewis, E. R., Leverenz, E. L., & Bialek, W. S. (1985). *The vertebrate inner ear.* Boca Raton, FL: CRC Press.

Liberman, M. C., & Kiang, N. Y. S. (1978). Acoustic trauma in cats. *Acta Otolarygnolgica. Supplement 358,* 1–63.

Martin, F. N. (1981). *Medical audiology.* Englewood Cliffs, NJ: Prentice-Hall.

Møller, A. R. (1973). *Basic mechanisms of hearing.* New York: Academic Press.

Møller, A. R. (1983). *Auditory physiology.* New York: Academic Press.

Møller, A. R. (2003). *Sensory systems: Anatomy and physiology.* New York: Academic Press.

Moroson, P., Rademacher, J., Palomero-Gallagher, N., & Zilles, K. (2005). Anatomical organization of the human auditory cortex: Cytoarchitecture and transmitter receptors. In R. Konig, P. Heil, E. Budinger, & H. Scheich (Eds.). *The auditory cortex* (pp. 27–50). Mahwah, NJ: Lawrence Erlbaum.

Musiek, F. E., & Baran, J. A. (2006). *The auditory system: Anatomy, physiology, and clinical correlates.* Glenview, IL: Allyn & Bacon.

Norton, S., & Neely, S. T. (1987). Tone-burst otoacoustic emissions from normal hearing adults. *Journal of the Acoustical Society of America, 81*(6), 1860–1872.

Parkins, C. W., & Anderson, S. W. (1983). Cochlear prostheses. *Annals of the New York Academy of Sciences, 405.*

Petkov, C. I., Kayser, C., Steudel, T., Whittingstall, K., Augath, M., & Logothetis, N. K. (2008). A voice region in the monkey brain. *Nature Neuroscience 11,* 367–374.

Pfeiffer, R. R. (1966). Classification of response patterns of spike discharges for units in the cochlear nucleus: Tone-burst stimulation. *Experimental Brain Research, 1,* 220–235.

Pickles, J. O. (1988). *An introduction to the physiology of hearing* (2nd ed.). London: Academic Press.

Rhode, W. W. (1985). The use of intracellular techniques in the study of the cochlear nucleus. *Journal of the Acoustical Society of America, 78,* 320–327.

Rossing, T. D. (2001). *The science of sound.* Reading, MA: Addison-Wesley.

Ryan, A., & Dallos, P. (1976). Physiology of the inner ear. In J. L. Northern, (Ed.), *Hearing disorders* (pp. 89–101). Boston: Little, Brown.

Sanford, C. A., & Feeney, M. P. (2008). Effects of maturation on tympanic wideband acoustic transfer function in human infants. *Journal of the Acoustical Society of America, 124*(4), 2106–2122.

Seixas, N. S., Kujawa, S. G., Norton, S., Sheppard, L., Neitzel, R., & Slee, A. (2004). Prediction of hearing threshold levels and distortion product otoacoustic emissions among noise-exposed young adults. *Occupational Environmental Medicine, 61*(11), 899–907.

Shaw, E. A. G. (1974). The external ear. In W. D. Keidel & W. D. Neff (Eds.), *Handbook of sensory physiology* (pp. 455–490). New York: Springer-Verlag.

Spicer, S. S., & Schulte, B. A. (1996). The fine structure of spiral ligament cells relates to ion return to the stria and varies with place-frequency. *Hearing Research, 100,* 80–100.

Syka, J., & Masterton, R. B. (1988). *Auditory pathway structure and function.* New York: Plenum Press.

Tobias, J. V., & Schubert, E. D. (1983). *Hearing research and theory* (Vol. 2). New York: Academic Press.

Tonndorf, J. (1958). The hydrodynamic origin of aural harmonics in the cochlea. *Annals of Otology, 67,* 754–774.

Tonndorf, J. (1960). Shearing motion in scala media of cochlear models. *Journal of the Acoustical Society of America, 32*(5), 238–244.

Von Békésy, G. (1960). *Experiments in hearing.* New York: McGraw-Hill.

Von Bohlen und Halbach, O., & Dermietzel, R. (2006). *Neurotransmitters and neuromodulators.* Weinheim, Germany: Wiley-VCH.

Wangemann, P. (2006). Supporting sensory transduction: cochlear fluid homeostasis and the endocochlear potential. *Journal of neurophysiology, 576*(1), 11-21.

Watson, S. R. D., Halmagyi, M., & Colebatch, J. G. (2000). Vestibular hypersensity to sound (Tullio phenomenon). *Neurology, 54*(3), 213–225.

Wever, E. G., & Bray, C. W. (1930). Action currents in the auditory nerve in response to acoustical stimulation. *Proceedings of the National Academy of Science, 16,* 344–350.

Winslow, R. L., & Sachs, M. B. (1988). Single tone intensity discrimination based on auditory nerve rate responses in backgrounds of quiet, noise, and with stimulation of the crossed olivocochlear nerve. *Hearing Research, 35*(2–3), 165–189.

Wilson, J. P., & Kemp, D. T. (1989). *Cochlear mechanisms: Structure, function, and models.* New York: Plenum Press.

Winans, S. S., Gilman, S., Manter, J. T., & Gatz, A. J. (2002). *Manter and Gatz's essentials of clinical neuroanatomy and neurophysiology* (10th ed.). Philadelphia, PA: F. A. Davis.

Yost, W. A. (2000). *Fundamentals of hearing: An introduction* (4th ed.). New York: Academic Press.

Yost, W. A., & Nielsen, D. W. (1977). *Fundamentals of hearing: An introduction.* New York: Holt, Rinehart & Winston.

Zemlin, W. R. (1998). *Speech and hearing science: Anatomy and physiology* (4th ed.). Needham Heights, MA: Allyn & Bacon.

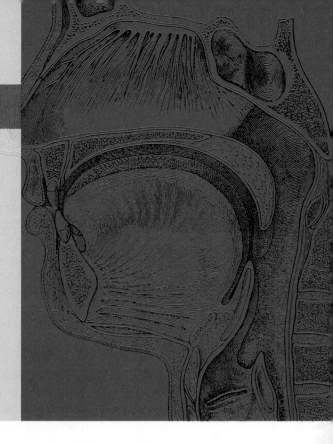

Chapter 11

NEUROANATOMY

There is nothing in nature so awe-inspiring as the nervous system. Despite centuries of study, humans have only begun to gain understanding of this extraordinarily complex system. The brain contains approximately 86 billion neurons, with the cerebral cortex being the home to 17 billion of them (Azevado et al., 2009; Karlsen & Pakkenberg, 2011). Neurons are densely interconnected, so that each neuron may communicate directly with as many as 2,000 other neurons: There are on the order of 190 trillion synapses (points of communication) within the brain. We tell you these extraordinary numbers so that you can get a notion of the vastness of the nervous system. The tremendous challenge of neuroscience is, and always has been, to figure out how these elements interact to produce all of the complex processes involved in thought, language, and speech. As before, we will discuss both the structure and function of this system.

OVERVIEW

During our discussion of human anatomy associated with speech and language, we have been quite concerned with the voluntary musculature and the supporting framework associated with it. Communication is, by and large, voluntary. Nonetheless, the term *voluntary* takes on new meanings when seen in the context of automaticity and background. **Automaticity** refers to the development of patterns of responses that no longer require highly specific motor control but rather are relegated to automated patterns. **Background** activity is the muscular contraction that supports action or movement, providing

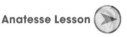

Anatesse Lesson

the form against which voluntary movement is placed. Voluntary activities are generally considered to be conscious activities, but they are, in reality, largely automated responses. To prove this to yourself, try washing the dishes and actually thinking about the act of dishwashing. The movements and responses to this act are so automated that you probably feel you do them "without thinking." In fact, your brain receives a vast number of signals from body sensors every second (including information about soap suds and water temperature), but you need not respond to all of it, because your brain will monitor and alert you to dangers. You can think about other things while your hands do the dishes.

Speech capitalizes on similar automaticity, as you can see in your ability to speak easily while riding a bike or while walking. You no more think of every movement of the extraordinary number of muscles contracting for the simple speech act than you do during dishwashing. This changes when the mechanism changes, however. When your mouth is numb from the dentist's anesthesia, you become very aware of your lack of feedback from that system, and inaccurate speech results. When an individual suffers a cerebrovascular accident, the result is often a loss of previously attained automaticity in speech. When a child is born with developmental apraxia of speech, a condition that limits the ability of a child to plan articulatory function, achieving automaticity may be a lifelong struggle. You might want to revisit our Chapter 7 discussion of motor control, feedback systems, and feed-forward systems as you think about these "automatic" functions of speech.

Automatic functions are supported by a background **tonicity**, a partial contraction of musculature to maintain muscle tone. All action occurs within an environment, and the environment of your musculature is the tonic contraction of supporting muscles. As you extend your arm to reach for a coffee cup, the action of your fingers to grasp the object is supported by the rotation of your shoulder and the extension of your arm. Without these background support movements, the act of grasping would not occur in the graceful, fluid manner to which you are accustomed. Your body works as a unit to meet your needs.

Voluntary functions are the domain of the **cerebral cortex** or **cerebrum**, a new structure by evolutionary standards that makes up the bulk of the human brain. It is the seat of consciousness, and sensory information that does not reach the level of the cerebrum does not reach consciousness. The cerebrum is also the source of voluntary movement, although many lower brain centers are involved in the execution of commands initiated by the cerebrum (see Figure 11-1).

Movement requires coordination, and that is one of the responsibilities of the **cerebellum**. Information from peripheral sensors is coordinated with the motor plan of the cerebrum to provide the body with the ability to make finely tuned motor gestures. The output from the cerebrum is modified by the **basal ganglia**, a group of nuclei (cell bodies) with functional unity deeply involved in background movement.

(A)

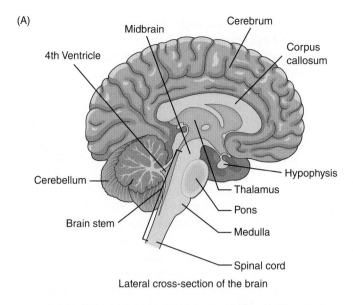

Lateral cross-section of the brain

(B)

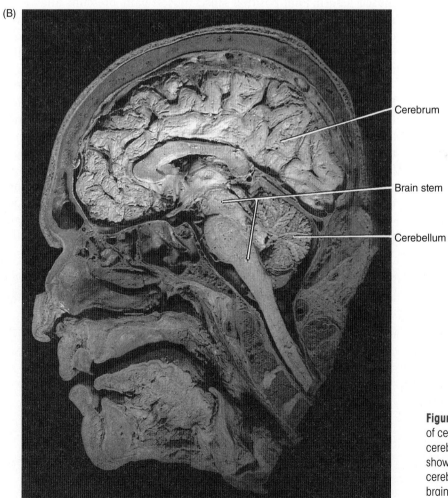

Figure 11-1. (A) Medial view of cerebrum, brain stem, and cerebellum. (B) Sagittal section showing relationship among cerebrum, cerebellum, and brain stem.
© Cengage Learning®.

Motor commands are conveyed to the periphery for execution by neural pathways termed **nerves** or **tracts**. Sensory pathways transmit information concerning the status of the body and its environment to the brain for evaluation. This information permits the cerebrum and lower centers to act on changing conditions to protect the systems of the body and to adjust to the body's environment. For instance, information that tells your brain that it is cold outside will be transmitted to the cerebrum and hypothalamus—the result will be shivering and goose bumps as well as a conscious effort to retrieve your ski parka from the car.

The brain can communicate with its environment only through sensors and effectors (see Tables 11-1 and 11-2). Sensors are the means by which your nervous system translates information concerning the internal and external environment into a form that is usable by the brain, whereas effectors are the means by which your body responds to changing conditions. Broadly speaking, **superficial sensation** (temperature, pain, touch) is a sensation arising from the stimulation of the surface of the body. **Deep sensation** includes muscle tension, muscle length, joint position sense, muscle pain, pressure, and vibration. **Combined sensation** integrates both multiple senses to process stimulation. This involves integration of many pieces of sensory information to determine a quality, such as **stereognosis** (the ability to recognize the form of an object through touch).

Within each of these broad classes are specific types of sensation. **Somatic sense** is that sensation related to pain, thermal sensation (temperature sense), and mechanical stimulation. Mechanical stimulation takes the form of light and deep pressure, vibration (which is actually pressure that is perceived to change over time), and changes in joints and muscles, particularly stretch. **Kinesthetic sense**, or *kinesthesia*, is the sense of the body in motion. **Special senses** are those designed to **transduce** (change one form of energy into another) specific exteroceptive information. For example, in the **visual sense**, light from external sources is transduced into electrochemical energy by

Table 11-1 **Classes of sensation**	
Superficial Senses	**Deep Senses**
Temperature	Muscle length and tension
Pain	Joint
Touch	Proprioception
	Muscle pain
	Pressure
	Vibration

© Cengage Learning®.

Table 11-2 **Sense, sensor, and stimulation**		
Sense	**Sensor Type**	**Stimulus**
Pain	Nerve ending	Aversive stimulation
Temperature	Thermosensor	Heat and cold
Mechanical stimulation	Pacinian corpuscle Golgi tendon organ Muscle spindle	Light and deep pressure Vibration Joint sense Muscle stretch
Kinesthetic sense	Labyrinthine (vestibular) hair cells	Motion of body
Vision	Photoreceptors	Light stimulation
Olfactory	Chemoreceptors	Chemical stimulation
Audition	Labyrinthine (cochlear) hair cells	Acoustical stimulation
Gustatory	Chemoreceptors	Chemical stimulation

© Cengage Learning®.

Coming to Your Senses

We have come to know the "five senses" as stereotypes: touch, taste, vision, hearing, and smell, thanks to Aristotle. The reality is far different, however. Physiologists now state that there are at least 21 senses, and some place the number much higher. Here is how they come to this conclusion.

There are certainly basic senses: vision, hearing, olfaction (smell), gestation (taste), tactile sense (touch), nociception (pain), mechanoreception, thermal sense, and interoception (senses associated with internal, subconscious processes such as blood pressure, CO_2 in the blood, etc.). That said, each of these basic senses can be further subdivided. For instance, vision can be divided into light and color, but some say it should be divided into light, red sense, green sense, and blue sense. This makes "sense," in that the receptors for these colors are mutually exclusive. You could make the same argument for taste. Taste consists of sweet, salty, bitter, sour, and umami. Smell is smell, right? Wrong. We can sense over 2,000 different and highly specific smells, and there is evidence that the olfactory receptors are highly specialized.

Mechanoreception diversifies in the same way. We have the sense of balance and acceleration (rotational and linear) mediated by the vestibular mechanism, but we also have joint sense (proprioception), body movement sense (kinesthesia), and muscle tension (Golgi tendon organs [GTO]), and stretch (muscle spindle) senses.

Finally, there are at least five basic interoceptors, including sensors for blood pressure, arterial pressure, venous pressure, oxygen content, acid balance of cerebrospinal fluid, and stomach distension. So, it looks as if Aristotle needs an update.

the photoreceptors of the retina; in **hearing**, acoustical disturbances in the air are transduced by the hair cells of the cochlea. Other special senses are **olfaction** (sense of smell), **tactile sense** (sense of touch), and **gustation** (sense of taste).

Sensor types vary by the stimulus to which they respond. Sensors communicate with the nervous system by means of dendritic connection with bipolar first-order sensory neurons. Axons of these first-order neurons **synapse** or make neurochemical connection within the central nervous system. A graded **generator potential** arises from adequate stimulation of the sensor, and adequate stimulation will cause the generation of an action potential.

Receptors may be mechanoreceptors, chemoreceptors, photoreceptors, or thermoreceptors. **Mechanoreceptors** respond to physical distortion of tissue. Pressure on the skin, for example, will result in the distension of **Pacinian corpuscles**, whereas hair follicles have mechanoreceptors to let you know that something has disturbed your hair. **Muscle spindle** and **Golgi tendon organs** and the **labyrinthine hair receptors** of the inner ear are also mechanoreceptors. In contrast, olfaction (smell) and gustation (taste) are mediated by

When Sensation Goes Bad

Sensations are processed by the nervous system as a means of relating the real world with our "inner world." These sensations are required for normal function, including motor coordination and protective action. When sensory systems fail, any valuable information required by the nervous system is lost. The most obvious sensory loss for those of us in the fields of speech-language pathology and audiology is those associated with hearing and vestibular function. Prenatal loss of hearing has a significant impact on the development of speech and language, whereas postnatal loss results in significant communication problems. Vestibular dysfunction, as in that seen in Meniere's disease (endolymphatic hydrops), results in significant balance difficulties and vertigo.

One can also have a disruption of sensory systems related to joint perception, which can cause errors in motor execution. Similarly, a deficit in sensory feedback drives the muscle spindle into hyperfunction when upper motor neuron lesion limits the inhibition of that reflexive system. Diseases such as diabetes can cause loss of pain sense, which may result in failure to recognize a wound until it has become seriously infected. Loss of appropriate sensory input to the cerebellum, which coordinates motor function (including correction of the motor plan), will result in cerebellar ataxia, which is reduction of coordinated movement.

Finally, sometimes our senses can fool us. There are well-known illusions that can be elicited relative to sensation. For instance, if you are seated so that you cannot see your right arm, but *can* see an artificial limb that could be your arm, you will perceive the artificial limb as your own arm if an experimenter stimulates both your hidden "real" arm and the visible artificial arm, an apparent function of the premotor cortex (Ehrsson, Spence, & Passingham, 2004). This very real and robust phenomenon is mirrored in several versions of the phantom limb phenomenon. In this condition, people who have undergone amputation of a limb sometimes perceive the presence of that limb, despite all evidence to the contrary. As Kandel (2012) notes, a person with phantom limb syndrome may feel the amputated limb move, and even perceive it extending to shake another person's hand.

Locked-in Syndrome

Locked-in syndrome is a condition that typically arises because of brain stem stroke or cerebrovascular accident (CVA). The condition results in complete paralysis of all musculature except the ocular muscles for eye movement. The condition typically has no effect on sensory or cognitive function, so the individual is left with intact mental function but no means of communication. A system of eye blinks is typically established with the individual as a means of alternative communication.

chemoreceptors because they depend on contact with molecules of the target substance. Visual stimulation by light is transduced by highly specialized **photoreceptors**, and temperature sense arises from **thermoreceptors**. Visual and auditory sensors are also termed **teleceptors** because their respective light and sound stimuli arise from a source that does not touch the body (olfactory sense is stimulated directly by molecules of the material being sensed).

Another way to categorize receptors is by the region of the body receiving stimulation. **Interoceptors** monitor events within the body, such as distention of the lungs during inspiration or blood acidity. **Exteroceptors** respond to stimuli outside of the body, such as tactile stimulation, audition, and vision. Contact receptors are exteroceptors that respond to stimuli that touch the body (e.g., tactile, pain, deep and light pressure, temperature). **Proprioceptors** are sensors that monitor change in a body's position or the position of its parts, and these include muscle and joint sensors, such as muscle spindles and Golgi tendon organs (GTOs). Vestibular sense falls into this category because it provides information about the body's position in space.

Despite our rich communicative ability, we can know our environment *only* by means of the sensory receptors of our skin, muscles, tendons, eyes, ears, and so forth. Without sensation, a perfectly functioning brain would be worthless as a communicating system. Likewise, communication *requires* some sort of muscular activity or glandular secretion. The absence of *all* motor activity would signal the end of communication. Fortunately, the extraordinary number of sensors in the human body permits us to use alternate pathways for receiving communication (e.g., tactile, or touch, communication) or for passing information to another person (e.g., use of eye-blink code). We are rarely completely cut off from communication with others. Let us now examine the components of this system.

DIVISIONS OF THE NERVOUS SYSTEM

The **nervous system** can be viewed and categorized in a number of ways. It is important to develop a framework for the discussion of this system, lest the volume of components become overwhelming. In the overview, we discussed an informal **functional view** of nervous system organization, assessing the components in terms

---

Table 11-3 **Divisions of the nervous system from anatomical and physiological perspectives**

Anatomical Divisions of the Nervous System:

Central Nervous System: Cerebrum, cerebellum, brain stem, spinal cord, thalamus, subthalamus, basal ganglia, etc.

Peripheral Nervous System: Spinal nerves, cranial nerves, sensors

Functional Divisions of the Nervous System:

Autonomic Nervous System: Involuntary bodily function

  Sympathetic nervous system: Expends energy (e.g., vasoconstriction when frightened)

  Parasympathetic nervous system: Conserves energy (e.g., vasodilation upon removal of feared stimulation)

Somatic Nervous System: Voluntary bodily function

© Cengage Learning®.

---

of their relationship to the systems of communication. We can view the nervous system as being composed of two major components (central nervous system and peripheral nervous system) or as having two major functions (somatic nervous system and autonomic nervous system) (see Table 11-3). We can also view the nervous system in developmental terms, differentiating based on embryonic structures.

Central Nervous System and Peripheral Nervous System

The nervous system may be divided anatomically into central and peripheral nervous systems (see Table 11-3). The **central nervous system (CNS)** includes the brain (cerebrum, cerebellum, subcortical structures, brain stem) and spinal cord. The **peripheral nervous system (PNS)** consists of the 12 pairs of cranial nerves and 31 pairs of spinal nerves as well as the sensory receptors. All the CNS components are housed within bone (skull or vertebral column), whereas most of the PNS components are outside of bone. We will spend a great deal of time within this organizational structure as we discuss the anatomy of the nervous system.

Autonomic and Somatic Nervous Systems

A functional view of the nervous system categorizes the brain into autonomic and somatic nervous systems (see Table 11-3). The **autonomic nervous system (ANS)** governs involuntary activities of the visceral muscles or **viscera**, including glandular secretions, heart function, and digestive function. You have little control over what happens to that triple chili cheeseburger once you make the commitment to eat it, although you will admit that occasionally you are *aware* of the digestive process. You can also view the enteric nervous system (ENS) as a subsystem of the ANS. The enteric nervous system governs how that cheeseburger is processed (Horn & Swanson, 2008). The ENS contains over 900,000 neurons (compared with 120,000 neurons in the spinal cord) that govern the stomach, heart, bladder, intestines, and vascular system all in the background.

The ANS may be further divided into two subsystems. The subsystem that responds to stimulation through energy expenditure is called the **sympathetic system** or **thoracolumbar system**, and the system that counters these responses is known as the **parasympathetic system** or **craniosacral system**. You feel the result of the sympathetic system when you have a close call in an automobile or hear a sudden, loud noise. Sympathetic responses include **vasoconstriction** (constriction of blood vessels), increase in blood pressure, dilation of pupils, cardiac acceleration, and goose bumps. If you attend for a few more seconds, you will notice the glandular secretion of sweat under your arms. All these fall into the category of "flight, fight, or fright" responses. Your body dumps the hormone norepinephrine into your system to provide you with a means of responding to danger, although the speed of modern emergencies such as automobile accidents clearly outstrips the rate of sympathetic responses (wear your seatbelt).

You may be less aware of the parasympathetic system response. This system is responsible for counteracting the effects of this preparatory act, because extraordinary muscular activity requires extraordinary energy. Parasympathetic responses include slowing of the heart rate, reduction of blood pressure, and pupillary constriction. While this view of the ANS as a pair of subsystems continually counteracting each other is useful, the reality is that the ANS is a system designed to create homeostasis rather than compensation. The ANS helps us respond to our internal and external environments in useful ways and is charged with maintaining an optimal "operating system" of the body. We do, however, encounter problems with this system when we live in highly charged, stressful environments, since our ANS will respond to those environments in a way to maximize our survival at the moment, even at the cost of our long-term viability. The CNS component of the ANS arises from the prefrontal region of the cerebral cortex, as well as from the hypothalamus, thalamus, hippocampus, brain stem, cerebellum, and spinal cord. The viscera are connected to these loci of control by means of **afferent** (ascending, typically sensory) and **efferent** (descending, typically motor) tracts.

The PNS components of the ANS include paired **sympathetic trunk ganglia** running parallel and in close proximity to the vertebral column, **plexuses** (networks of nerves), and **ganglia** (groups of cell bodies having functional unity and lying outside the CNS).

The **somatic** nervous system (voluntary component) is of major importance to speech pathology. This system involves the aspects of bodily function that are under our conscious and voluntary control, including control of all skeletal or **somatic muscles**. CNS control of

afferent: L., ad ferre, to carry toward

efferent: L., ex ferre, to carry away from

somatic: Gr., soma, body

muscles arises largely from the precentral region of the cerebral cortex, with neural impulses conveyed through descending motor tracts of the brain stem and spinal cord. Communication with the cranial nerves of the brain stem and with the spinal nerves of the spinal cord permits activation of the periphery of the body. Likewise, the sensory component of the somatic nervous system monitors information about the function of the skeletal muscles, their environment, and other "nonvisceral" activities.

The motor component of the somatic system may be subdivided into **pyramidal** and **extrapyramidal** systems, although defining all the anatomical correlates of this functional division is difficult. The pyramidal system arises from pyramidal cells of the motor strip of the cerebral cortex and is largely responsible for the initiation of voluntary motor acts. The extrapyramidal system also arises from the cerebral cortex (mostly from the premotor region of the frontal lobe) but is responsible for the background tone and movement supporting the primary acts. The extrapyramidal system is referred to as the **indirect system**, projecting to the basal ganglia and reticular formation.

There is one more important way of categorizing structures within the nervous system, and it is developmental in nature. The anatomical and developmental organizations overlap, and both sets of terminology are often used together.

Development Divisions

During the fourth week of embryonic development, the brain (**encephalon**) is composed of the **prosencephalon** (forebrain), **mesencephalon** (midbrain), and **rhombencephalon** (hindbrain). As the encephalon develops, further differentiation results in the telencephalon, rhinencephalon, diencephalon, metencephalon, and myelencephalon (see Table 11-4). The **telencephalon** refers to the "extended" or "telescoped" brain and includes the cerebral hemispheres, the white matter immediately beneath it, the basal ganglia, and the olfactory tract. The **rhinencephalon** refers to structures within the telencephalon. The name arises from the relationship of the structures to olfaction (remember that the combining form "rhino" refers to "nose"). These are parts of the brain that developed early in our evolution and include the olfactory bulb, tract, and striae; pyriform area; intermediate olfactory area; paraterminal area; hippocampal formation; and fornix. The **diencephalon** is the next descending level and includes the thalamus, hypothalamus, pituitary gland (hypophysis), and optic tract. The mesencephalon is the midbrain of the brain stem, and the **metencephalon** includes the pons and cerebellum. The **myelencephalon** refers to the medulla oblongata, the lowest level of the encephalon. The term **bulb** or **bulbar** refers technically to the pons and medulla but is nearly always used to refer to the entire brain stem, including the midbrain.

Phylogeny refers to the evolution of a species, whereas ontogeny is the development of an individual organism. The statement that "Ontogeny recapitulates phylogeny" refers to the notion that structures that are phylogenetically oldest tend to emerge earliest in the developing organism, whereas later evolutionary additions, such as the cerebral cortex, will emerge later in development.

telencephalon: Gr., telos enkephalos, end or distant brain

rhinencephalon: Gr., rhis enkephalos, nose brain

Table 11-4 **Development and elements of the encephalon**		
Development of Encephalon		
Prosencephalon	Telencephalon (including rhinencephalon)	
	Diencephalon	
Mesencephalon	Mesencephalon	
Rhombencephalon	Metencephalon	
	Myelencephalon	
Components of Levels of the Encephalon		
Telencephalon	Cerebral hemispheres	
	Basal ganglia	
	Olfactory tract	
	Rhinencephalon	
	Lateral ventricle, part of third ventricle	
Diencephalon	Thalamus	
	Hypothalamus	
	Pituitary gland (hypophysis)	
	Optic tract	
	Third ventricle	
Mesencephalon	Midbrain	
	Cerebral aqueduct	
	Cerebral peduncles	
	Corpora quadrigemina	
Metencephalon	Pons	
	Cerebellum	
	Portion of fourth ventricle	
Myelencephalon	Medulla oblongata	
	Portion of fourth ventricle and central canal	

© Cengage Learning®.

Let us examine the nervous system, beginning with the building block of the nervous system. The basic units of the nervous system are neurons, from which all larger structures arise.

ANATOMY OF THE CNS AND PNS

Although it is an understatement to say that the CNS is extremely complex, it may be a comfort to realize that there is a common denominator to all the structures of the nervous system: All structures are made up of neurons. Functionally, the smallest organizational unit of the nervous system is also the neuron, followed in complexity by the

Table 11-5 **Hierarchical order of complexity for the structures of the nervous system**	
Structure	**Function**
Glial cells	Nutrients to neurons, support, phagocytosis, myelin
Neuron	Communicating tissue
Reflexes	Subconscious response to environmental stimuli
Ganglia/nuclei	Aggregates of cell bodies with functional unity
Tracts	Aggregates of axons that transmit functionally united information; spinal cord
Structures of the brain stem	Aggregates of ganglia, nuclei, and tracts that mediate high-level reflexes and mediate the execution of cortical commands
Diencephalon	Aggregates of nuclei and tracts that mediate sensory information arriving at cerebrum and provide basic autonomic responses for body maintenance
Cerebellum	Aggregates of nuclei, specialized neurons, and tracts that integrate somatic and special sensory information with motor planning and command for coordinated movement
Cerebrum	All conscious sensory awareness and conscious motor function, including perception, awareness, motor planning and preparation, cognitive function, attention, decision making, voluntary motor inhibition, language function, speech function

© Cengage Learning®.

spinal arc reflex and higher reflexes (see Table 11-5). The brain stem provides the next level of complexity, followed by subcortical structures and the cerebellum, and finally the most complex aggregate of tissue, the cerebral cortex. Let us begin with the discussion of the most basic component of the nervous system, the neuron.

Neurons

Overview

The nervous system is comprised of the communicating elements, **neurons**, and support tissue, **glia** or **glial cells**. Neurons (nerve cells) are the functional building blocks of the nervous system and are unique among tissue types in that they are *communicating* tissue. Their function is to transmit information. Recently, however, the glial cell has come under close scrutiny, and it looks as if its original role as a support system for neurons grossly understates its function. Some scientists have demonstrated that without glial cells the neurons would be virtually incapable of storing information in long-term memory. Glial cells are also critical players in the development of synapses. Astrocytes secrete thrombospondin, which supports the development of synapses, so that without astrocytes there would be no communication between neurons.

The general structure of most neurons includes the **soma**, or cell body; a **dendrite**, which transmits information toward the soma; and an axon, which transmits information away from the soma (see Table 11-6 and Figure 11-2).

Neurons respond to stimulation, and the neuron's response is the mechanism for transmitting information through the nervous system. A neuron can have one of two types of responses: excitation or inhibition. **Excitation** refers to stimulation that causes an increase of activity of the tissue stimulated. That is, if a neuron is stimulated, it will increase its activity in response. It is as if you were at a traffic signal in your car, and when the light changed, the person behind you honked. Your response to this stimulation is to take off from the light (excitation). **Inhibition**, in contrast, refers to stimulation of a neuron that reduces the neuron's output. That is, when a neuron is inhibited, it will reduce its activity. Again, using the traffic analogy, if you hear a siren while at the traffic light, you know that there is an emergency vehicle coming. The siren inhibits your activity, and you decide *not to move* because of that stimulation. That is an inhibitory response. Neurons with excitatory responses give an active output when stimulated, whereas those with inhibitory responses *stop* responding when they are stimulated.

Table 11-6 **Basic components of the neuron**

Component	Function
Dendrite	Receptor region
Soma	Contains metabolic organelles
Axon	Transmits information from neuron
Hillock	Generator site for action potential
Myelin sheath	Insulator of axon
Schwann cells	Form myelin in PNS
Oligodendrocytes	Form myelin in CNS
Nodes of Ranvier	Permit saltatory conduction
Telodendria	Processes from axon
Terminal end boutons	Contain synaptic vesicles
Neurotransmitter	Substance that facilitates synapse
Synaptic cleft	Region between pre- and postsynaptic neurons

© Cengage Learning®.

Morphology Characteristics. There are several important landmarks of the neuron (see Figures 11-1 and 11-3). A neuron may have many dendrites, often referred to as the "dendritic tree" because it looks "bushy," but it will typically have only one axon. The **axon hillock** is the junction of the axon and the soma. Many axons are covered with a white fatty wrapping called the **myelin sheath**. Myelin is made up of **Schwann cells** in the PNS and of **oligodendrocytes** in the CNS, but in both cases myelin serves a very important function: It speeds up neural conduction. This means that axons (fibers) that have myelin wrapping around them are capable of conducting impulses at a much greater rate than those that do not have myelin. This will be very important when you study diseases that destroy the myelin, such as multiple sclerosis.

Myelin is segmented, so that it resembles a series of hot dog buns linked together. The areas between the myelinated segments are

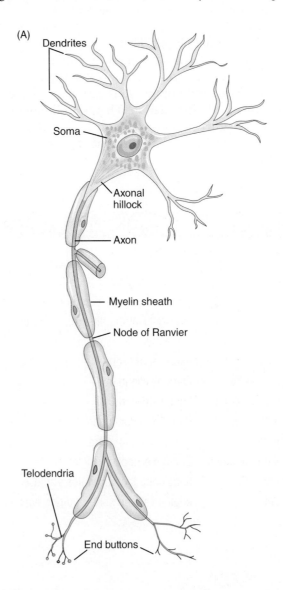

Figure 11-2. (A) Schematic of basic elements of a neuron. (continues).
© Cengage Learning®.

(B)

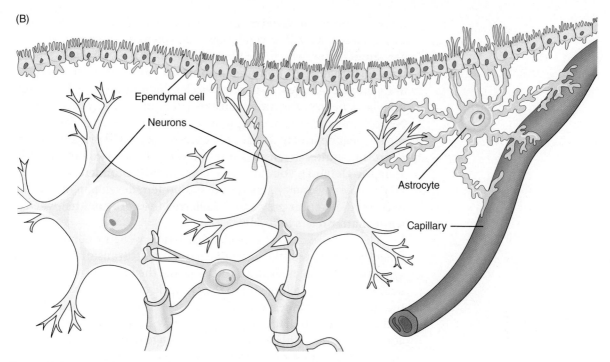

Ependymal cell

Neurons

Astrocyte

Capillary

Figure 11-2 continued. (B) The astrocyte is a glial cell that supports the transport of nutrients to the neuron while shielding it from toxins via the blood-brain barrier.
© Cengage Learning®.

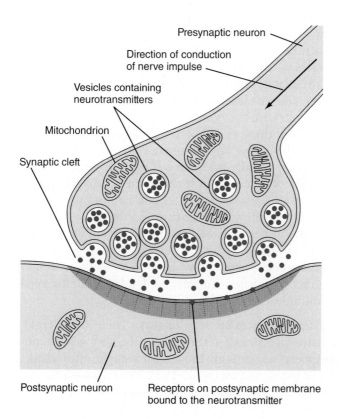

Presynaptic neuron

Direction of conduction of nerve impulse

Vesicles containing neurotransmitters

Mitochondrion

Synaptic cleft

Postsynaptic neuron

Receptors on postsynaptic membrane bound to the neurotransmitter

Figure 11-3. Schematic of elements of synapse. Note that the synapse consists of the terminal end bouton, synaptic cleft, and postsynaptic receptor sites.
© Cengage Learning®.

known as **nodes of Ranvier,** and we shall see that these are important in conduction as well. If you follow the axon to its end point, you will see **telodendria,** which are long, thin projections. The telodendria have **terminal (end) boutons** (or **buttons**), and within the boutons are **synaptic vesicles**. Synaptic vesicles contain a special chemical known as neurotransmitter substance (or simply *neurotransmitter*). **Neurotransmitters** are compounds that are responsible for activating the next neuron in a chain of neurons. As we will discuss later on, neurotransmitter is released into the gap between two neurons (the **synaptic cleft**). The boutons also contain **mitochondria,** organelles responsible for energy generation and protein development. Groups of cell bodies appear gray and are referred to as **gray matter,** whereas **white matter** refers to myelin.

The synapse deserves special discussion. When a neuron is sufficiently stimulated, the axon discharges neurotransmitter into the synaptic cleft. The neurotransmitter is like the key to your door: The neurotransmitter released into the synaptic cleft is the one to which the adjacent neuron responds. If some other class of neurotransmitter makes its way into that synaptic region, it will have no effect upon the adjacent neuron. This lock-and-key arrangement lets neurons have specific effects on some neurons while not affecting others.

We speak of the neurons in a chain as being either presynaptic or postsynaptic. **Presynaptic neurons** are those "upstream" from the synapse and are the ones that stimulate the **postsynaptic neurons** (the ones following the synapse). This makes sense when you realize that information passes in only one direction from a neuron: Information enters generally at the dendrite and exits at the axon.

Neurotransmitter released into the synaptic cleft stimulates **receptor sites** on the postsynaptic neuron. When the postsynaptic neuron is stimulated, ion channels in its membrane open up and allow ions to enter, and this leads to a discharge or "firing" of that neuron as well. Dendrites are the typical location for synapse on the receiving neurons, and these synapses are called **axodendritic synapses.** Synapse may also occur on the soma: These are called **axosomatic synapses** and are usually inhibitory. If synapse occurs on the axons of the postsynaptic neuron, it is called an **axoaxonic synapse** (see Figure 11-4), and these synapses tend to be modulatory in nature. Sometimes an axon stimulates a neuron secondarily on its way to the synapse with another neuron, and this is referred to as **en passant** ("in passing") synapse. Two other less common synapse formations are **somatosomatic synapse,** in which the soma of a neuron synapses with the soma of another neuron, and **dendrodendritic synapse,** in which communication is between two dendrites.

Morphological Differences between Neurons. There are several types or *forms* of neurons distributed throughout the nervous system. **Monopolar (unipolar) neurons** are those with a single, bifurcating process arising from the soma (see Figure 11-5). Neurons with two processes are called **bipolar neurons,** and **multipolar neurons** will have more

Synapse is a noun, but is often used as a verb, indicating the action of communication between two neurons.

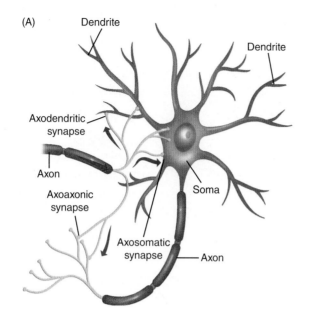

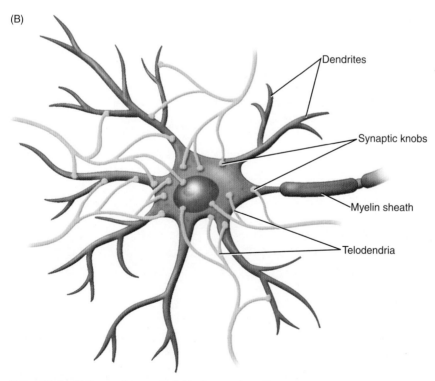

Figure 11-4. (A) Types of synapses, including axodendritic (excitatory), axosomatic (inhibitory), and axoaxonal (modulatory). (B) Illustration of excitatory and inhibitory synapses on a postsynaptic neuron. Note that excitatory axons synapse on the dendrite, while inhibitory axons synapse at the cell body.

© Cengage Learning®.

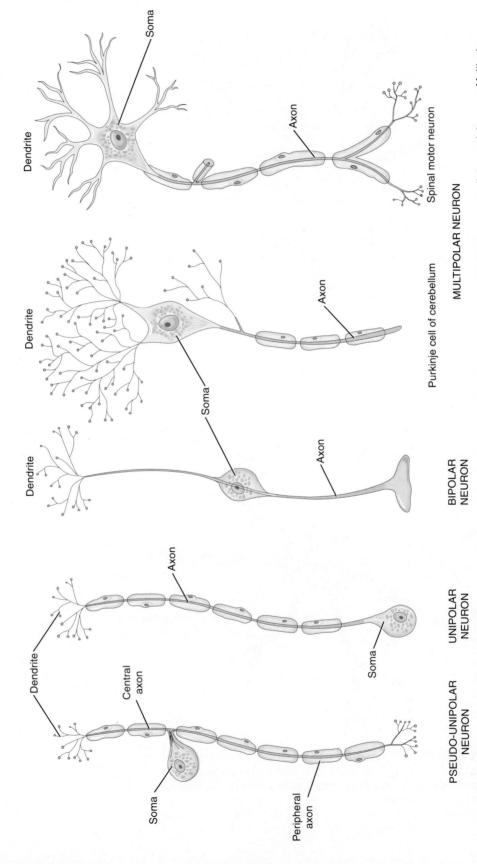

Figure 11-5. Types of neurons. Pseudo-unipolar and unipolar neurons are primarily somatic afferent neurons, whereas bipolar neurons mediate special senses. Multipolar neurons, which are primarily efferent, include pyramidal cells, spinal motor neurons, and Purkinje cells of the cerebellum.

© Cengage Learning®.

than two processes. Sensory neurons are generally monopolar or pseudomonopolar. The exception is neurons that transmit information about smell (olfaction), hearing (**audition**), and vestibular senses: these are bipolar.

Glial cells make up approximately half of the brain tissue (Azevado et al., 2009), providing support and nutrients to the neurons. **Astrocytes** appear to be largely structural, separating neurons from each other and adhering to capillaries. They appear to play a role in supplying nutrients to neurons, as well as in ion and neurotransmitter regulation at the synapse. Oligodendrocytes are glial cells that make up the CNS myelin, and **Schwann cells** are glia constituting the myelin of the PNS. Although technically not neurons, glial cells are an important component of the nervous system tissue. Astrocytes provide the primary support for neurons, aid in the suspension of neurons, and transport nutrients from the capillary supply. They also provide the important **blood–brain barrier**, a membranous filter system that prohibits some toxins from passing from the cerebrovascular system to neurons (de Vries, Kuiper, de Boer, Van Berkel, & Breimer, 1997).

Yet another type of glial cell, **microglia**, performs the housekeeping process known as *phagocytosis*. Microglia scavenge necrotic tissue formed by a lesion in the nervous system. Astrocytes will assist by forming scarring around necrotic tissue, effectively isolating it from the rest of the brain tissue.

Neuroscience is now taking a very hard look at the role of astrocytes. We have long known that they had an important role in support of neurons, including nutrient delivery, but only recently has evidence emerged to indicate that glial cells are critical to the creation of long-term memory, as well as to the formation of synapses (Suzuki et al., 2011).

Functional Differences between Neurons. There are *functional* differences between neurons as well. **Interneurons** make up the largest class of neurons in the brain. The job of interneurons is to provide communication between other neurons, and interneurons do not exit the central nervous system. Another type of neuron is the **motor neuron**. Motor neurons are efferent in nature, and they are typically bipolar neurons that activate muscular or glandular response. These neurons usually have long axons that are myelinated. Motor neurons are further differentiated based on size, **conduction velocity** (how fast they can conduct an impulse), and the degree of myelination. Generally speaking, a neuron with a wider axon and thicker myelin will have more rapid conduction of neural impulses.

Neuronal fibers are classified in terms of conduction velocity as being A, B, or C class fibers. The A and B fibers are myelinated. The **A fibers** are further broken down, based on conduction velocity, into **alpha, beta, gamma**, and **delta fibers** (see Table 11-7). **Alpha motor neurons** have high conduction velocities (between 50 and 120 m/s) and innervate the majority of skeletal muscle, called **extrafusal muscle fibers**. Slower-velocity **gamma motor neurons** innervate **intrafusal muscle fibers** within the muscle spindle, the sensory

Table 11-7 Type A, B, and C sensory and motor fibers

Fiber Class	Velocity (m/s)	Motor Function	Sensory
Class A			
A-α (Alpha)	50–120	Large alpha motor neurons innervating extrafusal muscle	
A-α Ia	120		Primary muscle spindle afferents
A-α Ib	120		Golgi tendon organs; touch and pressure receptors
A β (Betta)	70	Motor axons serving extrafusal and intrafusal fibers	
A β II	70		Secondary afferents of muscle spindles; secondary afferents for touch, pressure, vibration
A γ (Gamma)	40	Gamma motor neurons serving muscle spindles	
A δ III (Delta)	15		Touch, pressure, pain, temperature sensation
Class B			
B	14	Unmyelinated, pre-ganglion autonomic fibers	
Class C			
C	2	Unmyelinated post-ganglion autonomic fibers	
C IV	2		Unmyelinated pain, temperature fibers

Source: Data from Winans, Gilman, Manter, & Gatz (2002).

apparatus responsible for maintaining muscle length. Thus, alpha motor neurons activate the prime movers of the motor act; gamma motor neurons are responsible for maintaining muscle tone and muscle readiness for the motor act.

Sensory alpha fibers are identified by a Roman numeral and a lowercase letter (**type Ia, Ib, II, III, or IV fibers**), reflecting a different classification scheme. The Ia neurons are the primary afferent fibers from the muscle spindle, whereas the Ib neurons send sensory information generated at the Golgi tendon organs, sensors that respond to the stretching of the tendon. Type II afferent fibers are secondary muscle spindle afferents of the beta class and convey information from touch and pressure receptors. The type III afferent fibers are delta class, conducting pain, pressure, touch, and coolness sensation. Type IV fibers convey pain and warmth sense. Again, some sensory neurons are essential for movement, and these include types Ia, Ib, and II. Types III and IV are important for transmitting other body senses (pain, temperature, pressure) but are not essential to movement.

✔ *To summarize:*

- The **nervous system** is a complex, hierarchical structure made up of **neurons**.
- Many **motor functions** become automated through practice.
- **Voluntary movement**, **sensory awareness**, and **cognitive function** are the domain of the **cerebral cortex**, although we are capable of sensation and response without consciousness.
- The communication links of the nervous system are **spinal nerves**, **cranial nerves**, and **tracts** of the **brain stem** and **spinal cord**.
- The nervous system may be divided functionally as **autonomic** and **somatic nervous systems** serving involuntary and voluntary functions, respectively.
- It may be divided anatomically as **central** and **peripheral nervous systems** as well.
- **Developmental divisions** separate the brain into **prosencephalon** (which is further divided into telencephalon and diencephalon), the **mesencephalon** or midbrain, and the **rhombencephalon**, which includes the metencephalon and myelencephalon.
- **Neurons** are widely varied in morphology but may be broadly categorized as **monopolor**, **bipolar**, or **multipolar**.
- Neurons communicate through **synapse** by means of **neurotransmitter** substance, and the response by the postsynaptic neuron may be **excitatory** or **inhibitory**.
- The size and type of axon is related to the conduction of neural impulse.
- **Glial cells** provide the fatty sheath for **myelinated axons**, as well as support structure for neurons, and long-term memory potentiation.

Anatomy of the Cerebrum

Anatesse Lesson ▶

The cerebrum is the mostly highly evolved and organized structure of the human body. This is the largest structure of the nervous system, weighing approximately three pounds and made up of billions of neurons and glial cells. The cerebrum is divided into grossly similar left and right hemispheres and is wrapped by three meningeal linings that protect and support the massive structure of the brain. We will discuss those meningeal linings first and then introduce you to the most important structure of your body.

The brain remains one of the most complex structures in the known universe. The cells of the brain are packed to extraordinary density: one cubic centimeter (1 cm x 1 cm x 1 cm) contains on the order of 44 million neurons (Pakkenberg & Gunderson, 2011), and for every cubic centimeter of gray matter, there are nearly 90 billion synapses. This is some very dense tissue.

Meningeal Linings

The CNS is invested with a triple-layer meningeal lining serving important protective and nutritive functions. There are three meningeal linings covering the brain. The **dura mater** is a tough bilayered lining, which is the most superficial of the meningeal linings (see Figure 11-6). The dura mater itself is made up of two layers that are tightly bound together. The outer layer is more inelastic than the inner layer, and meningeal arteries course through this layer. Whereas the layers making up the dura mater are bound together,

dura mater: L., tough mother

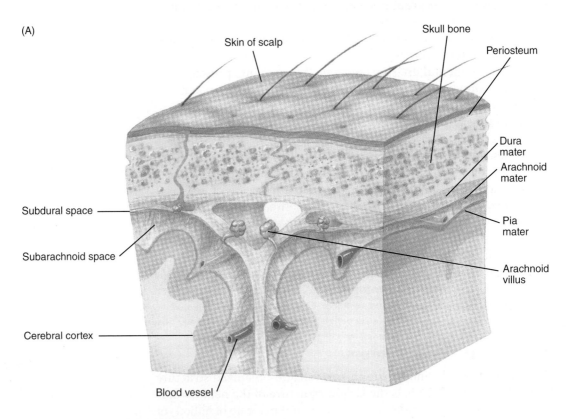

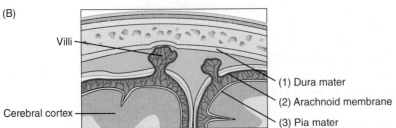

Figure 11-6. (A) Meningeal linings of the brain. (B) Schematic of meningeal linings.
© Cengage Learning®.

the potential space superficial to the dura mater is called the **epidural space**, a term that will gain meaning when discussing vascular lesions that can release blood into the areas of the brain (e.g., *epidural hematoma* is a hemorrhagic release of blood into the space between the two layers of the dura mater).

The **arachnoid mater** is a covering through which many blood vessels for the brain pass. The arachnoid lining is a lacey, spiderlike structure separating the dura mater from the innermost meningeal lining, the **pia mater**. The pia mater is a thin, membranous covering that closely follows the contour of the brain. The major arteries and veins serving the surface of the brain course within this layer.

The function of the meningeal linings is to protect the brain, holding structures in place during movement and providing support for those structures. To provide this protection, the linings must conform to the structure of the brain. As part of this support, the dura mater takes on four major infoldings, which separate the major structures of the brain, providing some isolation. The four infoldings are the falx cerebri, falx cerebelli, tentorium cerebelli, and diaphragma sella. The falx cerebri and falx cerebelli are sagittal dividers, separating left and right structures of the brain, while the tentorium cerebelli and diaphragma sella separate brain structures by means of a transversely posed membrane.

The **falx cerebri** separates the two cerebral hemispheres with a vertical sheath of dura, running from the crista galli of the ethmoid to the tentorium cerebelli. The falx cerebri completely separates the two hemispheres down to the level of the corpus callosum (to be discussed). The **falx cerebelli** performs the same function for the cerebellum, separating the left and right cerebellar hemispheres for protection and isolation (see Figure 11-7).

The **tentorium cerebelli** is a horizontal dural shelf at the base of the skull that divides the cranium into superior (cerebral) and inferior (cerebellar) regions. The **diaphragma sella** forms a boundary between the pituitary gland and the hypothalamus and optic chiasm. The dura mater encircles the cranial nerves as they exit the brain stem. Because of its placement, the tentorium cerebelli supports the cerebrum and keeps its mass from compressing the cerebellum and brain stem, as would most certainly happen if the dural lining was absent. The dural shelves can be liabilities when trauma results in **subdural hematoma**, a release of blood through hemorrhage beneath the dura that can push on the cerebrum, causing the temporal lobe to herniate under the tentorium. Subdural hematoma may also cause a life-threatening herniation of the brain stem into the foramen magnum.

There are meningeal linings of the spinal cord as well, paralleling the structure and function of the cerebral meninges. At the foramen magnum, the meningeal linings are continuous with the **spinal meningeal linings**. The spinal meninges are broadly similar to those of the brain, with some exceptions. The dura of the brain adheres to the bone, but the dura of the spinal cord does not adhere to the vertebrae. As with the brain meninges, cerebrospinal fluid flows through the

pia mater: L., pious mother; so named because of its gentle but faithful attachment to the cerebral cortex

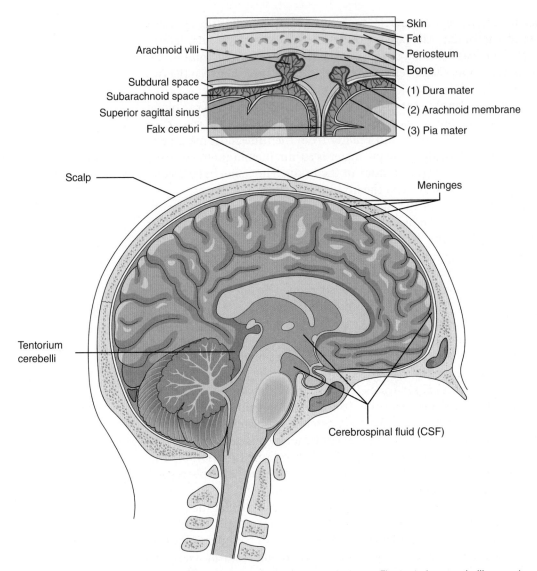

Figure 11-7. The falx cerebri separates the left and right cerebral hemispheres. The tentorium cerebelli separates the cerebellum from the cerebrum. The falx cerebelli (not shown) separates the cerebellar hemispheres.
Source: Data from Winans, Gilman, Manter, & Gatz, 2002.

Arnold–Chiari Malformation

Arnold–Chiari Malformation (or simply Chiari malformation) is a condition in which the space within the posterior skull is too small for the structures. Essentially, the cerebellum and the brain stem can herniate through the foramen magnum, causing a number of signs. Included in the problems associated with Chiari malformation is dizziness, ataxia (gait problems of cerebellar origin), hydrocephaly (increased cerebrospinal fluid pressure from the occlusion of the cerebral aqueduct), and muscular weakness.

subarachnoid space. Likewise, the pia mater closely follows the surface of the spinal cord but serves an anchoring function as well. The cord is attached to the dura by means of 22 pairs of **denticulate ligaments** arising from the pia. The dura extends laterally to encapsulate the dorsal root ganglion. At the inferior cord, the pia is continuous with the filum terminale, which is attached to the first segment of the coccyx (see Figure 11-8).

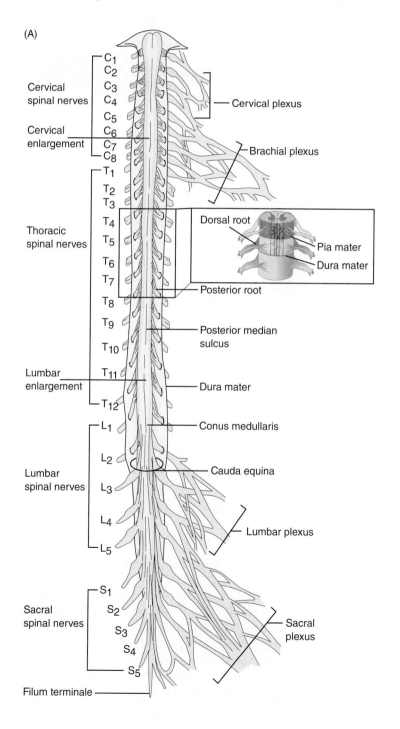

Figure 11-8. (A) Spinal cord and emerging spinal nerves. Note the inset showing the meningeal linings of the spinal cord. (continues).
© Cengage Learning®.

(B)

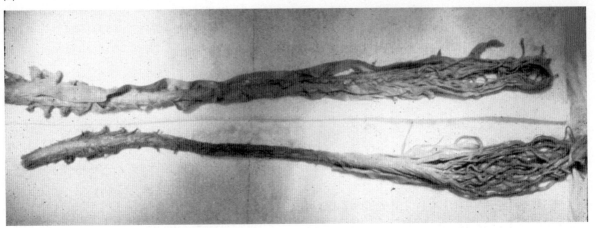

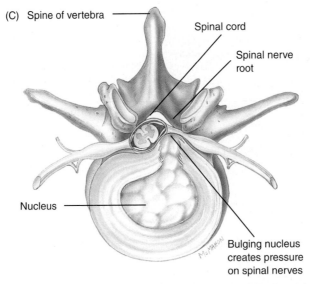

(C) Spine of vertebra

Spinal cord

Spinal nerve root

Nucleus

Bulging nucleus creates pressure on spinal nerves

Figure 11-8 continued. (B) Photograph of excised spinal cords. (C) Illustration of herniated vertebral disc and subsequent compression of spinal nerves.
© Cengage Learning®.

Together, the meningeal linings provide an excellent means of nurturing and protecting the CNS structures. The dura is a tough structure that provides a barrier between the bone of the skull and the delicate neural tissue, and to which blood vessels can be anchored as they pass to the cerebrum. The delicate pia mater completely envelopes the cerebrum, supporting the blood vessels as they serve the surface of the brain. Between the dura and pia is the arachnoid lining, through which a cushioning fluid, cerebrospinal fluid, flows (to be discussed). A similar network supports the spinal cord within the

Hematoma

Hematoma is a pooling of blood, typically arising from the breakage of a blood vessel. Subdural hematoma involves intracranial bleeding beneath the dura mater caused by the rupture of cortical arteries or veins, usually because of trauma to the head. Pressure from the pooling blood displaces the brain, shifting and compressing the brain stem, forcing the temporal lobe under the tentorium cerebelli, and compressing cerebral arteries. This critically dangerous condition may not be immediately recognized, because it may take several hours before pooling blood sufficiently compresses the brain to produce symptoms such as reduced consciousness, hemiparesis, pupillary dilation, and other symptoms associated with compressed cranial nerves. **Epidural hematoma**, hematoma occurring above the dura mater, may result in a patient being initially lucid but displaying progressively decreasing levels of consciousness, reflecting compression of the brain.

Hematomas are characterized by the location of insult. **Frontal epidural hematomas** arise from blows to the frontal bone and may result in personality changes. **Posterior fossa epidural hematomas** arise from blows to the back of the head, producing visual and coordination deficits.

vertebral column. Thus, the meninges support the brain, separate major structures, and maintain the brain in its fluid suspension. In this manner, the brain is able to overcome many otherwise dangerous shocks from external acceleration, such as those experienced during falls or blunt trauma. You may wish to read the Clinical Note on "An Ounce of Prevention" for a brief discussion of what happens when these protective measures are not enough.

The Ventricles and Cerebrospinal Fluid

The CNS is bathed in **cerebrospinal fluid (CSF)**, which provides a cushion for the delicate and dense neural tissue as well as some nutrient delivery and waste removal. Examining the system of ventricles and canals through which the CSF flows will help you as we describe the cerebral cortex and subcortical structures. You will want to refer to Figure 11-9 for this discussion.

The ventricles of the brain are spaces within the brain through which CSF flows. They are cavities that are, in reality, remnants of the embryonic neural tube. The system of ventricles consists of four cavities: the right lateral ventricle, the left lateral ventricle, the third ventricle, and the fourth ventricle. Within each ventricle is a **choroid plexus**, an aggregate of tissue that produces CSF. Whereas all ventricles produce CSF, the plexuses of the lateral ventricles produce the bulk of the fluid. The cavities are ideally suited to act as buffers for the delicate brain tissue. If you remember the discussion of the meningeal linings, you will recall that the cerebrum is supported by the tough dura and delicate pia and that CSF flows between these two linings within the arachnoid space. That CSF buffers the cerebral hemispheres and structures from sudden movements of the head

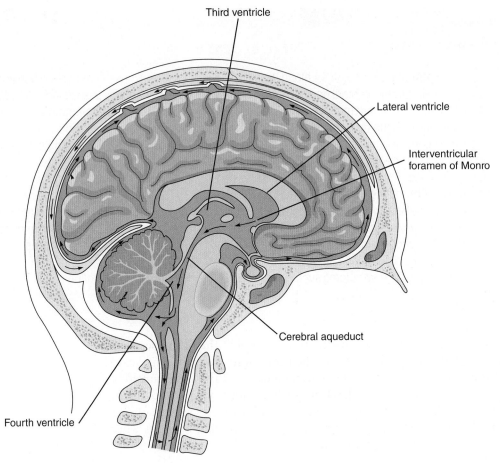

Figure 11-9. Ventricles of the brain.
© Cengage Learning®.

An Ounce of Prevention

Should you choose to work in a trauma center, a significant portion of your caseload will arise from traumatic brain injury (TBI). TBI is one of the leading causes of death in individuals under 24 years of age, with transportation-related brain injury far exceeding all other causes (falls, assaults, sport, firearms). The addition of seat and lap belts to automobiles has resulted in a reduction of death in automobile accidents arising from brain injury by nearly 50 percent. Unfortunately, use of alcohol is related to reduced seatbelt use and increased death arising from head injury during accidents. Mandatory use of helmets has reduced the frequency of brain injury in motorcycle accidents by 20 to 50 percent and up to 85 percent for bicycle riders.

Gunshot wounds to the head result in most deaths attributable to firearms, and handguns are involved in more than 60 percent of homicides. More than 40,000 people in the United States are killed by firearms annually. Whereas laws that restrict access to firearms are hotly debated as a constitutional issue, the ability to eliminate accidental firearm deaths through trigger lock systems could greatly reduce the carnage that occurs in the United States, a country in which nearly 50 percent of the households have firearms. You will want to refer to Mackay, Chapman, and Morgan (1997) for a thorough review of the causes and treatment in TBI.

(accelerations), and the addition of CSF within the brain by means of ventricles further buoys up the brain against trauma.

There are two **lateral ventricles**, which are the largest of the ventricles. These ventricles are composed of four spaces bounded superiorly by the corpus callosum that extend into each of the lobes of the cerebrum. The lateral ventricles are shaped somewhat like horseshoes opened toward the front, but with posterior horns attached. The **anterior horn** of the lateral ventricles projects into the frontal lobe to the genu of the corpus callosum. The medial wall is the septum pellucidum, and the inferior margin is the head of the caudate nucleus. The **central portion**, located within the parietal lobe, includes the region between the **interventricular foramen of Monro** and the splenium, with the superior border being the corpus callosum, the medial boundary being the septum pellucidum, and the inferior being portions of the caudate nucleus. The **posterior** or **occipital horn** extends into the occipital lobe to a tapered end, with its superior and lateral surfaces being the corpus callosum. The **inferior horn** extends into the temporal lobe, curving down behind the thalamus to terminate blindly behind the temporal pole. The hippocampus marks the lower margin of the inferior horn. The lateral ventricles communicate with the 3rd ventricle via the interventricular foramen of Monro.

The **3rd ventricle** is the unpaired medial cavity between the left and right thalami and hypothalami. The roof of the 3rd ventricle is the tela choroidea, and the ventricle extends inferiorly to the level of the optic chiasm. The prominent **interthalamic adhesion** (massa intermedia or intermediate mass) bridges the ventricle, connecting the two thalami. The CSF of the lateral ventricle passes into the 3rd ventricle by means of left and right interventricular foramina.

The **4th ventricle** is shaped roughly like a diamond, projecting upward from the central canal of the spinal cord and lower medulla. This ventricle is difficult to envision because it is the space between the brain stem and cerebellum. One must remove the cerebellum to see the 4th ventricle. The floor of the 4th ventricle is the junction of the pons and the medulla, and the cerebellum forms the roof and posterior margin. The 4th ventricle has three openings or **apertures**. The **median aperture (foramen of Magendie)** and the paired left and right **lateral apertures (foramina of Luschka)** permit CSF to flow into the subarachnoid space behind the brain stem and beneath the cerebellum (to be described).

Circulation of CSF. CSF is the clear, fluid product of the choroid plexus in each of the ventricles. It provides an excellent cushion to protect the brain against trauma and also serves a transport function, as mentioned previously. The volume of CSF in the nervous system is approximately 125 mL, which is replenished every seven hours. The fluid is under a constant pressure that changes with body position, and life-threatening conditions can develop should something occlude the pathway for CSF.

Circulation of CSF begins in each of the lateral ventricles, coursing through the interventricular foramina of Monro to the 3rd ventricle. From there, the fluid flows through the minute cerebral aqueduct to the 4th ventricle, where it drains into the subarachnoid space through the foramen of Luschka and the foramen of Magendie to the cerebellomedullary cistern beneath the cerebellum. From there it freely circulates around the brain and spinal cord. CSF then can course around the cerebellum and cerebrum to exit through the arachnoid granulation in sinuses of the dura mater and be absorbed by the venous system. Alternatively, the CSF will course downward through the foramen magnum and subarachnoid space around the spinal cord.

✔ *To summarize:*

- The **cerebral cortex** is protected from physical insults by **cerebrospinal fluid** and the **meningeal linings**, the **dura**, **pia**, and **arachnoid mater**.
- The meninges provide support for delicate neural and vascular tissue, with the dura dividing into regions that correspond to the regions of the brain supported.
- The **spinal meningeal linings** similarly protect the spinal cord from movement trauma.
- Cerebrospinal fluid originating within the **ventricles** of the brain and circulating around the spinal cord cushions these structures from trauma associated with rapid acceleration.

Cerebrum

Layers of Cerebrum. The cerebrum consists of two **cerebral hemispheres** or roughly equal halves of the brain (see Figure 11-11). The term **cortex** means "bark," referring to the bark or outer surface of a tree, and the cerebral cortex is the outer surface of the brain. The cortex is between 2 and 4 mm thick, being comprised of six cell layers.

The layers of the cerebrum consist of two basic cell types: pyramidal and nonpyramidal cells (see Figure 11-10). **Pyramidal cells** are large, pyramid-shaped cells that are involved in motor function. Pyramidal cells are oriented so that the apex of the pyramid is directed toward the surface of the cortex, with the base directed medially. A single apical dendrite projects through cortex layers toward the surface, whereas multiple basal dendrites course laterally through the layer in which the cell body resides. Axons of pyramidal cells typically project to the white matter beneath the cortex or beyond, although they will have branches within the cortex itself.

Nonpyramidal cells are small and often stellate (star shaped) and are involved in sensory function or intercommunication between brain regions. Their axons typically project only a short distance, either within a cortex layer or adjacent layers. Functionally, these nonpyramidal cells connect local regions, whereas pyramidal cells project to more distant regions, as will be discussed later.

The outermost layer of the cerebral cortex consists mostly of glial cells and axons from neurons of succeeding layers. The second and third layers consist of small and large pyramidal cells, respectively,

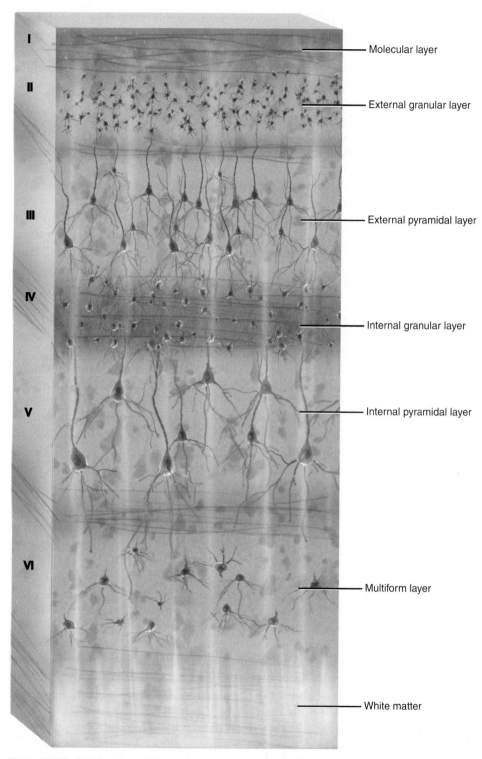

I — Molecular layer

II — External granular layer

III — External pyramidal layer

IV — Internal granular layer

V — Internal pyramidal layer

VI — Multiform layer

White matter

Figure 11-10. Cellular layers of the cerebral cortex. Layer I is termed the molecular layer, consisting of glial cells and axons from neurons. Layer II is the external granular layer, made up of small pyramidal cells. Layer III is the external pyramidal layer, made up of large pyramidal cells. Layer IV is the internal granular layer, which receives sensory input from the thalamus. Layer V is the internal pyramidal layer, and the cells from this layer project to distant motor sites. Layer VI is the multiform layer, consists of pyramidal cells that project to the basal ganglia, brain stem, and spinal cord.

© Cengage Learning®.

and are thus highly involved in motor function. The fourth layer receives sensory input from the thalamus and consists of nonpyramidal cells, whereas the fifth layer is made up of large pyramidal cells that project to motor centers beyond the cerebrum (basal ganglia, brain stem, and spinal cord). The sixth layer also consists of pyramidal cells, although these project to the thalamus.

The layers have varying densities within the cerebrum, corresponding to the dominant function for a specific region. For instance, the pyramidal layers will be thickest in the areas of the cortex responsible for motor function, whereas the granular layers will be most richly represented in the areas of the brain that process predominantly sensory input. The region of primary motor output (the motor strip, to be discussed) has extremely rich representation of the fifth layer, with a very thin fourth layer, while the primary sensory areas have a rich layer fourth with a few cells in the pyramidal layers. Areas involved in the association of sensory and motor functions will have representation of both sensory and motor layers.

Much of our early knowledge concerning the cell structure of the cortical layers arose from the work of Korbinian Brodmann in the early part of the twentieth century (Kandel, 2012). His microscopic examination of the cerebral cortex revealed the dominant cell types of the cortical layers, and his keen analysis showed that the localized areas of the brain were dominated by specific cell types, as discussed. From his work came what has become known as the "Brodmann map" of the cerebrum (see Figure 11-12), a tool that remains a mainstay for navigating the regions of the cerebrum. Brodmann's observations proved to be quite important, and his notation has served many decades of neuroscience study. You will want to refer to this figure as we discuss landmarks of the superficial cortex.

Landmarks of Cerebrum. The **cerebral longitudinal fissure** (also known as the **superior longitudinal fissure** and the **interhemispheric fissure**) separates the left and right cerebral hemispheres, as can be seen in Figure 11-11 and the photograph in Figure 11-13. You will remember from our discussion of the meningeal linings that the falx cerebri runs between the two hemispheres through this space. The cerebral longitudinal fissure completely separates the hemispheres down to the level of the corpus callosum, a major group of fibers providing communication between the two hemispheres, as will be discussed. Within the cerebral longitudinal fissure reside the anterior cerebral artery and its collaterals (to be discussed).

As you can also see in the photograph of Figure 11-13, the surface of the brain is quite convoluted. Early in development, the cerebral cortex has few of these furrows and bulges, but as the brain growth outstrips the skull growth, the cerebral cortex doubles in on itself. The result of this is greatly increased surface area, translating into more "neural horsepower." You can think of the surface as a topographical map with mountains and valleys. The mountains (**convolutions**) in

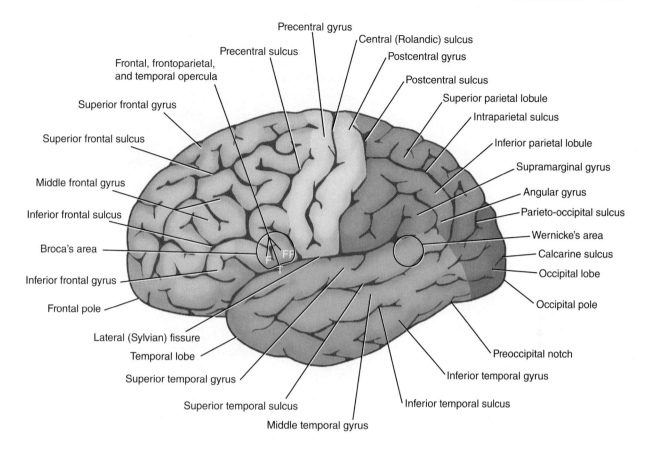

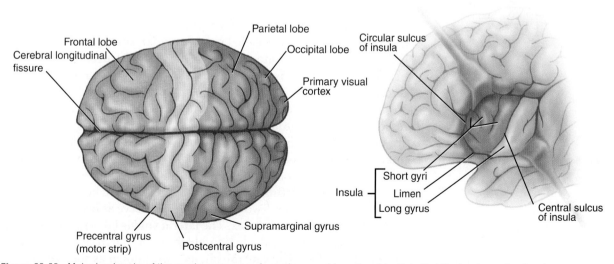

Figure 11-11. Major landmarks of the cerebrum as seen from above and from the side. Note that the insular cortex (insula, bottom left) is typically hidden from view.
© Cengage Learning®.

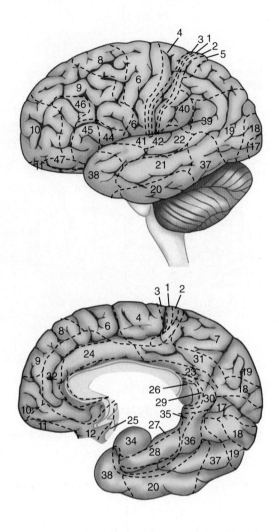

Figure 11-12. Brodmann map of lateral and medial cerebrum.
© Cengage Learning®.

insular: L., island

this case are called **gyri** (singular, **gyrus**) and the infolding valleys that separate the gyri are called **sulci** (singular, **sulcus**). If the groove is deeper and more pronounced, it is termed a **fissure**. These sulci, fissures, and gyri provide the major landmarks for navigating the cerebral cortex.

We divide the cerebral cortex into five lobes. Four of them are reasonably easy to see and are named after the bones with which they are associated (see Figures 11-13 and 11-14), but one of these lobes (**insular**) requires some thought and imagination. The five lobes are the frontal, parietal, occipital, temporal, and insular lobes.

Before differentiating the lobes of the brain, it will help to identify some major landmarks. Two prominent sulci serve as benchmarks in our study of the cerebral cortex. The **lateral sulcus** (also known as the **Sylvian fissure**) divides the temporal lobe from the frontal and anterior parietal lobes. The **central sulcus** (also known as the **Rolandic sulcus** or **Rolandic fissure**) separates the frontal and parietal lobes entirely. The central sulcus is the very prominent vertical groove running from the cerebral longitudinal fissure to the lateral sulcus,

(A)

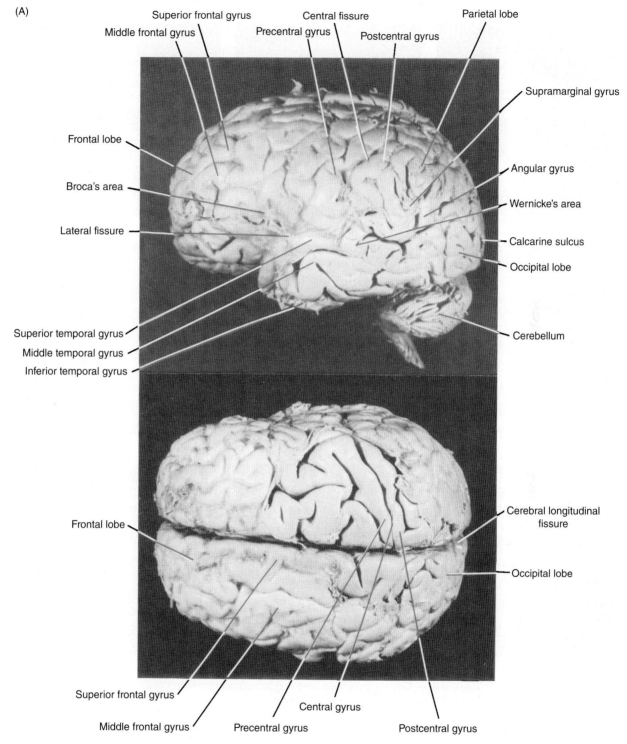

Superior frontal gyrus

Middle frontal gyrus

Central fissure

Precentral gyrus

Postcentral gyrus

Parietal lobe

Supramarginal gyrus

Frontal lobe

Broca's area

Lateral fissure

Angular gyrus

Wernicke's area

Calcarine sulcus

Occipital lobe

Superior temporal gyrus

Middle temporal gyrus

Inferior temporal gyrus

Cerebellum

Frontal lobe

Cerebral longitudinal fissure

Occipital lobe

Superior frontal gyrus

Middle frontal gyrus

Precentral gyrus

Central gyrus

Postcentral gyrus

Figure 11-13. (A) Lateral (upper) and superior (lower) views of cerebral cortex. Note that the pia mater may be seen in portions of both photographs. (continues).

© Cengage Learning®.

(B)

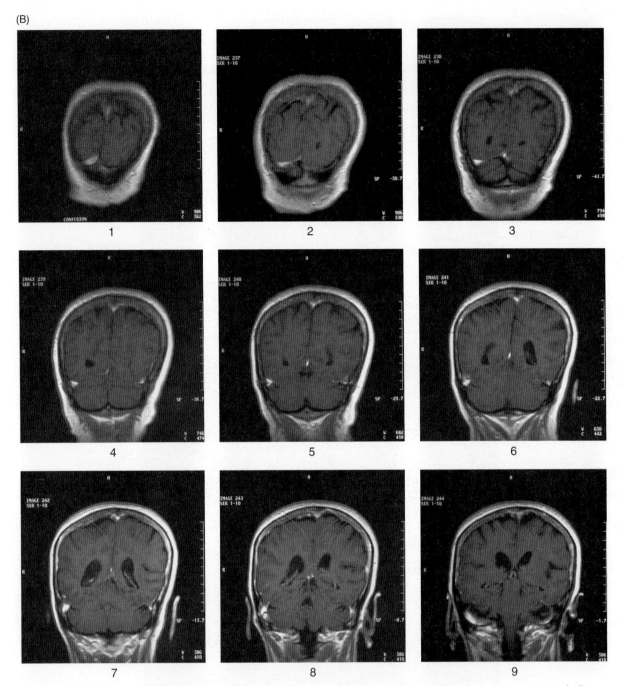

Figure 11-13 continued. (B) Magnetic resonance image of head, revealing brain structures. Note that a tumor emerges in the 12th slice, appearing lighter (denser) than the surrounding tissue. (continues).

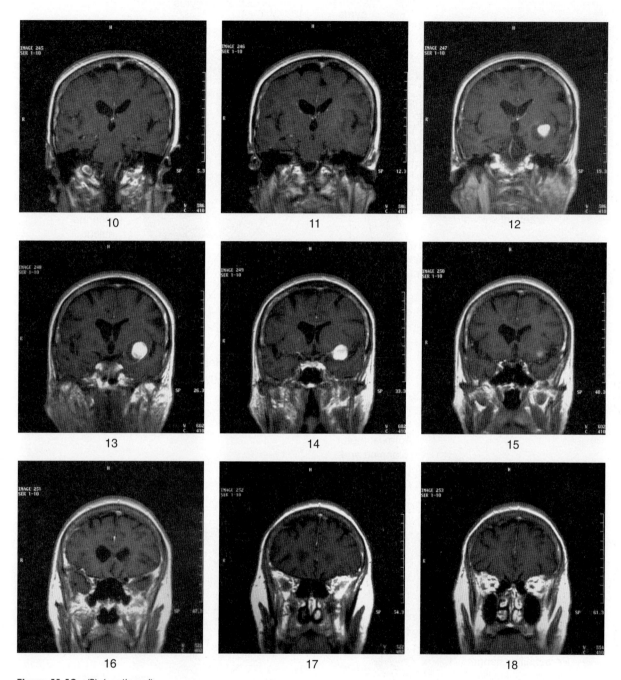

Figure 11-13. (B) (continued).
© Cengage Learning®.

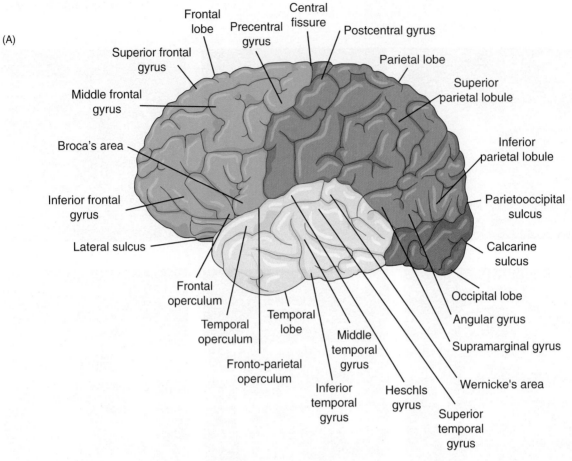

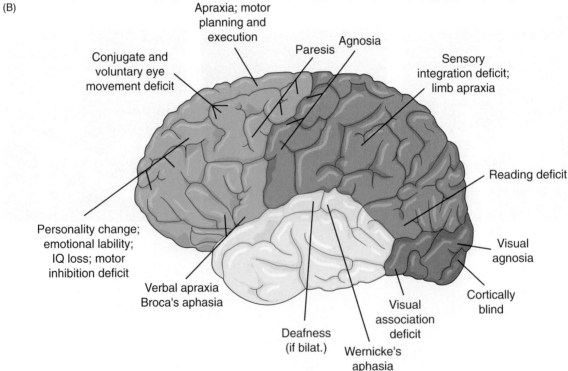

Figure 11-14. (A) Landmarks of the left cerebral hemisphere. (B) Effects of lesion at different cerebral locations.

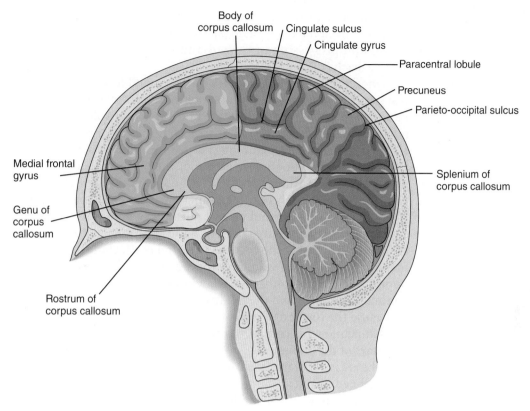

Figure 11-15. Medial surface of the cerebral cortex.
© Cengage Learning®.

terminating in the inferior parietal lobe. As you can see in the sagittal section of Figure 11-15, this sulcus does not extend far down the medial surface.

Frontal Lobe. The frontal lobe is the largest of the lobes, making up one-third of the cortex (see Figure 11-14). This lobe predominates in planning, initiation, and inhibition of voluntary motion, as well as cognitive function, as we shall see in Chapter 12. The frontal lobe is the anterior-most portion of the cortex and is bounded posteriorly by the central sulcus. The inferior boundary is the lateral sulcus, and the medial boundary is the longitudinal fissure.

Three gyri run parallel to the longitudinal fissure in the frontal lobe. The **superior frontal gyrus** borders the longitudinal fissure and is separated from the **middle frontal gyrus** by the superior frontal sulcus. The **inferior frontal gyrus** includes an extremely important region known as the **pars opercularis** or simply the **frontal operculum** (see Figure 11-14). This area overlies one of the "hidden lobes," the insular cortex. The frontal operculum is more commonly referred to as **Broca's area**, an extremely important region for speech motor planning within the dominant hemisphere, as will be discussed in Chapter 12. Another important region of the inferior frontal gyrus is the **pars orbitale** or **orbital region**, the region of the inferior frontal gyrus overlying the eyes. The pars orbitale and anterior regions of the upper frontal lobe are associated with memory, emotion, motor inhibition, processing of reward and punishment, and intellect (Kringelbach & Rolls, 2004).

Another important landmark of the frontal lobe is the **precentral gyrus** or **motor strip**. It is anterior to the central sulcus (thus the name "*pre*-central") and is the site of initiation of voluntary motor movement. Anterior to the motor strip is the premotor region, generally involved in motor planning (but see the note "When Sensation Goes Bad" for yet another function of the prefrontal cortex). The premotor cortex includes portions of the superior, middle, and inferior frontal lobes but is indicated functionally as area 6 on the Brodmann map. The upper and medial portions of area 6 are called the **supplementary motor area (SMA)**. Axons from the motor strip and the SMAs give rise to the corticospinal and corticobulbar tracts, the major motor tracts of voluntary movement on the side of the body opposite to the area of the cortex giving the command. That is, a command arising from the left hemisphere to move the little finger will cause the finger of the right hand to twitch. We will discuss the mechanism for this **contralateral innervation** when we discuss the pathways of the brain.

The areas of the motor strip serving regions of the body have been well mapped, thanks in large part to the pioneering direct brain stimulation work of Penfield and Roberts (1959) and Woolsey (Schaltenbrand & Woolsey, 1964). As you can see from Figure 11-16, different regions of the motor strip serve different regions of the body. The face, head, and laryngeal regions are on the far lateral edge, whereas the leg, thigh, and thorax are represented on the more medial surface of the superior cortex. If you compare this with the location of Broca's area on the side view of the hemisphere in Figure 11-14, you will see that these two regions are in close proximity. That is to say, you should begin to recognize that the area for motor function for the speech mechanisms (larynx, lips, facial muscles, and muscles of mastication) is immediately adjacent to Broca's area, the region responsible for planning the motor act for speech. We will say more about the organization of this region in Chapter 12.

Parietal Lobe. Look at the parietal lobe in Figure 11-14. The parietal lobe is the primary reception site for somatic (body) sense. That is, all senses that reach consciousness terminate within the parietal lobe. The anterior boundary of the parietal lobe is the central sulcus, and the inferior boundary is the lateral sulcus. To define the posterior boundary, one must identify the **parieto-occipital sulcus** and draw an imaginary line to the **preoccipital notch**.

The **postcentral gyrus** is the sensory counterpart to the motor strip. The motor strip is the site of motor output, and the postcentral gyrus is the primary site of sensory input. This area receives somatic sensation from various body regions. Remember that motor function is spatially arrayed along the motor strip: The same is true for

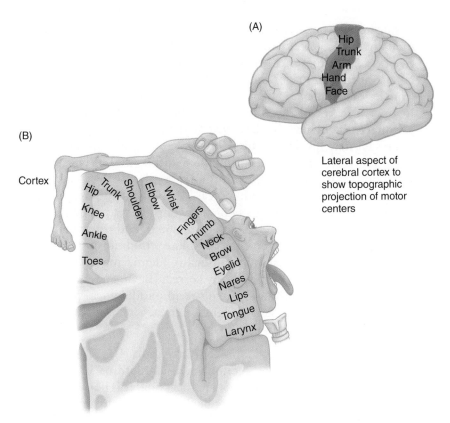

Figure 11-16. (A) Right hemisphere, displaying regions of motor strip governing activation of specific muscle groups. (B) Homunculus revealing areas of representation on the motor strip. Note that this represents a frontal section through the cerebral cortex. Size of structure drawn represents the degree of neural representation of the given structure (i.e., neural density).

© Cengage Learning®.

the postcentral gyrus. The distribution of sensory function by body region is quite close to that of the motor strip. Virtually all somesthetic sensation that reaches consciousness will terminate in this region, although the sensation from the left part of the body is projected to the right hemisphere.

Posterior to the postcentral gyrus is the **postcentral sulcus**, providing the anterior margin for the **superior** and **inferior parietal lobules**, separated by the **intraparietal sulcus**. The inferior parietal lobule is an important cortical **association area**, integrating information related to vision (from the occipital lobe), audition (from the temporal lobe), and somatic sense (from the parietal lobe). This inferior lobule is also quite important. It is divided into the **supramarginal** and **angular gyri**. The angular gyrus is particularly important in (but not solely responsible for) the comprehension of written material.

The angular gyrus has been shown to be involved in a number of critically important associative functions. It lies to the posterior of Wernicke's area (a critical language center, as we will discuss shortly) and receives input from visual and auditory centers, as well as somatosensory information from the parietal lobe, and is involved in mathematical calculation, as well as being a contributor to cognitive function. Agraphia (difficulty writing language), alexia (difficulty reading language), and semantic processing deficits can arise from lesions to the left angular gyrus, but this area is also implicated in a person's knowledge of who is completing an action. That is to say, there is evidence that knowing that I am involved in a specific motor act may involve circuitry of the right angular gyrus (Farrer, Frey, Van Horn, Tunik, Turk, Inati, & Grafton, 2007). The angular gyrus apparently collaborates with the supramarginal gyrus in reading and rhyming activity, with increased activity in children, perhaps reflecting development of the phonology during that period (Church, Coalson, Lugar, Petersen, & Schlaggar, 2008), and is important for comprehension of written material. The *supramarginal gyrus* is involved spatiomotor tasks in nonhumans (identifying if physical orientation of an object is functionally correct (Bach, Peelen, & Tipper, 2010), but appears intimately involved in phonological processing developmentally in humans (Sugiura, Ojima, Matsuba-Kurita, Dan, Tsuzuki, Katura, & Hagiwara, 2011).

Temporal Lobe. Find the temporal lobe on Figure 11-14. The temporal lobe is the site of auditory reception and is extraordinarily important for auditory and receptive language processing. It is bordered by the lateral sulcus medially, projecting back to the parietal and occipital lobes posteriorly.

The **superior temporal gyrus** runs posteriorly to the angular gyrus of the parietal lobe and is separated from the **middle temporal gyrus** by the **superior temporal sulcus**. The superior temporal gyrus is of profound importance in both speech-language pathology and audiology. If you look at the upper surface of the superior temporal lobe (area 41), you will see **Heschl's gyrus**, the location of the brain to which all auditory information is projected. The region actually includes a portion of the medial surface of the temporal lobe, as described in detail in Chapters 7 and 8. Lateral to Heschl's gyrus is area 42, a higher-order processing region for auditory stimulation. The posterior portion of the superior temporal gyrus is the

Bigger Is Better?

Size is not everything. We like to think that human brains are large, and they are in relation to, for instance, a chimpanzee. The human brain is about 1,600 grams, whereas that of a chimp is about 500 grams. Unfortunately, a bottlenose dolphin also has a 1,600-gram brain, and the sperm whale has an 8,000-gram brain. So, does size matter? Clearly, the size of the brain is directly related to the body size. Human brains are, remarkably, three times larger than our body size would predict, which does place us in a class of our own. Unfortunately, knowledge does not always imply wisdom, and the human brain seems capable of calculating ways to get in trouble that far outweigh the three-to-one advantage we have.

functionally defined region known as **Wernicke's area**. Damage to this area of the dominant hemisphere results in disturbances in spoken language decoding, often profound. The middle temporal gyrus and inferior temporal gyrus are regions of higher-level processing. The inferior temporal gyrus lies within the middle fossa of the skull.

Occipital Lobe. Identify the occipital lobe on Figure 11-14. The occipital lobe is the posterior limit of the brain. The occipital lobe is the region responsible for receiving visual stimulation, as well as some of the higher-level visual processing. The occipital lobe rests on the tentorium cerebelli discussed previously, with its anterior margin being the parieto-occipital sulcus. The regions surrounding the **calcarine sulcus** are the primary reception areas for visual information. The calcarine sulcus and parieto-occipital sulcus mark the boundaries of the wedge-shaped **cuneus**. Lateral to the calcarine sulcus is the **lingual gyrus**.

cuneus: L., wedge

Insula. Find the insular cortex on Figure 11-11. The insular lobe (also known as the insular cortex or the **island of Reil**, is located deep to a region of the cerebrum known as the operculum. The operculum consists of regions of the temporal lobe (medial areas 38, 41, 42), parietal lobe (inferior areas 1, 2, 3, and 40), and frontal lobes (areas 44, 45, and inferior 6) along the lateral sulcus. These regions, which overlie the insular cortex, are known as the **temporal operculum**, **fronto-parietal operculum**, and **frontal operculum**.

To see the insular cortex, you would have to pull the temporal lobe laterally and lift up the frontal and parietal opercula. Upon doing that, you would see the **circular sulcus** that surrounds the insula, deep in the lateral sulcus. The **central sulcus of the insula** divides the insula into anterior short gyri and a single posterior long gyrus. The insula is a fascinating structure that appears to be intimately involved in perception of taste (gustation: Kobayashi, 2006), processing emotion (Dalgleish, 2004), our perception of self (Craig, 2002), and even our development of compassion and empathy (Lutz, Greischar, Perlman, & Davidson, 2009). Damage to the insula has even been shown to completely disrupt craving cigarettes (Naqvi, Rudrauf, Damasio, & Bechara, 2007).

Limbic System. The limbic system is not an anatomically distinct region, but one arising from functional relationships associated with motivation, sex drive, emotional behavior, and affect. The limbic system includes the uncus (formed by the amygdala), parahippocampal gyrus, cingulate gyrus, and olfactory bulb and tract, as well as the hippocampal formation, orbitofrontal cortex, and the **dentate** gyrus, structures we shall discuss again (see Figure 11-17).

dentate: L., referring to tooth; notched; toothlike

✔ *To summarize:*

- The **cerebrum** is divided into two grossly similar, mirror-image **hemispheres** that are connected by means of the massive **corpus callosum**.
- The **gyri** and **sulci** of the hemispheres provide important landmarks for lobes and other regions of the cerebrum.

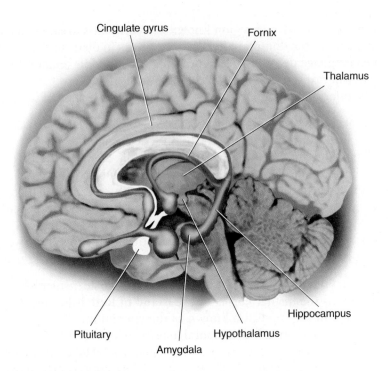

Figure 11-17. Schematic of components of the limbic system.
Source: (Modified from Carpenter, 1991.)

- The **temporal lobe** is the site of **auditory reception** and **Wernicke's area**.
- The temporal lobe is the prominent lateral lobe separated from the parietal and frontal lobes by the **lateral fissure**.
- The anterior-most region is the **frontal lobe**, the site of most voluntary **motor activation** and the important speech region known as **Broca's area**.
- Adjacent to the frontal lobe is the **parietal lobe**, the region of **somatic sensory reception**.
- The **occipital lobe** is the most posterior of the regions, the site of **visual input** to the cerebrum.
- The **insular lobe** is revealed by deflecting the temporal lobe and lies deep in the **lateral sulcus**.
- The **operculum** overlies the insula, and the functionally defined **limbic lobe** includes the **cingulate gyrus**, **uncus**, **parahippocampal gyrus**, and other deep structures.

Medial Surface of Cerebral Cortex

Viewing a sagittal section of the brain reveals a number of extremely important landmarks. As you can see from Figure 11-15, the **corpus callosum** is the large, dominating structure immediately inferior to the cerebral gray matter. It is the "information superhighway" of the brain. It provides communication concerning sensation and memory among the diverse regions of the two hemispheres by means of myelinated fibers. That is to say, any information arising in the left postcentral gyrus will be potentially shared by the right postcentral gyrus, so that each hemisphere "knows" what the other one knows.

corpus callosum: L., large (or hard) body

The corpus callosum makes up the roof of the lateral ventricles and the floor of the cerebral longitudinal fissure. The corpus callosum is divided into four major regions: rostrum, genu, body, and splenium. Fibers that course from one hemisphere to the other through the **genu** serve the anterior frontal lobes. Fibers of the posterior frontal lobes and parietal lobes course through the **body** (or **trunk**) of the corpus callosum. Information from the temporal and occipital lobes passes from one hemisphere to the other by means of the **splenium**.

Now look at the paracentral lobule in Figure 11-15. The **paracentral lobule** is in the superior aspect of the medial cortex. This landmark is the reflected union of the precentral and postcentral gyri of the frontal and parietal lobes, respectively. Posterior to the paracentral lobule is the **precuneus**, which is separated from the cuneus by the parieto-occipital sulcus. The **cingulate gyrus**, a major structure of the limbic system, dominates the region immediately superior to the corpus callosum.

genu: L., knee

Inferior Surface of Cerebral Cortex

Figure 11-18 shows the inferior cerebral cortex. The anterior portion is the **orbital surface** of the frontal lobe, so called because it is above the eyes and optic pathways. You can also see the inferior surface of the temporal lobe. In the posterior aspect is the inferior surface of the occipital lobe. Let us look at some of the landmarks of that region.

The **olfactory sulcus** is superior to the olfactory tract and bulb. As we will discuss, the olfactory mechanisms relay information concerning smell from the sensors within the nasal mucosa to the brain. The **parahippocampal gyrus** is the medial-most portion of the cerebral cortex. This gyrus and the prominence known as the **uncus** combine with the lateral olfactory stria to make up the primary olfactory cortex, also known as the **pyriform lobe**. Within the parahippocampal gyrus is the important **hippocampus**, a structure deeply involved in memory.

From this view, you can also see the undersurface of the inferior temporal gyrus and the calcarine sulcus of the occipital lobe. Visible also is the splenium of the corpus callosum, as well as the cerebral aqueduct (discussed with ventricles). Note also the pituitary gland or **hypophysis**, an important structure for autonomic regulation mediated by the hypothalamus.

Myelinated Fibers

The gray matter of the cortex is predominantly made up of neuron bodies, whereas the white matter of the brain represents myelinated axon fibers. These fibers make up the communication link between the neurons, and without them there would be no neural function. In diseases that cause **demyelination** of the fibers, dysfunction of the areas served is virtually guaranteed.

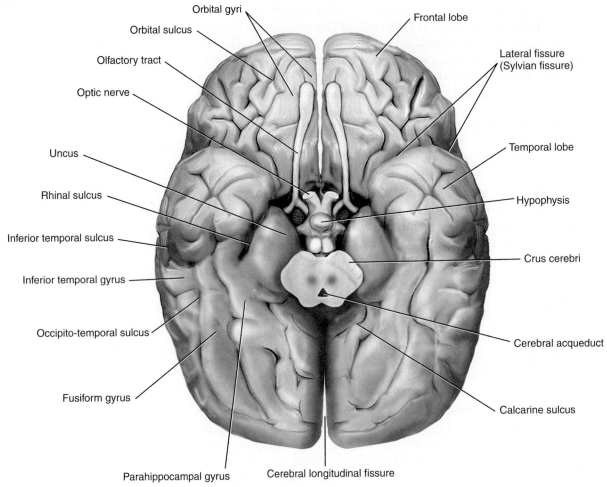

Figure 11-18. Inferior surface of the cerebral cortex.
© Cengage Learning®.

There are three basic types of fibers: projection fibers, association fibers, and commissural fibers.

Projection Fibers. The tracts running to and from the cortex to the brain stem and the spinal cord are made up of **projection fibers**. Projection fibers connect the cortex with distant locations. The **corona radiata** is a mass of projection fibers running from and to the cortex (see Figure 11-19). It condenses as it courses down, forming an "L" shape as it reaches a location known as the **internal capsule**. The **anterior limb** of the internal capsule separates the caudate nucleus and the putamen of the basal ganglia and serves the frontal lobe. The **posterior limb** includes the **optic radiation**, which is a group of fibers projecting to the calcarine sulcus for vision. Nearly all the *afferent* fibers within the corona radiata arise from the thalamus, the major sensory relay of the brain. The point of juncture of the anterior and posterior limbs is called the **genu**. *Efferent* fibers from the cortex make up the motor tracts. We will discuss these tracts shortly.

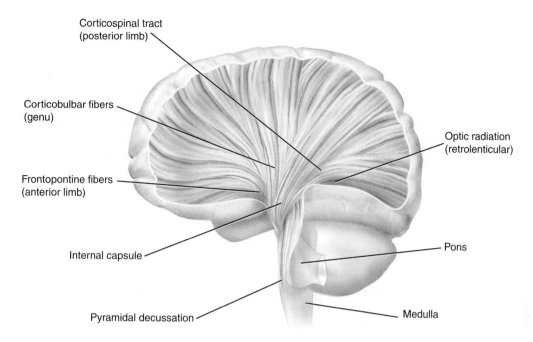

Corticospinal tract
(posterior limb)

Corticobulbar fibers
(genu)

Optic radiation
(retrolenticular)

Frontopontine fibers
(anterior limb)

Internal capsule

Pons

Pyramidal decussation

Medulla

Figure 11-19. Corona radiata as it passes through the internal capsule. The anterior limb of the internal capsule includes fibers from the frontal lobe, and the genu of the internal capsule includes fibers of the corticobulbar tract. The corticospinal tract passes through the posterior limb of the internal capsule.
© Cengage Learning®.

Association Fibers. The second group of fibers consists of **association fibers**. Association fibers provide communication between regions of the same hemisphere. For example, they may connect the superior temporal gyrus with the middle temporal gyrus within the left hemisphere.

There are both long and short association fibers. **Short association fibers** connect neurons of one gyrus to the next, traversing the sulcus. The **long association fibers** interconnect the lobes of the brain within the same hemisphere. The **uncinate fasciculus** connects the orbital portion, inferior, and middle frontal gyri with the anterior temporal lobe. The extremely important **arcuate fasciculus** permits the superior and middle frontal gyri to communicate with the temporal, parietal, and occipital lobes. The arcuate fasciculus has long been held to be the dominant pathway between Broca's and Wernicke's areas. We now know that the inferior parietal lobule connects the two portions of the arcuate fasciculus, apparently within the supramarginal gyrus (Ffytch, 2005). A lesion of the arcuate fasciculus can result in **conduction aphasia**, in which expressive language and receptive language remain essentially intact but the individual remains unable to repeat information presented auditorily. The **cingulum**, the white matter of the cingulate gyrus, connects the frontal and parietal lobes with the parahippocampal gyrus and temporal lobe. At birth only a small number of axons are myelinated. Myelination begins in earnest

Multiple Sclerosis

There are a number of demyelinating diseases, conditions that cause degeneration of the brain myelin. Multiple sclerosis (MS) is a disease in which an individual's immune system attacks the myelin of the brain. As the name indicates, multiple areas of the brain myelin are affected, causing diffuse symptoms. The myelin is damaged or destroyed, and replaced with a scarlike

plaque (sclerotic plaque), which greatly inhibits neural conduction. Early signs are often vestibular or balance dysfunction and optic neuritis (inflammation of the optic nerve). A subtype of MS is relapsing-remitting, in which an individual undergoes periods of disease activity followed by periods of remission in which signs and symptoms are greatly reduced.

after birth, and is completed around 30 years of age. It correlates well with the development of cognitive and motor functions in various parts of the brain, beginning in the posterior brain and working forward as you grow. Thus, the occipital and parietal lobes will have completed myelin before the frontal lobes, which are the final lobes to become myelinated. It has been hypothesized that this slow myelination process is responsible for the poor judgment shown by teenagers at times.

Commissural Fibers. The third group of fibers is the **commissural fibers**. The corpus callosum is the major group of commissural fibers. Commissural fibers run from one location on a hemisphere to the corresponding location on the other hemisphere, such as from the supramarginal gyrus of the left parietal lobe to that of the right parietal lobe. We have already discussed one of the groups of commissural fibers, the corpus callosum. Another important group of fibers makes up the **anterior commissure**. The anterior commissure crosses between hemispheres to connect the right and left olfactory areas as well as portions of the inferior and middle temporal gyri.

Anatomy of the Subcortex

Basal Ganglia. The basal ganglia (or basal nuclei) are a group of cell bodies intimately related to the control of background movement and initiation of movement patterns. The ganglia included under the broader term of basal ganglia include the **caudate nucleus** (including head, body, and tail), the **putamen**, and the **globus pallidus**. Some consider the **amygdaloid body** (or **amygdala**) to be part of the basal ganglia, but it is generally included within the limbic system. Functionally, the **subthalamic nuclei** and **substantia nigra** may be included as well, because of their central role in basal ganglia activity.

Visualizing the basal ganglia is a challenge. The relationship of the parts may be seen in Figure 11-20. The **head of the caudate nucleus** is anteriorly placed, the body courses up and back, and

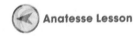 **Anatesse Lesson**

putamen: L., shell

globus pallidus: L., white (or pale) globe

amygdaloid body: L., amygdalinus, almond

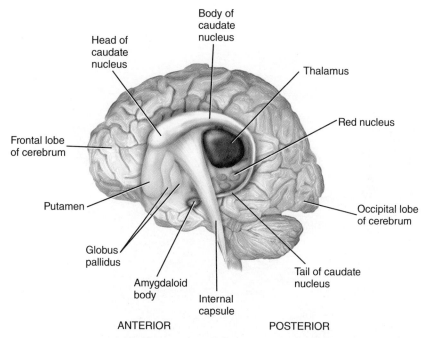

Figure 11-20. The basal ganglia consist of the caudate nucleus, amygdala, globus pallidus, and putamen. The basal ganglia are shown in relation to the other subcortical structures, including the diencephalic thalamus and hypothalamus, as well as the red nucleus and substantia nigra.

© Cengage Learning®.

the **tail** curves down. The amygdaloid body is adjacent to the tail but does not fuse with it. The globus pallidus and putamen attach to and reflect back on the caudate body.

The combination of globus pallidus and putamen is referred to as the **lentiform** or **lenticular nucleus** because their combined nuclei are lens shaped. The putamen and caudate nucleus together are referred to as the **striatum**. The **corpus striatum** includes the striatum (putamen and caudate) and globus pallidus. (The corona radiata forming the internal capsule perforates the caudate and putamen, giving a striped appearance—hence the term "striated body.")

Within the brain, the **lentiform nucleus** (globus pallidus and putamen) is lateral to the internal capsule, and the caudate is medial to the internal capsule. The head of the caudate protrudes into the anterior horn of the lateral ventricle. The body makes up a portion of the floor of the lateral ventricle and is lateral to the superior thalamus. The amygdaloid body lies in the roof of the inferior horn of the lateral ventricle. Lesions to the basal ganglia result in extrapyramidal dysfunction, including hyperkinetic and hypokinetic dysarthrias.

Hippocampal Formation. The hippocampal formation is strongly implicated in memory function and is part of the rhinencephalon. It communicates with the hypothalamus, which is related to visceral function and emotion, and to portions of the temporal lobe associated

corpus striatum: L., striped body

lentiform nucleus: L., lentis, lens , combined basal ganglia nuclei consisting of globus pallidus and putamen

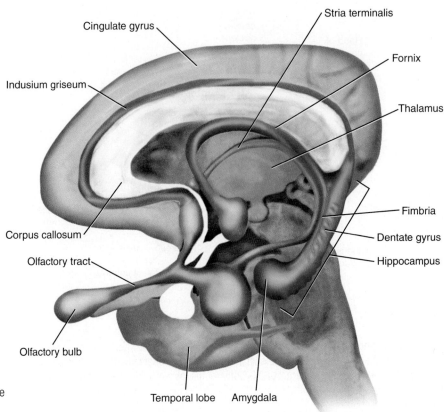

Figure 11-21. Orientation of the hippocampal formation.
© Cengage Learning®.

with memory function. As you can see from Figure 11-21, the hippocampal formation includes the parahippocampal gyrus and makes up a portion of the floor of the inferior horn of the lateral ventricle. Just lateral to the parahippocampal gyrus is the fusiform gyrus, also known as the fusiform face area. It appears to be specialized to recognize faces of individuals (Tsao, Feriwald, Tootell & Livingstone, 2006).

Figure 11-22 shows a cross section through the hippocampus. The hippocampal formation is a functionally related group of nuclei, including the hippocampus, dentate gyrus, entorhinal cortex, subiculum, presubiculum, and parasubiculum. There are three major subdivisions of the hippocampus: CA3, CA2, and CA1. The entorhinal cortex is, for the most part, the input gateway for the hippocampus, receiving input from subcortical (olfactory) and cortical (cingulate gyrus, insula, orbitofrontal cortex, and superior temporal gyrus) regions. Axons from the entorhinal cortex project to the dentate gyrus via the perforant pathway. Unlike most cortical areas, this projection is a one-way street. Most cortical regions have reciprocal connections: If the precentral gyrus projects to the postcentral gyrus, the postcentral gyrus will also project to the same area of the precentral gyrus. This unidirectional input is a unique feature of the hippocampal formation. In the same way, mossy fibers from the dentate nucleus project in one-way fashion to the pyramidal cells in CA3 of the hippocampus. The pyramidal cells then project to CA1, which

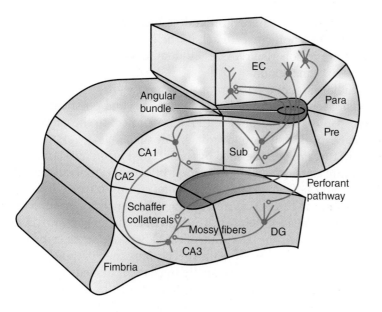

Figure 11-22. Cross section through the hippocampus. Note the following: CA1, (Cornu Ammonis) area 1; CA2, (Cornu Ammonis) area 2; CA3, (Cornu Ammonis) area 3; Para, Parasubiculum; Pre, Presubiculum; Sub, Subiculum; EC, Entorhinal cortex; and DG, Dentate gyrus.

© Cengage Learning®.

projects to the subiculum. It is not until the level of CA1 that there is reciprocal projection back to the entorhinal cortex. The hippocampus is made up of six cell layers, much as the cerebral cortex.

The **pes hippocampus** ("foot of the hippocampus") is the anterior projection of the hippocampus, and the **fimbria** of hippocampus is a medial layer of white fibers that are continuous with the fornix. The **fornix** is a near-circle of myelinated fibers terminating in the **mammillary body** and provides most of the communication between the hippocampus and the hypothalamus. It contains commissural fibers that permit communication with the opposite hippocampus.

The **dentate gyrus** (dentate fascia) lies between the fimbria of the hippocampus and the parahippocampal gyrus and continues as the indusium griseum. The **indusium griseum** is a layer of cell bodies that overlies the corpus callosum and becomes continuous with the cingulate gyrus.

Diencephalic Structures. The diencephalon is composed of the thalamus, epithalamus, hypothalamus, and subthalamus. This is a small and compact region.

Thalamus. The paired thalami are the largest structures of the diencephalon and are the final, common relay for sensory information directed toward the cerebral cortex. All sensation, with the exception of olfaction, passes through the thalamus, making it an exceedingly important region of the brain. Of those sensations, only pain (and possibly temperature) sense is consciously perceived at the thalamus, but pain cannot be localized without cortical function.

The **reticular activating system** that arises from the intralaminal nuclei of the thalamus is the functional system responsible for arousing the cortex and perhaps for focusing cortical regions to heightened awareness. In addition, the thalamus is the primary bridge for

pes hippocampus: L., foot of hippocampus

fimbria: L., fringe

fornix: L., arch

mammillary body: L., mamillia, nipple

information from the cerebellum and globus pallidus to the motor portion of the cerebral cortex. Each of the nuclei that communicate with a cortical region also receives efferent, corticothalamic projections from the same region.

The thalami form a portion of the lateral walls of the 3rd ventricle and are separated from the globus pallidus and putamen by the internal capsule. Fibers from the thalamus project to the cortex via the internal capsule and corona radiata. The thalamus is composed of 26 nuclei in three regions defined by the internal medullary lamina.

Thalamic nuclei may be organized into functional categories (see Figure 11-23). Specific thalamic nuclei communicate with specific regions of the cerebral cortex. **Association nuclei** communicate with association areas of the cortex. **Subcortical nuclei** have no direct communication with the cerebral cortex. There are some critically important nuclei for those of us in speech-language pathology and audiology. The **pulvinar** is a critically important nucleus related to language function, and damage to this nucleus can result in aphasia, an acquired language deficit. The **lateral geniculate body** is a visual relay, whereas **the medial geniculate body** is the last auditory relay of the auditory pathway before reaching the cerebral cortex.

Epithalamus. The most prominent structures of the epithalamus include the pineal body, which is a gland involved in the development of gonads, the **habenular nuclei** and habenular commissure, the

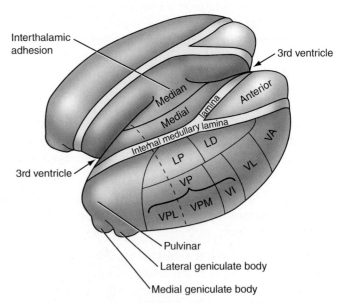

Figure 11-23. Major nuclei of the thalamus. Critical nuclei for speech-language pathology and audiology include the medial geniculate body (input to the core of the auditory cortex), lateral geniculate body (input to visual cortex), pulvinar (language function), ventral posteriomedial nucleus (input to anterolateral belt auditory cortex), and lateral dorsal nucleus (input to the parabelt of the auditory cortex). Note the following: LD, lateral dorsal nucleus; LP, lateral posterior nucleus; VA, ventral anterior nucleus; VI, ventral intermedial nucleus; VL, ventral lateral nucleus; VP, ventral posterior nucleus; VPL, ventral posterolateral nucleus; and VPM, Ventral posteromedial nucleus.
Based on Source: After view of Netter, 1988.

stria medullaris, and the posterior commissure. The habenular nuclei receive input from the septum, hypothalamus, brain stem, raphe nuclei, and ventral tegmental area via the habenulopeduncular tract and stria medullaris. Connections with the thalamus, hypothalamus, and septal area from the habenular nuclei are via the habenulopeduncular tract (fasciculus retroflexus), terminating in the interpeduncular nucleus, which projects to those structures. The posterior commissure consists of decussating fibers of the superior **colliculi**, nuclei associated with visual reflexes.

colliculi: L., mounds

Subthalamus. The major landmark of the subthalamus is the **subthalamic nucleus**, a lentiform structure on the inner surface of the internal capsule. Many fibers project through the subthalamus en route to the thalamus. The subthalamus receives input from the globus pallidus and the motor cortex and is involved in the control of striated muscle. Lesions to it have been known to produce the uncontrolled flailing movements of arms and legs known as **ballism** (e.g., Albin, 1995). Unilateral lesion produces **hemiballism** of the contralateral side.

Hypothalamus. The hypothalamus makes up the floor of the 3rd ventricle. Although it is comprised of numerous nuclei, it is generally divided into preoptic, mammillary, and tuberal regions (see Figure 11-24). The hypothalamus provides the organizational structure for the **limbic system**. Through interaction with the other components of this system (cingulate gyrus, septal area, parahippocampal gyrus, amygdala, and hippocampal formation), the hypothalamus regulates reproductive behavior and physiology, desire or perception of need for food and water, perception of satiation, control of digestive processes, and metabolic functions (including the maintenance of water balance and

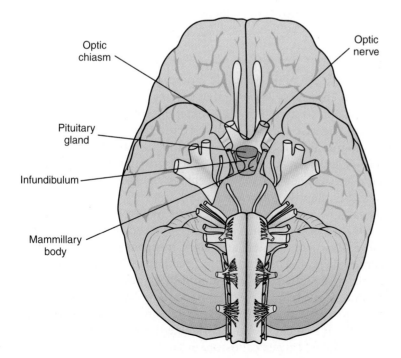

Optic chiasm

Optic nerve

Pituitary gland

Infundibulum

Mammillary body

Figure 11-24. Structures of the hypothalamus visible from an inferior view.
© Cengage Learning®.

body temperature). Damage to the hypothalamus can result in the loss of appropriate autonomic responses, such as heart-rate acceleration and sweating, shivering when cold, or even moving to a warmer environment when cold. Damage to the **satiety center** will result in voracious eating, whereas damage to the **feeding center** will result in starvation and dehydration. This structure is involved in the behavioral manifestations associated with emotion (tearing, heart-rate acceleration, sweating, gooseflesh, flushing, and mouth dryness), although it is assumed that cortical function is an important intermediary in normal emotional response.

✔ *To summarize:*

- The structures underlying the cerebral cortex are vital to the modification of information arriving at or leaving the cerebral cortex.
- The **basal ganglia** are subcortical structures involved in the control of **movement**, whereas the **hippocampal formation** of the inferior temporal lobe is deeply implicated in **memory** function.
- The **thalamus** of the **diencephalon** is the final relay for **somatic sensation** directed toward the cerebrum and for other diencephalic structures.
- The **subthalamus** interacts with the globus pallidus to control **movement**, and the **hypothalamus** controls many bodily functions and desires.
- The regions of the cerebral cortex are interconnected by means of a complex network of **projection fibers**, connecting the cortex with other structures; **association fibers**, which connect regions of the same hemisphere; and **commissural fibers**, which provide communication between the corresponding regions of the two hemispheres.

Cerebrovascular System

Although the brain makes up only 2 percent of the body weight, it consumes an enormous 20 percent of the oxygen transported by the vascular system to meet the high metabolic requirements of nervous tissue. The vascular system of the brain (the **cerebrovascular system**) maintains the constant circulation required by the nervous system (e.g., Jespersen & Ostergaard, 2012). Disruption of this supply for even a few seconds will lead to cellular changes in neurons, and longer vascular deprivation results in cell death.

The vascular supply of the brain arises from the carotid and vertebral branches, both of which originate from the aorta. The **carotid division** arises from the left and right **internal carotid arteries**, which enter the brain lateral to the optic chiasm. The internal carotid arteries give rise to the **anterior** and **middle cerebral arteries**.

The anterior cerebral artery courses along the superior surface of the corpus callosum within the medial longitudinal fissure (see Figure 11-25). It branches to supply the medial surface of the frontal and parietal lobes, corpus callosum, basal ganglia, and the anterior limb of the internal capsule.

cerebrovascular system: vascular supply of brain

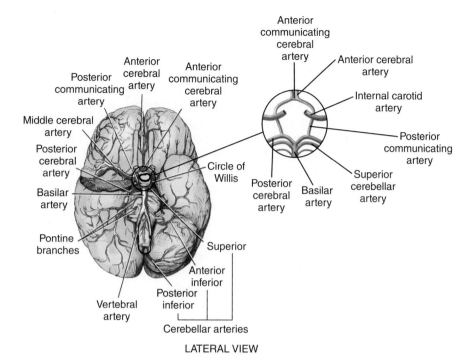

LATERAL VIEW

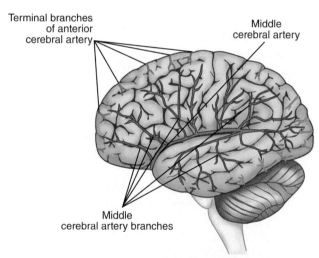

MEDIAL VIEW

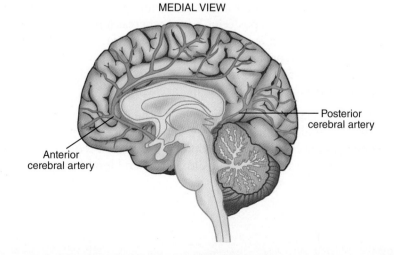

Figure 11-25. Major vascular supply of the cerebral cortex.
© Cengage Learning®.

The middle cerebral artery courses laterally along the inferior surface of the brain and through the lateral (Sylvian) fissure. It provides blood to the lateral surface of the hemispheres, including the temporal lobe, motor strip, Broca's area, Wernicke's area, sensory reception regions, and association areas. One branch of the middle cerebral artery serves the basal ganglia and internal capsule.

The **vertebral division** arises from the vertebral arteries that ascend on the anterior surface of the medulla oblongata. The vertebral artery branches, forming the descending **anterior** and **posterior spinal arteries**. The left and right vertebral arteries continue to ascend the ventral surface of the brain stem, joining at the superior medulla to form the **basilar artery**. The **superior cerebellar** and **anterior inferior cerebellar arteries** branch from the basilar artery to serve those locations of the cerebellum. (The **posterior inferior cerebellar artery** arises from the vertebral artery before this branching.) At the superior ventral pons, the basilar artery divides to become the left and right **posterior cerebral arteries**.

The posterior cerebral artery serves the inferior temporal and occipital lobes, the medial occipital lobe and primary visual cortex, upper midbrain, diencephalon, and cerebellum.

Circle of Willis. The cerebrovascular system of the brain contains many redundancies to ensure constant blood supply to the brain. The most prominent of these is the **circle of Willis**, a series of **anastomoses** (points of communication between arteries) that completely encircles the optic chiasm (e.g., Papantchev et al., 2007). If you will look again at Figure 11-25, you can see that the anterior cerebral arteries are connected by means of the **anterior communicating artery**, and the **posterior communicating artery** connects the middle cerebral artery with the posterior cerebral artery. This connects the vertebral and carotid systems, helps equalize locally high or low blood pressure, and promotes equal distribution of blood.

The anterior and posterior spinal arteries supply the spinal cord. The single anterior spinal artery descends in the anterior medial fissure of the spinal cord, giving off **radicular arteries** that serve the anterior spinal cord and anterior funiculus. The left and right posterior spinal arteries descend in similar fashion, also giving off radicular arteries. Blood from the posterior spinal arteries serves the posterior funiculi and posterior horns, whereas blood from the anterior spinal artery serves the anterior spinal cord. Radicular arteries from anterior and posterior arteries serve spinal nerves. Anastomoses with the vertebral, posterior intercostal, lumbar, and sacral arteries provide a safeguard against vascular accident.

Venous Drainage. The blood supply for the brain requires a return route for blood that has circulated and exchanged its nutrients. The **venous system** is the system of blood vessels called *veins* that provide the means of draining carbon-dioxide-laden blood to the lungs for reoxygenation.

Venous drainage is accomplished by means of a series of superficial and deep cisterns. Superficial drainage empties into the superior sagittal sinus and transverse sinus. Deep drainage is by means of the inferior sagittal sinus, the straight sinus, transverse sinuses, and the sigmoid sinus. Blood returns to the general bloodstream by means of the jugular veins, and spinal cord drainage is by means of radicular veins.

Obstruction of the cerebrovascular supply typically occurs in one of two ways. A **thrombus** is a foreign body (such as a blood clot or bubble of air) that obstructs a blood vessel, and such obstruction is called a **thrombosis**. If the thrombus breaks loose from its site of formation and floats through the bloodstream, it becomes an **embolus**, or floating clot. An **embolism** is an obstruction of a blood vessel by that foreign body brought to the point of occlusion by blood flow. **Aneurysm** is a dilation or ballooning of a blood vessel because of weak walls. When an intracranial aneurysm ruptures, the blood is released into the space surrounding the brain, in most cases, because most aneurysms occur in arteries rather than capillaries. The pressure associated with both the development of the ballooning aneurysm and the sudden release of blood into the cranial cavity is life threatening, with sites of neural damage being related to the location of the rupture.

Occlusion of the anterior cerebral artery is infrequent, but may result in hemiplegia, loss of some sensory function, and personality change. Occlusion of the middle cerebral artery is the most common and can result in severe disability because of the critical nature of the areas served. In addition to severe unilateral or bilateral motor and sensory deficit, left-hemisphere damage to Broca's area, Wernicke's area, and association areas may produce profound aphasia. Posterior cerebral artery occlusion produces variable deficit that may include memory dysfunction.

✔ *To summarize*:

- The **cerebrovascular system** is the literal lifeblood of the brain.
- The **anterior cerebral arteries** serve the medial surfaces of the brain, whereas the **middle cerebral artery** serves the lateral cortex, including the temporal lobe, motor strip, Wernicke's area, and much of the parietal lobe.
- The **vertebral arteries** branch to form the anterior and posterior spinal arteries, with ascending components serving the ventral brain stem.
- The **basilar artery** gives rise to the **superior** and **anterior inferior cerebellar arteries** to serve the cerebellum, whereas the **posterior inferior cerebellar artery** arises from the **vertebral artery**.
- The basilar artery divides to become the **posterior cerebral arteries**, serving the inferior temporal and occipital lobes, upper midbrain, and diencephalon.
- The **circle of Willis** is a series of communicating arteries that provides redundant pathways for blood flow to regions of the cerebral cortex, equalizing pressure and flow of blood.

- Obstruction of the blood supply is always critical. A foreign body within the blood vessel (**thrombus**) creates an obstruction to blood flow (**thrombosis**) or becomes an **embolus** when released into the bloodstream.
- An **aneurysm** is a ballooning of a blood vessel, and rupture of an aneurysm results in blood being released into the region of the brain.
- The **middle cerebral artery** is the most common site of occlusion; the result may be significant language and speech deficit if the occlusion involves the dominant cerebral hemisphere.

Cerebellum

The cerebellum is the largest component of the hindbrain, resting within the posterior cranial fossa, immediately inferior to the posterior cerebral cortex. The cerebellum is the heavy hitter of the nervous system in terms of neurons: While the cerebral cortex is home to 18 billion neurons, the cerebellum has 69 billion neurons, which is 80 percent of the total number in the brain (Azevado et al., 2009). Needless to say, this neuron density speaks to the critical nature of the cerebellum as an integration center. The cerebellum is responsible for coordinating motor commands with sensory inputs to control movement, and it communicates with the brain stem, spinal cord, and cerebral cortex by means of superior, middle, and inferior cerebellar peduncles. The cerebellum also plays a significant role as memory for motor function and even cognitive processing (Akshoomoff & Courchesne, 1992). It has connections with the limbic system, reticular activating system, and cortical association areas, and clinical studies of individuals with cerebellar lesions confirm its role in cognitive executive function and memory.

From behind, one can see that the cerebellum is composed of two hemispheres and is prominently invested with horizontal grooves. As you can see from the posterior view of Figure 11-26, the **primary fissure** separates the cerebellar cortex into two lobes (by the way, you now realize that the term "cortex" is not specific to the cerebral cortex). The **anterior lobe** is often referred to as the *superior lobe*, and the **middle lobe** is known also as the *inferior lobe*. The **vermis** separates the two hemispheres and aids in defining the **intermediate** and **lateral** cerebellar regions of the posterior surface.

To view the cerebellum from the front, you must remove it from the brain stem. The anterior surface reveals the third lobe of the cerebellum, the **flocculonodular lobe**, made up of the right and left **flocculi** and central **nodulus**. The prominent **middle cerebellar peduncle** is between the **superior** and **inferior cerebellar peduncles**.

The cerebellum may be divided functionally into three regions. The flocculonodular lobe is functionally referred to as the **vestibulocerebellum** (or **archicerebellum**), whereas the **spinocerebellum** (or **paleocerebellum**) is the anterior lobe and the portion of

vermis: L., worm

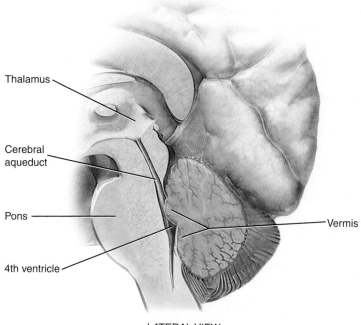

Thalamus

Cerebral
aqueduct

Pons

4th ventricle

Vermis

LATERAL VIEW

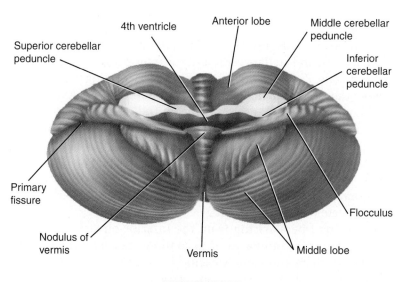

Superior cerebellar
peduncle

4th ventricle

Anterior lobe

Middle cerebellar
peduncle

Inferior
cerebellar
peduncle

Primary
fissure

Nodulus of
vermis

Vermis

Flocculus

Middle lobe

INFERIOR VIEW

Figure 11-26. Cerebellum as seen in sagittal section and from beneath.
© Cengage Learning®.

the posterior lobe associated with the arm and leg. The posterior lobes and the intermediate vermis make up the **neocerebellum** (or **pontocerebellum**).

The inner cerebellum is faintly reminiscent of the cerebral cortex. The outer cortex is a dense array of neurons, and beneath this is a mass of white communicating axons. At the center of the white fibers is a series of nuclei serving as relays between the cerebellum and the communicating regions of the body.

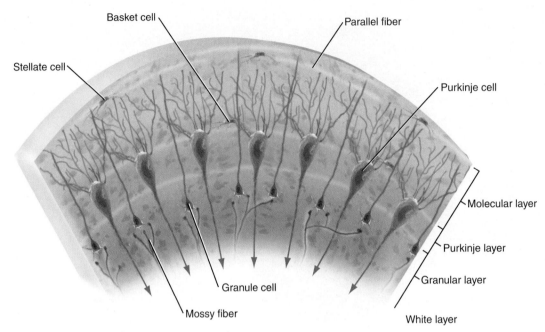

Figure 11-27. Cellular layers of the cerebellar cortex.
© Cengage Learning®.

The cerebellar cortex is composed of three layers: the outer **molecular layer**, the intermediate **Purkinje layer**, and the deep **granular layer** (see Figure 11-27). The outer molecular layer contains **Golgi**, **basket**, and **stellate cells**, and the intermediate layer contains **Purkinje cells**. Purkinje cells are large neurons forming the boundary between the molecular and granular layers of the cortex. Axons of the 15 million Purkinje cells project to the central cerebellar nuclei. Excitation of a Purkinje cell causes inhibition of the nucleus with which it communicates. Golgi cells project their dendrites into the molecular layer and their axons into the granular layer. Their soma receive input from both climbing fibers and Purkinje cells, and the axons synapse with granule cell dendrites. Basket cells and stellate cells arborize to communicate with Purkinje cells.

Climbing fibers arising from the inferior olivary nuclei pass through the inner granular layer to communicate with the Purkinje cells. These fibers are strongly excitatory to Purkinje cells. Granule cells within this inner layer project axons to the outer layer where they divide into a "T" form. The branches course at roughly right angles to the base of the axon, synapsing with the dendritic arborization of the Purkinje cells. Activation of these granule cells excites basket and stellate cells but inhibits Purkinje cells. Projections from noncerebellar regions (spinal cord, brain stem, cerebral cortex) terminate in mossy fibers.

There are four pairs of nuclei within the cerebellum, all of which receive input from the Purkinje cells of the cortex (see Figure 11-28). The **dentate nucleus** has the appearance of a serrated sac, opening medially. Projections from this nucleus route through the superior

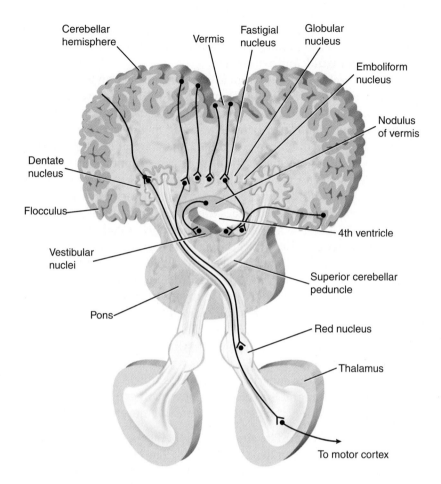

Cerebellar hemisphere

Vermis

Fastigial nucleus

Globular nucleus

Emboliform nucleus

Nodulus of vermis

Dentate nucleus

Flocculus

4th ventricle

Vestibular nuclei

Superior cerebellar peduncle

Pons

Red nucleus

Thalamus

To motor cortex

Figure 11-28. Schematic of cerebellar nuclei and interaction between cerebellum and cerebral cortex.
© Cengage Learning®.

cerebellar peduncle to synapse in the ventrolateral nucleus of the thalamus and from there ascend to the cerebral cortex by means of thalamocortical fibers. The **emboliform** and **globose nuclei** (collectively referred to as the **nucleus interpositus**) project to the red nucleus, providing input to the **rubrospinal** tract. The **fastigial nucleus** communicates with the vestibular nuclei of the brain stem, the reticular formation of the pons and medulla, and the inferior olive.

Tracts of the Cerebellum. The **dorsal spinocerebellar tract** communicates sensation of temperature, proprioception (muscle spindle), and touch from the lower body and legs to the ipsilateral cerebellum. Afferents arise from the nucleus dorsalis (Clarke's column) in the spinal cord and project to both the anterior and posterior lobes of the cerebellum. The **cuneocerebellar tract** serves the same function for the arms and upper trunk, originating in the external cuneate nucleus of the cervical region and entering the cerebellum through the inferior cerebellar peduncle.

The **ventral spinocerebellar tract** transmits proprioception information (GTOs) and pain sense from the legs and lower trunk to the ipsilateral cerebellar cortex. Fibers decussate within the spinal cord, ascend, enter through the superior cerebellar peduncle, and then

rubrospinal: L., ruber spina, red thorn, referring to the tract arising from the red nucleus

decussate again to project to the cortex. The **rostral spinocerebellar tract** is the cervical parallel of the ventral spinocerebellar tract, serving the upper trunk and arm region.

Pontocerebellar fibers from the pontine nuclei provide the greatest input to the cerebellum as they cross midline and ascend as the middle cerebellar peduncle to terminate as mossy fibers. **Olivocerebellar fibers** from the inferior olivary and medial accessory olivary nucleus of the medulla project to the contralateral cerebellum, terminating as climbing fibers. The olive receives input from the spinal cord, cerebral cortex, and red nucleus, as well as visual information. All other tracts of the cerebellum terminate on mossy fibers. The **vestibulocerebellar** tract provides input from the vestibular nuclei to the flocculonodular lobe via the inferior cerebellar peduncles.

The **corticopontine** projection is an important feedback system for the control of voluntary movement. Projections from parietal, occipital, temporal, and frontal lobes (including the motor cortex) synapse on the pontine nuclei, projecting via pontocerebellar fibers to the opposite cerebellar cortex. The mossy fiber terminations synapse with granule cells, the branches of which synapse with Purkinje cell dendrites. The Purkinje cells synapse with the dentate nucleus, which projects back to the cerebellar cortex as well as to the motor cortex of the cerebrum via the superior cerebellar peduncle and thalamus. In this way, the command for voluntary movement can be modified relative to body position, muscle tension, muscle movement, and so on.

Cerebellar Peduncles. The superior cerebellar peduncle (brachium conjunctivum) arises in the anterior cerebellar hemisphere, coursing through the lateral wall of the 4th ventricle to decussate within the pons at the level of the inferior colliculi. Many tracts are served by this peduncle. **Dentatothalamic** fibers arise from the dentate nucleus and synapse in the opposite red nucleus and thalamus. The ventral spinocerebellar tract ascends within this peduncle, and fibers from the fastigial nucleus descend in conjunction with this peduncle as they course to the lateral vestibular nucleus. The **middle cerebellar peduncle** (brachium pontis) is made up of fibers projecting from the contralateral pontine nuclei. The inferior cerebellar peduncle (restiform body) communicates input from the spinocerebellar tracts to the cerebellum, exiting the brain stem at the upper medulla.

Cerebellar Control Function. Cerebellar control function may be reasonably partitioned according to the portions of the cerebellum. The flocculonodular lobe (archicerebellum) is the oldest component and is responsible for the perception of orientation of the body in space. It receives input from the vestibular nuclei of the brain stem. Damage to this portion of the cerebellum will result in trunk ataxia, staggering, and generally reduced response to motion (as in reduced vestibular responses or motion sickness).

The newer anterior (superior) lobe (the paleocerebellum) exerts moderating control over antigravity muscles. Damage can result in increased stretch reflexes of support musculature. The "young" posterior (inferior) lobe (neocerebellum) is responsible for stopping or damping movements, especially those of the hands. Damage to this lobe will result in problems with fine movements, dysmetria (inability to control the range of movement), tremor associated with voluntary movement, and trouble with performing alternating movement tasks (such as oral diadochokinetic tasks). One can see gait deficits and hypotonia as well. Cognitive function appears to involve the neocerebellum, whereas emotion control is affected by lesions to the vermis (Akshoomoff & Courchesne, 1992; Marien et al., 2008).

The cerebellum is a vital "silent partner" in the integration of body movement with the internal and external environment of the body. Although it is incapable of initiating movement, it is intimately related to the control of the rate and range of movement, as well as the force with which that movement is executed.

✔ *To summarize:*

- The **cerebellum** is responsible for **coordinating motor commands** with sensory inputs, communicating with the brain stem, cerebrum, and spinal cord.
- The cerebellum is divided into **anterior**, **middle**, and **flocculonodular lobes** and communicates with the rest of the nervous system via the **superior**, **middle**, and **inferior cerebral peduncles**.
- The **flocculonodular** lobe coordinates position in space via the **vestibular nuclei**.
- The **anterior lobe** coordinates **postural adjustment** against gravity, and the **posterior lobe** mediates **fine motor** adjustments.
- The **cerebellar cortex** consists of an **outer molecular layer**, a **Purkinje layer**, and a deep **granular layer**.
- The **Golgi**, **basket**, **stellate**, and **Purkinje cells** are responsible for coordinating input received from the nervous system.

Four pairs of nuclei are found in the cerebellum.

- The sacklike **dentate nucleus** projects output through the **superior cerebellar peduncle** to the **red nucleus, thalamus,** and ultimately the **cerebral cortex**.
- The **emboliform** and **globose nuclei** project to the **inferior olive** via the **red nucleus**, with information ultimately reaching the **contralateral cerebellar hemisphere**.
- The **fastigial nucleus** communicates with the **vestibular nuclei**.

Several tracts provide conduit to and from the cerebellum.

- The **dorsal spinocerebellar** and **cuneocerebellar tracts** communicate proprioception (muscle spindle), temperature, and touch sense from the lower and upper body to the cerebellum.
- The **ventral spinocerebellar** and **rostral spinocerebellar tracts** mediate ipsilateral proprioceptive information (GTO) and pain sense from the lower and upper body.

- The **olivocerebellar tract** mediates information received at the olivary complex from the spinal cord, cerebral cortex, red nucleus, and visual and cutaneous senses and provides communication between cerebellar hemispheres.
- The **superior cerebellar peduncle** enters the pons at the level of the inferior colliculi, serving the dentate nucleus, red nucleus, and thalamus.
- The **middle cerebellar peduncle** consists of projections from the pontine nuclei, and the **inferior cerebellar peduncle** receives input from the spinocerebellar tracts, exiting at the upper medulla.

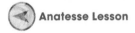 Anatesse Lesson

Anatomy of the Brain Stem

The brain stem consists of the medulla oblongata, pons, and midbrain. The brain stem reflects an intermediate stage of organization, between the simple reflexive responses seen at the level of the spinal cord and the exquisitely complex responses generated by the cerebral cortex. Cranial nerves and their nuclei arise from the brain stem, and basic bodily functions for life are maintained here. We will work from the superficial to deep structures of the brain stem. It will be helpful to refer to Figures 11-29 through 11-31 as we do this.

Superficial Brain Stem Landmarks

Viewing the brain stem "from the outside" provides useful hints as to the structures housed within it. This is a good time to take a tour of the external form of this amazing part of the brain, before examining the internal structures. To do this, let us work from the lower reaches of the brain stem (medulla oblongata) to the upper portion (midbrain).

Superficial Medulla Oblongata. The **medulla oblongata**, or medulla, is the inferior-most segment of the brain stem. It looks like an enlargement of the upper spinal cord and is about 2.5 cm long and 1 cm in diameter. This is a small but mighty structure: Damage to the medulla is imminently life threatening.

Take a look at Figure 11-29 as we begin our discussion of the medulla. The **anterior (ventral) median fissure** of the spinal cord (to be discussed) continues through the medulla. There is an interruption in it, however, that marks a very important point for us. If you can find the **pyramidal decussation**, you will see the point within the medulla at which fibers of the corticospinal tract cross from one side to the other. That is, most of the axons carrying motor commands from the left hemisphere cross to the right side of the medulla to continue down through the spinal cord on the right side, and this is where that happens. The significance of this will not be lost on you if you remember meeting an individual with left-hemisphere stroke who had right-side hemiparesis. That is, unilateral paralysis signals a

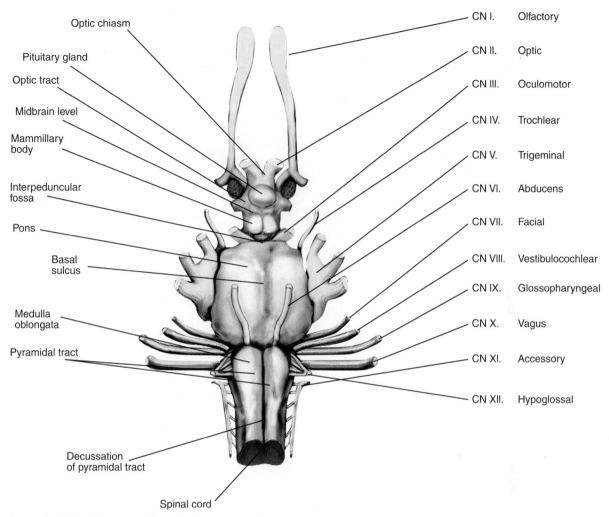

Optic chiasm

Pituitary gland

Optic tract

Midbrain level

Mammillary body

Interpeduncular fossa

Pons

Basal sulcus

Medulla oblongata

Pyramidal tract

Decussation of pyramidal tract

Spinal cord

CN I.   Olfactory

CN II.   Optic

CN III.   Oculomotor

CN IV.   Trochlear

CN V.   Trigeminal

CN VI.   Abducens

CN VII.   Facial

CN VIII. Vestibulocochlear

CN IX.   Glossopharyngeal

CN X.   Vagus

CN XI.   Accessory

CN XII.   Hypoglossal

Figure 11-29. Anterior view of the brain stem.
© Cengage Learning®.

neuropathology on the side opposite the lesion. The point of decussation marks the lower border of the medulla, roughly at the level of the foramen magnum.

Now look at Figure 11-30 for a side view of the medulla. This is a good time to remind you that we are just looking at the external brain stem and that there are myriad structures within it that have a great impact on function (see Figure 8-13). For instance, the sides of the medulla are marked by two prominent sulci. The **ventrolateral sulcus** marks the lateral margin of the pyramid and is also the groove from which the **XII hypoglossal nerve** exits the medulla to innervate the muscles of the tongue (to be discussed). The **dorsolateral sulcus** is the groove from which the **XI accessory**, **X vagus**, and **IX glossopharyngeal nerves** exit. You can see from Figure 11-30 the spinal portion of the XI accessory nerve arising from the C2 through C5 spinal segments. If you recall the discussion of the auditory pathway in Chapter 7,

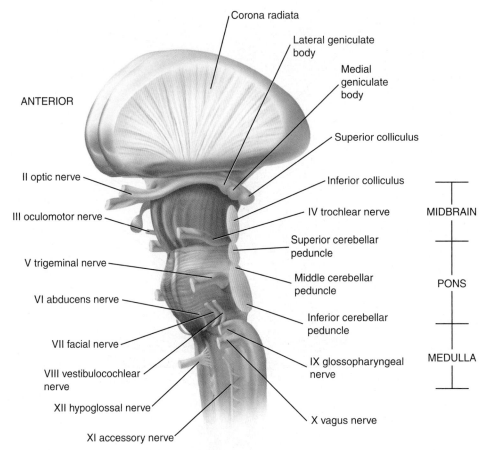

ANTERIOR

Corona radiata

Lateral geniculate body

Medial geniculate body

Superior colliculus

II optic nerve

Inferior colliculus

III oculomotor nerve

IV trochlear nerve

MIDBRAIN

Superior cerebellar peduncle

V trigeminal nerve

Middle cerebellar peduncle

VI abducens nerve

PONS

Inferior cerebellar peduncle

VII facial nerve

IX glossopharyngeal nerve

VIII vestibulocochlear nerve

MEDULLA

XII hypoglossal nerve

X vagus nerve

XI accessory nerve

Figure 11-30. Lateral view of the brain stem.
© Cengage Learning®.

you may remember the inferior olivary complex. The **olive** is the bulge between the ventrolateral and dorsolateral sulci, caused by the **inferior olivary nuclear complex**, which consists of nuclei serving to localize sound in space.

Now let us look at the posterior surface of the medulla. In Figure 11-31, the cerebellum has been removed, revealing the 4th ventricle. As you recall, the ventricles provide a means for CSF to be produced and to circulate through the CNS, and the 4th ventricle is the last of the series of ventricles. The 4th ventricle is the space between the cerebellum and the brain stem, and by removing the cerebellum, we can see several structures on the ventricle (dorsal) side of the brain stem that are otherwise hidden from view.

On Figure 11-31 you can see that the inferior-most point on the ventricle is the **obex**. The obex is a point that marks the beginning of a region known as the **calamus scriptorius**, so named because it looks like the point of a calligraphy pen. Lateral to the obex is the **clava** or **gracilis tubercle**, a bulge caused by the **nucleus gracilis**. As you shall see, one of the important afferent pathways is the fasciculus gracilis, and it terminates in the brain stem at the nucleus gracilis. To the side

obex: L., band

calamus scriptorius: L., reed cane (calligraphy) pen

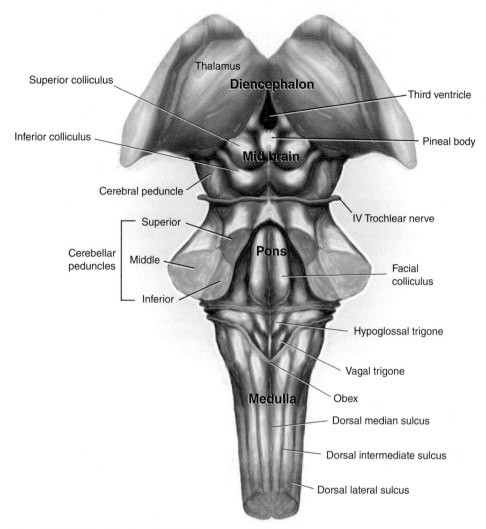

Figure 11-31. Posterior view of the brain stem.
© Cengage Learning®.

and a little above the clava is the **cuneate tubercle**, which is the prominence that marks the end point of the fasciculus cuneatus (to be discussed). Information concerning touch pressure, vibration, muscle stretch, and tension from the upper and lower extremities terminates at these two locations in the brain stem. As you can well imagine, focal damage to this region would affect sensation for the entire body.

The calamus scriptorius includes the **vagal trigone**, a bulge marking the dorsal vagal nucleus of the X vagus nerve, as well as the **hypoglossal trigone**, a prominence caused by the XII hypoglossal nucleus. You will remember the importance of the vagus nerve for phonation, because this is the nerve responsible for adducting, abducting, tensing, and relaxing the vocal folds (and so much more). You will also remember that the hypoglossal nerve activates the tongue muscles. A little reflection is all that is needed to realize the importance of the medulla for speech.

Superficial Pons. The pons is above the medulla, serving as the "bridge" between medulla and midbrain, as well as to the cerebellum. The significant anterior bulge of the pons is an obvious landmark for this structure. The pons is the site of four cranial nerve nuclei and is the origin of the middle and superior cerebellar peduncles, as we mentioned earlier. These peduncles serve as "superhighways" for communication with the cerebellum. At the junction of the medulla and the pons, the inferior cerebellar peduncle has expanded in diameter to its maximum and is entering the cerebellum.

Look once again at Figure 11-29. The anterior pons is marked by a prominent band of transverse fibers that provide communication between the cerebellum and the pons, the **pontocerebellar tract**. The **basal sulcus** is a prominent anterior landmark, because it marks the course of the vital basilar artery. The VI abducens nerve exits at the inferior border of the pons, from the **inferior pontine sulcus**. As you will learn, this nerve is important for rotating the eye outward, and a deficit in that ability serves as an indication to neurologists of the location of a lesion of the brain stem.

Now let us look at the lateral surface of the pons (Figure 11-30). You can see the middle **cerebellar peduncle (brachia pontis)**, which is the intermediate communicating attachment of the pons to the cerebellum. You may remember from your audiology coursework that one of the important functions of an audiologist is to help diagnose cerebellopontine angle tumors. The **cerebellopontine angle** is the space created by the cerebellum, the middle cerebellar peduncle, and the medulla oblongata. The VII facial and VIII vestibulocochlear nerves emerge from the cerebellopontine angle, so tumors at this location may cause sensorineural hearing loss as well as facial paralysis. Also you will notice that the V trigeminal nerve exits the pons from the middle cerebellar peduncle of the lateral pons. You will recall that the trigeminal nerve is responsible for facial sensation and the activation of the muscles of mastication.

The surface of the posterior pons marks the upper limit of the 4th ventricle. As can be seen in Figure 11-31, the **superior cerebellar peduncles (brachia conjunctiva)** form the upper lateral surface of the 4th ventricle, and the **superior** and **inferior medullary veli** and cerebellum provide the superior border. On either side of the median sulcus are the paired **facial colliculi**. The facial colliculus represents the location of the nucleus of the VI abducens nerve as well as the place where the fibers of the VII cross that nucleus.

Superficial Midbrain. The superior-most structure of the brain stem is the midbrain. As you can see in Figure 11-31, the lower surface of the midbrain is dominated by the prominent paired **crus cerebri**. These crura represent the **cerebral peduncles**, which house the communicating pathways leading to and from the cerebrum. Again, if you stop and think about it, a lesion to a small area in the midbrain could have devastating effects on the function of the entire body, because all the motor fibers must pass through this crus.

Between the cerebral peduncles is an indentation known as the **interpeduncular fossa**. The III oculomotor nerve exits from this fossa, at the juncture between the pons and midbrain. The **optic tracts**, an extension of the optic nerve, course around the crus cerebri following the decussation at the **optic chiasm**. Once again, problems in visual function following stroke provide vital information to the neurologist about the site of a lesion, as we will discuss shortly.

Now turn your attention to the posterior midbrain (Figure 11-31). The posterior midbrain is the **tectum**. The tectum is behind the cerebral aqueduct, which is the upper extension of the 4th ventricle. There are four important landmarks on the tectum, known as the **corpora quadrigemina**. The corpora quadrigemina (literally "four bodies") are made up of the **superior** and **inferior colliculi**. As shown in this figure, the IV trochlear nerve emerges near the inferior colliculus and courses around the crus cerebri.

corpora quadrigemina: L., body of four parts

Deep Structure of the Brain Stem

An examination of the deep structure of the brain stem requires some patience and a good imagination. Similar to the spinal cord, the brain stem is organized vertically. It is made up of columnar nuclei and tracts that serve the periphery, spinal cord, cerebral, cerebellar, and subcortical structures. Referring to Figure 11-32 may help you with orientation as we discuss the brain stem. We will once again take you from the medulla to the level of the midbrain, this time looking at the deep structures of the brain stem.

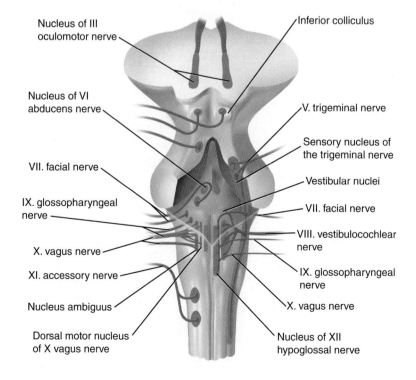

Figure 11-32. Posterior view of the brain stem revealing orientation of major nuclei and cranial nerves supplied by those nuclei.
© Cengage Learning®.

Deep Structures of Medulla Oblongata. The deep structure of the medulla represents an expansion on the developments that started in the spinal cord (see Figure 11-33). At the lowest regions of the medulla, the central canal makes a good reference point. This canal expands in the upper medulla to become the lower part of the 4th ventricle. Surrounding this canal is a zone of central gray matter containing nuclei, which expands to the **reticular formation**. The reticular formation is an important mass of nuclei that spans the medulla, pons, and midbrain. It is a composite of brain stem nuclei, forming the "oldest" part of the brain stem and representing our first evolutionary effort at complex processing. This formation begins above the level of the decussation of the pyramids and makes up the central

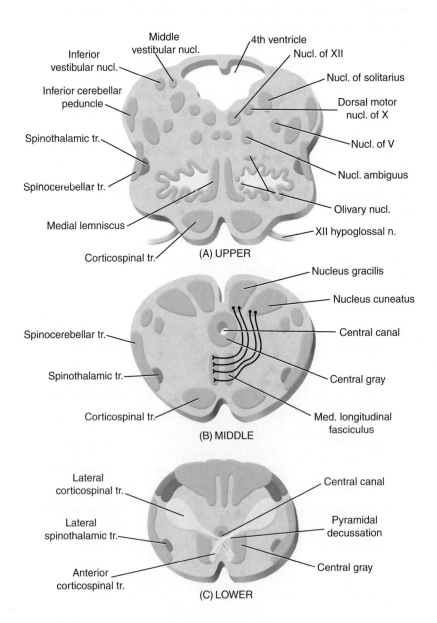

Figure 11-33. Low, mid, and upper medulla levels in a transverse schematic view.
© Cengage Learning®.

structure of the brain stem. The reticular formation is extraordinarily important for life function, as it contains nuclei associated with respiration and the maintenance of blood pressure (see Figure 8-13).

At this lower level, you can also see the **decussation of the pyramids**. As mentioned earlier, the pyramids represent the bundle of fibers that forms the corticospinal tracts. You will remember that the corticospinal tract is responsible for the activation of skeletal muscle of the extremities and commands to move those muscles arise from the cerebrum. Look again at Figure 11-28 to remind yourself that the pyramidal decussation is a visible blur on the anterior surface of the medulla. At the decussation, the fibers divide into **lateral** and **anterior corticospinal tracts**: The lateral tract forms after the fibers cross the midline, and the much smaller anterior tract is made up of uncrossed nerve fibers. This is also a good time to remember that motor commands originating in the left cerebrum activate muscles on the right side of the body. This decussation is the manifestation of that.

Looking again at Figure 11-33, you can see that the prominent fasciculus gracilis and cuneatus and their nuclei are in the posterior medulla. Information concerning kinesthetic sense, muscle stretch, and proprioceptive sense arrives from the lower body to the **accessory cuneate nucleus**. That information is relayed to the cerebellum by means of the cuneocerebellar tract passing through the inferior cerebellar peduncle. Also in the posterior portion of the medulla are the trigeminal nerve nucleus and the spinal tract of the trigeminal.

The complexity of the upper medulla reflects the importance of this region (upper portion of Figure 11-33). The corticospinal tract arising from the cerebrum has yet to divide into anterior and lateral components, so it appears as a single pathway. The central canal has now expanded to become the 4th ventricle. Lateral to the hypoglossal and dorsal vagal nuclei is the **nucleus solitarius**, an important nucleus of the X vagus nerve. The **hypoglossal nucleus** gives rise to the XII hypoglossal nerve, and the IX glossopharyngeal, X vagus, and XI accessory nerves arise from the **nucleus ambiguus**, dorsal vagal nucleus, and solitary tract nucleus. We will discuss these cranial nerves in detail.

You can quickly find the **inferior olivary complex** in the anterolateral aspect of the medulla as a structure looking like an intestine doubled over on itself. A number of fibers from this complex decussate and enter the cerebellum via the inferior cerebellar peduncle. Parts of this structure appears like a bag with a drawstring (the **principal inferior olivary nucleus**), and axons from the nuclei within the complex decussate at the **median raphe** to ascend to the cerebellum as the major component of the inferior cerebellar peduncle. The lateral medulla is dominated by the inferior cerebellar peduncle, with the trigeminal spinal tract and nucleus medial to it. The nucleus ambiguus may be seen in the anterolateral medulla, marking the anterior boundary of the reticular formation.

Look closely at the posterior margin of the upper medulla, and you can see the **medial** and **inferior vestibular nuclei**. You may remember these from your audiology course, because they are important nuclei associated with knowing and maintaining one's position in space (vestibular sense). Projections from the vestibular portion of the VIII vestibulocochlear nerve reach these nuclei. If you can locate the lateral spinothalamic tracts, you can identify the region that carries pain and touch information from the spine to the thalamus.

Clearly, a lesion to the medulla would have devastating impact on all motor and sensory function. We have just mentioned the nuclei associated with balance, motor function for the larynx, respiration, cardiac function, movement of the tongue and muscles of mastication, as well as pathways mediating the vestibular sense, all motor function in the periphery, and all sensations that reach the cerebrum or cerebellum. Take just an instant to realize that all these extraordinarily important functions and processes are housed within an area about the size of the first joint of your thumb. Once again, ponder the danger associated with a lesion to this region, and we promise to tell you a story with a surprisingly happy ending related to a brain stem stroke.

Deep Structures of the Pons. The pons is classically divided into two parts: the posterior **tegmentum** and the anterior **basilar portion**. Look at Figures 11-34 and 11-35 as we discuss the pons.

First, let us examine the basilar (anterior) portion of the pons. Orient yourself by finding the corticospinal and corticobulbar tracts. At the level of the lower pons, the tracts are beginning to become organized for their medulla decussation and course through the spine. At higher levels of the pons, you would see that the tracts are less well defined and more diffusely distributed. Near these tracts are the **pontine nuclei**. The pontine nuclei are important because they receive

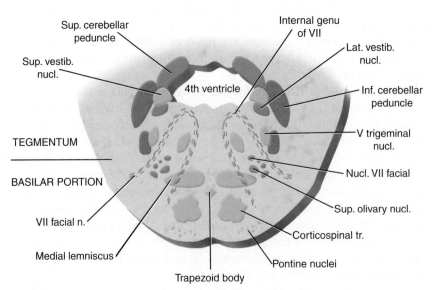

Figure 11-34. Schematic of a transverse section through the pons.
© Cengage Learning®.

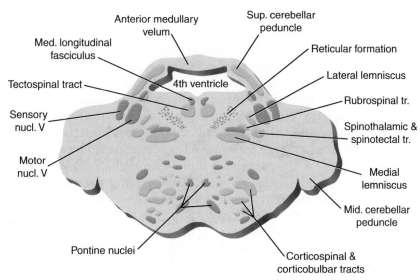

Figure 11-35. Schematic of a transverse section through the middle pons.
© Cengage Learning®.

input from the cerebrum and spinal cord, with that information being relayed to the cerebellum by means of the axons of the pontine nuclei that make up the pontocerebellar tract. This tract ascends to the cerebellum as the middle cerebellar peduncle. The transmission of information from the cerebrum to the pontine nuclei and pontocerebellar tract is an extremely important conduit between the cerebrum and cerebellum.

Locate the **medial lemniscus** on Figure 11-34. The lemniscal pathway begins to coalesce within the medulla, becoming the medial lemniscus within the pons. This is an important pathway for somatic (body) sense.

In the section on spinal cord anatomy, we will discuss the medial longitudinal fasciculus (MLF), which is responsible for the maintenance of flexor tone. Most of the ascending fibers of the MLF shown in Figure 11-35 arise from the vestibular nuclei and project to muscles of the eye for the regulation of eye movement with relation to head position in space. Note the relationship between the vestibular nuclei (Figure 11-34) and the MLF (Figure 11-35) and you will see the important interaction between the vestibular system and ocular tracking: Without the vital information from the vestibular system, the eyes would interpret every movement as external to the body. As it is, the vestibular system can notify the visual system of how the head is moving (for instance, bumping up and down on a country road) so that the ocular muscles can adjust for these changes in head position.

You will also certainly remember that we discussed the vestibular nuclei as being part of the medulla. In reality, only the inferior vestibular nucleus is within the medulla. The lateral and superior vestibular nuclei are shown in Figure 11-34, although the medial vestibular nucleus is not visible in this view. Another center of the auditory system, the **trapezoid body**, is a mass of small nuclei and fibers seen at this level. The trapezoid body is a relay within the auditory pathway. Lateral and posterior to the trapezoid body is the **superior olivary complex**, containing auditory relays associated with the localization of sound in space, as well as with the efferent component of the auditory pathway. We discuss this further in Chapter 12.

The posterior **pontine tegmentum** is actually a continuation of the reticular formation of the medulla. Projections from the reticular formation ascend to the thalamus and hypothalamus. As you can see from Figure 11-34, the tegmentum houses nuclei for cranial nerves V, VI, VII, as well as relays of the VIII. To remind you, within this small space are the control centers for mastication, ocular abduction, facial musculature, and portions of the auditory pathway. The ventral pons is made up largely of fibers of the corticospinal, corticobulbar, and corticopontine tracts. At this level, those fibers are less compactly bundled than they are at the level of the medulla. Notice that the motor nucleus of the VII facial nerve is found near the superior olive. Axons from the facial nucleus course around the nucleus of the VI abducens nerve at the internal genu before exiting the brain stem.

If you examine the basilar portion of the pons in Figure 11-35, you can see that the corticospinal tract is broken into small bundles, as mentioned previously. Fibers of the **corticopontine tract** (not shown) course with the corticospinal tract but synapse with the pontine nuclei, which surround the corticospinal tract. Axons of these nuclei decussate to make up the middle cerebellar peduncle. The superior cerebellar peduncle of the tegmental region is dorsal to the nuclei of the trigeminal nerve. The superior cerebellar peduncle forms the lateral margin of the 4th ventricle, and the anterior medullary velum forms the roof of the ventricle, as mentioned earlier.

Deep Structures of Midbrain. Look at Figure 11-36 as we discuss the midbrain. The midbrain may be divided into three areas: the posterior tectum (also known as the *quadrigeminal plate*); the medial tegmentum, which is a continuation of the pontine tegmentum; and the crus cerebri, the prominent anterior structure.

In the posterior midbrain, the tectum is dominated by the **inferior colliculus**, an important auditory relay. This nucleus receives input from the lateral lemniscus and those fibers encapsulate it. Within the tegmentum you can see the decussation of the superior cerebellar peduncle (tegmental decussation). Remember that the crus cerebri are the efferent pathways from the cerebrum serving the body. Included within the crus cerebri are the corticobulbar and corticospinal tracts, and the **frontopontine** fibers that will terminate in the pons. Between the crus cerebri and tegmentum is the **substantia nigra**, a dark brown mass of cells that manufactures dopamine, a neurotransmitter essential for normal movement. Destruction of this substance results in Parkinson's disease, a debilitating neuromuscular disease.

The **cerebral aqueduct** is an extremely narrow tube connecting the 4th ventricle with the 3rd ventricle, as previously discussed.

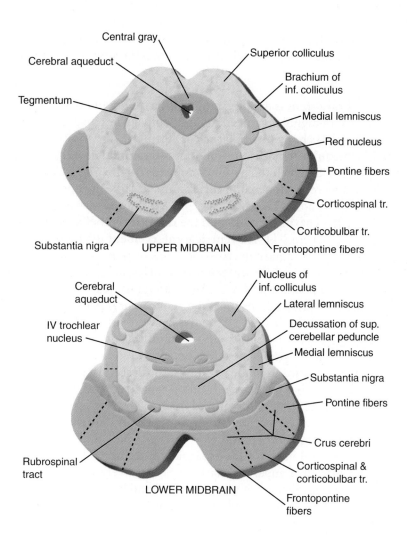

Figure 11-36. Transverse section through the upper and lower midbrain.
© Cengage Learning®.

Surrounding it is a mass of cells known as the **periaqueductal** or **central gray**, where the nucleus of the IV trochlear nerve can be found.

The **superior colliculus** can be found in the superior midbrain within the tectum. This nucleus receives input from the cerebral cortex, optic tract, inferior colliculus, and the spinal cord and appears to be responsible for eye and head movements relative to visual stimuli. Perhaps because of the inferior colliculus connection, it may also serve as a point of integration of auditory localization and visual orientation.

Also within the tegmentum lies the massive **red nucleus**. The red nucleus receives input from the cerebral cortex and cerebellum and gives rise to the **rubrospinal tract**. Input from the red nucleus is from the cerebellum and cerebral cortex, and it is an important component of flexor control. Near the red nucleus is the **Edinger–Westphal nucleus**, controlling accommodation of the eye to light by the iris. Also medially placed is the III oculomotor nerve nucleus. The dorsolaterally placed **medial geniculate body** is actually a nucleus of the thalamus and is the final subcortical relay of the auditory pathway.

✔ *To summarize:*

- The **brain stem** is divided into **medulla**, **pons**, and **midbrain**. It is more highly organized than the spinal cord, mediating higher-level body function such as vestibular responses.
- The **medulla** contains the important **pyramidal decussation**, the point at which the motor commands originating in one hemisphere of the cerebral cortex cross to serve the opposite side of the body. The **IX, X, XI,** and **XII cranial nerves** emerge at the level of the medulla, and the **inferior cerebellar peduncle** arises there. The **4th ventricle enlargement** is a prominent brain stem landmark in cross-section. The **pons** contains the **superior** and **middle cerebellar peduncles**, as well as four cranial nerve nuclei, the **V, VI, VII,** and **VIII** nerves.
- The **midbrain** contains the important **cerebral peduncles** and gives rise to the **III** and **IV cranial nerves**.
- The deep structure of the brain stem reflects the level of the brain stem's phylogenetic development.
- At the **decussation** of the pyramids, the **descending corticospinal tract** has condensed from the less-structured form at higher levels to a well-organized tract.
- The **reticular formation** is a phylogenetically old set of nuclei essential for life function.
- In the rostral medulla, the expansion to accommodate the **4th ventricle** is apparent, marking a clear divergence from the minute central canal of the spinal cord and lower medulla.
- The levels of the pons and midbrain set the stage for communication with the higher levels of the brain, including the cerebellum and cerebrum.
- This communication link permits not only complex motor acts but also consciousness, awareness, and volitional acts.

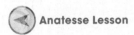 Anatesse Lesson

Cranial Nerves

Working knowledge of the cranial nerves is vital to the speech-language pathologist or audiologist. You may wish to refer to Appendixes F and G as we discuss them. Although not all cranial nerves are involved with speech or hearing, knowledge of cranial nerves is of great assistance in assessment. Figure 11-37A might help you organize these nerves.

Cranial Nerve Classification

Cranial nerves are referred to by name, number, or both. By convention, roman numerals are used when discussing cranial nerves, and the number represents inverse height in the brain stem. Cranial nerves I through IV are found at the level of the midbrain, V through VIII are pons-level cranials, and IX through XII are found in the medulla. When we discussed the spinal cord, we pointed out that the nuclei of sensory neurons resided in dorsal root ganglia and that their axons entered the spinal cord for synapse. This pattern is followed in the brain stem as well, in which axons of sensory nuclei enter the brain stem for synapse and motor nuclei are within the brain stem.

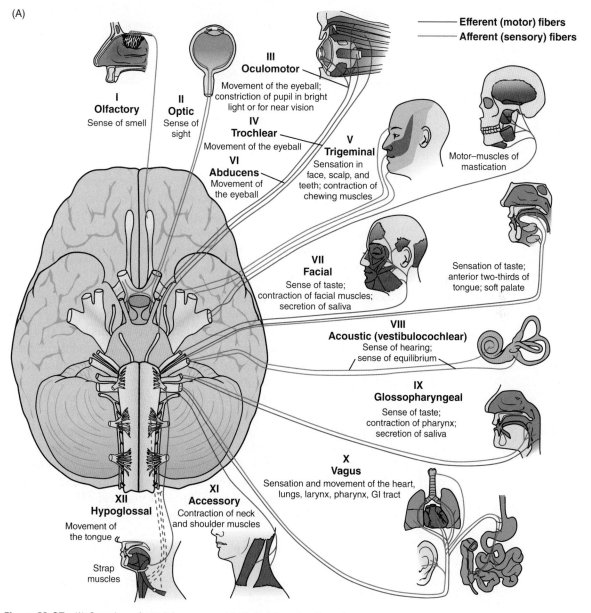

Figure 11-37. (A) Overview of cranial nerves and their function. (continues).
© Cengage Learning®.

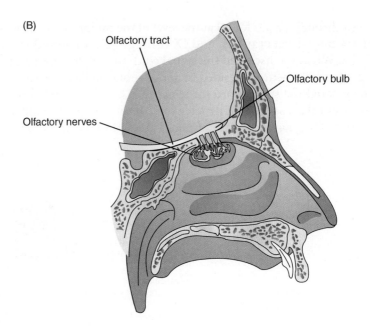

Figure 11-37 continued.
(B) Olfactory bulb, nerves, and tract.
© Cengage Learning®.

Unlike spinal nerves, cranial nerves are differentiated based upon seven defining characteristics or categories. Cranial nerve functions are divided into *general* and *special*, with areas of service being *somatic* and *visceral*. Nerves can be efferent, afferent, or mixed efferent/afferent as well. Thus, you will see the notation *general somatic afferent* for one component of the V trigeminal nerve that combines all three functional categories.

General somatic afferent (GSA) nerves are sensory nerves involved in communicating the sensory information from skin, muscles, and joints, including pain, temperature, mechanical stimulation of skin, length and tension of muscle, and movement and position of joints. That is, GSA nerves provide general information about body function, and this information usually reaches consciousness (although the fact that this information reaches the level of consciousness does not necessarily mean that you attend to it). **Special somatic afferent** (SSA) nerves, in contrast, serve the special body senses such as vision and hearing. **General visceral afferent** (GVA) nerves transmit sensory information from receptors in visceral structures, such as the digestive tract; this information only infrequently reaches conscious levels. **Special visceral afferent** (SVA) nerves provide information from the special visceral senses of taste and smell.

Efferent nerves follow parallel form. **General visceral efferent** (GVE) nerves are the autonomic efferent fibers serving viscera and glands. **General somatic efferent** (GSE) nerves provide the innervation of skeletal muscle and are quite important for speech production. The "wild cards" in this mixture are the **special visceral efferent** (SVE) nerves, which are involved with the innervation of striated muscle of branchial arch origin, including the larynx, pharynx, soft palate, face, and muscles of mastication.

Specific Cranial Nerves

I Olfactory Nerve (SVA)

The olfactory nerve is not a true cranial nerve because it reaches the brain without passing through the thalamus first. This *special visceral afferent* nerve mediates the sense of smell (olfaction), which developed quite early in our phylogenetic development. The olfactory sensors are embedded in the epithelium of the nasal cavity, including the superior conchae and the septum.

Dendrites of the bipolar cells that make up this nerve pass superiorly through the cribriform plate of the ethmoid bone to enter one of the paired **olfactory bulbs**, the nuclei of the nerve that resides within the cranium, at the base of the brain (see Figure 11-37). The olfactory nerve divides into medial and lateral branches. The lateral branches communicate with the olfactory cortex, which is made up of the pyriform lobe and hippocampal formation.

II Optic Nerve (SSA)

Although not technically related to speech, hearing, or language, the optic nerve provides valuable clinical insight into the extent of damage arising from cerebrovascular accident. The optic nerve is the *special somatic afferent* component associated with the visual system. Motor function of the eye is accommodated through other nerves.

The retinal cells receive stimulation from light, and output from the rod and cone cells of the retina (first-order neurons) is relayed to bipolar cells and modified by horizontal interneuron cells (second-order neurons). The output of these cells is transmitted by alterations of membrane potential, but in the absence of an action potential. The result of this complex process of inhibition and excitation is transmitted to the dendrite of the bipolar ganglion cells of the optic nerve (third-order neurons) whose cell bodies lie in the **lateral geniculate body (LGB)**, a nucleus of the thalamus.

Visual information can take three different paths following synapse at the LGB (Mackay, Chapman, & Morgan, 1997). Eighty percent of information passes from the retina to the lateral geniculate body, and then to the calcarine sulcus. It is thought that this pathway is involved in spatial discrimination and form analysis. Information used for motor response passes from the retina to the thalamus and subsequently to the cerebrum, whereas the final pathway passes

Damage to the I Olfactory Nerve

Trauma to the nasal region can result in the loss of CSF through the nose **(cerebrospinal fluid rhinorrhea)**, which alternatively becomes a route for **meningeal infection** (infection of the meningeal linings of the brain). The most common trauma resulting in **anosmia** (loss of sense of smell and taste) is an injury involving frontal impact, probably because of damage to the sensory apparatus itself, especially because of shearing forces applied to the nerve at the cribriform plate.

to the brain stem to mediate reflexes associated with vision, such as the pupillary responses to light. See the Clinical Note on this cranial nerve for an interesting insight into the different responses that can be manifested because of damage to one component of this pathway.

The paired optic nerves converge on the optic chiasm. Information from the medial half of the retina decussates there, whereas information from the lateral half of each retina remains uncrossed (see Figure 11-38).

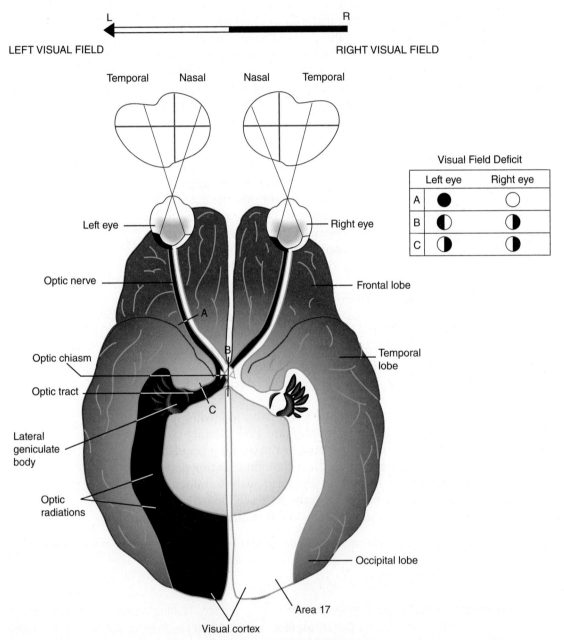

Figure 11-38. Representation of the visual pathway and effect of site of lesion. A cut in the optic nerve at point A would eliminate both left and right visual fields of the left eye. A lesion at point B would cause loss of information from the right and left temporal fields (heteronymous bitemporal hemianopsia). A lesion at point C on the optic tract will result in loss of information from the right visual field of both eyes (homonymous hemianopsia).

Lesions of the II Optic Nerve and Tract

Function provides a window on the site of a lesion. In the visual system, the degree of visual **cut** or loss will give clues about the location of damage to the nerve or tract. Figure 11-38 illustrates the pathway, with reference to a visual image presented to the eyes. The image will reverse as it passes through the lens, so that it is inverted both vertically and horizontally when projected upon the retina.

Information is sensed and transduced such that light reaching the medial portion of the retina (area nearest the nose) crosses at the chiasm, whereas that on the lateral portion of the retina (near the temples) remains ipsilateral. Thus, light from the left **visual field** strikes the left medial and right lateral retinae, combining in the right hemisphere of the brain. Likewise, information from the right visual field strikes the right medial and left lateral retinae and courses to the left cerebral hemisphere. In this manner, left visual field enters the right hemisphere, and right visual field enters the left hemisphere.

Difficulties occur when part of the pathway is damaged. Definition of an individual's visual impairment is always with reference to the damage to the visual field. If a lesion to the optic tract occurs behind the optic chiasm, the result will be loss of vision of the opposite field. Right optic tract damage will result in loss of left visual field, as in point C on the figure. This is referred to as left **homonymous** ("having the same name," or more appropriately, same side) **hemianopia** (blindness in half of the field of vision).

A lesion arising at the chiasm (point B), such as a tumor compressing the nerve, will result the in loss of decussating information. In this case, the right eye will lose right visual field and the left eye will lose the left visual field. This is termed **heteronymous** (different side) **bitemporal** (affecting both temporal regions) **hemianopia**. A patient with a chiasm lesion may also lose olfaction, because of the close proximity of the olfactory nerve.

Traumatic injury to the optic nerve and tract can have devastating and seemingly paradoxical effects. A blow to the region of the eyebrow frequently results in unilateral optic neuropathy by compressing the optic nerve at the optic canal. Visual impairment resulting from trauma may also arise from occipital lobe damage, resulting in cortical blindness or inability to process higher-level visual information. Because of the separate pathways mediating visuo-spatial information and movement, cortical blindness arising from trauma or cerebrovascular accident may leave the individual responsive to moving visual stimulation because of sparing of the retinal-thalamic-cortical pathway associated with oculomotor function (see Mackay, Chapman, & Morgan, 1997).

Crossed and uncrossed information passes through the optic tract to the LGB. Dendrites of fourth-order neurons synapse and course via the optic radiation (geniculostriate projection) to the occipital lobe (Brodmann's area 17), the primary receptive area of the cerebral cortex. Branches from the LGB course to the **superior colliculus** of the midbrain, an apparent point of interaction between visual and auditory information received at the inferior colliculus and the relay involved in orienting to visual stimuli. The image from the retina is neurally projected onto the occipital lobe, inverted from the real-world object it represents.

III Oculomotor Nerve (GSE, GVE)

The III oculomotor is comprised of two components. The *general somatic efferent* component serves the extrinsic ocular muscles ipsilaterally, including the superior levator palpebrae; superior, medial, and inferior rectus muscles; and inferior oblique muscle. The only ocular muscles not innervated by the III oculomotor nerves are the superior oblique and lateral rectus muscles (see Figure 11-39). The oculomotor nuclei are found within the midbrain at the level of the superior colliculus, an important relay for the visual system.

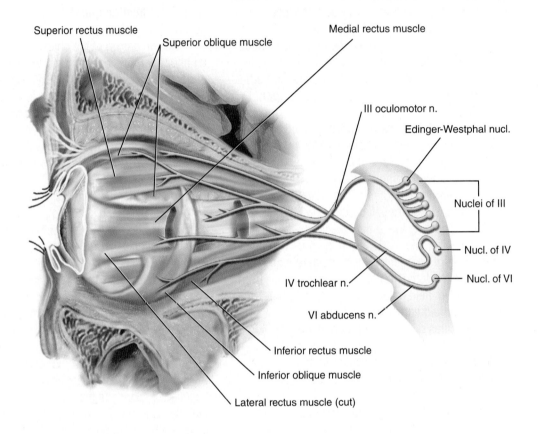

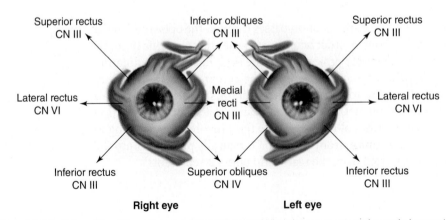

Figure 11-39. Schematic of III oculomotor, IV trochlear, and VI abducens nerve and muscle innervated.
© Cengage Learning®.

Axons from the nuclei course through the red nucleus and medial to the cerebral peduncles, exiting the brain stem to differentiate into inferior and superior branches. Activation of muscles served by the oculomotor nucleus results in the eye being turned up and out (temporally), inward (nasally), or down and out.

The *general visceral efferent* component arising from the Edinger–Westphal (accessory oculomotor) nucleus provides light and accommodation reflexes associated with pupil constriction and focus. The nuclei reside ventral to the cerebral aqueduct, emerge medial to the cerebral peduncle, and pass into the orbit via the superior orbital fissure.

IV Trochlear Nerve (GSE)

The IV trochlear is broadly classed as a *general somatic efferent* nerve. It arises from the trochlear nucleus of the midbrain and innervates the ipsilateral superior oblique muscle of the eye, which turns the eye down and slightly out. Fibers of the trochlear nerve course around the cerebral peduncles and enter the orbit.

Lesion to the III Oculomotor, IV Trochlear, and VI Abducens Nerves

These three nerves provide motor control of the eye, eyelid, and iris. The III oculomotor nerve passes near the circle of Willis and is subject to compression from tumors, aneurysms, or hemorrhage. It serves the muscles responsible for adducting the eye (superior rectus, medial rectus, inferior rectus, and inferior oblique muscles), for elevating the eyelid (levator palpebrae), and for pupil constriction. A left motor neuron (LMN) lesion of one of the oculomotor nerves will result in ipsilateral paralysis, because decussation occurs before this level. Because of the unopposed activity of the lateral rectus (which rotates the eye out) oculomotor paralysis will result in abduction (outward deviation, or **divergent strabismus**) of the eye and inability to turn the eye in, **ptosis** (drooping of the eyelid), and **mydriasis** (abnormal dilation of the pupil). Control of the III nerve arises predominantly from area 8 of the frontal lobe, with a projection to the superior colliculus, and from there to the contralateral pontine reticular formation and nuclei for the III, IV, and VI nerves. Because of the extreme coordination of movements of the two eyes for **convergence** (bringing the eyes together) and **conjugate movement** (moving the eyes together to look toward the same side), hemispheric damage affecting ocular movements will result in contralateral involvement. That is, right hemisphere damage results in an inability to turn the eyes to the left side, because the right hemisphere controls movements of the eyes to the left. In other words, the patient with UMN lesion will "look at the lesion."

LMN lesion of the IV trochlear nerve affects the superior oblique muscle. When an eye rotates medially, the superior oblique is able to pull the eye down, and paralysis will result in loss of this ability. The VI abducens nerve controls the lateral rectus, which rotates the eye out. An LMN lesion to this nerve results in **internal strabismus** (eye is rotated in). The concomitant inability to fuse the visual images from both eyes is called **diplopia**, or double vision.

Traumatic injury to the IV trochlear and VI abducens is more frequent than damage to the III oculomotor nerve. Surgical intervention to remedy the diplopia is typically attempted after nine months, giving the nerves an opportunity to recover function and stabilize. Surgery is performed to eliminate double vision in the reading position (see Mackay, Chapman, & Morgan, 1997).

V Trigeminal Nerve (GSA, SVE)

The V trigeminal nerve is an extremely important mixed nerve for speech production, as it provides motor supply to the muscles of mastication and transmits sensory information from the face. As Figure 11-40 indicates, the nerve arises from the motor trigeminal nucleus and sensory nucleus of the trigeminal within the upper pons, emerging from the pons at the level of the superior margin of the temporal bone. An enlargement in the nerve indicates the trigeminal ganglion containing pseudounipolar cells, and there the nerve divides into three components: the ophthalmic, maxillary, and mandibular nerves.

The **ophthalmic nerve** is the small, superior nerve of the trigeminal, and is entirely sensory. The *general somatic afferent* component of the ophthalmic branch transmits general sensory information from the skin of the upper face, forehead, scalp, cornea, iris, upper eyelid, conjunctiva, nasal cavity mucous membrane, and lacrimal gland.

The **maxillary nerve** is only sensory, being *general somatic afferent* in nature (see Figure 11-41). It transmits information from the lower eyelid, skin on the sides of the nose, upper jaw, teeth, lip, mucosal lining of buccal and nasal cavities, maxillary sinuses, and nasopharynx.

The **mandibular nerve** is both *general somatic afferent* and *special visceral efferent*. This largest branch of the trigeminal nerve exits the skull via the foramen ovale of the sphenoid and gives rise to a number of branching nerves. The afferent component conducts general somatic afferent information from a region roughly encompassing the mandible, including the skin, lower teeth, gums, and lip; a portion of the skin and mucosal lining of the cheek; the external auditory meatus and auricle; the temporomandibular joint; and the region of the temporal bone, as well as kinesthetic and proprioceptive sense of muscles of mastication. The **lingual nerve** conducts somatic sensation from the anterior two-thirds of the mucous membrane of the tongue and floor of the mouth.

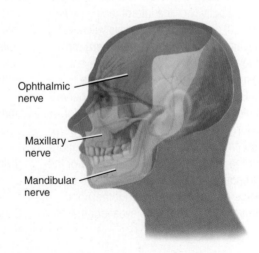

Ophthalmic nerve

Maxillary nerve

Mandibular nerve

Figure 11-40. Areas served by the nerves arising from the V trigeminal nerve.
© Cengage Learning®.

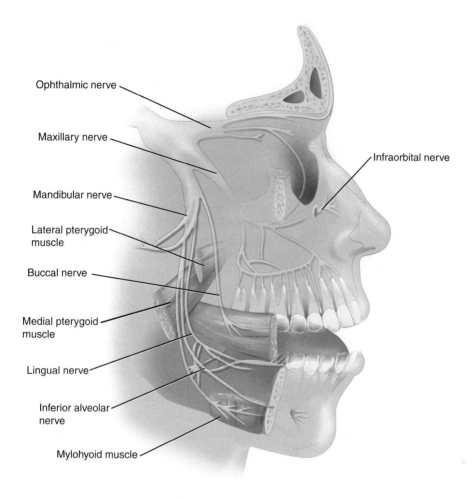

Ophthalmic nerve

Maxillary nerve

Mandibular nerve

Lateral pterygoid muscle

Buccal nerve

Medial pterygoid muscle

Lingual nerve

Inferior alveolar nerve

Mylohyoid muscle

Infraorbital nerve

Figure 11-41. Ophthalmic, maxillary, and mandibular branches of the V trigeminal nerve.
© Cengage Learning®.

The *special visceral efferent* component arises from the trigeminal motor nucleus of the pons, innervates the muscles of mastication (masseter, medial and lateral pterygoids, temporalis), the tensor tympani, the mylohyoid, the anterior digastricus, and the tensor veli palatini muscles. Note that taste is *not* mediated by the trigeminal, but the pain from biting the tip of your tongue is.

VI Abducens Nerve (GSE)

As the name implies, the **VI abducens** (or **abducent**) is an abductor, providing *general somatic efferent* innervation to the lateral rectus ocular muscle. It arises from the abducens nucleus of the pons, which is embedded in the wall of the 4th ventricle and emerges from the brain stem at the junction of the pons and medulla. The abducens enters the orbit via the superior orbital fissure to innervate the lateral rectus.

Lesions of the V Trigeminal Nerve

The V trigeminal nerve has both motor and sensory components, and all have the potential to be affected by lesions. UMN damage to the V trigeminal will result in minimal motor deficit because of strong bilateral innervation by each hemisphere. With UMN lesion, you may see increased **jaw jerk reflex** (elicited by pulling down on the passively opened mandible). LMN damage will result in **atrophy** (wasting) and weakness on the affected side. When your patient closes his or her mouth, the jaw will deviate toward the side of the lesion because of the action of the intact internal pterygoid muscle. The jaw will hang open with bilateral LMN damage, which has an extreme effect on speech. The tensor veli palatini is also innervated by the trigeminal, and weakness or paralysis may result in hypernasality because of the role of this muscle in maintaining the velopharyngeal sphincter.

Damage to the sensory component of the V cranial nerve will result in loss of tactile sensation for the anterior two-thirds of the tongue, loss of the corneal blink reflex elicited by touching the cornea with cotton, and alteration of sensation at the orifice of the Eustachian tube, external auditory meatus, tympanic membrane, teeth, and gums. Sensation of the forehead, upper face, and nose region will be lost with ophthalmic branch lesion, and the sensation to the skin region roughly lateral to the zygomatic arch and over the maxilla will be lost with maxillary branch lesion. Damage to the mandibular branch will affect sensation from the side of the face down to the mandible. **Trigeminal neuralgia (tic douloureux)** may also arise from damage to the V cranial nerve. The result of this is severe and sharp shooting pain along the course of the nerve, which may be restricted to areas served by only one of the branches.

VII Facial Nerve (SVE, SVA, GVE)

The facial nerve is quite important to any discussion of speech musculature. This nerve supplies efferent innervation to the facial muscles of expression and tear glands, as well as sense of taste for a portion of the tongue. It communicates with the X vagus, V trigeminal, VIII vestibulocochlear, and IX glossopharyngeal nerves.

The *special visceral efferent* component arises from the motor nucleus of the facial nerve within the reticular formation of the inferior pons. As you may see in Figure 11-42, fibers from both hemispheres of the cerebral cortex terminate on this nucleus. The motor nucleus is divided, so that not all muscles are innervated bilaterally. The upper facial muscles receive bilateral cortical input, whereas those of the lower face receive only contralateral innervation. Unilateral damage to the cerebral cortex will produce contralateral deficit in the lower facial muscles, but no noticeable deficit of the upper muscles, because those receive innervation from both cerebral hemispheres. That is, left hemisphere damage could result in right facial paralysis of the oral muscles, but spare the ability to wrinkle the forehead, close the eye, and so forth.

The nerve exits the pons at the cerebellopontine angle to enter the internal auditory meatus (see Figure 11-43), coursing laterally through the facial canal of the temporal bone. At the geniculate ganglion, the nerve turns to continue as a medial prominence in the

RIGHT HEMISPHERE   LEFT HEMISPHERE

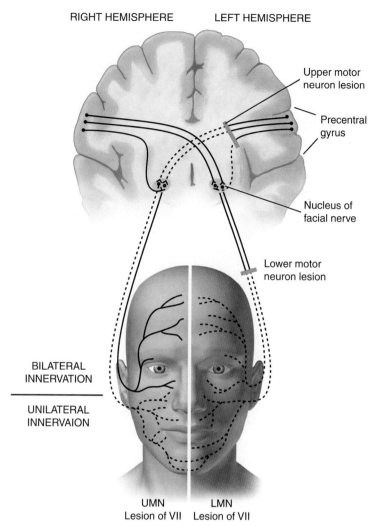

Figure 11-42. Effects of upper and lower motor neuron lesion of the VII facial nerve on facial muscle function.

Based on Source: After view of Gilman & Winans, 2002.

middle ear cavity. A twig of the facial nerve, the **chorda tympani**, enters the cavity and passes medial to the malleus and tympanic membrane. It ultimately joins the lingual nerve of the V trigeminal.

The facial nerve exits at the stylomastoid foramen of the temporal bone, coursing between and innervating the stylohyoid and posterior digastricus muscles. The nerve branches into **cervicofacial** and **temporofacial** divisions. The cervicofacial division further gives off the buccal, lingual, marginal mandibular, and cervical branches, whereas the temporofacial division gives rise to the temporal and zygomatic branches.

The *general visceral efferent* component of the facial nerve arises from the **salivatory nucleus** of the pons, forming the **nervus intermedius**. Fibers from the nervus intermedius innervate the **lacrimal**

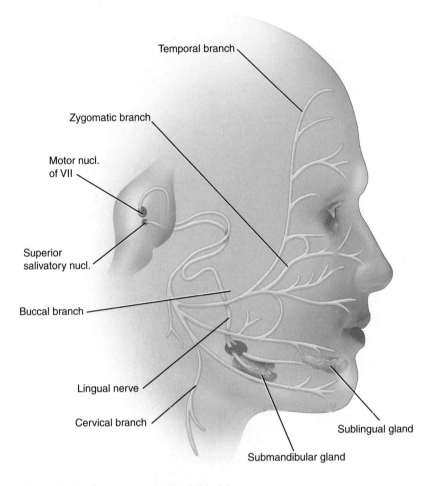

Figure 11-43. General course of the VII facial nerve.
© Cengage Learning®.

gland (for tearing), the **sublingual gland** beneath the tongue, and the **submandibular gland**.

The *special visceral afferent* sense of taste (gustation) arising from the anterior two-thirds of the tongue is mediated by the facial nerve. Information is transmitted via the chorda tympani to the nervus intermedius, and ultimately to the **solitary tract nucleus**.

VIII Vestibulocochlear Nerve (SSA)

This nerve is extremely important for both the speech-language pathologist and the audiologist because it mediates both auditory information and sense of movement in space. The nerve consists of both afferent and efferent components. The *special somatic afferent* portion mediates information concerning hearing and balance, whereas the efferent component appears to assist in selectively damping the output of hair cells (see Figures 11-44 and 10-11).

Lesions of the VII Facial Nerve

Lesions of the facial nerve may significantly affect articulatory function. Because the upper motor neuron supply to the upper face is bilateral, unilateral UMN damage will not result in upper face paralysis. It may, however, paralyze all facial muscles below the eyes. Even then, muscles of facial expression (**mimetic muscles**) may be contracted involuntarily in response to emotional stimuli, because these motor gestures are initiated at regions of the brain that differ from those of speech.

LMN damage will cause upper- and lower-face paralysis on the side of the lesion. This may involve the inability to close the eyelid and will result in muscle sagging, loss of tone, and reduction in wrinkling around the lip, nose, and forehead. When the individual attempts to smile, the affected corners of the mouth will be drawn toward the unaffected side.

Your patient may drool because of loss of the ability to impound saliva with the lips, and the cheeks may puff out during expiration because of a flaccid buccinator.

Bell's palsy (palsy means "paralysis") may result from any compression of the VII nerve, or even from cold weather. It results in the paralysis of facial musculature, which remits in most cases within a few months.

Damage to the facial nerve following penetrating facial or cranial trauma is quite common. Damage to the middle ear or skull fractures involving the temporal bone will both result in facial nerve damage. Most fractures of the temporal bone occur along the long axis of the temporal bone, although facial paralysis is much more likely if the fracture is transverse (see Mackay, Chapman, & Morgan, 1997).

Acoustic Branch. Information concerning acoustic stimulation at the **cochlea** is transmitted via short dendrites to the spiral ganglion within the modiolus of the bony labyrinth. The spiral ganglion consists of bodies of bipolar cells whose axons project through the internal auditory meatus, where the nerve joins with the vestibular branch of the VIII nerve. The nerve enters the medulla oblongata at the junction with the pons to synapse with the **dorsal cochlear nucleus (DCN)** and the **ventral cochlear nucleus (VCN)**, lateral to the inferior cerebellar peduncle.

Vestibular Branch. The vestibular branch of the VIII cranial nerve transmits information concerning acceleration and position in space to the bipolar cells of the **vestibular ganglion** within the internal auditory meatus. From within the pons, fibers branch to synapse in the nuclei of the pons and medulla, as well as directly to the flocculonodular lobe of the cerebellum. Within the pons and medulla, the vestibular branch communicates with the superior, medial, lateral, and inferior vestibular nuclei. Vestibular nuclei project to the spinal cord, cerebellum, thalamus, and cerebral cortex.

Efferent Component. Although considered to be a sensory device, the cochlea is served by efferent fibers of the **olivocochlear bundle**. Despite the fact that this pathway has only about 1,600 fibers (compared with the 30,000 fibers of the afferent VIII), activation of the bundle has a significant attenuating effect on the output of the hair cells with which they communicate.

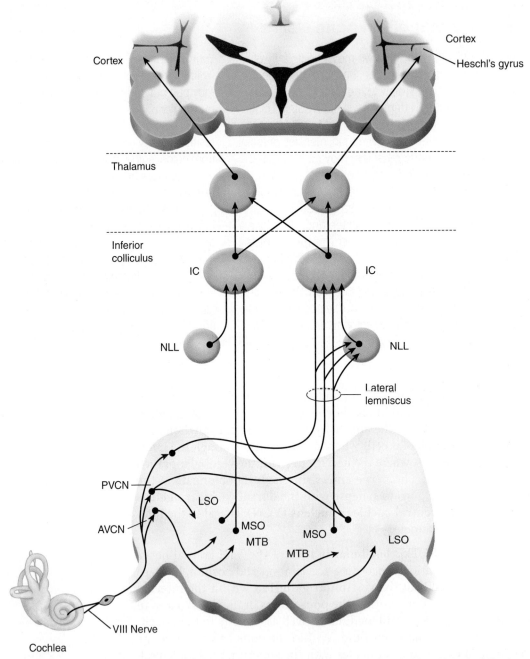

Figure 11-44. The auditory pathway, showing the nuclei of the brain stem involved in audition. Note the following: AVCN, Anteroventral Cochlear Nucleus; PVCN, Posteroventral Cochlear Nucleus; DCN, Dorsal Cochlear Nucleus; LSO, Lateral Superior Olive; MSO, Medial Superior Olive; MTB, Medial Nucleus of Trapezoid Body; NLL, Nucleus of Lateral Lemniscus; IC, Inferior Colliculus; MGB, Medial Geniculate Body.

Based on Source: Pickles, J. O. (2012). An Introduction to the physiology of hearing. Bingley, UK: Emerald Group Publishing.

Lesions of the VIII Vestibulocochlear Nerve

Clearly, damage to the VIII nerve will result in ipsilateral hearing loss, reflecting the degree of trauma. Damage to the VIII nerve may arise from a number of causes, including physical trauma (skull fracture), tumor growth compressing the nerve (benign but life-threatening tumors of the myelin sheath will result in slow-onset unilateral hearing loss and other symptoms as compression of the brain stem increases), or vascular incident. Damage to the vestibular component of the VIII nerve may result in disturbances of equilibrium arising from the loss of information concerning position in space.

Traumatic injury to the VIII vestibulocochlear nerve usually arises from fracture of the temporal bone or penetrating injury, such as that from gunshot wounds. A fracture along the long axis of the temporal bone will often result in sensorineural loss and vertigo without VIII nerve compression or apparent damage to the labyrinth. If the fracture is in the transverse dimension, the VII and VIII nerves may well be sheared or compressed. Vertigo and nystagmus in head injury often occur when the head position is changed (as in turning the head, looking up or down, or turning a corner when walking): In the absence of evidence of physical damage to the labyrinth, it is hypothesized that the vertigo and nystagmus arise from the disturbance of calcium particles used within the sensory mechanisms of the vestibular system. Fortunately, most trauma-induced vertigo remits over time (see Mackay, Chapman, & Morgan, 1997).

The **crossed olivocochlear bundle (COCB)** arises from a region near the **medial superior olive** (MSO) of the olivary complex. Fibers descend, and most of them decussate near the 4th ventricle and communicate with **outer hair cells**. The **uncrossed olivocochlear bundle (UCOB)** originates near the **lateral superior olive** of the olivary complex, with most of the fibers projecting ipsilaterally to the **inner hair cells** of the cochlea. It is believed that the olivocochlear bundle can be controlled through cortical activity and may be active in signal detection within noise.

Auditory Pathway. The auditory pathway to the cerebral cortex is illustrated in Figure 11-44 (see also Chapter 10, Figures 10-11 and 10-13): Dendrites of VIII nerve fibers synapsing on cochlear hair cells become depolarized following adequate mechanical stimulation via the cochlear traveling wave. Axons of the bipolar cells of the VIII vestibulocochlear nerve project to the cochlear nucleus, which is functionally divided into the dorsal cochlear nucleus (DCN), anteroventral cochlear nucleus (AVCN), and posteroventral cochlear nucleus (PVCN) of the pons. (Some anatomists distinguish only two nuclei, the DCN and the ventral cochlear nucleus.) Projections from the VIII nerve are arrayed **tonotopically** within the cochlear nucleus, reflecting the organization of the cochlear partition. That is, there is an orderly array of fibers representing the information processed within the cochlea, from low to high frequency. This order is maintained throughout the auditory nervous system.

Projections from the cochlear nucleus take the form of **acoustic striae**. The **dorsal acoustic stria** arises from the DCN, coursing around the inferior cerebellar peduncle. It decussates, bypasses the superior olivary complex (SOC) and lateral lemniscus, and makes synapse at the inferior colliculus (IC). Fibers of the **ventral acoustic stria** course anterior to the inferior cerebellar peduncle and terminate in the contralateral superior olivary nuclei. The **intermediate acoustic stria** arises from the PVCN and terminates at the ipsilateral superior olivary complex.

The medial superior olive (MSO) and lateral superior olive (LSO, also known as the **s-segment**) are major auditory nuclei of the superior olivary complex within the pons. Localization of sound in the environment is processed primarily at this level. High-frequency information at the LSO provides the binaural intensity cue for the location of sound in space, whereas low-frequency information projected to the MSO provides the interaural phase (frequency) cue for localization. In addition, the crossed and uncrossed olivocochlear bundles arise from cells peripheral to the MSO and LSO nuclei.

As you can see from the schematic of the auditory pathway, fibers from the SOC ascend to the lateral lemniscus and inferior colliculus, structures apparently involved in localization of sound. You may also notice that there are ample decussations throughout the pathway, following cochlear nucleus synapse. Indeed, the auditory pathway is primarily crossed, although a small ipsilateral component is retained. Unilateral deafness will result from cochlea or VIII nerve damage, but not from unilateral damage to the auditory pathway above the level of the auditory nerve. Although much hearing function will be retained because of the redundant pathway, interaction of the two ears is essential for localization of sound in space, and damage to the brain stem nuclei will result in loss of discrimination function. Of course, complete bilateral sectioning of the pathway would result in complete loss of auditory function.

The medial geniculate body (MGB), a thalamic nucleus, is the final auditory relay. The **auditory radiation** (also known as the **geniculotemporal radiation**) projects from the MGB to Heschl's gyrus (area 41) of the temporal lobe. This segment of the dorsal surface of the superior temporal convolution is partially hidden in the Sylvian fissure, and projections to the auditory cortex retain tonotopic organization. The adjacent area 42 is an auditory association area, which projects to other areas of the brain, as well as to the contralateral auditory cortex via the corpus callosum (see Chapter 10 for a discussion of the architecture of the auditory reception region.)

IX Glossopharyngeal Nerve (GSA, GVA, SVA, GVE, SVE)

The IX glossopharyngeal nerve serves both sensory and motor functions (see Figure 11-45). The motor component arises from the nucleus ambiguus and inferior salivatory nucleus of the medulla, whereas axons of the sensory component terminate in the medulla at

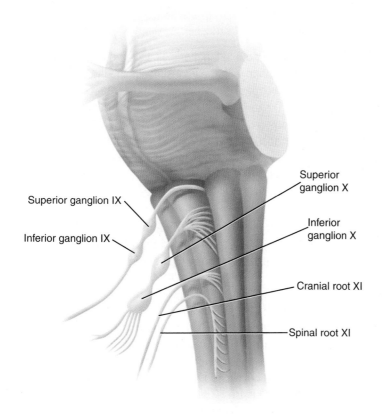

Superior ganglion IX

Inferior ganglion IX

Superior ganglion X

Inferior ganglion X

Cranial root XI

Spinal root XI

Figure 11-45. Relation of glossopharyngeal nerve to vagus and accessory nerves.
© Cengage Learning®.

the **solitary tract nucleus** and **spinal tract nucleus** of the V trigeminal. The rootlets emerge in the ventrolateral aspect of the medulla, converge, and exit the skull through the jugular foramen of the temporal bone. The nerve courses deep to the styloid process of the temporal bone and beside the stylopharyngeus muscle. It enters the base of the tongue after penetrating the superior constrictor muscle. The nerve has **superior and inferior (petrosal) ganglia**.

The *special visceral afferent* function of the nerve mediates sensation from taste receptors of the posterior one-third of the tongue and a portion of the soft palate, with this information delivered to the solitary tract nucleus. Impulses from **baroreceptors** within the carotid sinus convey information concerning arterial pressure within the common carotid artery to the same nucleus. The *general visceral afferent* component provides sensation of touch, pain, and temperature from the posterior one-third of the tongue, as well as from the faucial pillars, upper pharynx, and Eustachian tube to the inferior ganglion.

General somatic afferent information from the region behind the auricle and external auditory meatus is transmitted by the superior branch of the IX glossopharyngeal to the nucleus of the spinal trigeminal via the superior ganglion.

Efferent innervation by the IX glossopharyngeal includes *special visceral efferent* activation of the stylopharyngeus and superior

Lesions of the IX Glossopharyngeal Nerve

The IX glossopharyngeal nerve works in concert with the X vagus, making its independent function difficult to determine. Damage to the IX nerve will result in paralysis of the stylopharyngeus muscle and may result in the loss of general sensation (**anesthesia**) for the posterior one-third of the tongue and pharynx, although the vagus may support these functions as well. The cooperative innervation with the vagus results in little effect on the pharyngeal constrictors, although reduced sensation of the auricle and middle ear may indicate IX nerve damage. IX nerve damage may also cause reduced or absent gag reflex, although absence of the reflex does not guarantee that a lesion exists.

constrictor muscles by means of the nucleus ambiguus. *General visceral efferent* innervation of the parotid gland for salivation arises from the inferior salivatory nucleus via the otic ganglion.

X Vagus Nerve (GSA, GVA, SVA, GVE, SVE)

The vagus nerve is both complex and important. Let us examine both motor and sensory components of this nerve. The vagus arises from the lateral medulla oblongata and exits from the skull through the jugular foramen along with the IX glossopharyngeal and XI accessory nerves (see Figure 11-46).

The vagus is served by several nuclei and ganglia. The dorsal vagal nucleus (dorsal motor nucleus) gives rise to visceral efferent fibers for parasympathetic innervation and receives information from the inferior vagal ganglion. The solitarius tract and nucleus serve taste, whereas the nucleus ambiguus provides motor innervation to laryngeal musculature and mucosa. As with the glossopharyngeal nerve, the vagus has inferior (nodose) and superior ganglia.

The *general visceral efferent* component of the vagus arises from the dorsal motor nucleus of the X vagus, providing parasympathetic motor innervation of intestines, pancreas, stomach, esophagus, trachea, and bronchial smooth muscle and mucosal glands, kidneys, liver, and the heart. This branch is responsible for inhibiting heart rate. The striated muscles of the larynx, as well as most pharyngeal and palatal muscles, are innervated by the *special visceral efferent* portion of the vagus, served by the nucleus ambiguus.

The *general somatic afferent* component of the vagus delivers pain, touch, and temperature sense from the skin covering the ear drum, posterior auricle, and external auditory meatus to the superior vagal ganglion, and subsequently to the spinal nucleus of the V trigeminal. It is this innervation that triggers nausea or vomiting when the ear drum is touched by external stimuli.

Pain sense from the mucosal lining of the lower pharynx, larynx, thoracic and abdominal viscera, esophagus, and bronchi is conveyed by means of the *general visceral afferent* component, with soma in the

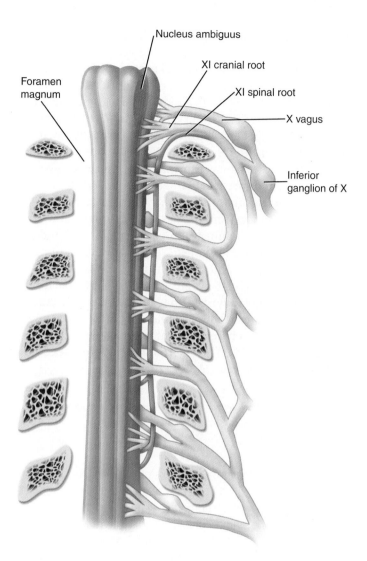

Nucleus ambiguus

XI cranial root

XI spinal root

X vagus

Inferior
ganglion of X

Foramen
magnum

Figure 11-46. Spinal accessory
nerve origins.
© Cengage Learning®.

inferior ganglion, and with axons terminating in the caudal nucleus
solitarius and dorsal vagal nucleus. Sensations of nausea and hunger
are mediated by the vagus. This GVA component supports the maintenance of heartbeat, blood pressure (via baroreceptors), respiration
(stretch receptors in the lung signal fully distended tissue to terminate inspiration), and digestion.

Taste sense from the epiglottis and valleculae is mediated by the
special visceral afferent component of the vagus, with some of these
afferent fibers residing in the inferior ganglion (Gilman & Winans,
2002). Axons from this component terminate in the caudal nucleus
solitarius.

These functions are served through four important branches of
the vagus. The auricular branch arises from the superior ganglion,
whereas the pharyngeal, recurrent laryngeal, and superior laryngeal
branches arise from the inferior ganglion.

The right **recurrent laryngeal nerve** courses under and behind the subclavian artery and ascends between the trachea and the esophagus. The left recurrent laryngeal nerve loops under the aortic arch to ascend between the trachea and esophagus. After entering the larynx between the cricoid and thyroid cartilages, tracheal and esophageal branches provide GVA innervation to the laryngeal mucosa beneath the vocal folds, and SVE innervation serves the intrinsic muscles of the larynx and the inferior pharyngeal constrictor. The auricular branch conveys sensory information from the tympanic membrane and external auditory meatus.

The **pharyngeal branch** of the vagus mediates the SVA taste sense and GVA sensation from the base of the tongue and upper pharynx. It also mediates SVE innervation of the upper and middle pharyngeal constrictors, palatopharyngeus, palatoglossus, salpingopharyngeus, levator veli palatini, and musculus uvulae. The only soft-palate muscle not innervated by the vagus is the tensor veli palatini.

The **superior laryngeal nerve** has both internal and external branches. The internal branch enters the larynx through the thyrohyoid membrane, receiving GVA information from the laryngeal region above the vocal folds. The external branch provides SVE innervation of the cricothyroid muscle.

Lesions of the X Vagus Nerve

The X vagus is the most extensive of the cranial nerves, presenting an important constellation of clinical manifestations. Damage to the pharyngeal branch will result in deficit in swallowing, potential loss of gag through interaction with the IX glossopharyngeal nerve, and hypernasality arising from weakness of the velopharyngeal sphincter (all velopharyngeal muscles are innervated by the vagus, with the exception of the tensor veli palatini, which is innervated by the trigeminal). Unilateral pharyngeal branch damage will result in failure to elevate the soft palate on the involved side (asymmetrical elevation), producing hypernasality. Bilateral lesion will produce absent or reduced (but symmetrical) movement of the soft palate, causing hypernasality, **nasal regurgitation** (loss of food and liquid through the nose), dysphagia, and paralysis of the pharyngeal musculature.

Lesions of the superior laryngeal nerve may result in loss of sensation of the upper larynx mucous membrane and stretch receptors, as well as paralysis of the cricothyroid muscle. Recurrent laryngeal nerve damage will alter sensation below the level of the vocal folds and stretch receptor information from the intrinsic muscles. Unilateral recurrent laryngeal nerve lesion typically results in a flaccid vocal fold on the side of the lesion, accompanied by hoarse and breathy voice. In bilateral lesion, the vocal folds may rarely be paralyzed in the adducted position, which is life threatening because of airway occlusion. More commonly, the vocal folds are paralyzed in the paramedian position, compromising the airway by risk of aspiration. Paralysis in the adducted position will result in **laryngeal stridor** (harsh, distressing phonation upon inspiration and expiration). Paralysis in the paramedian position may permit limited breathy and hoarse phonation with limited pitch range arising from loss of tensing ability of the vocalis. Vocal intensity range will be extremely limited by the loss of adductory ability.

XI Accessory Nerve (SVE)

The XI accessory nerve consists of both cranial and spinal components. It provides *special visceral efferent* innervation directly to the sternocleidomastoid and trapezius muscles and works in conjunction with the vagus to innervate the intrinsic muscles of the larynx, pharynx, and soft palate. The exceptions to this are the tensor veli palatini, which is innervated by the V trigeminal, and the cricothyroid muscles, which are innervated by the superior laryngeal nerve of the vagus (Figure 11-45).

The cranial root arises from the caudal portion of the nucleus ambiguus, where it is joined by the spinal root, to exit through the jugular foramen with the vagus. On exiting the skull, the internal branch of the accessory nerve joins the inferior ganglion of the vagus. The accessory nerve serves both recurrent laryngeal and pharyngeal nerves of the vagus.

The spinal root emerges from the first five spinal segments between the dorsal and ventral rootlets, ascends to enter the skull through the foramen magnum, and joins the cranial accessory nerve before exiting the skull (see Figure 11-45). The spinal root makes up the external root of the accessory nerve and innervates the sternocleidomastoid and trapezius muscles.

XII Hypoglossal Nerve (GSE)

As the name implies, this nerve provides the innervation to motor function of the tongue. *This general somatic efferent* nerve arises from the hypoglossal nucleus of the medulla, exits the skull through the hypoglossal canal, and courses with the vagus. The hypoglossal nerve descends and branches to innervate all intrinsic muscles of the tongue, and all the extrinsic muscles of the tongue except the palatoglossus, which is innervated via the XI accessory nerve through the pharyngeal plexus.

Each hypoglossal nucleus is served primarily by the contralateral corticobulbar tract, which means that *left* upper motor neuron (UMN) damage will result in *right* tongue weakness. Damage to the lower motor neurons (LMNs) will result in ipsilateral deficit, because

Lesions of the XI Accessory Nerve

Lesion to the XI accessory nerve may have an effect on the trapezius and sternocleidomastoid muscles. Unilateral lesion affecting the sternocleidomastoid will result in the patient being unable to turn his or her head away from the side of the lesion. (The left sternocleidomastoid rotates the head toward the right side when contracted.) Lesions resulting in the paralysis of trapezius will result in restricted ability to elevate the arm and a drooping shoulder on the side of the lesion.

Lesions of the XII Hypoglossal Nerve

Lesions affecting the XII hypoglossal will have a profound impact on articulation function and speech intelligibility. This nerve provides efferent innervation of intrinsic and extrinsic muscles of the tongue, as well as afferent proprioceptive supply. Unilateral LMN lesion will result in loss of movement on the side of the lesion. Muscular weakness and atrophy on the affected side will result in deviation of the tongue toward the side of the lesion (function of the normal contralateral genioglossus will cause this). **Fasciculations**, or abnormal involuntary twitching or movement of muscle fibers, may occur before atrophy, arising from damage to the cell body. At rest the tongue may deviate toward the unaffected side before because of the tonic pull of the normal styloglossus muscle. Upper motor lesion may result in muscle weakness and impaired volitional movements with accompanying spasticity.

Cranial Nerve 0: The Terminal Nerve

The final nerve we wish to discuss is also the first one. The terminal nerve (cranial nerve 0) was first discovered in sharks in the early twentieth century and is known to mediate pheromones that are used for sexual-partner selection and identification. Recent discussion reveals that it may be functional in humans. Cranial nerve 0 terminates in the vomeronasal organ, located on either side of the nasal septum. It is clearly evident in sharks and other animals, but the field is divided on whether it exists *functionally* in humans. Fuller and Burger (1990) found positive evidence of the terminal nerve in adult humans, and recent studies indicate that, indeed, humans may use this nerve as a subconscious but very real means of mate selection. Although many feel that it is most likely vestigial, it is found in almost half of humans, dependent upon the study. An article by Fields (2007) shows strong evidence that not only is the terminal nerve present in humans, but we use that information for mate selection.

the fibers of the corticobulbar tract decussate before reaching the hypoglossal nucleus. Thus, left UMN damage or right LMN damage will affect muscles of the right side of the tongue. When the tongue is protruded, it will point to the side of the paralyzed muscles, because contraction of the posterior genioglossus is bilaterally unequal.

✔ *To summarize:*

- **Cranial nerves** are extremely important to the speech-language pathologist.
- Cranial nerves may be **sensory, motor,** or **mixed sensory-motor** and are categorized based on their function as being **general** or **specialized** and as serving **visceral** or **somatic** organs or structures.
- The **I olfactory nerve** serves the sense of smell, and the **II optic nerve** communicates visual information to the brain.

- The **III oculomotor**, **IV trochlear**, and **VI abducens nerves** provide innervation for eye movements.
- The **V trigeminal nerve** innervates muscles of **mastication** and the **tensor veli palatini** and communicates sensation from the face, mouth, teeth, mucosal lining, and tongue.
- The **VII facial nerve** innervates muscles of **facial expression**, and the sensory component serves taste of the anterior two-thirds of the tongue.
- The **VIII vestibulocochlear nerve** mediates auditory and vestibular sensation.
- The **IX glossopharyngeal nerve** serves the **posterior tongue taste** receptors, as well as somatic sense from the tongue, fauces, pharynx, and Eustachian tube.
- The **stylopharyngeus** and **superior pharyngeal constrictor** muscles receive motor innervation via this nerve.
- The **X vagus nerve** is extremely important for autonomic function as well as somatic motor innervation.
- Somatic sensation of **pain**, **touch**, and **temperature** from the region of the **ear drum** is mediated by the vagus, as well as pain sense from **pharynx**, **larynx**, **esophagus**, and many other regions.
- The **recurrent laryngeal nerve** and **superior laryngeal nerves** supply motor innervation for the intrinsic muscles of the larynx.
- The **XI accessory nerve** innervates the **sternocleidomastoid** and **trapezius** muscles and collaborates with the vagus in the activation of palatal, laryngeal, and pharyngeal muscles.
- The **XII hypoglossal nerve** innervates the **muscles of the tongue** with the exception of the **palatoglossus**.

Anatomy of the Spinal Cord

Anatesse Lesson

The spinal cord is the information lifeline to and from the periphery of the body. Movement of axial skeletal muscles occurs by means of information passed through this structure, and sensory information from the periphery must pass through it as well. The spinal cord is a long mass of neurons, with both cell bodies and projections from (and to) those neurons. If you can imagine taking many long lengths of rope, stretching them out and banding them together so it made a long cable, you will have the basic concept of the spinal cord. The spinal cord is the aggregation of many single-nerve fibers into bundles (called tracts) of fibers. These bundles provide communication between the peripheral body and the brain, and each bundle has unique properties. Because of this, the spinal cord can be viewed in its length (vertical anatomy) and in cross-section (transverse anatomy). Both of these views are important, because discussion of the spinal cord provides an understanding of how the brain communicates with the rest of the body. Without that communication, there would be no reason to have a brain.

Vertical Anatomy

The spinal cord is a longitudinal mass of columns. The columns consist of neurons: Gray portions are neuron cell bodies within the spinal cord, whereas white portions are the myelinated fibers of tracts that communicate information to and from the brain. The spinal cord is wrapped in **meningeal linings** (meninges), which are thin coverings that were discussed earlier in this chapter (see Figure 11-8).

The spinal cord begins at the foramen magnum of the skull (the superior margin of the atlas or C1) and courses about 46 cm through the vertebral canal produced by the vertebral column (you may want to refresh your memory of the vertebral column by reviewing Figure 2-4). You can think of the spinal cord as being safely contained within a long tube made up of connective tissue (the meningeal linings). The spinal cord is suspended within the tube by means of denticulate ligaments that pass through the meningeal linings and attach the spinal cord to the vertebral column. The lower portion of the spinal cord ends in a cone-shaped projection known as the **conus medullaris**, so that the spinal cord is present down to the level of the first lumbar vertebra. There is a fibrous projection from the conus medullaris called the **filum terminale** ("end filament"), and this joins with the toughest part of the tube surrounding the spinal cord (the **dural tube**) and then becomes the **coccygeal ligament** (see Figure 11-8). The coccygeal ligament attaches to the posterior coccyx. Thus, the spinal cord is wrapped in meningeal linings, is attached to the vertebral column laterally by denticulate ligaments, and is firmly attached to the coccyx by means of the coccygeal ligament.

What you can also see from Figure 11-47 is that there are nerves arising at regular intervals along the cord. The 31 pairs of **spinal nerves** arise from regions related to each vertebra, with the first (spinal nerve C1) arising from the spinal cord on the superior surface of the atlas (C1 vertebra). Thus, there are eight pairs of cervical spinal nerves instead of seven (the number of cervical vertebrae), 12 pairs of thoracic nerves, five pairs of lumbar and sacral nerves, and one pair of coccygeal nerves. The spinal nerves are referred to in the abbreviated manner of vertebrae, with the first thoracic spinal nerve being T1, and so forth.

During embryonic development, the spinal cord is of the same length as the vertebral column, but as the brain and body develop, the spinal cord moves up in the canal so that the adult spinal nerves course downward before exiting the vertebral column. (We have seen this same developmental configuration in the relationship between the thorax and the lungs, as you will recall.) When a child is born, the conus medullaris is at the L3 vertebral level, but it will be at the L1 level by adulthood. This changing size relationship is reflected in the relationship between the location of **spinal cord segment** (the functional unit representing the spinal nerve) and vertebra as well. The vertebrae will have a higher number than the cord segment at that vertebral level, as you can see in Figure 11-47. This becomes most marked in the caudal end, where the segment from which the

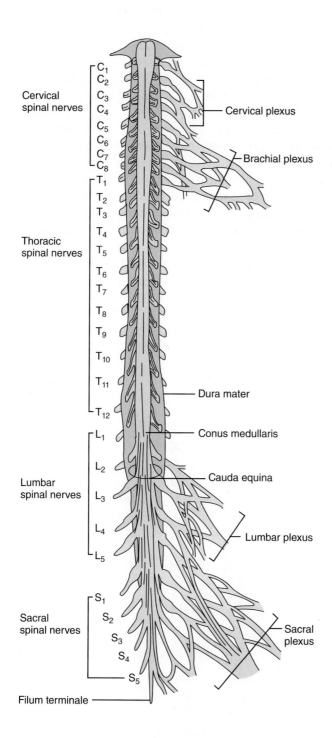

Figure 11-47. Arrangement of spinal nerves relative to vertebral segment.
© Cengage Learning®.

L5 nerve arises corresponds to the L1 vertebra. This relationship gives rise also to a rather descriptive term for the lowermost nerves. The **cauda equina** ("horse's tail") is the tail-like region beneath the filum terminale in which no spinal cord segments will be found. This is, by the way, the region chosen for a lumbar puncture to sample cerebrospinal fluid for medical testing.

Spinal nerves have both sensory (afferent) and motor (efferent) components. The distribution of sensory function is generally related to the segment level, such that upper nerves serve upper body regions, and so forth. A mapping of regions served by spinal nerve afferents reveals a fairly consistent pattern of innervation, with each region served by a nerve being functionally referred to as a **dermatome**. There is overlap of innervation, one of the safeguards of nature against complete loss of sensation. This relationship, shown in Figure 11-48, is not as clear-cut for motor function, which is mediated by cooperatives of nerves, referred to as plexuses. A plexus is a network of nerves that physically communicate with other nerves.

If you think again of the spinal cord as a series of ropes lashed together, then each of these ropes is a columnar tract, which is a collection of nerve fibers with functional unity (see Figure 11-49). If you were to cut the spinal cord transversely, you might see a segment that looked like that in Figure 11-50. In the center of the transverse section, you would see a gray "H" shape, with white matter surrounding the gray matter. The peripheral white segment is made up of myelinated ascending and descending pathways. The central matter is gray

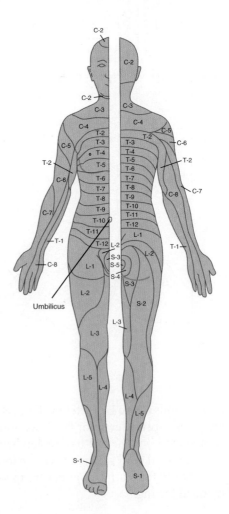

Figure 11-48. Dermatomes reflecting sensory innervation by spinal afferents.
© Cengage Learning®.

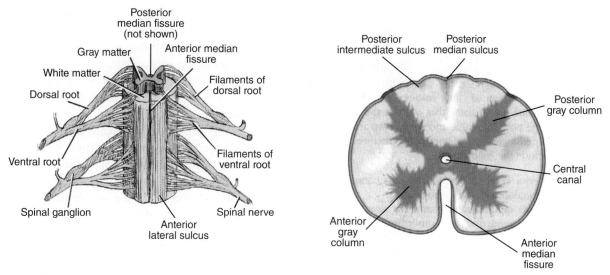

Figure 11-49. Transverse section through spinal cord, with landmarks.
© Cengage Learning®.

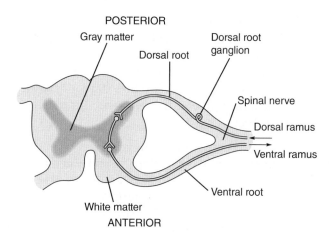

Figure 11-50. Transverse section through spinal cord and vertebral segment. Note the dorsal root ganglion and ventral root.
© Cengage Learning®.

because of the concentration of neuron bodies there. Thus, the tracts that we referred to are within the white matter, whereas the gray matter consists of neuron cell bodies that provide input to the afferent tracts or receive input from efferent tracts.

Transverse Anatomy

Several important landmarks of the sectioned spinal cord are shown in Figure 11-49. At the center of the cell mass is the **central canal**. This central canal is continuous with the 4th ventricle, a space we discussed when we talked about the cerebrum. The anterior surface of the spinal cord has a deep longitudinal **anterior median fissure** that continues through the medulla. Lateral to that is the **anterior lateral sulcus**. In the dorsal aspect you can see the **posterior median sulcus**.

Lateral to the posterior median sulcus at the cervical and upper thoracic levels is the **posterior intermediate sulcus**.

The internal spinal cord itself can be divided into gross regions. The **posterior gray column** (or **horn**) is a mass of nuclei directed posteriorly. The **anterior gray column** makes up the anterior portion of the gray matter. The white matter is divided into funiculi, which are further divided into fasciculi, as will be discussed.

Sensory information enters the spinal cord by means of the afferent neurons, the **dorsal root fibers**. The cell bodies of these sensory neurons combine into the **dorsal root ganglia**, which lie outside the spinal cord (Figures 11-49 and 11-50). Motor information leaves the spinal cord through the ventral root, but there are no "ventral root ganglia" because the cell bodies of motor neurons are housed within the spinal cord instead of outside of the cord. The dorsal and ventral roots combine to form the spinal nerve, so that each spinal nerve has both a sensory and a motor component. The spinal nerves divide into posterior and anterior parts (**dorsal** and **ventral rami**) to serve posterior and anterior portions of the body, respectively. Branches of the ventral rami course anteriorly to communicate with the sympathetic ganglia, nuclei of the autonomic nervous system. Efferent neurons of the dorsal and ventral rami communicate with muscle by means of a **motor endplate**. The motor endplate is analogous to the synapse seen as the communication between two neurons. Afferent fibers that enter the spinal cord receive their stimulation from sensors that are peripheral to the spinal cord. We now have all the elements in place for the most basic unit of interaction with the environment, the single-segment reflex arc.

The Reflex Arc. The **segmental spinal reflex arc** is the simplest stimulus–response system of the nervous system and is the most basic means that the nervous system has of responding to its environment (see Figure 11-51). Although we use the term *basic* to imply simplicity, it is not too early to let you know that many speech-language pathologists involved in oral motor therapy recognize that this "basic" response is an essential element of their therapy, because it is a critical component of adequate muscle tone.

Muscle length and tension must be continually monitored by the nervous system. Your brain needs to know where its muscles are in space and what degree of tone the muscle has. As importantly, a muscle that is supposed to hold a static or stable posture for long periods of time needs to have a system that keeps its length constant. The nervous system has a means of monitoring length and tension that fulfills both of these important functions. The muscle spindle unit senses muscle length and that information is transmitted to the brain for the purposes of programming movement. The muscle spindle also provides a way to monitor muscle length without having to bother the brain with that piece of detail.

Look at Figure 11-51. Sensory information concerning the length of the muscle is transmitted by means of dorsal root fibers to the

(A)   (B)   (C)   (D)

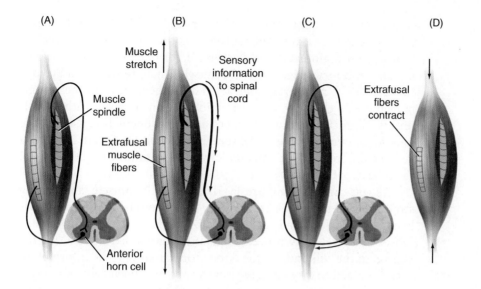

(E)

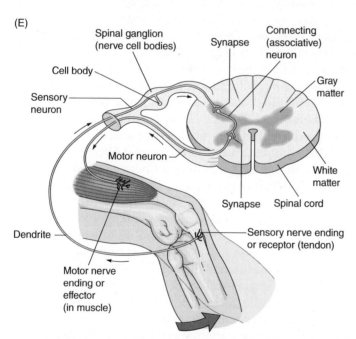

Figure 11-51. Schematic of segmental spinal reflex arc. (A) The muscle is in a stable state. (B) The muscle has been passively stretched. Information from the muscle spindle concerning muscle length is transmitted to the spinal cord via the dorsal root ganglion. (C) Synapse with motor neuron causes efferent activation of muscle fiber. (D) Extrafusal muscle contracts, shortening the muscle to its original length. (E) Patellar tendon reflex.
© Cengage Learning®.

spinal cord. The dorsal root fibers synapse with the motor neuron in the ventral cord, and the motor fiber exits the cord to innervate muscle fibers that are being sensed by the muscle spindle. Therefore, if the muscle spindle senses that a muscle has been passively stretched, that information causes the muscle that became longer passively to contract to its original length. The purpose of this reflex is to maintain the length of a muscle fiber that is not being actively contracted, typically for maintenance of posture. If, for instance, you are standing and lean forward slightly, the muscles that are stretched by your leaning will be reflexively contracted until they return to their original length. In this way, you can maintain tonic posture without voluntary effort. This is not a trivial or academic detail, because we have muscle spindles in some of the speech musculature, and that makes a very big difference in neuropathology. Let us examine the sequence of the reflex arc in detail.

As you can see in Figure 11-51B, at rest the muscle is not being stretched and the reflex arc is quiet. In Figure 11-51E, the muscle is being stretched, and a highly specialized sensor, the muscle spindle, senses that stretching process. This information is passed along the neuron to the cell body in the dorsal root ganglion. The information is then passed to a synapse within the anterior horn cells of the spinal cord. The axon synapses with the cell body of a motor neuron in the dorsal gray area of the spinal cord, and that causes the muscle it innervates to contract. Thus, when a muscle is passively stretched, it contracts to return to its original length.

To make this muscle contract, an efferent neuron had to be excited. This neuron within the gray matter of the ventral gray matter is known as the **final common pathway** or **LMN**, a very functional unit to remember (scc Figure 11 52). The LMN consists of the dendrites and soma within the spinal cord as well as the axon and components that communicate with the muscle fiber. In contrast, upper motor neurons (**UMNs**) are efferent fibers descending from upper brain levels. UMNs bring commands from the upper brain levels that activate or inhibit muscle function by synapsing with LMNs.

Damage to LMNs results in muscle weakness or complete paralysis, just as if you cut the power line leading to your radio. Damage to the UMNs will cause muscle weakness or paralysis because the information from the brain to the LMN is lost, but this UMN damage will leave reflexes intact because the spinal arc reflex is an LMN process. This has great clinical significance, which will become clearer in Chapter 12 when we examine function.

These reflexive responses are certainly important and provide a basic response to the environment. For instance, you reflexively withdraw your hand upon touching the hot burner on a stove. However, for you to make *decisions* about the information, it must reach the cerebral cortex, the seat of conscious thought. You might recall that when you touched the burner on that stove, you retracted your hand well before you felt the heat and pain. This is the hallmark of interaction between the cerebrum and the reflex. Reflexes "put out the brush fire," but neural circuitry also lets the cerebrum know that something has happened so that other action may be taken (such as putting ice on the burn). The time lag between retracting your hand and feeling the burn is an important reminder that reflexes provide nearly instant,

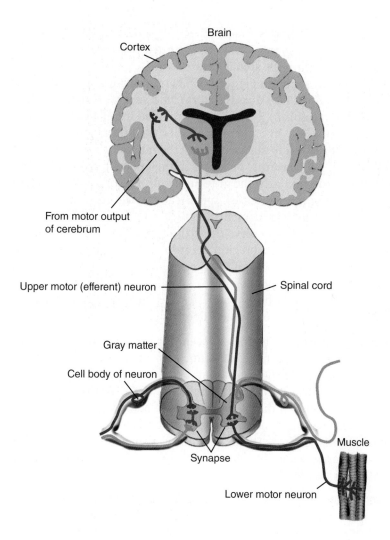

Brain

Cortex

From motor output
of cerebrum

Upper motor (efferent) neuron

Spinal cord

Gray matter

Cell body of neuron

Synapse

Muscle

Lower motor neuron

Figure 11-52. Schematic representation of UMN arising from precentral gyrus of cerebral cortex and projecting through corticospinal tract.
© Cengage Learning®.

automated response well before the cortex could ever respond. On the other hand, the simple reflex is never going to win you the Nobel Prize. These neurons will not produce conscious thought or mediate cognitive processes.

There must be a system of pathways for information to reach the higher centers or to come from those centers. Within the CNS, such pathways are referred to as tracts. Tracts are groups of axons with a functional and anatomical unity (i.e., they transmit generally the same information to generally the same locations).

Pathways of the Spinal Cord

The spinal cord is a conduit of information, and the channels are built along the longitudinal axis. The spinal cord is compartmentalized, so that it is actually subdivided into functionally and anatomically distinct areas. The gray matter of the spinal cord is divided into nine **laminae** or regions, based on cell-type differences. These laminar regions correspond well with the nuclei and regions identified anatomically within the spinal gray.

As you can see from Figure 11-53, a transverse section of the spinal cord is divided into **dorsal, lateral,** and **ventral funiculi** (a *funiculus* is a large column), which are subdivided into **fasciculi** or tracts of white matter. The size and presence of a tract depend on the level of the spinal cord. Tracts that must serve the muscles of the entire body, for instance, will certainly be larger in the upper spinal cord than in the lower cord. Similarly, the gray matter of the cord will be wider in regions serving more muscles, specifically in the cervical (segments C3 to T2) and thoracic segments (segments T9 to T12). Those regions have more cell bodies to serve the extremities. Tracts of white matter are widest in the cervical region because all descending and ascending fibers must pass through those segments. Sensory pathways tend to be in the posterior portion of the spinal cord, and motor pathways tend toward the anterior aspect, reflecting the dorsal and ventral orientation of the spinal roots (see Table 11-8).

Ascending Pathways. The major ascending sensory pathways include the fasciculus gracilis, fasciculus cuneatus, anterior and lateral spinothalamic tracts, and the anterior and posterior spinocerebellar tracts (see Figure 11-54). Neurons are referred to as first-order, second-order, and so on to indicate the number of neurons in a chain. Thus, the afferent neuron transmitting information from the sensor will be the first-order neuron, the next neuron in the chain following synapse will be the second-order neuron, and so forth up to the terminal point in the neural chain.

Posterior Funiculus. The **fasciculus gracilis** and **fasciculus cuneatus** are separated by the posterior intermediate septum of the posterior funiculus. These tracts convey information concerning touch

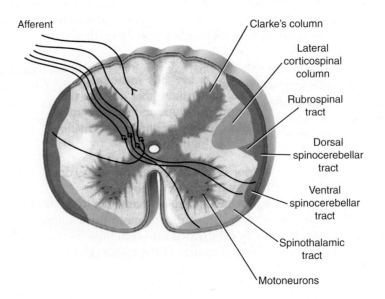

Figure 11-53. Transverse section of a spinal cord segment revealing dorsal, lateral, and anterior funiculi and major ascending tracts.
© Cengage Learning®.

Table 11-8 **Major ascending and descending pathways**

Afferent Pathways

Tract	Origin	Termination	Function
Fasciculus gracilis (lemniscal pathway)	Posterior funiculus	Nuc. gracilis	Touch pressure, vibration, kinesthetic sense, muscle stretch (spindles), muscle tension (GTOs), proprioceptionfor lower extremities
Fasciculus cuneatus (lemniscal pathway)	Posterior funiculus	Nuc. cuneatus	Touch pressure, vibration, kinesthetic sense, muscle stretch (spindles), muscle tension (GTOs), proprioception for upper extremities
Anterior spinothalamic (anterior white commissure and medial lemniscus)	Anterior funiculus	Ventral posterolateral nucleus of thalamus	Light touch
Lateral spinothalamic	Anterior funiculus	Ventral posterolateral nucleus of thalamus	Pain, thermal sense
Anterior spinocerebellar	Lateral funiculus	Vermis of cerebellum	Muscle tension from Golgi tendon organ
Posterior spinocerebellar	Lateral funiculus	Vermis of cerebellum	Muscle tension from Golgi tendon organ

Efferent Pathways

Tract	Origin	Termination	Function
Corticospinal	Frontal lobe, cerebrum	Spinal cord	Activation of skeletal muscle of extremities
Corticobulbar	Frontal lobe, cerebrum	Brain stem	Activation of muscles served by cranial nerves
Tectospinal	Superior colliculus, midbrain	C1–C4 spinal cord	Orienting reflex to visual input
Rubrospinal	Red nucleus, midbrain	Spinal cord	Flexor tone
Vestibulospinal	Lateral vestibular nuclei, pons, and medulla	Spinal cord	Extensor tone, spinal refl exes
Pontine reticulospinal	Medial tegmentum, pons	Spinal cord	Voluntary movement
Medullary reticulospinal	Medulla oblongata	Spinal cord	Voluntary movement

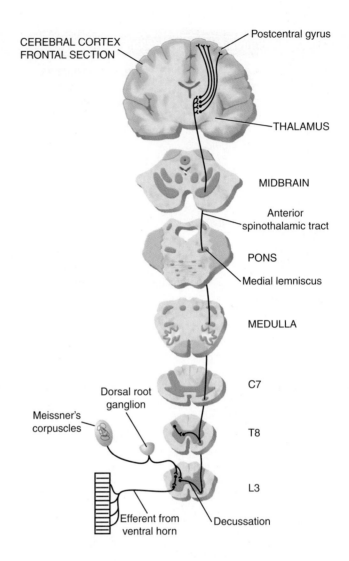

CEREBRAL CORTEX
FRONTAL SECTION

Postcentral gyrus

THALAMUS

MIDBRAIN

Anterior
spinothalamic tract

PONS

Medial lemniscus

MEDULLA

C7

Dorsal root
ganglion

Meissner's
corpuscles

T8

L3

Efferent from
ventral horn

Decussation

Figure 11-54. Anterior spinothalamic tract, transmitting information concerning the sense of light touch.
© Cengage Learning®.

pressure and **kinesthetic sense** (sense of movement), as well as vibration sense, which is actually a temporal form of touch pressure. These columns convey information from group Ia muscle spindle sensors and GTOs as well. The Ia spindle fibers convey information about rate of muscle stretch, whereas the GTOs appear to respond to stretch of the tendon.

Information concerning sensation in the periphery is conducted by the unipolar, first-order neuron of the dorsal root ganglion to the spinal cord. The axons of those neurons ascend on the same side of entry, so that the information is conveyed toward the brain. (The same information remains at the level of entry to form the spinal reflex.) The fasciculus gracilis serves the lower extremities, whereas the fasciculus cuneatus arises from the cervical regions.

The fibers of these tracts ascend **ipsilaterally** (on the same side they entered the cord) until they reach the level of the medulla oblongata of the brain stem to synapse with the nucleus gracilis and **nucleus cuneatus**. The axons of the second-order neuron arising from those nuclei combine and **decussate** (cross the midline) to ascend **contralaterally** (on the other side) as the medial lemniscus to the **thalamus**, and from the thalamus to the precentral gyrus, which is the major sensory relay of the brain (for this reason, the pathway is also referred to as the **lemniscal pathway**). **Spatiotopic** information (information about the specific region of the body stimulated) is maintained throughout the process.

Damage to these pathways will cause problems in touch discrimination, especially in the hands and feet. Patients may lose **proprioceptive sense** (sense of body position in space), which can greatly impair gait.

Anterior Funiculus. The **anterior spinothalamic tract** conveys information concerning light touch, such as the sense of being stroked by a feather, conveyed from the *spinal cord* to the *thalamus* (see Figure 11-55). Afferent axons of the first-order neuron synapse with anterior spinothalamic tract neurons, the axons of which decussate in the **anterior white commissure** of the spine at the level of entry, or perhaps two or three segments higher. The second-order tract neurons ascend to the pons of the brain stem, where fibers enter the **medial lemniscus** to terminate at the ventral posterolateral (VPL) nucleus of the thalamus.

Lateral Funiculus. The last time you stubbed your toe, the information concerning that pain traveled through the **lateral spinothalamic tract**. This important tract transmits information concerning pain and thermal sense. Dorsal root fibers synapse with second-order interneurons that subsequently synapse with third-order tract neurons. These decussate in the anterior white commissure to ascend to the VPL of the thalamus and reticular formation. If the spinal cord is cut unilaterally, the result will be *contralateral* loss of pain and thermal sense beginning one segment below the level of the trauma.

Anterior and Posterior Spinocerebellar Tracts. These important tracts convey information concerning muscle tension to the cerebellum. The **posterior spinocerebellar tract** is an uncrossed tract, meaning that information from one side of the body remains on that side during

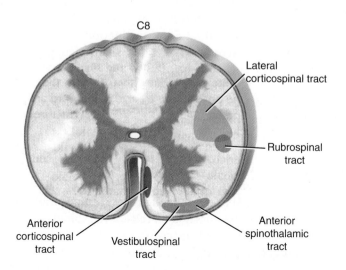

C8

Lateral corticospinal tract

Rubrospinal tract

Anterior corticospinal tract

Vestibulospinal tract

Anterior spinothalamic tract

Figure 11-55. Major efferent tracts of the spinal cord as seen in a transverse segment of the cervical spinal cord.
© Cengage Learning®.

its ascent through the pathway. Afferent information from GTOs and muscle spindle stretch receptors enters the spinal cord via the dorsal root ganglion where axons of these neurons synapse with the second-order tract fibers. Branches of these first-order neurons ascend and descend, so that synapse occurs at points above and below the site of entry as well. The second-order neurons arise from the dorsal nucleus of Clarke, located in the posterior gray of the cord. Upon reaching the medulla oblongata, the second-order neurons enter the inferior cerebellar peduncle, the lower pathway to the cerebellum. These axons terminate in the rostral and caudal vermis of the cerebellum.

None of the information transmitted by this tract reaches consciousness, although the result of damage to the pathway would. Information from muscles concerning length, rate of stretch, degree of muscle and tendon stretch, and some pressure and touch sense would all be impaired, causing deficit in movement and posture.

The **anterior spinocerebellar tract** is a crossed pathway. Information from Ib afferent fibers serving the Golgi apparatus enters the spinal cord via the dorsal root, where it synapses with the second-order tract neurons. Tract fibers decussate at the same level and ascend through the anterolateral portion of the spinal cord. The tract enters the superior cerebellar peduncle, the superior pathway to the cerebellum from the brain stem. Most of the fibers cross to enter the cerebellum on the opposite side of the tract (but the same side as initial stimulation), with the information presumably serving the same function as that of the posterior spinocerebellar tract.

Descending Pathways. Descending motor pathways are the conduits of information commanding muscle contraction that will result in voluntary movement, modification of reflexes, and visceral activation. The most important of these arise from the cerebral cortex, although there are tracts originating in the brain stem as well. The major pathways include the **pyramidal pathways** (the corticospinal and corticobulbar tracts), and the tectospinal, rubrospinal, vestibulospinal, pontine reticulospinal, and medullary reticulospinal tracts (see Figure 11-56).

Corticospinal Tract. As the name implies, this extraordinarily important tract runs from the cortex to the *spine*, providing innervation of skeletal muscle (see Figure 11-56). Myelination of the axons of these fibers occurs after birth and is normally complete by a child's second birthday. The corticospinal tract is made up of more than 1 million fibers, about half of which arise from cells in each frontal lobe of the cerebral cortex (Brodmann areas 4 and 6, areas known as the motor strip and premotor region, to be discussed in Chapter 12). The remainder of the neurons supplying the corticospinal tract arise from the region anterior to the motor strip, the premotor region, and from the supplementary motor area on the superior and medial surface of the cerebrum. In addition, some fibers from the parietal sensory cortex (areas 1, 2, and 3) project through the corticospinal tract, generally terminating on the dorsal horn cells of the spinal cord. The fibers from the cortex descend as the corona radiata, through the internal capsule and crus cerebri at the level of the midbrain.

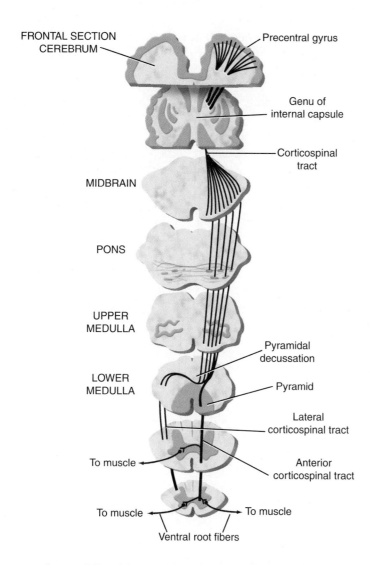

FRONTAL SECTION
CEREBRUM

Precentral gyrus

Genu of
internal capsule

Corticospinal
tract

MIDBRAIN

PONS

UPPER
MEDULLA

LOWER
MEDULLA

Pyramidal
decussation

Pyramid

Lateral
corticospinal tract

To muscle

Anterior
corticospinal tract

To muscle

To muscle

Ventral root fibers

Figure 11-56. Corticospinal pathway as traced from cerebral cortex to spinal cord.
© Cengage Learning®.

At the medulla oblongata, the fibers enter the pyramids (so called because of the pyramidal column shape), where they undergo the important pyramidal decussation. Seventy-five to 90 percent of corticospinal tract fibers cross to descend as the lateral corticospinal tract in the lateral funiculus. This tract becomes increasingly smaller as it descends through the cord to serve skeletal muscles.

The fibers that do not decussate at the pyramids descend uncrossed as the **anterior corticospinal tract**. On reaching the point of innervation, the axons decussate to synapse with LMNs. This arrangement of partial decussation is a safeguard. Incomplete damage to this pathway may result in the retention of voluntary motor function.

The corticospinal tract is responsible not only for the activation of muscles but also for the inhibition of the reflexes. Corticospinal tract lesions (UMN lesion) result in muscle weakness, loss of voluntary use of musculature, and initial loss of muscle tone. Reduced muscle tone will return to the antigravity muscles and hyperactive tendon reflexes will be seen. The **Babinski reflex** will be elicitable in many individuals with UMN lesion. When the sole of a relaxed foot

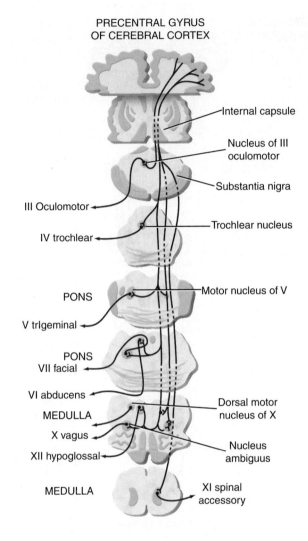

PRECENTRAL GYRUS
OF CEREBRAL CORTEX

Internal capsule

Nucleus of III
oculomotor

Substantia nigra

III Oculomotor

Trochlear nucleus

IV trochlear

Motor nucleus of V

PONS

V trigeminal

PONS
VII facial

VI abducens

Dorsal motor
nucleus of X

MEDULLA

X vagus

XII hypoglossal

Nucleus
ambiguus

Figure 11-57. Corticobulbar tract as traced from cerebral cortex to cranial nerve nuclei.
© Cengage Learning®.

MEDULLA

XI spinal
accessory

is stroked, a positive Babinski sign would be extension of the great toe and spreading of the outer toes. This reflex is normally present in infants but diminishes through cortical control arising from progressive myelination of the corticospinal tract.

Corticobulbar Tract. Although the corticobulbar tract is not a tract of the spinal cord, it is included here because it is extraordinarily important for speech production, paralleling the importance of the corticospinal tract for muscles of the trunk and extremities (see Figure 11-57). The corticobulbar tract acts also on sensory information, both facilitating and inhibiting its transmission to the thalamus.

The corticobulbar tract arises from cortical cells in the lateral aspects of the precentral gyrus of the frontal lobe, in the region of the motor strip serving the head, face, neck, and larynx. It arises also from the premotor and **somesthetic** (body sense) regions of the parietal lobe of the cortex. Fibers from these areas follow a descent pattern similar to those of the corticospinal tract, passing through the corona radiata and genu of the internal capsule, and entering the brain stem.

These axons branch and decussate at various levels of the brain stem, synapsing with nuclei of cranial nerves to provide bilateral innervation to many muscles of the face, neck, pharynx, and larynx.

Other Descending Pathways. The **tectospinal tract** arises in the superior colliculus ("little hill") of the midbrain, crosses midline in the dorsal tegmental decussation, and descends to the first four cervical spinal cord segments. Because the superior colliculus is a visual relay, it is assumed that this efferent pathway is associated with reflexive postural control arising from visual stimulation, perhaps orienting to the source of visual stimulation.

The rubrospinal tract arises from the red nucleus of the midbrain tegmentum. Fibers of this tract cross in the ventral tegmental decussation of the midbrain and descend with the **medial longitudinal fasciculus (MLF)** of the spinal cord (see Figures 11-53 and 11-55). Most fibers from this tract serve the cervical region, although they descend the length of the spinal cord. The red nucleus receives input from the cerebral cortex and the cerebellum and appears to be responsible for the maintenance of tone in flexor muscles.

The **vestibulospinal tract** arises from the lateral vestibular nucleus of the pons and medulla and descends ipsilaterally the length of the spinal cord. Fibers of this tract facilitate spinal reflexes and promote muscle tone in extensor musculature.

The **pontine reticulospinal tract** arises from nuclei in the medial tegmentum of the pons and descends, primarily ipsilaterally, near the MLF in the spinal cord. The **medullary reticulospinal tract** is formed in the medulla oblongata near the inferior olivary complex and descends in the lateral funiculus. Activity of these neurons have both facilitating and inhibiting effects on motor neurons and hence on voluntary movement.

Terms of Paralysis

Paralysis refers to temporary or permanent loss of motor function. Paralysis is **spastic** in nature if the lesion causing it is of an UMN. In this type of paralysis, voluntary control is lost through the lesion, but hyperactive reflexes will remain, producing seemingly paradoxical **hyperreflexia** (brisk and overly active reflex responses) and **hypertonia** (muscle tone greater than appropriate) coupled with muscular weakness. **Flaccid** paralysis arises from lesion to the LMN, and results in **hypotonia** (reduced muscle tone) and **hyporeflexia** (reduced or absent reflex response), with co-occurring muscle weakness.

Paralysis of the lower portion of the body, including legs, is termed **paraplegia**. **Quadriplegia** refers to the paralysis of all four limbs, usually arising from damage to the spinal cord above C5 or C6. Spinal cord cut above C3 causes death. If lesions produce paralysis of the same part on both sides of the body, it is referred to as **diplegia**, whereas **triplegia** involves three limbs. **Monoplegia** refers to paralysis of only one limb or group of muscles. **Hemiplegia** arises from UMN damage, resulting in loss of function in one side of the body.

✔ *To summarize:*

- The **spinal cord** is comprised of tracts and nuclei.
- The 31 pairs of **spinal nerves** arise from spinal segments, serving sensory and voluntary motor function for the limbs and trunk.
- **Sensory nerves** have their cell bodies within the dorsal root ganglia, whereas **motor neuron** bodies lie within the gray matter of the spinal cord.
- The **spinal reflex arc** is the simplest motor function, providing an efferent response to a basic change in muscle length.
- Several landmarks of the transverse cord assist in identifying the **funiculi** and **fasciculi** of the spinal cord.
- **Upper motor neurons** have their cell bodies rostral to the segment at which the spinal nerve originates, whereas **lower motor neurons** are the final neurons in the efferent chain.
- **Efferent tracts**, such as the corticospinal tract, transmit information from the brain to the spinal nerves.
- **Afferent tracts**, such as the spinothalamic tract, transmit information concerning the physical state of the limbs and trunk to higher brain centers.
- The **corticobulbar tract** is of particular interest to speech-language pathologists because it serves the motor **cranial nerves** for speech.

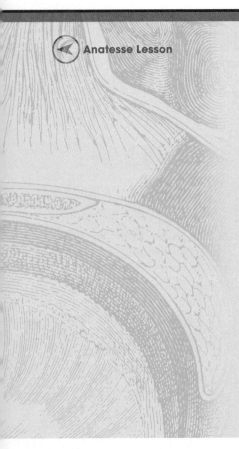

◀ **Anatesse Lesson**

CHAPTER SUMMARY

The nervous system is a complex, hierarchical structure. Voluntary movement, sensory awareness, and cognitive function are the domain of the cerebral cortex. The communication links of the nervous system are spinal nerves, cranial nerves, and tracts of the brain stem and spinal cord. Several organizational schemes characterize the nervous system. The autonomic and somatic nervous systems control involuntary and voluntary functions. We may divide the nervous system into central and peripheral nervous systems. Developmental characterization separates the brain into prosencephalon (telencephalon and diencephalon), the mesencephalon (midbrain), and the rhombencephalon (metencephalon and myelencephalon). Monopolar, bipolar, or multipolar neurons communicate through synapse by means of neurotransmitter substance. Responses may be excitatory or inhibitory. Glial cells provide the fatty sheath for myelinated axons, as well as support structure for neurons. They also are implicated in long-term memory facilitation.

The cerebral cortex is protected from physical insult by cerebrospinal fluid and the meningeal linings, the dura, pia, and arachnoid mater. Cerebrospinal fluid originating within the ventricles of the brain and circulating around the spinal cord cushions these structures from trauma associated with rapid acceleration. The cerebrum is divided into two hemispheres connected by the corpus callosum. The gyri and sulci of the hemisphere provide important landmarks for lobes and other regions of the cerebrum. The temporal lobe is the site of auditory reception and auditory comprehension; the frontal lobe is responsible for most voluntary motor activation and use of the important speech region known as Broca's area. The parietal lobe is the region of somatic sensory reception. The occipital lobe is the site of visual input to the cerebrum. The insular lobe is revealed by deflecting the temporal lobe and lies deep in the lateral sulcus. The operculum overlies the insula. The functionally defined limbic lobe includes the cingulate gyrus, uncus, parahippocampal gyrus, and other deep structures.

The basal ganglia are subcortical structures involved in the control of movement, and the hippocampal formation of the inferior temporal lobe is deeply implicated in memory function. The thalamus of the diencephalon is the final relay for somatic sensation directed toward the cerebrum and other diencephalic structures. The subthalamus interacts with the globus pallidus to control movement, and the hypothalamus controls many bodily functions and desires. The regions of the cerebral cortex are interconnected by means of a complex network of projection fibers that link the cortex with other structures; association fibers, which connect regions of the same hemisphere; and commissural fibers, which provide communication between corresponding regions of the two hemispheres.

The anterior cerebral arteries serve the medial surfaces of the brain, and the middle cerebral artery serves the lateral cortex, including the temporal lobe, motor strip, Wernicke's area, and much of the parietal lobe. The vertebral arteries branch to form the anterior and posterior spinal arteries, with ascending components serving the ventral brain stem. The basilar artery gives rise to the superior and anterior inferior cerebellar arteries to serve the cerebellum, whereas the posterior inferior cerebellar artery arises from the vertebral artery. The basilar artery divides to become the posterior cerebral arteries, serving the inferior temporal and occipital lobes, upper midbrain, and diencephalon. The circle of Willis is a series of communicating arteries that provide redundant pathways for blood flow to regions of the cerebral cortex, equalizing pressure and flow of blood.

The cerebellum coordinates motor and sensory information, communicating with the brain stem, cerebrum, and spinal cord. It is divided into anterior, middle, and flocculonodular lobes and communicates with the rest of the nervous system via the superior, middle, and inferior cerebellar peduncles. Position in space is coordinated via the flocculonodular lobe, and adjustment against gravity is mediated by the anterior lobe. The posterior lobe mediates fine motor adjustments. The superior cerebellar peduncle enters the pons and serves the dentate nucleus, red nucleus, and thalamus. The middle cerebellar peduncle communicates with the pontine nuclei, whereas the inferior cerebellar peduncle receives input from the spinocerebellar tracts.

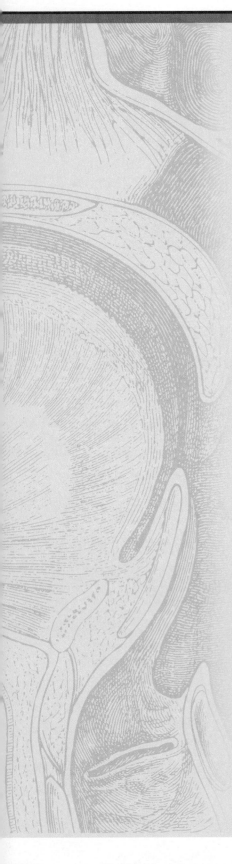

The brain stem is divided into medulla, pons, and midbrain. It is more highly organized than the spinal cord and mediates higher-level body functions such as vestibular responses. The pyramidal decussation of the medulla is the point at which the motor commands originating in one hemisphere of the cerebral cortex cross to serve the opposite side of the body. The IX, X, XI, and XII cranial nerves emerge at the level of the medulla. The pons contains four cranial nerve nuclei, the V, VI, VII, and VIII nerves. The midbrain contains the important cerebral peduncles and gives rise to the III and IV cranial nerves. The reticular formation is a phylogenetically old set of nuclei essential for life function. The pons and midbrain set the stage for communication with the higher levels of the brain, including the cerebellum and cerebrum. This communication link permits not only complex motor acts but also consciousness, awareness, and volitional acts.

Cranial nerves are extremely important to the speech-language pathologist. Cranial nerves may be sensory, motor, or mixed sensory-motor and are categorized based on their function as being general or specialized, and as serving visceral or somatic organs or structures. The V trigeminal innervates muscles of mastication and the tensor veli palatini, and communicates sensation from the face, mouth, teeth, mucosal lining, and tongue. The VII facial nerve innervates muscles of facial expression, and the sensory component serves taste of the anterior two-thirds of the tongue. The VIII vestibulocochlear nerve mediates auditory and vestibular sensation. The IX glossopharyngeal nerve serves the posterior tongue taste receptors, as well as somatic sense from the tongue, fauces, pharynx, and Eustachian tube. The stylopharyngeus and superior pharyngeal constrictor muscles receive motor innervation via this nerve. The X vagus serves autonomic and somatic functions, mediating pain, touch, and temperature from the ear drum and pain sense from the pharynx, larynx, and esophagus. The recurrent laryngeal nerve and superior laryngeal nerves supply motor innervation for the intrinsic muscles of the larynx. The XI accessory nerve innervates the sternocleidomastoid and trapezius muscles and collaborates with the vagus in the activation of palatal, laryngeal, and pharyngeal muscles. The XII hypoglossal nerve innervates the muscles of the tongue with the exception of the palatoglossus.

The spinal cord is comprised of tracts and nuclei. The 31 pairs of spinal nerves serve the limbs and trunk. Sensory nerves have cell bodies in dorsal root ganglia and motor neuron bodies lie within the spinal cord. Upper motor neurons have their cell bodies above the segment at which the spinal nerve originates. Lower motor neurons are the final neurons in the efferent chain. Efferent tracts, such as the corticospinal tract, transmit information from the brain to the spinal nerves. Afferent tracts, such as the spinothalamic tract, transmit information concerning the physical state of the limbs and trunk to higher brain centers. The corticobulbar tract is of particular interest to speech-language pathologists because it serves motor cranial nerves for speech.

This overview of neuroanatomy should give you some feel for the complexity of this system. The interaction of these systems provides us with the smooth motor function required for speech, as well as the cognitive and linguistic processes required for the comprehension of the spoken word and formulation of a response. Chapter 12 examines some of those processes.

Media Connection

Go to the accompanying online resources at CengageBrain.com and have fun learning! Study with the Anatesse software program, play games, view animations and videos, and take practice tests to help reinforce the key concepts you learned in this chapter.

Study Questions

1. The _____ governs voluntary actions.

2. The _____ is responsible for coordinating movement.

3. _____ is the sense of muscle and joint position.

4. _____ are groups of cell bodies in the PNS with functional unity.

5. _____ sense is the sense of the body in motion.

6. Special senses include _____, _____, _____, and _____.

7. The _____ system includes the cerebrum, cerebellum, subcortical structures, brain stem, and spinal cord.

8. The _____ consists of the 12 pairs of cranial nerves and 31 pairs of spinal nerves, as well as the sensory receptors.

9. The _____ governs involuntary activities of involuntary muscles.

10. The _____ governs voluntary activities.

11. Information directed toward the brain is termed _____ whereas information directed from the brain is termed.

12. Developmental divisions: Identify the division referred to by each statement.

  a. _____ refers to the "extended" or "telescoped" brain and includes the cerebral hemispheres, the white matter immediately beneath it, the basal ganglia, and the olfactory tract.

  b. _____ refers to the olfactory bulb, tract, and striae; pyriform area; intermediate olfactory area; hippocampal formation; and fornix.

  c. _____ includes the thalamus, hypothalamus, pituitary gland (hypophysis), and optic tract.

  d. _____ refers to the midbrain.

  e. _____ includes the pons and cerebellum.

  f. _____ refers to the medulla.

13. On the figure below, identify the parts of the neuron indicated.

a. _____

b. _____

c. _____

d. _____

e. _____

f. _____

g. _____

h. _____

i. _____

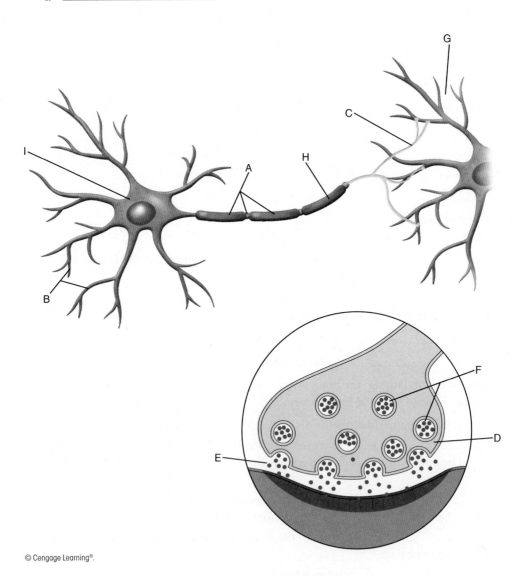

14. On the figure below, identify the parts of the cerebrum indicated.

a. _____ lobe

b. _____ lobe

c. _____ lobe

d. _____ lobe

e. _____ gyrus

f. _____ gyrus

g. _____ sulcus

h. _____ sulcus

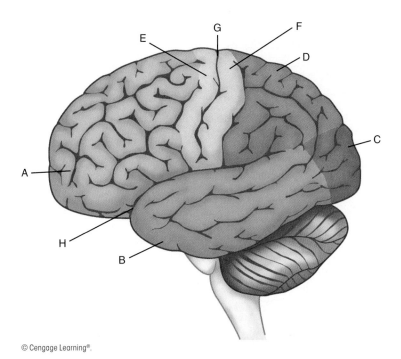

© Cengage Learning®.

15. On the figure below, identify the parts of the surface of the cerebrum.

a. _____ gyrus

b. _____

c. _____ gyrus

d. _____ area

e. _____ area

f. _____ area

g. _____ gyrus

h. _____ gyrus

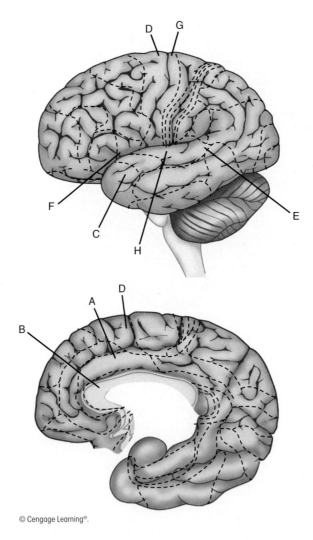

© Cengage Learning®.

16. On the figure below, identify the components of the ventricle system indicated.

a. _____

b. _____

c. _____

d. _____

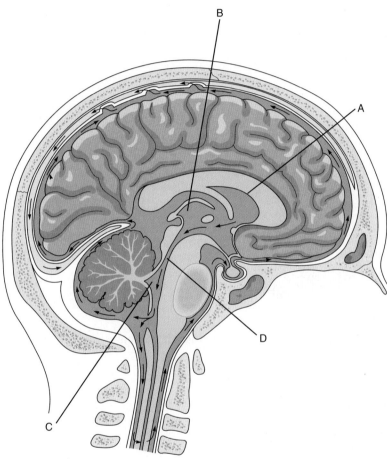

17. On the figure below, identify the arteries and the structure indicated.

a. _____ artery

b. _____ artery

c. _____ artery

d. _____ artery

e. _____ artery

f. _____ artery

g. _____ artery

h. _____ artery

i. _____

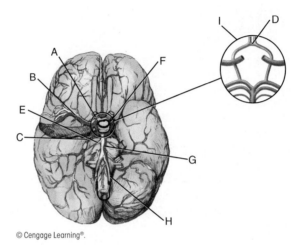

© Cengage Learning®.

18. Redundancy is nature's safety net. Identify as many redundant systems as you can within the nervous system.

Study Question Answers

1. The **CEREBRUM** governs voluntary actions.

2. The **CEREBELLUM** is responsible for coordinating movement.

3. **PROPRIOCEPTION** is the sense of muscle and joint position.

4. **GANGLIA** are groups of cell bodies in the PNS with functional unity.

5. **KINESTHETIC** sense is the sense of the body in motion.

6. Special senses include **OLFACTION, VISION, GUSTATION**, and **AUDITION**.

7. The **CENTRAL NERVOUS SYSTEM** includes the cerebrum, cerebellum, subcortical structures, brain stem, and spinal cord.

8. The **PERIPHERAL NERVOUS SYSTEM** consists of the 12 pairs of cranial nerves and 31 pairs of spinal nerves, as well as the sensory receptors.

9. The **AUTONOMIC NERVOUS SYSTEM** governs involuntary activities of involuntary muscles.

10. The **SOMATIC NERVOUS SYSTEM** governs voluntary activities.

11. Information directed toward the brain is termed **AFFERENT** whereas information directed from the brain is termed **EFFERENT**.

12. Developmental divisions: Identify the division referred to by each statement.
    a. **TELENCEPHALON** refers to the "extended" or "telescoped" brain, and includes the cerebral hemispheres, the white matter immediately beneath it, the basal ganglia, and the olfactory tract.
    b. **RHINENCEPHALON** refers to the olfactory bulb, tract, and striae; pyriform area; intermediate olfactory area; hippocampal formation; and fornix.
    c. **DIENCEPHALON** includes the thalamus, hypothalamus, pituitary gland (hypophysis), and optic tract.
    d. **MESENCEPHALON** refers to the midbrain.
    e. **METENCEPHALON** includes the pons and cerebellum.
    f. **MYELENCEPHALON** refers to the medulla.

13. On the figure below, identify the parts of the neuron indicated.
    a. **AXON**
    b. **DENDRITE**
    c. **TELODENDRIA**
    d. **TERMINAL END BOUTON**
    e. **SYNAPTIC CLEFT**
    f. **SYNAPTIC VESICLES**
    g. **POSTSYNAPTIC NEURON**
    h. **MYELIN SHEATH**
    i. **SOMA**

14. On the figure below, identify the parts of the cerebrum indicated.
    a. **FRONTAL** lobe
    b. **TEMPORAL** lobe
    c. **OCCIPITAL** lobe
    d. **PARIETAL** lobe
    e. **PRECENTRAL** gyrus
    f. **POSTCENTRAL** gyrus
    g. **CENTRAL** sulcus
    h. **LATERAL** sulcus

15. On the figure below, identify the parts of the surface of the cerebrum.
    a. **CINGULATE** gyrus
    b. **CORPUS CALLOSUM**
    c. **SUPERIOR TEMPORAL** gyrus
    d. **SUPPLEMENTARY MOTOR** area
    e. **WERNICKE'S** area
    f. **BROCA'S** area
    g. **PRECENTRAL** gyrus
    h. **HESCHL'S** gyrus

16. On the figure below, identify the components of the ventricle system indicated.
    a. **LATERAL VENTRICLE**
    b. **3RD VENTRICLE**
    c. **4TH VENTRICLE**
    d. **CEREBRAL AQUEDUCT**

17. On the figure below, identify the arteries and the structure indicated.
   a. **ANTERIOR CEREBRAL** artery
   b. **MIDDLE CEREBRAL** artery
   c. **POSTERIOR CEREBRAL** artery
   d. **ANTERIOR COMMUNICATING** artery
   e. **SUPERIOR CEREBELLAR** artery
   f. **INTERNAL CAROTID** artery
   g. **BASILAR** artery
   h. **VERTEBRAL** artery
   i. **CIRCLE OF WILLIS**

18. Redundancy takes many forms within the nervous system. One of the most obvious is the presence of two cerebral hemispheres, although they are not functionally equal, as we will see in Chapter 12. The fact that the corticospinal tract divides into anterior and lateral corticospinal tracts indicates some safety in spreading the "risk" around. Likewise, the circle of Willis within the cerebrovascular system is an important safety valve. What about the fact there are identical nuclei within each half of the brain stem? How about the fact that the upper face is bilaterally innervated? Can you think of any other redundancies?

Bibliography

Adams, R. D., Victor, M., & Ropper, A. H. (1997). *Principles of neurology* (6th ed.). New York: McGraw-Hill.

Akshoomoff, N. A., & Courchesne, E. (1992). A new role for the cerebellum in cognitive operations. *Behavioral Neuroscience, 106*(5), 731–738.

Albin, R. L. (1995). The pathophysiology of chorea/ballism and Parkinsonism. *Parkinsonism and Related Disorders, 1*(1), 3–11.

Amaral, D., & Lavenex, P. (2007). Hippocampal anatomy. In P. Andersen, R. Morris, D. Amaral, T. Bliss, & J. O'Keefe (Eds.), *The hippocampus book* (pp. 37–114). New York: Oxford University Press.

Andersen, P., Morris, R., Amaral, D., Bliss, T., & O'Keefe, J. (2007). The hippocampal formation. In P. Anderson, R. Morris, D. Amaral, T. Bliss, & J. O'Keefe (Eds.), *The hippocampus book* (pp. 3–6). New York: Oxford University Press.

Aronson, A. E. (2000). *Aronson's neurosciences pocket lectures*. San Diego, CA: Singular Publishing Group.

Azevado, F. A. C., Carvalho, L. R. B., Gringberg, L. T., Farfel, J. M., Ferretti, R. E. L., Leite, R. E. P., Filho, W. J., Lent, R., & Herculano-Houzel, S. (2009). Equal numbers of neuronal and non-neuronal cells make the human brain an isometrically scaled-up primate. *The Journal of Comparative Neurology, 513*, 532–541.

Bach, P., Peelen, M. V., & Tipper, S. P. On the role of object information in action observation: An fMRI study. (2010). *Cerebral Cortex, 20*(12), 2798–2809.

Bateman, H. E., & Mason, R. M. (1984). *Applied anatomy and physiology of the speech and hearing mechanism.* Springfield, IL: Charles C. Thomas.

Bear, M. F., Connors, B. W., & Paradiso, M. A. (1996). *Neuroscience: Exploring the brain*. Baltimore, MD: Williams & Wilkins.

Berkovitz, B. K. B., & Moxham, B. J. (2002). *Head and neck anatomy*. London: Martin Dunitz Ltd.

Bhatnagar, S. C., & Andy, O. J. (2002). *Neuroscience for the study of communicative disorders* (2nd ed.). Baltimore, MD: Williams & Wilkins.

Bly, L. (1994). *Motor skills acquisition in the first year*. Tucson, AZ: Therapy Skill Builders.

Bowman, J. P. (1971). *The muscle spindle and neural control of the tongue*. Springfield, IL: Charles C. Thomas.

Carpenter, M. B. (1991). *Core text of neuroanatomy* (4th ed.). Baltimore, MD: Williams & Wilkins.

Church, J. A., Coalson, R. S., Lugar, H. M., Petersen, S. E., & Schlaggar, B. L. (2008). A developmental fMRI study of reading and repetition reveals changes in phonological and visual mechanisms over age. *Cerebral Cortex, 18*, 2054–2065.

Chusid, J. G. (1985). *Correlative neuroanatomy and functional neurology* (17th ed.). Los Altos, CA: Lange Medical Publications.

Cotman, C. W., & McGaugh, J. L. (1980). *Behavioral neuroscience*. New York: Academic Press.

Craig, A. D. (2002). How do you feel? Interoception: The sense of the physiological condition of the body. *Nature Reviews Neuroscience, 3*, 655–666.

Crossman, A. R. (2008). Overview of the nervous system. In S. Standring (2008). *Gray's anatomy: The anatomical and clinical basis of practice* (40th ed., pp. 225–236). London: Churchill Livingstone.

Dalgleish, T. (2004). The emotional brain. *Nature Reviews Neuroscience, 5*, 582–589.

Darley, F. L., Aronson, A. E., & Brown, J. R. (1975). *Motor speech disorders*. Philadelphia, PA: W. B. Saunders.

de Vries, H. E., Kuiper, J., de Boer, A. G., Van Berkel, T. J. C., & Breimer, D. D., (1997). The blood–brain barrier in neuroinflammatory disease. *Pharmacological Reviews, 49*(2), 143–156.

Edvinsson, L., & Krause, D. N. (2002). *Cerebral blood flow and metabolism*. Philadelphia, PA: Lippincott/Williams & Wilkins.

Ehrsson, H. H., Spence, C., & Passingham, R. E. (2004). That's my hand! Activity in the premotor cortex reflects feeling ownership of a limb. *Science, 305*(5685), 875–877.

Farrer, C., Frey, S. H., Van Horn, J. D., Tunik, E., Turk, D., Inati, S., & Grafton, S. T. (2007). The angular gyrus computes action awareness representations. *Cerebral Cortex, 18*, 254–261.

Ffytch, D. H. (2005). Perisylvian language networks of the human brain. *Annals of Neurology, 57*, 8–16.

Fields, D. (2004, April). The other half of the brain. *Scientific American*, 53–61.

Fields, R. D. (2007). Sex and the Secret Nerve. *Scientific American Mind, 18*, 20–27.

Filskov, S. B., & Boll, T. J. (1981). *Handbook of clinical neuropsychology*. New York: John Wiley & Sons.

Fiorentino, M. R. (1973). *Reflex testing methods for evaluating CNS development*. Springfield, IL: Charles C. Thomas.

Fuller, G. N., & Burger, P. C. (1990). Nervus terminalis (cranial nerve zero) in the adult human. *Clinical Neuropathology, 9*(6), 279–283.

Ganong, W. F. (1981). *Review of medical physiology*. Los Altos, CA: Lange Medical Publications.

Gelfand, S. A. (1990). *Hearing*. New York: Marcel Dekker.

Gelfand, S. A. (2001). *Essentials of audiology* (2nd ed.). New York: Thieme Medical Publishers.

Gilman, S., & Winans, S. S. (2002, 10th edition). *Manter and Gatz's essentials of clinical neuroanatomy and neurophysiology*. Philadelphia, PA: F. A. Davis.

Gilroy, A. M., MacPherson, B. R., & Ross, L. M. (2012). *Atlas of anatomy* (2nd ed.). New York: Thieme.

Gilroy, J. (2000). *Basic neurology* (3rd ed.). New York: McGraw-Hill.

Gray, H., Bannister, L. H., Berry, M. M., & Williams, P. L. (Eds.). (1995). *Gray's anatomy*. London: Churchill Livingstone.

Horn, J. P., & Swanson, L. W. (2008). The autonomic motor system and the hypothalamus. In Kandel, E. R., Schwartz, J. H., Jessell, T. M., Siegelbaum, S. A. & Hudspeth, A. J. (2012). *Principles of neural science* (5th ed., pp. 1056–1078). New York: McGraw Hill.

Jespersen, S. N., & Ostergaard, L. (2012). The roles of cerebral blood flow, capillary transit time heterogeneity, and oxygen tension in brain oxygenation and metabolism. *Journal of Blood Flow and Metabolism, 32*(2), 264–277.

Kandel, E. R. (1991). Brain and behavior. In E. R. Kandell, J. R. Schwartz, & T. M. Jessell (Eds.), *Principles of neural science* (3rd ed., pp. 9–48). Norwalk, CT: Appleton & Lange.

Kandel, E. R. (2012). From nerve cells to cognition: The internal representation of space and action. In K. R. Kandel, J. H. Schwartz, T. M. Jessell, S. A. Siegelbaum, & A. J. Hudspeth *Principles of neural science* (5th ed., pp. 370–392). New York: McGraw Hill.

Kandel, E. R., Schwartz, J. H., Jessell, T. M., Siegelbaum, S. A. & Hudspeth, A. J. (2013). *Principles of neural science* (5th ed.) New York: McGraw Hill.

Kanwisher, N., McDermott, J., & Chun, M. M. (1997). The fusiform face area: A module in human extrastriate cortex specialized for face perception. *The Journal of Neuroscience, 17*(11), 4302–4311.

Karlsen, A. S., & Pakkenberg, B. (2011). Total numbers of neurons and glial cells in cortex and basal ganglia of aged brains with Down syndrome-a sterological study. *Cerebral Cortex, 21*(11), 2519–2524.

Kaufman, D. M. (2000). *Clinical neurology for psychiatrists* (5th ed.). Philadelphia, PA: W. B. Saunders.

Kobayashi, M. (2006). Functional organization of the human gustatory cortex. *Oral Bioscience, 48*(4), 244–260.

Kringelbach, M. L., & Rolls, E. T. (2004). The functional neuroanatomy of the human orbitofrontal cortex: evidence from neuroimaging and neuropsychology. *Progress in Neurobiology, 72*, 341–372.

Kuehn, D. P., Lemme, M. L., & Baumgartner, J. M. (1989). *Neural bases of speech, hearing, and language*. Boston: College-Hill Press.

Lutz, A., Greischar, L. L., Perlman, D. M., & Davidson, R. J. (2009). BOLD signal in insula is differentially related to cardiac function during compassion meditation in experts vs novices. *Neuroimage, 47*, 1038–1046.

Mackay, L. E., Chapman, P. E., & Morgan, A. S. (1997). *Maximizing brain injury* recovery. Gaithersburg, MD: Aspen Publishers.

Marien, P., Baillieux, H., De Smet, H. J., Engelborghs, S., Wilssens, I., Paquier, P., & De Deyn, P. P. (2009). Cognitive, linguistic and affective disturbances following a right superior cerebellar artery infarction: A case study. *Cortex 45*(4): 527–536.

McMinn, R. M. H., Hutchings, R. T., & Logan, B. M. (1994). *Color atlas of head and neck anatomy*. London: Mosby-Wolfe.

Mcller, A. R. (2003). *Sensory systems: Anatomy and physiology*. New York: Academic Press.

Moore, K. L. (1988). *The developing human*. Philadelphia, PA: W. B. Saunders.

Naqvi, N. H., Rudrauf, D., Damasio, H., & Bechara, A. (2007). Damage to the insula disrupts addiction to cigarette smoking. *Science, 315*(5811), 531–534.

Netsell, R. (1986). *A neurobiologic view of speech production and the dysarthrias*. San Diego, CA: College-Hill Press.

Netter, F. H. (1983a). *The CIBA collection of medical illustrations. Vol. 1. Nervous system. Part I. Anatomy and physiology*. West Caldwell, NJ: CIBA Pharmaceutical.

Netter, F. H. (1983b). *The CIBA collection of medical illustrations. Vol. 1. Nervous system. Part II. Neurologic and neuromuscular disorders*. West Caldwell, NJ: CIBA Pharmaceutical.

Netter, F. H. (1997). *Atlas of human anatomy*. Los Angeles: Icon Learning Systems.

Noback, C. R., Demarest, R. J., & Strominger, N. L. (1991). *The nervous system: Introduction and review*. Philadelphia: Williams & Wilkins.

Nolte, J. (2002). *The human brain* (5th ed.). St. Louis, MO: Mosby Year Book.

Pakkenberg, B. & Gunderson, H. J. G. (2011). Total number of neurons and glial cells in human brain nuclei estimted by the disector and tracionator. *Journal of microscopy, 10*(1), 1-20.

Papantchev, V., Hristov, S., Todorova, D., Naydenov, E., Paloff, A., Nikolov, D., Tschirkov, A., & Ovtscharoff, W. (2007). Some variations of the Circle of Willis, important cerebral protection in aortic surgery—A study in Eastern Europeans. *European Journal of Cardiothoracic Surgery, 31*(6), 982–989.

Parker, J., Mitchell, A., Kalpakidou, A., Walshe, M., Jung, H. Y., Nosarti, C., Santosh, P., Rifkin, L., Wyatt, J., Murray, R. M., & Allin, M. (2008). Cerebellar growth and behavioural and neuropsychological outcome in preterm adolescents. *Brain, 131*(5), 1344–1351.

Penfield, W., & Roberts, L. (1959). *Speech and brain mechanisms*. Princeton, NJ: Princeton University Press.

Pickles, J. O. (2012). An introduction to physiology of hearing, 4th edition. Bingley, UK: Emerald Group Publishing.

Poritsky, R. (1992). *Neuroanatomy: A functional atlas of parts and pathways*. St. Louis, MO: Mosby Year Book.

Rohen, J. W., & Yokochi, C. (1993). *Color atlas of anatomy*. New York: Igaku-Shoin.

Schaltenbrand, G., & Woolsey, C. N. (1964). *Cerebral localization and organization*. Madison, WI: University of Wisconsin Press.

Schuenke, M., & Ross, L. M., (2010). *Thieme atlas of anatomy*. New York: Thieme.

Standring, S. (2008). *Gray's anatomy: The anatomical and clinical basis of practice* (40th ed.). London: Churchill Livingstone.

Sugiura, L., Ojima, S., Matsuba-Kurita, H., Dan, I., Tsuzuki, D., Katura, T., & Hagiwara, H. (2011). Sound to language: Different cortical processing of the first and second language in elementary school children as revealed by a large scale study using fNIRS. *Cerebral Cortex, 21*(10), 2374–2393.

Suzuki, A., Stern, S. A., Bozdagi, O., Huntley, G. W., Walker, R. H., & Alberini, C. M. (2011). Astrocyte-neuron lactate transport is required for long-term memory formation. *Cell, 4*(5), 810–823.

Tsao, D. Y., Freiwald, W. A., Tootell, R. B. H., & Livingstone, M. S. (2006). A cortical region consisting entirely of face-selective cells. *Science, 311*, 670–674.

Twietmayer, A., & McCracken, T. (1992). *Coloring guide to regional human anatomy*. Philadelphia, PA: Lea & Febiger.

Webster, D. B. (1999). *Neuroscience of communication* (2nd ed.). San Diego, CA: Singular Publishing Group.

Whitlock, K. E. (2004). Development of the nervus terminalis: Origin and migration. *Microscopic Research Techniques, 65*(1–2), 2–12.

Williams, P., & Warrick, R. (1980). *Gray's anatomy* (36th British ed.). Philadelphia, PA: W. B. Saunders.

Winans, S. S., Gilman, S., Manter, J. T., & Gatz, A. J. (2002). *Manter and Gatz's essentials of clinical neuroanatomy and neurophysiology* (10th ed.). Philadelphia: F. A. Davis.

Wood, P. J., & Criss, W. R. (1975). *Normal and abnormal development of the human nervous system*. Hagerstown, MD: Harper & Row.

Yost, W. A. (2000). *Fundamentals of hearing: An introduction* (4th ed.). New York: Academic Press.

Zemlin, W. R. (1998). *Speech and hearing science: Anatomy and physiology* (4th ed.). Needham Heights, MA: Allyn & Bacon.

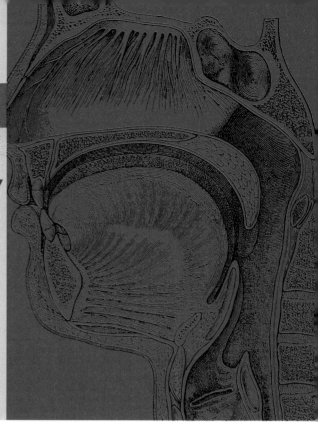

Chapter 12

NEUROPHYSIOLOGY

Although extraordinary advances over the past 30 years have vastly expanded our understanding of the workings of the brain, we still have a great deal to learn. We will set out in this chapter to provide at least some of the pieces of the puzzle. Knowledge of how the nervous system functions is the key to successful treatment by speech-language pathologists. All speech-language therapy works within the limits of the client's nervous system, because behavior, motivation, learning, and especially speech and language function depend on the ability to process information and respond to it. We hope that this introduction to nervous system physiology will tempt you to spend your life examining it.

We will approach our discussion of nervous system function from the "bottom up," looking first at the simplest responses of the system (communication between neurons) and working our way up to the all-important functions of the cerebral cortex (see Table 12-1). The **single neuron response** and the **reflex arc** associated with the spinal cord represent the basic level of information processing, and the brain stem structures provide control of balance and other **high-level reflexes**. The diencephalon supports attention to stimulation and basic (but highly organized) responses to danger. The cerebellum provides exquisite **integration of sensory information** and **motor planning**, and participates in cognitive processing and learning (Akshoomoff & Courchesne, 1992), but the cerebrum is the site of **consciousness**, **planning**, **ideation**, and **cognition**. When you are caught off guard by a loud noise, your lower (primary) neural processes will register the noise, cause you to orient to it, cause you to flinch, and even possibly cause you to move away from it. Only your

Table 12-1 **Structures of nervous system and general functions**	
Structure	**General Function**
Spinal arc reflexes	Subconscious response to environmental stimuli
Tracts	Transmission of information to cerebrum or periphery
Brain stem	Mediation of high-level reflexes and maintenance of life function; activation of cranial nerves
Diencephalon	Mediation of sensory information arriving at cerebrum and provision of basic autonomic responses for body maintenance
Cerebellum	Integration of somatic and special sensory information with motor planning and command for coordinated movement
Cerebrum	Processing of conscious sensory information, planning and executing voluntary motor act, analyzing stimuli, performing cognitive functions, decoding and encoding linguistic information

© Cengage Learning®.

cerebrum evaluates the input to determine the nature and meaning of the noise. Your eyes can receive light reflected off of the Mona Lisa; your brain stem's visual pathways can process information concerning shapes, forms, textures, and colors—but it takes your cerebrum to wonder why she is smiling.

INSTRUMENTATION IN NEUROPHYSIOLOGY

The physiology of the nervous system is extraordinarily complex, the structures we are attempting to measure are exquisitely tiny, and the number of structures we want to examine boggle the mind. A wide array of instruments and techniques have been developed to help us peer into this marvelous system.

Many methods attempt to view the structure and function of the brain in a macroscopic way. These methods will have resolution down to the millimeter level (i.e., the level that we would have with the naked eye, were we to have the opportunity to view the tissue itself). We are all familiar with the beautiful display of the brain presented through the lens of magnetic resonance imaging (MRI). This method uses very strong magnets to align nuclei of the atoms of your body, and the results can be analyzed to produce two- or three-dimensional images that far exceed those available through X-ray radiographic techniques. MRI is particularly useful for soft tissue, such as that found in the brain, and contrast agents can help physicians identify different structures (such as tumors, or characteristics of the blood supply). A positive benefit of MRI is that it does not use radiation, and therefore has significantly reduced risk for the patient. A modification of the MRI is functional MRI (fMRI), which measures blood flow to tissue. The notion of fMRI is that blood flowing to tissue reflects increased metabolic activity, which implies function of the tissue. Thus, if you are hearing words and the left-hemisphere Wernicke's area is active ("lights up"), researchers imply that Wernicke's area is important for listening to words. If the same subject is given warble tones to listen to and the right superior temporal gyrus is active, the researcher may conclude that these two types of stimuli are processed differentially by the brain. fMRI summates information over of a 2- to 3-second period, so that temporal resolution is limited (they are also very, very noisy, which reduces their functionality for intricate psychoacoustical studies). Specific pathways of the brain can be visualized using diffusion tensor imaging, providing striking evidence of tracts within the brain (e.g., Mueller et al., 2013). MRI and fMRI provide resolution down to about 1 mm, which is remarkable. (Realize, also, that the cortex is between 1 and 5 mm thick, has a volume of 11,300 cubic millimeters, and holds 17,000,000,000 neurons. That 1-mm resolution will include the activity of between 1.5 million and 7.5 million neurons.)

Another macroscopic view is provided by computer aided tomography (CT or CAT) scans. CT scans use low-dose irradiation to create three-dimensional images of the tissue under study. The patient may swallow a contrast medium that enhances aspects of the tissue, such as the vascular supply. CT scans are quite useful for imaging problems with the cerebrovascular supply, and can show evidence of hemorrhage or ischemia (blockage) that has caused a cerebrovascular accident. Density of tissue will cause differences in the image, so tumors can be more readily seen through CT scans than MRI. Variants of the CT scan include single photon emission computed tomography (SPECT) and positron emission tomography (PET). PET is similar to fMRI, in that it reveals blood flow, albeit requiring use of ionizing radiation. PET allows researchers to label neurotransmitters and observe active sites, which is a significant advantage over fMRI.

Magnetoenceophalography (MEG) measures the magnetic fields generated by the brain, and provides excellent temporal resolution (but poor spatial resolution). The most common implementation of MEG is through superconducting quantum interference devices (SQUID).

There are many microscopic methods available to researchers, some of which we have discussed in Chapter 10. Time-honored electroencephalography (EEG) remains a clinical and research staple. EEG measures the brainwave activity over the scalp, revealing frequencies of activity at a significant distance from the generator source. Auditory brain stem responses (ABR) are an example of evoked EEG activity, wherein audiologists measure the brain's EEG relative to an auditory stimulus, specifically brain stem activity. Event-related potentials (ERP) record cortical activity using a large array of electrodes. Unlike ABR, ERP allows researchers and clinicians to more accurately define the neural generator for responses to stimuli (Johnson, 2009). Using these methods, for instance, a researcher can produce verbal or visual stimuli that differ in some strategic way (e.g., verb versus noun) and identify the primary sites of activation and changes that occur over time relative to the stimuli. Single-cell measurement has been a staple of neurophysiological research for decades, and recent advances in microvisualization methods have allowed researchers to view the activity of small volumes of the brain in laboratory animals (e.g., Andermann, ,Kerlin, Roumis, Glickfeld, & Reid, 2012; Martinez et al., 2005). A creative variation on this theme is placement of a grid of electrodes over a portion of the brain of an individual undergoing assessment to identify the locus of seizure activity (electrocorticography [ECoG], also known as intracranial EEG [iEEG]). The electrodes remain in place on the surface of the brain (frequently on the temporal lobe, which is prone to seizure activity), often for many days as the patient and physician await the onset of a seizure (Keene, Whiting, & Ventureyra, 2000). During that time researchers can present stimuli to patients and make direct measurements from human brains. This method has allowed researchers to directly measure complex activity in the human brain for the first time (e.g., Miller, denNijs, Shenoy, Miller, Rao & Ojemann, 2007). There are many instrumental variations on these macroscopic and microscopic measures. Many are very invasive (requiring direct measurement of neural tissue), while others are indirect methods. We will call on many of these methods as we examine the physiology of the nervous system.

THE NEURON
Neuron Function

The nervous system is composed of billions of neurons with trillions of synapses whose singular function is to communicate. The communication between neurons occurs at the **synapse**, the point of union of two neurons. The synapse consists of the end *bouton* and the synaptic vesicles, the synaptic cleft, and the region of the postsynaptic neuron that contains the ion channels. You will recall from Chapter 11 that when a neurotransmitter is released into the synaptic cleft, the postsynaptic neuron (the neuron after the synapse) will either be inhibited from acting or be excited to act. Let us examine the transmission of information at the neuronal level. To do that, we must address energy gradients, electrical charge, and membrane permeability.

Gradients

The analogy of a water tower will help explain gradients. Engineers build water towers to hold water so that you can turn on your tap for a drink or a shower. Water is pumped up into the tower using electrical energy, and the energy expended to do that is stored in the elevated water. Because the energy has the potential of being expended, it is referred to as *potential energy*. There is a gradient of pressure between the tank and your faucet, and the water will flow from the point of higher pressure to the point of lower pressure. You know that water will not naturally flow up the pipe to the tower, but it will flow quite freely if you break a pipe in your house. That sets the stage for discussing the passage of ions through the membranous wall of a neuron. Gradients are established between the inside and outside of the cell, and ions have a tendency to flow to equalize that "pressure." We have pumps that move ions to increase that gradient, and we have faucets that we turn on to let those ions flood in. There are two basic forms of gradient that drive ion transport: electrochemical and concentration gradients.

Electrochemical Gradient. In neurons, a gradient is established using electrical charge and molecule density rather than gravity, but the analogy with the water tower holds. You may remember from playing with magnets that the positive poles of two magnets repel each other, but opposite poles attract. **Ions** are atoms that have either lost or gained an **electron** (negative particle), causing them to acquire either a positive or a negative charge, much like your magnet. Just as with your magnets, positive ions will be repelled by other positive ions but will be attracted to negative ions.

Concentration Gradient. A second type of gradient is derived from the concentration of ions. If there is a high concentration of molecules on one side of a membrane (a high **concentration gradient**), the molecules will tend to migrate until there are equal numbers of molecules on either side of the membrane. When charged particles move, the movement produces an electrical current. That is to say, if ions move across a membrane to enter or leave a cell, the very act of moving creates an electrical current. This is important for several reasons. First, current is a prime mover in activating the cell membrane, in that it activates ion channels, which open to promote more movement, as will be discussed. Second, this is the electrical activity that physicians record when they perform electroencephalography: EEG traces are the sum of much neural activity within the brain, produced by "generators." More importantly, for our field, the electrical activity of neurons is recorded by the audiologists when they perform **auditory brain stem response (ABR)** testing. This permits the audiologists to determine whether the auditory pathway is intact by measuring EEG emanations that have been time-locked to a stimulus such as a pure-tone source or a click. While you will learn more of this in your study of audiologic procedures, you must know for now that the ABR and similar measures of brain function are extremely important tools used by audiologists.

Ions cannot pass through membranous walls unless those walls are **permeable**. **Permeability** is the property of a membrane that determines the ease with which ions may pass through a membrane. Given appropriate circumstances, the wall of a neuron is considered to be semipermeable, meaning that *some* ions may pass through it. Ions may pass into or out of a healthy neuron wall through two mechanisms: passive and active transport.

Passive Transport. Ions in higher concentrations are held back from crossing the neural membrane by special proteins that serve as gatekeepers. **Voltage-sensitive proteins** are those gatekeepers that open when they receive adequate electrical stimulation. There also are **channel proteins** that allow specific ions to pass through the membrane. Essentially, these proteins prohibit ions from passing across the membrane until specific circumstances occur. When the circumstances of transport are met, these proteins will let specific ions pass through the membrane wall. The movement is considered to be passive transport because no energy is expended to move the ions across the barrier; rather, the gradient established by the inequalities between the two sides of the membrane causes ion movement.

Active Transport. The second mechanism for moving ions (**ion transport**) is active pumping. You will recall that in the water tank analogy, something had to pump water up into the tank. To do so required an *active* process that used energy. There are ion pumps to move sodium (Na^+) and potassium (K^+) ions against the gradient (i.e., pump them "uphill"). The energy used by these **sodium–potassium pump** proteins is in the form of adenosine triphosphate (ATP), a product of the mitochondria of the cell. The pumps operate continually, moving three sodium ions out for every two potassium ions moved in. Active transport is required to readjust the balance of ions across the membrane so that there is a gradient between the outside and inside of a neuron. Ions move passively across a membrane as a result of a gradient, but when that gradient is eliminated, active transport is responsible for reestablishing it. We now have the pieces to fire a neuron.

Figure 12-1 shows a neuron at rest. The minus signs inside the neuron indicate a negative charge, arising from the relatively smaller number of positive ions within the **intracellular space** (the space within individual cells) than outside in the **interstitial space** (the space between cells). At rest, there is a potential difference of 120 mV, a gradient that will promote ion movement if a channel opens to permit that movement. This charge is referred to as the **resting membrane potential (RMP)**. At rest, there are 30 times as many K^+ ions inside as outside, and 10 times as many Na^+ ions outside as inside. K^+ is continually leaking out of the cell and is continually being pumped back in by the sodium–potassium pumps. There are also markedly more negatively charged chloride ions (Cl^-) outside the cell than within. If the membrane were to permit free ion flow, the chemical gradient would drive Na^+ into the cell and K^+ out of the cell. The smaller number of charged particles within the cell would drive the potential difference to –70 mV.

An **action potential (AP)** is a change in electrical potential that occurs when the cell membrane is stimulated adequately to permit ion exchange between intra- and extracellular spaces. When a critical threshold of stimulation is reached, the Na^+ ion gates open up, causing the large number of ions to flood the intracellular space and thus raising the intracellular potential to +50 mV over the course of about

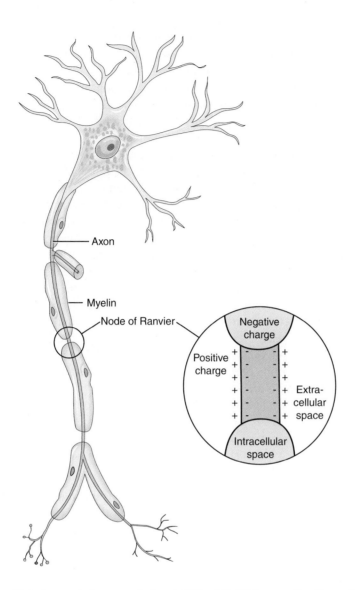

Axon

Myelin

Node of Ranvier

Negative charge

Positive charge

Extra-cellular space

Intracellular space

Figure 12-1. A quiescent neuron, showing equilibrium of membrane potential.
© Cengage Learning®.

1 ms (this is a net change of about 120 mV). This equalization of the ion gradient is called **depolarization**. For about 0.5 ms, no amount of stimulation of that region of the membrane will cause it to depolarize again. This phase of depolarization is termed the **absolute refractory period**, largely accomplished by the clamping effect of the introduction of Cl⁻. The absolute refractory period is the time during which the cell membrane cannot be stimulated to depolarize. During the absolute refractory period, the K^+ channels open up and K^+ ions flow out of the intracellular space. The sodium gates will spontaneously close and become inactivated (**sodium inactivation**), and the sodium–potassium pump removes most of the Na^+ ions while increasing the intracellular concentration of K^+ ions. Potassium channels are slower than sodium channels, and the outflow of K^+ ions actually promotes restoration of the RMP, because it increases the relative positivity of the extracellular fluid and, thus, the negativity of the intracellular fluid.

There is a period after the absolute refractory period during which the membrane may be stimulated, but stimulation will have to be much greater than that required to depolarize it initially. The **relative refractory period** is a period during which the membrane may be stimulated to excitation again, but only with greater than typical stimulation. This period follows the absolute refractory period. The relative refractory period lasts from 5 to 10 ms.

For APs to be generated, the membrane channels must break down. Portions of the cell membrane may be depolarized, but other parts of the membrane will not be depolarized until a critical threshold has been reached. The critical limit at which the membrane channels break down is approximately −50 mV. That is, portions of cell membrane may be depolarized, but an AP is not generated until ion movement is sufficient to elevate the membrane potential from −70 to −50 mV. If the membrane receives sufficient stimulation to cause the potential difference to drop to −50 mV, an AP will be generated, causing a cascade of ion movement and total depolarization of the neuron. If stimulation does not result in sufficient ion transfer to reach this level, an AP will not be triggered and the RMP will be restored by the ongoing action of the ion pump. This is an important modulating function of neurons, as we will see: It keeps neurons from firing until there is an adequate stimulus.

This whole cycle from RMP to AP and back to RMP takes about 1 ms in most neurons, and this is a defining time period. This means that a neuron may respond every 1/1,000 of a second, or 1,000 times per second. Even if it is stimulated 2,000 times per second, it will not be able to respond more often.

Propagation. An AP would do no good at all if it did not propagate, because no information would be passed to the next neuron or to a muscle fiber. **Propagation** refers to the spreading effect of wave action, much as the ripple generated by throwing a rock in a pond spreads out from the stone's point of contact with the water. The AP is propagated in a wave of depolarization. When the membrane undergoing the local polarization reaches the critical limit, ions flow rapidly across the membrane, as we discussed. Because the adjacent membrane contains voltage-sensitive protein channels, the current flow stimulates those regions to depolarize as well. In this manner the depolarization spreads along the membrane, ultimately reaching the terminal of the axon. This regeneration of the AP along the entire length of the axon will produce precisely the same voltage difference.

The neuron responds in an all-or-nothing manner. That is, it either depolarizes or it does not. If it fails to depolarize, no AP is generated and no information is conveyed. If the critical threshold for depolarization is reached, an AP will be produced and information will be transmitted. The neuron acts like a light switch in this sense, and the only variation in information is caused by the frequency with which the neuron is "turned on," referred to as **spike rate** or **rate of discharge**.

Propagation of the AP is facilitated by axon diameter and the presence of myelin. Fibers with larger diameters propagate at a much higher rate than those with smaller diameters, and myelin further speeds up propagation. Figure 12-2 shows that myelin is laid down on the axon in "donuts" with nodes of exposed membrane between them, called the nodes of Ranvier. Voltage-sensitive channels are found within the membrane of the **nodes of Ranvier** but generally are absent in the myelinated regions. The myelin insulates the fiber so that even if there were channels they would serve no function, because ions cannot pass through them. The nodes of Ranvier are precisely spaced, based upon the diameter of the axon, to promote maximum conduction time.

Thus, the membrane becomes depolarized at one node, and the effect of that depolarization is felt at the next node where the membrane depolarizes as well. The propagating action potential is "passed" from node to node, and this jumping is referred to as **saltatory conduction**. Clearly, in long fibers, many precious milliseconds can be saved by skipping from node to node.

The node of Ranvier is described inChapter 11.

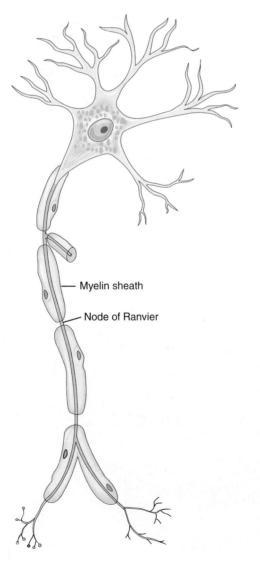

Myelin sheath

Node of Ranvier

Figure 12-2. Myelin sheath and nodes of Ranvier.
© Cengage Learning®.

When the impulse reaches the terminal point on an axon, a highly specialized process begins. The synaptic vesicles within the terminal end boutons release a neurotransmitter substance that will permit communication between two neurons. A **neurotransmitter** is a substance that causes either the excitation or inhibition of another neuron or the excitation of a muscle fiber. When the AP reaches the terminal point, the vesicles are stimulated to migrate to the membrane wall, where they will dump their neurotransmitter through the membrane into the synaptic cleft (see Figure 12-3 and Table 12-2).

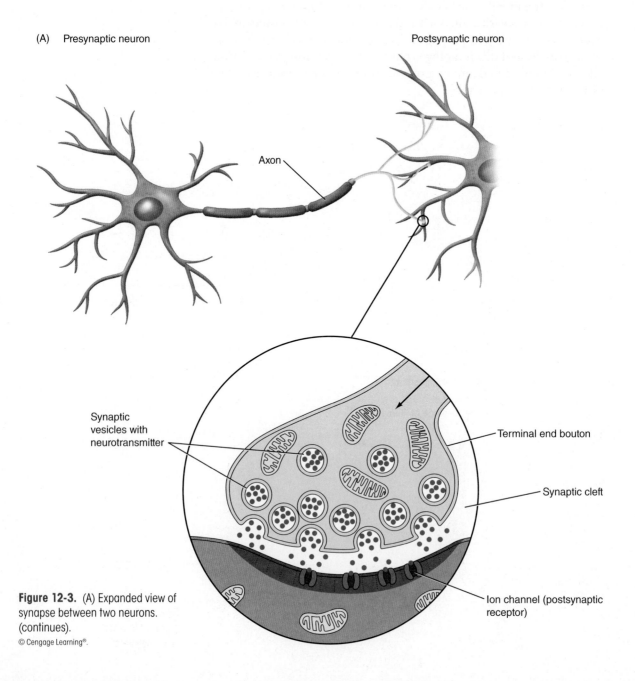

(A) Presynaptic neuron

Postsynaptic neuron

Axon

Synaptic vesicles with neurotransmitter

Terminal end bouton

Synaptic cleft

Ion channel (postsynaptic receptor)

Figure 12-3. (A) Expanded view of synapse between two neurons. (continues).

© Cengage Learning®.

(B)

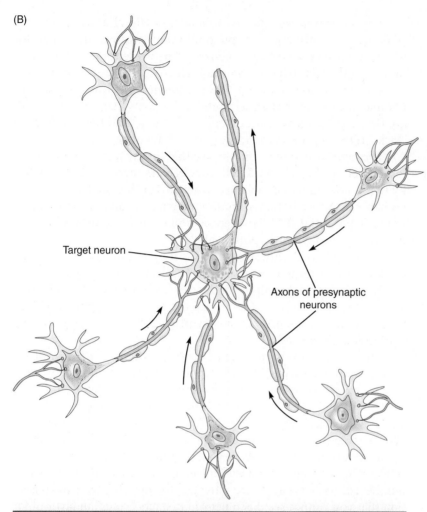

Target neuron

Axons of presynaptic neurons

Figure 12-3 continued.
(B) Convergence of multiple neurons upon a single postsynaptic neuron.
© Cengage Learning®.

Table 12-2 **Some neurotransmitters of the peripheral and central nervous system**

Neurotransmitter	Site	Specific Region (Function)
Acetylcholine	PNS	Myoneural junction (excitatory)
	CNS	Forebrain, brain stem (modulatory), basal ganglia (inhibitory)
Dopamine	CNS	Limbic system (modulatory), basal ganglia (excitatory)
Norepinephrine	CNS	Brain stem reticular formation (regulatory)
Serotonin	CNS	Brain stem, limbic system (regulatory)
Gamma-aminobutyric	CNS	Basal ganglia, other CNS structures (GABA) (inhibitory)
Endorphins	CNS	Throughout CNS (pain regulation)

Source: See Bhatnagar, 2007 and Cotman & McGaugh, 1980, for further discussion.

The neurotransmitter travels across the cleft very quickly (100 microseconds) and is emptied into the cleft to activate receptor proteins on the **postsynaptic neuron**. The presence of neurotransmitters in the cleft triggers ion channels to open. Neurotransmitters fit into specific ion channels, and if a given neurotransmitter does not match a receptor channel protein, the postsynaptic neuron will not fire. That is, the neurotransmitter is a "key" and the receptor is a "lock." If the key does not fit, the gate will not open.

The neurotransmitter may have either an excitatory or an inhibitory effect on the neuron. **Excitatory effects** increase the probability that a neuron will depolarize, whereas **inhibition** decreases that probability. An excitatory stimulation generates an **excitatory postsynaptic potential (EPSP)**, whereas inhibitory stimulus produces an **inhibitory postsynaptic potential (IPSP)**. Excitation causes depolarization, whereas inhibition causes **hyperpolarization**, greatly elevating the threshold of firing. Generally, inhibitory synapses are found on the soma. Synapses on the dendrites are usually excitatory. Synapses on the axon tend to reduce the amount of neurotransmitter substance released into the synaptic cleft, thereby modulating neurotransmitter flow.

The EPSP actually begins as a **micropotential** or **miniature postsynaptic potential (MPSP)**, depolarizing the membrane by only about 3 mV. If there is a sufficient number of MPSP depolarizations, the sum of their depolarization will reach the critical threshold and an AP will be generated, as before. You may think of this as voting by neurons. Hundreds or even thousands of neurons form synapses on a given neuron, and that means that the output of that single neuron reflects the "conventional wisdom" of all those neurons. If sufficient numbers of those synapses are activated, the majority wins in an election that you cannot see: Each neuron casts its "votes" in favor of (or against) activation, in the form of activation of a small portion of the receptive membrane. If there are sufficient numbers of depolarizations, there will be an AP. This is called spatial summation. **Spatial summation** refers to the phenomenon of many near-simultaneous synaptic activations, representing many points of contact arrayed over the surface of the neuron. Likewise, there can be **temporal summation**, in which a smaller number of regions depolarize virtually simultaneously. To stretch our voting analogy to fit temporal summation, votes would have to be cast at approximately the same time to be counted (late-arriving mail-in ballots would not help make the decision).

Single neurons may take input from thousands of other neurons to produce a single response, a process called **convergence**. In this configuration, a volume of information is distilled into a single response. In contrast, **divergence** occurs when the axon of one neuron makes synapse with many thousands of other neurons. Its single piece of information is transmitted to a vast array of other neurons.

The neurotransmitter substance released into the synaptic cleft does not go to waste. As soon as it is released, enzymes specific to it break it down for its resynthesis within the neuron.

Myasthenia Gravis

Myasthenia gravis is a neuromuscular disease; its primary effect is on the neuromuscular junction. It appears that an affected individual's autoimmune system develops an immune response to the neurotransmitter receptor of the neuromuscular junction, building antibodies that block the receptor. Blocked receptors are unable to respond to neurotransmitter substances, so that, as the disease progresses, greater numbers of receptors become blocked and increasingly fewer ion channels can be utilized to activate a muscle. The result is a progressive loss of strength in the muscle that is activated by the myoneural junction.

An individual with myasthenia gravis will complain of extreme fatigue as the day progresses: He or she may feel reasonably well in the morning but become exhausted by noon. Speech-language pathologists are quite often the first to suspect myasthenia gravis because they notice when speech has become more difficult and when people are having difficulty understanding what they say. Reduced velar function is often an early sign, producing hypernasal speech with reduced intelligibility.

✔ *To summarize:*

- Communication between neurons of the nervous system occurs at the **synapse**.
- **Neurotransmitters** passing through the **synaptic cleft** will either **excite** or **inhibit** the postsynaptic neuron.
- If a neuron is excited sufficiently, an **action potential** will be generated.
- Stimulation of a neuron membrane to **depolarize** the neuron causes exchange of ions between the extracellular and intracellular spaces, and the ion movement results in a large and predictable change in voltage across the membrane.
- The **resting membrane potential** is the electrical potential measurable prior to excitation.
- The **absolute refractory period** after excitation is an interval during which the neuron cannot be excited to fire, whereas it may fire during the **relative refractory period**, given adequate stimulation.
- Because an **action potential** always results in the same neural response, the neuron is capable of representing differences in input only through its rate of response.
- Myelinated fibers conduct the wave of depolarization more rapidly than demyelinated fibers, primarily because of **saltatory conduction**.

Muscle Function

A similar process occurs at the **neuromuscular junction**, the point where a nerve and muscle communicate. In this case, the product of the communication will be a muscle twitch rather than an AP. The basic unit of skeletal muscle control is the **motor unit**, consisting of the motor neuron, its axon, and the muscle fibers it innervates.

Figure 12-4 shows a neuromuscular junction, which looks very much like a synapse. In this case, however, there is a **terminal endplate** on the axon, with a synaptic cleft as before. The neurotransmitter **acetylcholine** is released into the active zone, and a **miniature end plate potential (MEPP)** will be generated. If there are sufficient numbers of MEPPs, a muscle action potential will be generated. This is directly analogous to that of a synapse, in that it takes many activated regions to excite a muscle fiber. In addition, we will see that we have to activate many muscle fibers to actually move a muscle and do work.

You know that movement requires muscular effort, and that muscles can only contract, shortening the distance between two points. This is a good opportunity to examine that function at a microscopic level.

If you were to look at a cotton rope, you would see that the rope is actually made up of smaller ropes, wrapped in a spiral. If you were to look closer, you could see that those smaller spiral ropes are made up of individual strings, and your microscope would show you that those strings were made of cotton fibers that had been spun into thread. There are successively smaller elements from which the rope is made, and they all have a similar orientation and structure. The same is true for the muscle.

As you can see from Figure 12-5, the skeletal (striated) muscle is a long ropelike structure made up of strands of muscle fiber, each running the length of the muscle and having many nuclei. Each muscle fiber is made up of long **myofibrils**, and myofibrils are composed of either **thin** or **thick myofilaments**.

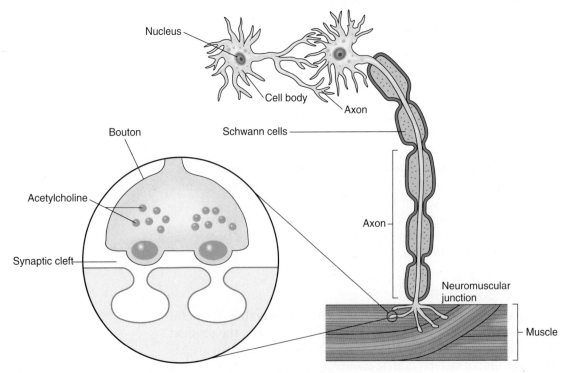

Figure 12-4. Neuromuscular junction between neuron and muscle fiber.
© Cengage Learning®.

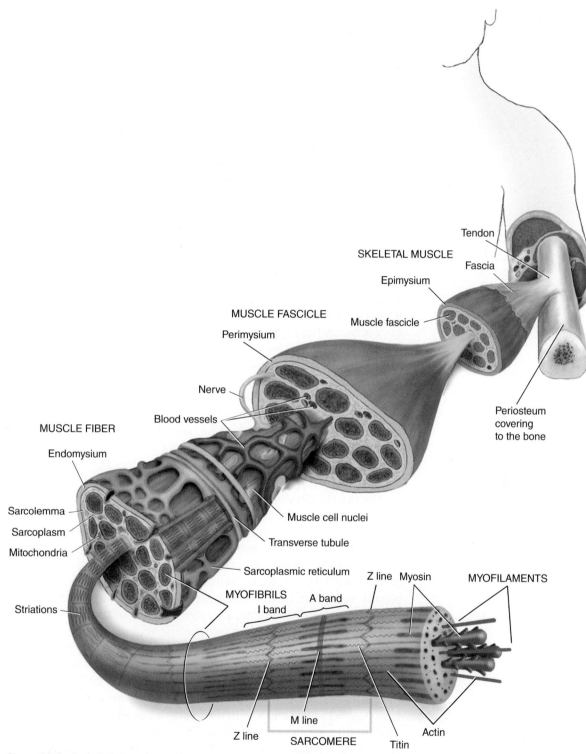

Figure 12-5. Exploded view of muscle fiber components. Each muscle fiber is made up of thin and thick filaments.

© Cengage Learning®.

Thin myofilaments are composed of a pair of **actin** protein strands coiled around each other to form a spiral or helix. Double strands of tropomyosin that are laced with molecules of troponin wrap around this helix. Thick myofilaments are composed of myosin molecules arranged in a staggered formation. These two components (actin and myosin) are key players in movement: The actin and myosin filaments slide past each other during muscle contraction, with **bridging arms** reaching from the myosin to the actin. The tropomyosin and troponin facilitate the bridging arms, as you shall see.

When the myofilaments group together to form muscle myofibrils, a characteristic striated appearance is seen. This is the product of alternating dark and light myofilaments. Each of these combined units is known as a **sarcomere**. The sarcomere is the building block of striated muscle. An area known as the **Z line** marks the margin of the sarcomere, and the thin filaments are bound at this point. The thick filaments are centered within the sarcomere, much like overlapping bricks in a wall. The **A band** is the region of overlap between thin and thick fibers at rest, and the **H zone** in the center of the sarcomere is a region with only thick filaments. The two myofilaments slide across each other as the muscle shortens, bringing the centers of the thin and thick filaments closer together. Here is how that happens.

When the muscle is at rest, the regulatory proteins of tropomyosin on the thin filaments block the binding sites, prohibiting the formation of cross-bridges. The regulatory proteins are guards that prohibit the myosin and actin from interacting. For a cross-bridge to form, the tropomyosin must be moved out of the way to free up the binding sites, and that function is performed by calcium. When calcium is present in the environment, it changes the configuration of the proteins, revealing the binding site on the thin filaments and facilitating the development of cross-bridges. Calcium has the "password" that causes the tropomyosin "guards" to move away from the binding sites and to permit cross-bridges to form. What causes the calcium to enter the environment, though?

Calcium is found within the sarcoplasmic reticulum of the muscle cytoplasm. (Sarcoplasmic reticulum is a form of the cellular endoplasmic reticulum.) An AP generated at the neuromuscular junction is conveyed deep into the muscle cell by a series of transverse tubules that are in contact with the sarcoplasmic reticulum. The AP depolarizes the membrane of the sarcoplasmic reticulum, permitting calcium ions to be released. Tropomyosin and troponin are critical to the formation of bridges that causes the muscle fibril to shorten in length. When the tropomyosin and tropinin are activated by calcium they change shape, which reveals the binding site for myosin. This, in turn, allows myosin to form a bridge with the thin filaments. Adenosine triphosphate (ATP) provides the energy to the bridging arm (that is the same energy that you run out of when you become fatigued from overwork), which reaches across to a binding site on the thin filaments, pulls, and releases even as other arms are pulling and releasing. When the AP terminates, calcium is taken back up into the sarcoplasmic reticulum, the binding site is once again hidden, and contraction ceases. That is, an AP at the neuromuscular junction causes the release of calcium into the environment of actin and myosin. Calcium causes the binding sites to be revealed so that crossbridges can be formed between the two molecules—at that point, muscle contraction begins.

It seems like a lot of work to contract a muscle, and it is. Work requires energy, and ATP supplies it. The actual contraction is much like pulling yourself up a mountainside using a rope. You grab the rope (cross-bridge) and pull, hand-over-hand, drawing yourself upward. Your arms are like the myosin arms, the rope is like the thin filament of actin, and you are the thick filament. This is the **sliding filament model** of muscle contraction.

In this process, the center of the sarcomere (the H zone) will disappear as the sarcomere shortens. There are about 350 heads on each thick filament that can bridge across to the thin filaments, and each bridge can perform its "hand-over-hand" act five times per second. If you remember that it takes many myofilaments to make up one muscle fiber, and that a muscle bundle is made up of many muscle fibers, you will begin to realize the magnitude of activity involved in moving your little finger.

Muscle Control

This still does not tell us how a muscle does its job. When the AP is generated and the sarcoplasmic reticulum releases calcium, there is an all-or-none response, and the muscle twitches. From your study, you already know that muscles come in all sizes, from the massive to the minute. In addition, muscles must perform vastly different functions, ranging from gross, slow movement to quick, precise action. How do we manage this?

The answer lies largely in the allocation of resources. For fine movement, only a limited number of muscle fibers need be recruited, because you are not trying to move as much mass. In contrast, heavy lifting requires the recruitment of many muscle fibers. This makes sense if you consider the effort involved in moving objects. It takes only one person to move a chair, but it might take four or five individuals to lift a piano.

Neuromotor innervation accounts for much of the allocation of resources: Each muscle fiber is innervated by one motor neuron, but each motor neuron may innervate a large number of muscle fibers. The more motor neurons that are activated, the greater the number of fibers that will contract. The use of many motor nerves to activate a muscle is called **multiple motor unit summation**.

Another mechanism of control comes from a functional difference between how various muscles act. There are two basic types of muscle fibers: slow twitch fibers and fast twitch fibers. As their name implies, **slow twitch fibers** take a longer time to move, whereas fast twitch fibers are capable of much more rapid movement. Slow twitch muscle fibers remain contracted five times longer than do fast twitch fibers, perhaps because calcium remains in the cytoplasm for longer periods. Slow twitch fibers are typically found in muscles that must contract for long periods of time, such as those used to support your body against gravity. Fast twitch muscles, in contrast, are used to meet rapid contraction requirements. Now remember our discussion of the tongue anatomy and physiology: Recall that the tongue tip moves much more rapidly than the massive dorsum, but it is not *only* the mass of the musculature that determines the speed of response. The rapidly moving tongue tip is supplied with *fast twitch fibers*, but the slow-moving deep tongue muscles have *slow twitch fibers*.

There is another significant difference between slow and fast twitch fibers. One neuron may innervate thousands of slow twitch fibers, but neurons serving fast twitch fibers may innervate only 10 or 20 muscle fibers. With this difference in innervation ratio you can get extremely fine control: If you need to tense the vocal folds quickly for pitch change, you want to be able to control precisely the fraction of a millimeter required to keep your voice from going sharp while singing. This control comes from being able to activate progressively more motor units in fine steps. In contrast, maintaining an erect posture requires less precision and more stamina.

✔ *To summarize:*

- Activation of a muscle fiber causes the release of calcium into the environment of **thick myofilaments**, revealing the binding sites on the **thin filaments** that permit **cross-bridging** from the thick filaments.
- The action of the bridging causes the myofilaments to slide past each other, thereby shortening the muscle.
- **Slow twitch** muscle fibers remain contracted longer than **fast twitch** fibers, with the former being involved in the maintenance of posture and the latter in fine and rapid motor functions.

Muscle Spindle Function

We touched upon the activities of the muscle spindle in Chapter 11, but let us discuss its function more thoroughly. If you examine Figure 12-6, you will see the major players in posture and motor control in general. It is sobering to realize that the lowest level of motor response (the stretch reflex) is intimately related to the highest levels of motor response requiring extraordinary skill and dexterity, such as the fine motor control of the fingers. Discussion of the muscle spindle will provide the background necessary to talk about higher-level motor control.

The role of the muscle spindle is to provide feedback to the neuromotor system about muscle length and thus information about motion and position. Before we explain that function, let us examine the structure of this important sensory element.

There are two basic types of striated muscle fibers with which we must be concerned. **Extrafusal muscle** fibers make up the bulk of the muscles discussed over the past several chapters. Deep within

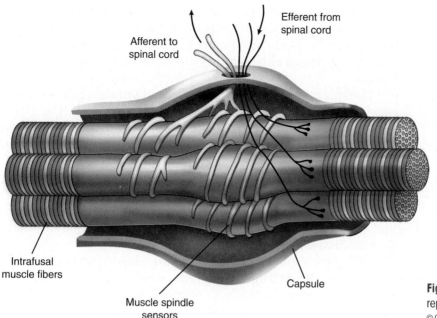

Efferent from
spinal cord

Afferent to
spinal cord

Intrafusal
muscle fibers

Muscle spindle
sensors

Capsule

Figure 12-6. Schematic
representation of a muscle spindle.
© Cengage Learning®.

the structure of the muscle is another set of muscle fibers, referred
to as **intrafusal muscle fibers**. These fibers have a parallel course to
the extrafusal fibers and would not really be obvious on gross examination of a muscle. Close examination would reveal short intrafusal
fibers that attach to the muscle and are capable of sensing changes
in the length of the muscle. At or near the **equatorial region** of the
intrafusal muscle fiber are the stretch sensors themselves, with the
combination of muscle and sensor known as the **muscle spindle**, so
named because of its spindle shape.

The intrafusal fibers may be classified as being either thin or
thick. Thick muscle fibers are typically outfitted with a capsule that
contains nuclear bag fibers, and thin muscle fibers house nuclear
chain fibers. **Nuclear bag fibers** are groups of stretch receptors col-
lected in a cluster at the equatorial region of the intrafusal muscle
fiber. **Nuclear chain fibers**, in contrast, are a row of stretch sensors in the equatorial region. These two configurations serve different functions, as we shall see. The placement of the capsules in the
equatorial region is important, because that portion of these fibers is
noncontractile.

The muscle spindle has both afferent and efferent innerva-
tions. The afferent component conveys the sensation of muscle
length change to the central nervous system (CNS), while the efferent system conveys nerve impulses that cause the intrafusal fibers
to contract. The innervation pattern is important. Nuclear bag
fibers send information to the CNS by means of **Group Ia primary**
afferent fibers, which wrap around the capsule in a spiral formation. Group Ia fibers are large, and when a muscle is stretched, the
nuclear bag changes shape. That distortion causes the nerve to fire,

The term nuclear bag fiber
refers to the portion of the
muscle spindle that is formed
by a cluster of stretch sensors
situated on the equatorial
region of the muscle fiber.

sending information to the spinal cord. Bags surrounding nuclear chain fibers may have either primary Ia or Group II secondary afferent fibers. These are smaller fibers conveying a functionally different response, although they also respond to stretching of the muscle.

Extrafusal (general skeletal muscle) and intrafusal (muscle spindle) muscle fibers have distinctly different innervation. The extrafusal muscle is innervated by **alpha motor neuron** fibers, which are larger in diameter than the **gamma** (or **fusimotor**) efferent fibers of the intrafusal muscle.

As you can see, there is a great deal of physical differentiation going on with this sensorimotor system. There are two types of sensors, two types of afferent fibers delivering information to the CNS, and a specialized efferent system (gamma efferents) that can cause the intrafusal muscle to contract.

The muscle spindle responds to both phasic and tonic muscle lengthening. **Phasic lengthening** refers to the process of *change* in a muscle length. This information is transduced by the nuclear bag fibers and conveyed via Group Ia afferents to the CNS. **Tonic lengthening** refers to activity of *maintaining* a muscle in a lengthened condition, and this information is conveyed via the nuclear chain fibers by means of either type of afferent. It turns out that both pieces of information are essential for motor control.

Figure 12-7 will help you discuss how this system helps you control your muscles. A useful way to describe how the spindle works is to think of posture control. If you were to pay close attention to your

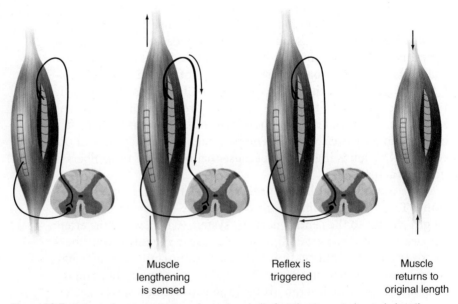

| Muscle lengthening is sensed | Reflex is triggered | Muscle returns to original length |

Figure 12-7. Schematic representation of muscle spindle function to control muscle length.
© Cengage Learning®.

body as you stand in line to buy a ticket, you would notice that you sway ever so slightly. That slight movement you feel is a trigger for the intrafusal system.

When you lean a little, some of your leg muscles stretch. When they do so, the spindle sends notice to the motor neuron within the spinal column that the muscle has changed position. The motor neuron with which it synapses immediately activates the extrafusal muscle mass, causing it to contract, thereby counteracting that "accidental" stretching that occurred in response to gravity. Notice that you passively stretched the muscle spindle fibers and then the muscles of your leg with which those spindles are associated contracted to return the muscle to its original length.

One more thing to note in Figure 12-7 is that this afferent synapses with another neuron. In the figure, the spindle within the flexor is sending its information centrally. The afferent makes an **inhibitory synapse** with extensors associated with the same joint, so that you are not only actively contracting flexors but also actively inhibiting the contraction of extensors.

There are hosts of reflexive responses, mediated by the spinal cord and brain stem, and even through cortical response. While it is clearly beyond the scope of this review to discuss those, you may wish to examine Table 12-3 for a sampling of some of those reflexes.

Lesions and the Gamma Efferent System

To appreciate the effects of lesions to the extra-pyramidal system, it might help to do a quick exercise. Do this: Reach across the desktop to pick up a pencil. As you do this, pay attention to what your muscles are doing. Even as you reach for the pencil, your elbow rotates to accommodate the needs of your arm and hand to make contact with the object. As you get close to the target, your fingers start to close and the rate of movement of your arm slows down. For all of this to happen, your brain must know how fast your muscles are changing length, as well as where the target is located in space relative to your hand and body. Contraction of extensors obviously is important, but your brain must also contract flexors to help control extensor contraction, lest the movement be ballistic.

Damage to the cerebellum will reduce activation of the fusimotor system. Because this system maintains muscle tone through mild, constant muscle contraction, muscles in a patient with lesions to the cerebellum will lose tone and become flaccid. In contrast, loss of the moderating control by the cerebrum through lesions will cause hypertonia in antigravity musculature and extensors, because the stretch reflexes are unrestrained. In this condition, the alpha system is either disabled or not well coordinated with the gamma system due to the lesion, and spasticity results.

Lesions or conditions of the basal ganglia will have various effects, one among them being the rigidity of Parkinson's disease. In this condition, intrafusal systems for both extensors and flexors are unrestrained, resulting in the simultaneous contraction of antagonists and rigidity. Other basal ganglia lesions will result in general hypertonicity or fluctuating muscle tone, resulting in extraneous movement.

Table 12-3 **A sample of reflexes mediated by the spinal cord and the brainstem. Note that several variations have been eliminated for brevity, as have specific stimulus conditions**

Spinal Reflexes

Palmar grasp reflex	Placing object on ventral surface of fingers causes fingers to flex (up to 3 to 4 months).
Sucking reflex	Stroking lips laterally causes sucking action (ends at 6 months to 1 year).
Knee-jerk tendon	Rapid stretching of patellar tendon by tapping on knee at tendon causes extension of leg (present after 6 months).
Flexor withdrawal	In supine position, head in mid position; leg flexes when sole of foot is stimulated (ends at 2 months).
Extensor thrust	In supine position with head in mid position, one leg extended and one leg flexed; leg remains flexed when sole is stimulated (ends at 2 months).
Crossed extension	In supine position with head in mid position, one leg extended and one leg flexed; when extended leg is flexed, the opposite leg will extend (before 2 months) or remain flexed (after 2 months).
Crossed extension	In supine position with head in mid position and legs extended; stimulation of medial leg surface causes adduction (ends at 2 months).

Brain Stem Reflexes

Asymmetrical tonic neck reflex (ATNR)	In supine position with arms and legs extended and head in mid position; if head is turned, arm on face side extends, arm on opposite side flexes (ends 4–6 months).
Symmetrical tonic neck reflex	In quadrupeds, on tester's knee; ventroflex (toward belly), no change in arm/leg tone (before 6 months) or arms flex or increase tone and legs extend or increase tone (after 6 months).
Tonic labyrinthine supine reflex	In supine position with arms and legs extended; passive flexing of arms and legs does not increase tone (before 6 months) or does increase tone (after 6 months).
Tonic labyrinthine prone reflex	In prone position with head in mid position; no increase in flexor tone (before 4 months) or cannot dorsiflex head, retract shoulders, or extend arms and legs (after 4 months).
Associated	In supine position, have individual squeeze object; increases tone in opposite arm and hand (before 6 months) or produces no change in opposite-side tone (after 6 months).
Positive supporting reactions	In standing position, bounce individual on soles of feet; no increase in leg tone (up to 8 months) or increase in extensor tone (after 8 months).
Neck righting reflex	In supine position with head in mid position and arms and legs extended; rotate head, and body will rotate (before 6 months) or not rotate (after 6 months).
Body righting; acting on the body	In supine position with head in mid position, arms and legs extended; rotate head to one side, and body rotates as a whole (before 6 months), or head turns, then shoulders, and finally pelvis (after 6 months).

Labyrinthine righting; acting on the head	Blindfolded and suspended in prone; head does not rise (before 2 months) or rises with face vertical and mouth horizontal (after 1 month).
Optical righting	Held in space in prone, head does not rise (before 2 months) or rises to face vertical and mouth horizontal (after 2 months).
Moro reflex	In semireclined position, drop head backward; arms extend, arms rotate, fingers extend and abduct (under 4 months).
Landau reflex	Held in space supported at thorax in prone; raise head and spine, and legs extend and remain in flexed position (from 6 months).
Positive extensor thrust (parachute reaction)	In prone position with arms extended overhead, suspended in space by pelvis; move suddenly downward; arms extend, fingers abduct and extend to protect head (after 6 months).
Rooting reflex and sucking reflex	Stroke the side of the mouth at the corner of the lips laterally; the infant will orient toward the fingers with a sucking motion of the lips (before 6 months).
Jaw reflex	Pull down on the mandible briskly, or draw down on the masseter with deep pressure and the mandible will snap to close (before 6 months).

Source: For a thorough review of reflexes, elicitation procedures, and normal and pathological responses, see Bly (1994) and Fiorentino (1973).

What if you move your legs purposefully? How do the muscle spindles oppose *that* movement? When a new posture is reached, the intrafusal muscle contracts to adjust the tension on the spindle, accommodating the new posture. Likewise, the muscle spindle afferent information is delivered to the cerebral cortex and cerebellum. When voluntary movement is initiated, both alpha and gamma systems are activated. There is speculation that the gamma system receives information from the cortex concerning the desired or *target* muscle length, and thus the gamma system provides feedback to the cortex when this length has been achieved. Thus, the gamma system may be a regulatory mechanism for voluntary movement: Damage to this system has devastating effects.

Golgi Tendon Organs

Another type of sensor, which is less well understood, is the Golgi tendon organ (GTO), a sensor located at the tendon and sensitive to the degree of tension on the muscle. If the muscle is passively stretched, it takes a great deal to excite a GTO. However, if a muscle is contracted, the GTO is quite sensitive to the tension placed on it.

The GTO probably works in close conjunction with the muscle spindle. The muscle spindle is active any time a muscle is lengthened, while the GTO is sensitive to the *tension* placed on the muscle. If a muscle is tensed the isometrically, the lengthening will be minimal but the GTO will react to the tension placed on it by contraction. Likewise, if a muscle is passively stretched, the muscle spindle will respond but the tendon organ will not.

Other Sensation and Sensors

There are a host of other receptors, as we discussed in Chapters 8 and 11. Sensory receptors are nerve endings that have become specialized to **transduce** (change) energy from one form to another.

When one of these sensors is stimulated, it sends information concerning that stimulation to the CNS for processing. You will not be aware of stimulation unless a threshold of stimulation is reached. This threshold varies from sensor to sensor, and even from individual to individual. A stimulus capable of eliciting a response from a given receptor is termed the **adequate stimulus**. The receptor converts the excitatory energy (e.g., tactile pressure) into electrochemical energy by the creation of a receptor potential that stimulates a dendrite. The magnitude of the potential is related to that of the stimulus and will typically be constant until the stimulus is removed.

Sensors vary in morphology and function, but fall into the general classes of encapsulated and nonencapsulated. Encapsulated sensors tend to be pressure sensitive, transducing pressure applied to the skin into electrochemical energy sensed by the nervous system. Some sensors are **rapidly adapting**, in that they respond only to change in stimulation. These sensors are particularly well suited for transduction of vibration, whereas **slowly adapting** sensors respond better to long-duration stimulation. Pain, temperature, and some mechanoreceptors are simply unshielded nerve endings that respond when stimulated by one or several different stimuli. The sensation of joint position in space apparently is the product of many of these encapsulated and nonencapsulated sensors.

✔ *To summarize:*

- **Muscle spindles** provide feedback to the neuromotor system about muscle length, tension, motion, and position.
- Muscle spindles running parallel to the intrafusal muscle fibers sense lengthening of muscle, whereas **Golgi tendon organs** sense muscle tension.
- **Nuclear bag fibers** convey information concerning acceleration, whereas the **nuclear chain fibers** are responsive to sustained lengthening.
- When a muscle is passively stretched, a **segmental reflex** is triggered; this in turn activates the **extrafusal muscles** paralleling the muscle spindles, thereby shortening the muscle.
- **Golgi tendon organs** apparently respond to the tension of musculature during active contraction.
- There are many other receptor types, but the common thread is that they all transduce internal or external environment information into electrochemical impulses.
- When a sensor is stimulated beyond its threshold for response, it sends information concerning that stimulation to the CNS for processing.

HIGHER FUNCTIONING

We have been discussing responses that occur at the lowest levels of the nervous system and often do not even reach consciousness. Although it is essential for your brain to know what your tongue muscles are doing, it is obvious that there is more to speech than the movement of muscles.

A lively debate concerning localization of function within the brain has been going on for well over 100 years. **Localizationists**, on the one hand (or "materialists" as they were called in the 1860s), held that, given sufficiently sensitive tools, specific functions could be localized to specific brain regions. The opposing view, held by "**spiritualists**," was that it was degrading to think that the human body (much less the brain) could be so mechanically dissected, and that functions such as language or mathematics could not be isolated to a single brain region. Perhaps the first localizationist was Joseph Gall, who also proposed that a properly knowledgeable individual could identify specific cognitive traits of an individual by reading the bumps on that person's head (**phrenology**) (Kandel, Schwartz, & Jessell, 2000).

While phrenology did not retain many followers, one admirer of Gall, Paul Broca, was the first to identify the region for expressive language within the dominant hemisphere of the brain (Kandel, Schwartz, & Jessel, 2000; Schuell, Jenkins, & Jiménez-Pabon, 1964). Others provided counterevidence, including patients whose acquired language deficit clearly arose from another region distal from the area identified by Broca. Such notables as Sigmund Freud refuted the notion of localization of function, saying that although some specific locations for basic processes might be found, that still did not explain complex cognitive function (Schuell, Jenkins, & Jiménez-Pabon, 1964).

Carl Wernicke entered the battle, clearly identifying a language center within the temporal lobe, distinct from that identified by Broca. Indeed, as the twentieth century dawned, localization of function was demonstrated through ablation studies of the occipital and temporal lobes of dogs, which eliminated visual and auditory recognition, respectively. Researchers found that they could stimulate specific locales of a dog's cerebrum and cause single, replicable movements of the limbs (Schuell, Jenkins, & Jimenez-Pabon, 1964).

Although such notable researchers as Karl Lashley countered the growing body of evidence, research that examined brain-damaged soldiers during the First and Second World Wars revealed a great deal of "regional" consistency of symptoms, and these findings led us into the study and treatment of acquired language disorders (Kandel, Schwartz, & Jessell, 2000).

Parallel work by microbiologists such as Nobel laureates David Hubel and Torsten Wiesel, dealing with monkeys (Hubel, 1979), and Colin Blakemore and Grahame Cooper (1970), studying cats, revealed a degree of specificity in the nervous system that must have surpassed even Broca's dreams. Researchers have found neurons within the

Synaptic Pruning

A normal and natural process, called synaptic pruning, involves elimination of synapses that are no longer needed. This pruning, which results in a massive loss of synapses, axons, and neurons, occurs at three significant points in a person's life: prenatally, during childhood, and at puberty. All of these prunings occur as a direct result of experience. You may have heard the statement "use it or lose it." This is the starkest manifestation of it, because literally if you do not use a synapse, you will lose it. This is not bad, mind you, because if you never pruned back on connections in your brain, your thought processes would be overwhelmed by the noise of those residual connections. As it is, the process of learning (experiencing stimuli) causes synapses to increase in strength, and the process of deprivation (not experiencing stimuli) causes synapses to die off. This is an elegant process that supports memory and learning, and keeps our brain from becoming overwhelmed.

Neuroscience has long held that the blood–brain barrier, arising from the protective function of astrocytes, kept the immune system from operating within the brain. Research by Chun and Schatz (1999) has shown that not only are there identity markers for neural tissues (major histocompatibility complex [MHC] markers) within the brain, but it now appears that these MHC markers team up with a molecule (C1q) secreted by neurons to prune synapses that are not needed. Astrocytes secrete thrombospondin to support development of synapses. The C1q marks the synapses as "junk," and macrophages collect and dispose of them.

This synaptic pruning poses some interesting and intriguing questions about neurogenic disorders. It is possible that aberrant C1q function is at the root of demyelinating diseases such as multiple sclerosis. Indeed, individuals who have early signs of Alzheimer's dementia have already lost over half of their synapses, and the C1q molecule is present in overwhelming numbers. Similarly, it is hypothesized that children with autism may have excessive numbers of synapses, as demonstrated by increased cerebral volume. One research group (Belmonte et al., 2004) posited that maternal infection during prenatal development may trigger an immune dysfunction in the brain of the fetus that may later result in inadequate synaptic pruning. One of the long-held observations about autism is the extraordinary response of the individual to sensory overload, and this would be supported by the pruning hypothesis.

nervous system that respond to exactly one form of stimulation (e.g., vertical lines presented to the visual system) and no other stimulation. These findings revealed extremes of localization of function.

That having been said, there appears no end to the complexity of the nervous system. As an example, the fusiform gyrus is just lateral to the parahippocampal gyrus. It is also known as the fusiform face area and appears to be specialized in recognizing faces of individuals (Tsao, Feirwald, Tootell, & Livingstone, 2006). Indeed, there is mounting evidence that *single neurons* within this area are dedicated to specific faces of people. That is to say, there are neurons that recognize, for instance, your grandmother (indeed, they have been called "grandmother neurons"). They recognize the canonical version of your grandmother, however, and not just a single picture of her. For instance, if you were to see a picture of your grandmother that you had never seen before, the same neuron would fire in response to it. (Let's be careful here, however: That single neuron has received input from a large number of other neurons, so its development of that canonical version of your grandmother arises from many inputs.) Evidence of the "grandmother neuron" emerged from physiological, single neuron studies of individuals undergoing craniotomy (open skull surgery) for epileptic seizures. In this treatment (electrocorticography), individuals are fitted with a grid of electrodes that are placed on the surface of the brain and that record electrical discharge. Patients must be hospitalized as they wait for a seizure to be recorded. Since many epileptic seizures focus upon the temporal lobe, researchers recognized that this population would be ideal for studying the face-sensitive neurons. These face-sensitive neurons are the localizationist's dream because they represent the type of specificity that defines that model of neural processing.

We will take a regional approach to review of the function of the cerebral cortex. Although it is clear that regions of the cerebral cortex, such as the motor strip, are highly specialized for specific functions, other regions of the cortex are less well defined. To further confound things is the fact that the developing brain is **plastic**. The brains of infants who receive trauma are more likely to overcome damage to function than those of adults receiving the same trauma. This and other evidence have led to theories of **equipotentiality**, which state that the brain functions as a whole. One could strike a balance with the notion of **regional equipotentiality**. According to this theory there seems to be a functional unity by regions, but the degree of functional loss to an individual receiving trauma is also related to the total volume of damaged tissue. Our discussion will focus on the functional regions and association pathways of the brain, and on the interconnections among regions. The current view of neural function is a system-wide view, where regions of the brain are activated or entrained to complete a task or function. Thus, for instance, the task of concentration may include the temporo-parietal junction, the dorsolateral prefrontal cortex, and the orbitofrontal cortex, but the preparation to act on information derived through attention will involve entraining the premotor cortex, supplemental motor area, and other areas.

Lead Exposure

We have known for many years that lead exposure is bad for children. Excessive exposure to lead causes permanent brain damage, resulting in mental retardation, learning disability, attention deficit, and memory problems. Recently, however, researchers have found an even more insidious route for lead effects. Basha et al. (2005) found that when infant monkeys were given milk with low levels of lead, at 23 years of age they developed the plaques associated with Alzheimer's disease. If the monkeys had the genetic markers for Alzheimer's susceptibility they were twice as likely to develop the plaques.

The cortex appears to be organized around regions of **primary activity of a cortical region**, such as the primary receptive area for somatic sense, primary motor area, primary auditory cortex, and primary region of visual reception (see Figure 12-8). Adjacent to these are **higher-order areas of processing**. That is, there are secondary, tertiary, and even quaternary areas of higher-order processing adjacent to the primary receptive areas for sensation. There are also higher-order areas of processing for motor function, as we shall see. Beyond the higher-order areas of processing are **association areas** in which the highest form of human thought occurs. That is, we receive information from our senses at primary reception areas and we extract the information received and put it together with other information associated with the modality at higher-order areas of processing. This information is passed to association areas for the highest level of cognitive processing.

The **primary reception area for vision (VI)** is located within the calcarine fissure of the occipital lobe (area 17). At that location, precise maps of information received at the retinae are projected. The secondary visual processing region is considered to be area 18

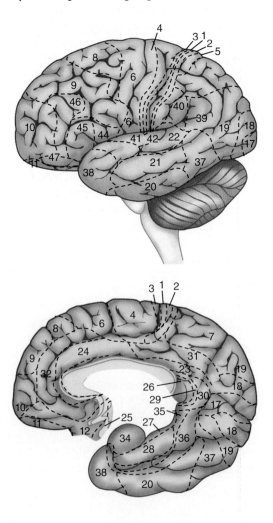

Figure 12-8. Brodmann's area map of lateral and medial cerebrum.

© Cengage Learning®.

of the occipital lobe, with even **higher-level processing regions for vision** found in the temporal lobe (areas 20 and 21) and the occipital lobe (area 19 and the region anterior to it). Area 7 of the parietal lobe performs higher-level processing of visual information. Because higher-level processing sites seem to be concerned with feature extraction, the precise visual field map projected onto the primary cortex is generally not found at those higher-level processing sites.

Somatic sense is received by the parietal lobe, with the primary reception area (SI) being the postcentral gyrus (areas 1, 2, and 3). Again, studies have repeatedly demonstrated that body sense is projected somatotopically along this strip, but this projection is much less apparent at the secondary sites. The opercular portion of the parietal lobe is considered to be the higher-order processing region, as is area 5 of the parietal lobe (Kupferman, 1991). **Auditory information** is tonotopically projected at Heschl's gyrus (area 41) of the temporal lobe (AI), whereas the superior temporal gyrus (area 22) performs higher-level processing of the auditory input. There is some retention of the tonotopic nature of the received signal at the higher-level processing region. You may want to refer to our discussion of higher-level auditory processing at the end of Chapter 10 to gain some insight into these processes.

Three regions of the brain play central roles in **motor function**, but to discuss these areas we must clarify the three phases of the voluntary motor act. First, to perform a voluntary motor task, you must identify a target, such as making the tongue tip contact the alveolar ridge. Next, you must develop a plan to achieve the target behavior. Finally, you must execute the plan, a process requiring the movement of muscles with accurate timing, force, and rate.

These three functions appear to be governed by three different regions of the cerebral cortex. First, the identification of a target is a function of the posterior parietal lobe. The posterior parietal lobe (areas 5, 7, 39, and 40) processes information about somatic sensation related to **spatial orientation**, including the integration of information about the position of body parts in space and visual information. Inputs to these parietal regions arise from the thalamus: The venteroposterolateral thalamic nucleus (VPLo) projects body sense information from distant receptors; the caudal ventrolateral thalamic nucleus (VLc) and VPLo project cerebellar information to the posterior parietal regions; and the VLc and ventral anterior nucleus (VA) project information from the basal ganglia to the posterior parietal lobe. In this way, the posterior parietal lobe receives a complete "body map" of the location and condition of all body parts, including the speech articulators.

The second area, the **premotor region** (area 6), anterior to the motor strip, appears to be involved in action planning. The premotor region takes information from the parietal lobe (areas 1, 2, and 3) concerning the immediate location of muscles and joints and integrates that information with as action plan. In addition, the **supplementary motor area** (**SMA**; superior and medial portions of area 6) is

The cochlea and the brain stem nuclei serving it have a tonotopic array, which is the correlate of the spatiotopic array seen in the motor strip. High-frequency sounds are resolved at the basal end of the cochlea, whereas low-frequency sounds are resolved at the cochlea apex. Frequency is spread out in an orderly, sequential array along the basilar membrane of the cochlea, and this tonotopic arrangement is seen in the projections at nearly all levels of the auditory pathway.

involved in even more complex acts, including speech initiation. The SMA is strongly involved in the preparatory speech act, as well as in the decision to initiate the act. If an individual is told only to mentally rehearse, the SMA will be activated without the premotor region becoming involved.

Finally, the precentral gyrus or **motor strip** (MI) found in area 4 is responsible for the execution of voluntary movement. The motor strip neurons make up half of the pyramidal tract, the major motor pathway. Commands to muscles from the motor strip include information concerning the degree of force and timing of contraction.

Motor System Lesions

Damage to specific regions of the brain has been used repeatedly to infer the function of those regions. Clearly, if a portion of the brain is damaged and a specific dysfunction can be consistently identified, that portion of the brain can be assumed to be intimately involved in the lost function. That having been said, specific regions of function for higher cognitive processes are difficult to specify, precisely because the processes involved are so complex and require multiple subsystems to function. In the same vein, removing the knob of a radio may make it impossible to receive a radio signal, but that does not mean that the knob was the *only* component involved in receiving a signal. It is important to realize that speech, language, and cognitive processes are exceedingly complex, and our understanding of localized function is revised continuously. Nonetheless, it is fruitful to examine the information we have gleaned from years of observing the results of brain damage.

A lesion in the motor strip will result in muscular weakness and loss of motor function on the side of the body opposite the lesion. **Dysarthria** is a speech disorder arising from paralysis, muscular weakness, and dyscoordination of speech musculature. The type of dysarthria is broadly defined by the site of the lesion.

Flaccid dysarthria arises from damage to lower motor neurons (LMNs) or their cell bodies. Thus, flaccid dysarthria generally reflects damage to the cranial nerves serving speech muscles. As we discussed in Chapter 11, focal lesions to the cranial nerves have focal effects on the musculature they serve, and this is manifested in the various subtypes of flaccid dysarthria that one sees clinically. For instance, damage to the VII facial nerve will result in facial paralysis, whereas damage to the V trigeminal will produce paralysis of the muscles of mastication. Damage to the recurrent laryngeal nerve of the X vagus will result in flaccid dysphonia. In all cases, the result will be a flaccid paralysis, manifested as a muscular weakness and **hypotonia** (low muscle tone). If the cell body is involved in the lesion, there may also be **fasciculations** or twitching movements of the affected articulator. In addition, because the damage occurs distal to the interneurons serving the reflex arc (which is a central phenomenon within the brainstem or spinal cord), reflexive responses

Specific cranial nerve functions and disorders are discussed in Chapter 11.

Sleep Apnea

Sleep apnea comes in two major forms. Obstructive sleep apnea is a condition in which individuals stop breathing during deep sleep because some structure, such as the posterior pharyngeal wall, occludes the airway. The condition can be life threatening, as it induces significant cardiac stress. It has been linked to significant sleep deprivation, as it never allows a person to gain full, deep sleep.

The second type of apnea is termed *central apnea*. It may be the cause of death for individuals who die in their sleep (McKay, Janczewski, & Feldman, 2005). It was found in rats that when cells within the brain stem known as preBotzinger-complex neurons are damaged, as could happen in neurodegenerative disease. They stop breathing entirely during rapid eye movement sleep (REM).

mediated by the nerve are either reduced or absent. You can normally elicit a jaw jerk reflex by pulling down on a slack jaw, but this reflex may be reduced or absent in patients with flaccid dysarthria if the V trigeminal is involved.

Spastic dysarthria arises from bilateral damage to the upper motor neurons (UMNs) of the pyramidal (direct) and extrapyramidal (indirect) motor pathways. The direct pathway is generally excitatory, being involved in the execution of skilled motor acts. The indirect pathway is generally inhibitory, controlling background activities such as maintenance of muscle tone, posture, and agonist contraction to control the trajectory for movement.

Bilateral UMN damage results in an inability to execute skilled movements (paralysis) and muscle weakness. Damage to the extrapyramidal system results in the loss of inhibition of reflexes, or **hyperreflexia**, as well as increased muscle tone, or **hypertonia**. Thus, the jaw jerk reflex mentioned in the discussion of flaccid dysarthria would now be very easily triggered, to the point that the individual cannot control the response.

The person with spastic dysarthria demonstrates reduced force of contraction of muscles due to the pyramidal lesion, and this condition is further confounded by easily elicited reflexive contractions arising from attempting to use the articulators. That is, attempts by the affected individual to lower his or her jaw will result in the reflexive contraction of the muscles that elevate the jaw, thereby foiling the attempt. Therapy obviously will be directed toward regaining control over those reflexes.

When a unilateral lesion occurs in the region of facial muscle control, the result is **unilateral upper motor neuron** (UUMN) **dysarthria** (Duffy, 2005). The effects of UUMN dysarthria are less devastating than those of a bilateral lesion. UUMN results in spastic signs on the side contralateral to the lesion for the tongue and lower facial muscles, because they have unilateral (contralateral) innervation, whereas other articulatory muscles are bilaterally innervated.

Ataxic dysarthria arises from damage to the cerebellum or to the brain stem vestibular nuclei, or both. Because the cerebellum is responsible for coordination of motor activity, ataxic dysarthria is characterized by the loss of coordination; deficits in achieving an articulatory target; and problems in coordinating rate, range, and force of movement. Speech in ataxic dysarthria will be distorted because irregular articulation results from **overshoot** (moving an articulator beyond its target) and **undershoot** (moving an articulator insufficiently to reach the target). **Dysdiadochokinesia**, a deficit in the ability to make repetitive movements, is a dominant characteristic, as is **dysprosody**, or deficit in the maintenance of the intonation and linguistic stress of speech.

Hyperkinetic and hypokinetic dysarthria are the result of damage to different regions of the extrapyramidal system. **Hyperkinetic dysarthria** is characterized by extraneous, involuntary movement of speech musculature in addition to the movement produced voluntarily. That is, in hyperkinetic dysarthria, articulators move without voluntary muscular contraction, and this is overlaid on the speech act. Hyperkinesias are seen primarily in instances of damage to the basal ganglia circuitry, especially that responsible for inhibiting movement.

Damage to the subthalamic nucleus, which inhibits the globus pallidus, results in uncontrolled flailing known as **ballism**. If damage to the basal ganglia results in a decrease in the neurotransmitter acetylcholine (ACh) or an increase in dopamine (DA), extraneous **choreiform** movements (involuntary twitching and movement of muscles) will result, such as those seen in Huntington's disease. Hyperkinesias take a number of forms, ranging from **tics** (rapid movement of small groups of muscle fibers) and **tremors** (rhythmic contractions) to **athetosis** (slow, writhing movements) and **dystonia** (involuntary movement to a posture, with the posture being held briefly).

Hypokinetic dysarthria is characterized by a paucity of movement, most often seen in Parkinson's disease. The disease arises from damage to the substantia nigra, the cell mass responsible for the production of DA. DA is used by the basal ganglia to balance ACh, and a shortage of DA results in inhibited initiation of motor function, reduction in range of movements, co-contraction of agonists and antagonists (resulting in **rigidity**), and a characteristic pill-rolling tremor of the hands. Speech in Parkinson's disease will be rushed, with reduced duration of speech sounds, reduced vocal intensity, and reduced fluctuation in fundamental frequency.

Mixed dysarthrias arise from damage to more than one of the controlling systems. **Mixed spastic-flaccid dysarthria** is found in amyotrophic lateral sclerosis, a disease that attacks the myelin of the UMN and LMN fibers. **Mixed spastic-ataxic dysarthria** results from damage to the UMN and cerebellar control circuitry, as often seen in multiple sclerosis. **Mixed hypokinetic-ataxic-spastic dysarthria** occurs with the degeneration of Wilson's disease (hepatolenticular degeneration). Generally, one may see any combination of dysarthrias, based on the systems involved in the disease process (Duffy, 2005).

The dysarthrias are all characterized by some degree of loss of motor function accompanied by muscular weakness and dyscontrol. In contrast, **dyspraxia** is a dysfunction of motor planning in the absence of muscular weakness or muscular dysfunction.

Damage to the premotor region results in gross dyspraxia of the motor function mediated by the area broadly served by the adjacent motor strip neurons. With damage to the SMA, an individual will have difficulty initiating speech, and the effect is bilateral. Verbal dyspraxia appears to be directly related to damage of the precentral region of the dominant insular cortex. This region is deep to **Broca's area**, an area intimately involved in expressive language function. Verbal dyspraxia is characterized by significant loss of fluency and groping behavior associated with even the simplest articulations. Dyspraxia occurs in the absence of the muscular weakness typical of an individual with motor strip damage, but the ability to contract the musculature voluntarily is impaired. One may also experience **oral apraxia**, which is a deficit in the ability to perform nonspeech oral gestures, such as imitatively puffing up the cheeks or blowing out a candle. A word of caution is due, however: Lesions are rarely so focal; it is much more often the case that frontal lobe damage that causes dyspraxia will be of a magnitude to also include regions of the motor strip. That is, dyspraxia and dysarthria very often co-occur.

If an individual has damage to the posterior parietal cortex, the result will be difficulty focusing on the target of an action. This individual will have difficulty locating objects in space and may even ignore or neglect the side of the body served by the damaged parietal

Parkinson's Disease

Parkinson's disease is a neuromuscular disease that results in tremors, muscular rigidity, difficulty initiating movement, and dementia. The physical cause of the disease is known to be the loss of cells in the substantia nigra, the "black substance" within the cerebral peduncles of the midbrain. While researchers are comfortable with the cause of the disease, the cause of the damage to the substantia nigra is elusive. It has long been felt that some sort of environmental etiology was at work, but evidence is emerging to show that Parkinson's is caused through pesticides. In a five-country study of Parkinson's patients, Betarbet et al. (2000) found that the use of pesticides was strongly related to a later development of Parkinson's disease.

There is good news regarding Parkinson's disease, however, in that the injection of glial line neurotrophic factor (GDNF) into the brain tissue of Parkinson's patients resulted in significant and long-term gains in motor function. All patients injected showed remarkable benefits in motor and cognitive functions. Unfortunately, the company that owns the patent for GDNF removed the drug from clinical trials because of fears concerning safety. Prior treatments using neural tissue transplants have also been quite successful but remain experimental because of ethical dilemmas concerning the source of the tissue (aborted fetuses).

Deep brain stimulation has been beneficial in the treatment of Parkinson's disease, reducing tremor and increasing motor function for speech, ambulation, and swallowing.

lobe tissue, because he or she cannot use that information. In addition, the *supramarginal gyrus* is involved spatiomotor tasks in nonhumans (identifying if physical orientation of an object is functionally correct (Bach, Peelen, & Tipper, 2010), but appears intimately involved in phonological processing developmentally in humans (Sugiura, Ojima, Matsuba-Kurita, Dan, Tsuzuki, Katura, & Hagiwara, 2011).

Afferent Inputs

The motor strip is populated by giant Betz cells, and this area receives input from the thalamus, sensory cortex, and premotor area. Regions involved in fine motor control (such as those activating facial regions or the fingers) are very richly represented. There is heavy sensory input to this motor region, underscoring the notion that the control of movement is strongly influenced by information about the ongoing state and position of the musculature. Some muscle spindle afferents terminate in the motor strip, and spinal reflexes are modified and controlled, at least in part, by activity from this region. The portion of the motor strip serving a particular part of the body will receive tactile and proprioceptive information from the same body region, providing an effective path for modification of the motor plan even as it is being executed.

The premotor region appears to be involved in the preparation for movement, anticipation of movement, and organization of skilled movement. It receives somatic sensory information from the parietal lobe, as well as sensory information from the thalamus, and projects its output to the motor strip. Afferent parietal information to the supplementary motor area also supports its involvement in the active planning and rehearsal of the motor act, as well as decision making about movement. Broca's area (regions 44 and 45 of the frontal lobe) uses parietal lobe information to perform a high-level planning function for the movement of the speech articulators for speech function, as will be discussed.

Association Regions

Association areas are considered to provide the highest order of information processing of the cerebral cortex. It appears that higher-order integration areas extract detailed information from the signal input to the primary areas, whereas association areas permit that information to flow among the various processing sites, effectively connecting modalities. These regions are involved in intellect, cognitive functions, memory, and language.

There are three major association areas of interest: the **temporal-occipital-parietal (TOP) association cortex**, the **limbic association cortex**, and the **prefrontal association cortex**.

The **TOP region** is of the utmost importance to speech-language pathologists, because it includes the areas associated with language in humans. This region includes portions of the temporal, parietal, and

The Amygdala and Limbic Function

The amygdala has fascinating responsibilities. It is involved in the processing of fearful stimuli, such as fearful faces. When you see a fearful face (such as that of a grizzly bear during your hike), your limbic system properly engages to help you recognize the danger (fear) and make a quick exit. If a person has a damaged amygdala, he or she may not recognize the fearful stimulus. If that person has a hypertrophied (large) amygdala, on the other hand, he or she may have an exceptionally large rage response (Whittle et al., 2008), particularly if the person is an adolescent. The amygdala interacts with the cerebral cortex by means of the cingulate gyrus. Whittle et al. found that not only were amygdalas bigger in aggressive adolescents, but their connection with the cerebral cortex was smaller, as was the cortical region to which it would connect. The cerebral cortex and limbic system work together to monitor emotion-laden information and to moderate it. The limbic system is responsible for quickly screening stimuli for their emotional content (fear, joy, etc.) and formulating a basic response (running, fighting, etc.). At the same time the cerebral cortex, particularly the orbitofrontal cortex, is also charged with assessing the information. The frontal lobe can perform higher cognitive processing of the stimulus and can modulate the output of the limbic system, so an initial fear response (grizzly bear head) might be modulated to simple interest (grizzly bear in a cage at a zoo) based upon cognitive processes not available directly to the limbic system.

occipital lobes (areas 39 and 40; and portions of 19, 21, 22, and 37). It receives input from the auditory, visual, and somatosensory regions, permitting the integration of this information into language function.

The **limbic association area** (regions 23, 24, 38, 28, and 11) includes regions of the parahippocampal gyrus and temporal pole (temporal lobe), cingulate gyri (parietal and frontal lobes), and orbital surfaces (inferior frontal lobe). The limbic system is involved with motivation, emotion, and memory, making it an ideal association area. Clearly, memory function is served by the reception of information from diverse sensory inputs.

The **prefrontal association area** (anterior to area 6) is involved with the integration of information in preparation for the motor act, as well as higher-level cognitive processes. The premotor regions, consisting of the premotor gyrus and supplemental motor area, appear to be vital to the initiation of motor activity, whereas the prefrontal region anterior to these regions is involved in the motor plan. According to Kupferman (1991), the premotor region receives input from the primary sensory reception areas or low-order processing regions, whereas the prefrontal regions derive their input from the higher-order regions. Both premotor and prefrontal regions project to the motor strip, permitting both low-order and abstract sensory perceptions to influence the motor act. Broca's area (regions 44 and 45), the frontal operculum, and the insula are also involved in motor programming. These regions share qualities of both the prefrontal association region and the premotor gyrus, because damage to them results in both motor-planning and higher-level language deficits, including word retrieval problems.

Alcohol and the Brain

Alcohol is a toxin to neural tissue, hence the name *intoxication*. Alcohol use is widespread throughout the world and in all cultures, as are the effects of alcohol on the brain. Acute alcohol intoxication results in the disabling of the hippocampus, which effectively removes the ability to learn or memorize, including the ability to learn from aversive responses. Thus, attempting to discuss meaningful information with an intoxicated person is a futile activity. Chronic alcohol use has a more sinister effect. The frontal lobes of individuals who chronically abuse alcohol deteriorate, reducing the patients' ability to make cognitive judgments and process information. Alcohol consumption over time results in liver damage (sclerosis of the liver) that causes the body to be unable to metabolize vitamin B (thiamin). A vitamin B deficiency results in reduced function of neurons and glial cells, as well as the inability to process iron, which in turn results in the reduced oxygen carrying capacity of blood. The result is permanent brain damage due to the chronic anemic condition. Individuals who chronically abuse alcohol and who are genetically predisposed to Alzheimer's develop the disease at twice the rate of the average population. Finally, thiamine deficiency ultimately results in Wernicke–Korsakoff syndrome, a permanent dementia characterized by confusion, confabulation, memory loss, inability to encode new memory, and various motor signs such as nystagmus and ataxia.

Meditation and Brain Change

Meditation has been practiced for thousands of years, and it now appears that those practitioners were onto something. Zen Buddhist monks have been shown to have strong synchronization of gamma brain waves (Lutz et al., 2004). Unlike only slightly trained meditators, the monks showed extreme synchronization of brain waves, indicative of highly coordinated neural structures. Disease states such as schizophrenia show highly disorganized (asynchronous) brain wave activity, and some neuroscientists feel that this type of a synchrony is the hallmark of consciousness.

Tibetan monks and Catholic nuns also show increased blood flow to the frontal lobes (particularly the dorsolateral prefrontal cortex), most likely due to the concentration involved in meditation. They both revealed reduced blood flow to the parietal lobe. Meditators experience differences not only in function but also in structure. Apparently meditation increases the density of neurons within the right insular lobe, as well as in the frontal lobe (Lazar et al., 2005; Treadway et al., 2005). Interestingly, the right insula was also recently implicated in addiction: Lesion in this area caused long-term smokers to have no interest in cigarettes. See Navqui et al. (2007) for the story on that.

In addition to this, the orbitofrontal region (the region on the underbelly of the cerebrum that overlies the orbit region) is involved in the limbic system function, as well as in the motor planning memory associated with delayed execution.

✔ *To summarize:*

- The complexity of higher functions of the brain is reflected in the inability to assign precise locations for specific functions.
- General regions can be assigned broad functions, and this view facilitates the examination of brain function and dysfunction.
- A broad view of brain function classifies regions of the cerebrum as primary, higher-order, and association regions.
- **Primary** sensory and motor regions include the **primary reception area** for somatic sense, **primary motor area, primary auditory cortex**, and **primary** region of **visual reception**.
- Adjacent to these are the higher-order areas of processing, apparently responsible for extracting features of the stimulus.
- **Association areas** are the regions of highest cognitive processing, where sensory information is integrated with memory.
- The **prefrontal area** appears to be involved in a higher function related to motor output (such as inhibition of motor function and the ability to change motor responses), whereas the **temporal-occipital-parietal association area** is involved in the language function.
- The limbic association area integrates information related to affect motivation, emotion, and memory.
- **Flaccid dysarthria** results from damage to the LMNs, whereas UMN lesions result in **spastic dysarthria**.
- **Ataxic dysarthria** arises from cerebellar damage.
- **Hyperkinetic dysarthria** is the result of damage to inhibitory processes of the extrapyramidal system, whereas **hypokinetic dysarthria** results from lesions to areas modulating the excitatory mechanisms.
- **Apraxia** arises from lesions to the regions associated with preparation and planning for a motor act: specifically Broca's area, insula, and the SMA.

Hemispheric Specialization

Despite the gross similarities between the two cerebral hemispheres, the brain is functionally asymmetrical, and the functional and anatomic asymmetries underlie basic processing differences of extreme importance to speech-language pathologists. When researchers have examined large numbers of brains, they have found that the lateral fissure is slightly longer on the left hemisphere than on the right. The area of primary auditory reception (the planum temporale, or Heschl's gyrus) is larger on this side as well. This anatomical asymmetry supports an extremely rich body of functional asymmetry between the two hemispheres.

decussate: L., decussare, to make an X; to decussate means to cross over

If you write with your right hand, you may count yourself among the broad majority of individuals who exhibit functional dominance for language and speech in the left hemisphere. Motor pathways **decussate** as they descend, and auditory pathways decussate in ascension, with the result being that your right hand (and right ear) are dominated by activities of the left hemisphere.

The two hemispheres continually work in concert with each other, being anatomically connected via the corpus callosum. Virtually all right-handed individuals show language function in the left hemisphere, whereas 30 percent of left-handers either have their language function within the right hemisphere or have it shared between the two hemispheres. Thus, one will speak of the "dominant hemisphere" for language as being, typically, the left hemisphere, knowing full well that there is a group for whom the reverse is true. With that in mind, let us examine some of the hemispheric differences that have been found.

A great deal of the information we have gained concerning hemispheric specialization has come from the treatment of seizure disorders. These disorders often involve the temporal lobe, which, as you shall soon see, is intimately involved with language function. When surgical procedures are planned to alleviate seizures, the neurosurgeon does everything possible to spare the speech and language regions. To learn where these regions are, he or she may electrically stimulate regions of the brain to determine their location prior to removing a portion of the cortex, in a procedure known as **brain mapping**. The physician may also inject the carotid artery of one or the other of the hemispheres with amytal sodium, a barbiturate, thereby incapacitating the hemisphere. In this way the surgeon can determine which hemisphere is dominant for language function. Among the surgical procedures used to terminate seizures is severing of the communication link between the two cortices, the corpus callosum.

Individuals in whom the corpus callosum has been severed have provided a great deal of the evidence concerning hemispheric specialization. Auditory information presented to the right ear is processed predominantly by the left hemisphere, and left-ear information is received by the right hemisphere. By careful examination of responses, researchers have found that short-duration acoustic information (such as consonants, transitions, and stop consonant bursts) is processed most efficiently by the left hemisphere in right-handed individuals. The left hemisphere seems to be specialized for the process of analysis, favoring discrete, sequential, rapidly changing information. Spoken and written language perception and production are clearly favored by this hemisphere, whereas the nondominant right hemisphere favors more spatial and holistic elements, such as face recognition, speech intonation, melody, and perception of form. This is not to say that the right hemisphere has nothing to say. It has been demonstrated that the right hemisphere has a reasonably large vocabulary (dominated by nouns), but rudimentary grammar. Although expressive abilities are quite limited, the right hemisphere can follow commands and demonstrate knowledge of verbal information through gesture and pointing using the left hand.

Thus, in the majority of individuals, language processing is lateralized to the left hemisphere, and speech production is controlled by the same hemisphere. Interpretation of the speaker's intention, as presented through intonation and facial expression, is processed by the right hemisphere. As you shall soon see, damage to the two hemispheres produces markedly different deficits.

Lesion Studies

Damage to the nervous system can arise from many sources. **Cerebrovascular accident (CVA)** refers to events that cause cessation of blood flow (**ischemia**) to neural tissue, either through hemorrhaging (rupturing of a blood vessel), thrombosis (closure of a blood vessel by means of a foreign object, such as a blood clot), or embolism (closure of a blood vessel by a floating clot). Hemorrhage can occur when an aneurysm (ballooning of a blood vessel due to a weak wall) is subjected to increased blood pressure (hypertension). Aneurysms can be repaired if discovered prior to hemorrhaging (see Figure 12-9). Chronic high blood pressure can lead to lacunar (hypertensive) strokes, which are insidious in onset but which can further lead to aphasia, dysarthria, and dementia.

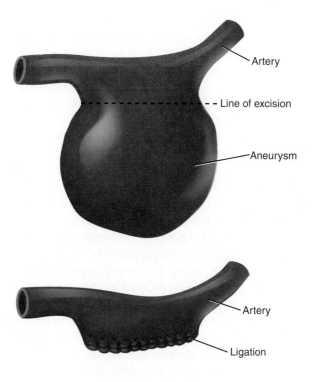

Artery

Line of excision

Aneurysm

Artery

Ligation

Figure 12-9. Repair of an aneurysm to prevent hemorrhage.
© Cengage Learning®.

CVA and Micropollutants

Certainly there is a significant relationship between lifestyle and cerebrovascular (CVA) accident. We already know that accumulation of plaques within the vascular system can cause CVA. Now it has been found that the small particles present in pollutants may also trigger stroke. Particles of smoke in pollution measuring 2.5 microns or less apparently become "cement-like," forming plaques within arteries. These particles are found near highways in large cities.

Damage can also occur from traumatic brain injury (TBI). Injuries depend on the type of trauma (see Figure 12-10). Open injury occurs from trauma that fractures the skull, including gunshot wounds. Closed head injury (CHI) can be translational (front-back or side-side) or angular (rotatory). Translational injuries occur when an object strikes the skull, or more likely, when the skull strikes an object. Being thrown from a car as a result of a motor vehicle accident (MVA) often damages the frontal lobe (Figure 12-10A), while rotational injury causes diffuse axonal damage (Figure 12-10C).

CVA is the most frequent cause of aphasia, and TBI is the most frequent cause of acquired cognitive deficit. That having been said, either class of disorder can cause a wide spectrum of language and cognitive dysfunction.

Aphasia

A primary source of information concerning function of the cerebral cortex in humans is lesion studies. Researchers have examined the behavioral outcome of accidental or surgical lesions in individuals, thus contributing to our understanding of cortical function.

Of particular interest to our field are the regions associated with speech and language. We have long known that damage to Wernicke's area (posterior area 22) typically results in a disruption of language known as receptive or fluent **aphasia**. Similarly, we have come to recognize that damage to Broca's area (areas 44 and 45) severely disrupts the oral manifestation of language (speech). Through cortical mapping and precise lesion studies, researchers have described these conditions and the sites of lesions more precisely, providing us with some insight into how the cerebral cortex functions.

As you know, Heschl's gyrus of the temporal lobe has the primary responsibility of auditory reception; the region adjacent to it in the superior temporal gyrus is a higher-order processing region; and the hippocampus is involved with memory. Portions of the inferior and middle temporal gyri are regions of higher-level integration of visual information. Wernicke's area is posterior to this, technically comprised of the posterior superior gyrus of the temporal lobe, but we know that language function involves a markedly larger area, generally including the temporal-occipital-parietal association areas.

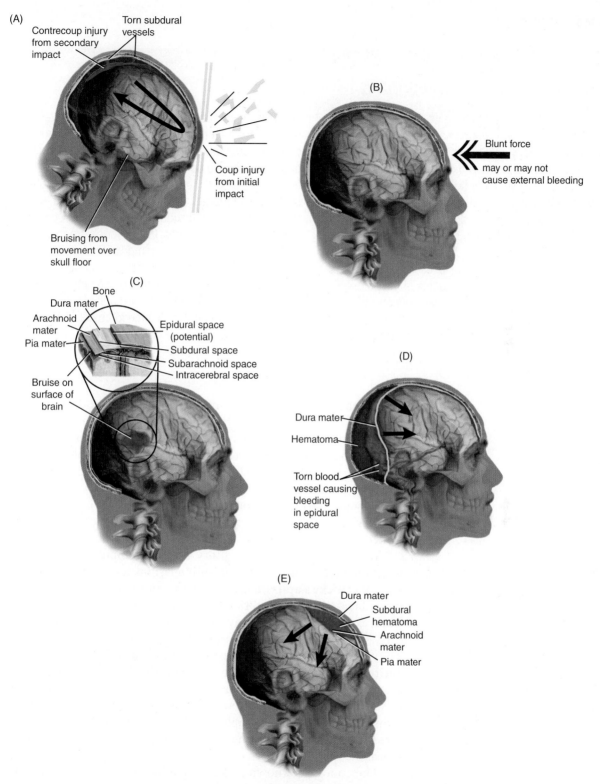

Figure 12-10. Effects of trauma on the cerebrum and related structures. (A) Closed head injury (CHI) producing a direct effect (coup) on frontal region and a rebound effect (contracoup) in the occipital region. (B) Blunt force trauma to the frontal region causing neural damage, but which may not manifest as external damage. (C) Cerebral contusion (bruising of the brain). (D) Subdural hematoma arising from broken blood vessels deep to the dura mater. (E) Epidural hematoma, arising from broken blood vessels superficial to the dura mater.

A Story with a Happy Ending

We promised that we would tell you a story of aneurysm and hemorrhage with a happy ending. While at a public event one Saturday, a dear friend developed a debilitating headache. When her headache did not improve after an hour of nursing it in the cab of her truck, her husband began the long drive home. Her husband wisely decided that a stop by the local hospital to check if everything was in order, and the emergency physician suggested magnetic resonance imaging (MRI) to help determine the source of the pain. As the MRI was activated, she became unconscious.

As we later learned, she had a history of aneurysms in her family and had been examined frequently and repeatedly to ensure that there were no surprises in her future. Despite these precautions, an aneurysm had developed at the base of her brain and hemorrhaged as the MRI was activated. Life-flight took her to a metropolitan center that specialized in the management of hemorrhage, and friends and family watched anxiously as she slowly became aware of her surroundings. To everyone's great joy and relief, her recovery was remarkably complete, and she was able to return to her life and work unencumbered. The quick action of the emergency room medical team and the stroke unit at the receiving hospital gave her the chance to be called the "miracle woman" by all who know her.

Damage to Heschl's gyrus may result in cortical deafness, the inability to hear information that has passed through the lower auditory nervous system. Lesions of the higher-order processing region adjacent to AI will produce a deficit in processing complex auditory information, and if the lesion involves the inferior temporal lobe (area 28), the individual may experience a memory deficit associated with visual information. You may wish to review the information in Chapter 10 on the auditory pathway and higher cortical functioning related to auditory stimuli.

With the notion of the auditory and visual input function of the temporal lobe in mind, let us examine lesions involving Wernicke's area. **Wernicke's aphasia** is referred to as a *fluent aphasia*, because individuals with this condition have relatively normal flow of speech. Their expressive language may have relatively normal syntactic structure, but the content of their productions will be markedly reduced. They will often substitute words (**verbal paraphasias**) or create entirely new words (**neologisms**). If you think of the proximity of Wernicke's area to the auditory reception areas and the discussion of auditory integration, you will not be surprised to learn that the individual with Wernicke's aphasia will have a great deal of difficulty understanding what he or she hears and will not be able to accurately repeat the speech of others.

The condition known as **Broca's aphasia** is a stark contrast to Wernicke's aphasia. Broca's aphasia arises not only from lesions to Broca's area (areas 44 and 45) but also from lesions to the operculum of the frontal and parietal regions, and the insula, and the white matter beneath these regions. Broca's area is involved with the planning of speech, and the aphasia associated with it makes speech far from fluent. Although the individual with Broca's aphasia generally demonstrates comprehension of auditory or visual input, the patient's expressive abilities may be severely impaired. Length and complexity of utterances will be markedly reduced, and speech may require extreme effort.

Wernicke's and Broca's areas communicate directly with each other by means of the arcuate fasciculus, providing a very strong link between the receptive component of language and its expressive component. When these fibers or the supramarginal gyrus of the parietal lobe have been damaged, a patient will show signs of **conduction aphasia**. This individual will have a good comprehension of speech or written material and relatively fluent spontaneous speech, but have an impaired ability to repeat utterances heard. There will also be phoneme substitutions (**literal paraphasias**).

If damage to the brain includes Wernicke's and Broca's areas and areas below the cortex, the result may be **global aphasia**. In this condition, both expressive and receptive abilities are severely impaired. Speech is halting and nonfluent at best, with a poverty of grammatical structures and significant comprehension deficit. Gestures and facial expressions may be the primary means of communication for this individual.

You can see how these areas of deficit fit together. Damage to regions of the temporal lobe tends to cause receptive language problems, depending on the location of the lesion, whereas damage to the frontal speech regions may leave receptive abilities intact but cause a deficit in the expression of language (speech).

We have been conveniently ignoring the fact that the cerebral cortex is firmly attached to subcortical structures, including the basal ganglia and thalamus. Improvement in brain imaging techniques has revealed that damage to many of these areas results in language impairment, although these reports emphasize the importance of not assuming a strict localizationist stance. Damage to the thalamus may have a significant impact on attention, but also has resulted in a type of aphasia that includes difficulty in naming objects (**anomia**), in the generation of novel words (neologisms), and the condition of word or sound substitutions. Damage to the basal ganglia has resulted in nonfluent aphasia as well if there is damage to the putamen or caudate nucleus. It is likely that the hierarchical nature of the brain involves using these phylogenetically older structures to integrate information necessary for expression and reception, and that the disruption of these pathways always results in some deficit.

Although damage to the posterior language area (TOP) always results in receptive deficit, *any* individual with aphasia will have some degree of receptive impairment. Similarly, word-finding problems are universal in individuals experiencing aphasia. Both of these deficits should remind you that strict localization of function is not always demonstrable.

Impact of Aphasia

The life of an individual with aphasia is significantly changed by a cerebrovascular event. With the brain lesion comes an instant change in how the individual can interact with his or her environment, how readily linguistic information can be used to process information and to communicate, and how easily cognitive processes can be performed.

The individual with a left-hemisphere stroke of the frontal lobe faces difficulty in output that leaves her or him dysfluent and very aware of the jumble of verbal output. If the lesion is in the posterior regions, speech will be more fluent, but may be "empty" of content, and the person may have difficulty with comprehension, not realizing that his or her speech is not doing what was intended.

It is extremely important to enlist the help of your client's spouse or close friend very early in the process. This "significant other" will be most able to extend your therapy into every aspect of the client's life, and will become the client's most valuable communication partner. Including a partner early on will give you the opportunity to move your client back into the world of communication.

Dyspraxia

Sometimes lesions can result in **primary oral** or **primary verbal dyspraxia**, a deficit in the ability to program the articulators for nonspeech (oral dysapraxia) or speech production (verbal dyspraxia) in the absence of muscular weakness or paralysis. Dyspraxia often co-occurs with aphasia and is viewed by many to be a component of Broca's aphasia. Errors in dyspraxia tend to be phoneme substitution errors, although they are much less predictable than articulation errors arising from other causes. Because the person with dyspraxia often has good comprehension, he or she may be quite aware of the errors and will struggle to correct them. This struggle will result in the loss of speech fluency (and a great deal of frustration for the speaker). As the desired articulatory configuration becomes more complex (as in producing consonant clusters instead of singletons), the client's speech difficulty will increase.

At least two regions are involved in dyspraxia. If damage is restricted to the frontal lobe in the insular cortex (Dronkers, 1996), the individual will have difficulty producing even the simplest movements with the articulators.

Other Deficits

Not all lesions affect language directly. Left-frontal lobe lesions often result in deficits in cognitive functions. *Cognition* can be defined as the ways in which we perceive and process information: Cognitive processes include such diverse functions as memory, attention, and perception. The frontal lobe appears to be the primary site for cognitive functions, as well as the locus of the **executive functions** with which we exercise control over cognitive processes. Executive functions include the ability to set goals, sequence motor behaviors, and self-monitor behavior. Through the interplay of cognitive processes and the control of the executive functions, we are able to perceive information that is projected from myriad areas of the body and cerebrum, compare it with our stored memories or with previous analyses, evaluate those stimuli, and plan an appropriate response. In the same vein, our executive functions help us to control those responses so that we do not impulsively say or do something inappropriate.

Although individuals experiencing CVAs may demonstrate a loss of cognitive functions, the fact that these functions appear to be localized predominantly to the prefrontal region explains why clients who have suffered TBI more often have deficits in these areas. Because most TBI arises from vehicle accidents, the most frequently injured region is the frontal lobe. TBI frequently results in impaired decision-making ability and difficulty changing strategies in problem solving. There is often a loss of response inhibition, and the ability to evaluate the context of communication, which results in the loss of social communication ability, also known as a deficit in pragmatics or use of language. Control of emotion may be compromised by frontal lobe lesions, resulting in **emotional lability** (excessive and uncontrollable emotional response not necessarily related to the stimulus) or reduced emotion. Personality characteristics are often altered by frontal lobe lesion.

If the parahippocampal region of the cerebral cortex is involved, the client may have difficulty learning complex tasks and remembering information received through sensory modalities. Penfield and Roberts (1959) found that the removal of both hippocampi produced profound long-term memory deficit, whereas much milder problems arose from unilateral lesion. Removal of the left hippocampus results in difficulty remembering verbal information.

Although right-hemisphere lesions generally do not result in aphasia, they do have linguistic and social significance. Lesions in this hemisphere may result in a deficit in the ability to process information contained in the intonation of speech, so that nuance is lost. Communication of emotion, intent, and humor may be impaired in this individual. Individuals with right-hemisphere lesions often make linguistically inappropriate responses, most likely arising from the inability to process these pragmatic functions. Because the right hemisphere appears to be responsible for getting the "big picture," individuals who have suffered right-hemisphere damage lose some of their ability to get the gist of information and to recognize that they need to provide background contextual information during conversation ("given-new" violation), and have difficulty interpreting emotional and paralinguistic information. They often have

When Memory Fails

Memory is one of the most important of the cognitive processes, as it serves as the critical element in most executive functioning. We know that the hippocampus is essential for the processing of short-term memory into long-term storage, but nowhere has it been more dramatically shown than in the case of H.M.

H.M. had suffered seizures since childhood, and no treatment had succeeded in reducing this problem. When he was 27 years old, in 1953, he underwent bilateral temporal lobectomy, wherein the anterior 8 cm of both medial-temporal lobes were removed, including the amygdale and the anterior 2/3 of the hippocampus.

The seizures were finally controlled, but at a terrible cost. H.M. suffered little or no executive function deficit as a result of the lobectomy, and his language function was intact. The startling outcome of the surgery, however, was the H.M. forever remained in the day of his surgery. Up until the day he died in December, 2008, he was unable to remember anything that happened to him after the surgery, although his memory of events leading up to it is unaffected. This means that, to H.M., the president is still Dwight Eisenhower, and the Korean War has not reached a cease fire. H.M. can remember new information for a few minutes, but this memory trace quickly fades. He is faintly aware that something is amiss, but cannot really relate the nature of his problem. For fascinating reading, examine *Memory's Ghost* by Phillip Hilts. A recent technical report on H.M. can be found in Corkin (2002).

difficulty making inferences from details (such as interpreting the many parts of a picture by inferring the relation of the parts). The left hemisphere tends to be the residence of canonical or "dictionary" meanings, while the right hemisphere has the alternative or less-frequently used meanings for words. Thus, the left hemisphere can quickly access the stereotypical meaning of a word, but if that does not match the context, it can poll the right hemisphere for a word that might better suit the intent. For instance, if someone says "The fan is running," the left hemisphere will picture a device for moving air through a room. If, on the other hand, the television picture shows a football field with police trying to catch someone on the field who should not be there, the sentence "The fan is running" takes on a different meaning, and the right hemisphere will be called upon to disambiguate the sentence and context. With right hemisphere dysfunction (RHD) an individual may only have very concrete representations and may not be able to appropriately disambiguate sentences such as that discussed earlier. Indeed, the person with RHD may not recognize that there is any problem with his or her interpretation, since the concreteness includes a lack of recognition of contextual mismatch. Similarly, the concreteness of RHD makes idioms (e.g., "do not beat around the bush") seem irrelevant or even irritatingly unimportant. Alternative meanings are intrinsic to humor, so the concreteness of RHD can lead to a loss of the ability to see the humor in cartoons or jokes. (For an excellent review of right-hemisphere dysfunction, see Myers [1999].)

✔ *To summarize:*

- The **hemispheres** of the brain display clear functional differences.
- The **left hemisphere** in most individuals is dominant for language and speech, processes brief-duration stimuli, and performs detailed analysis.
- The **right hemisphere**, in contrast, appears to process information in a more holistic fashion, preferring spatial and tonal information.
- **Face recognition** appears to be a right-hemisphere function.
- Lesion studies have shown that damage to **Wernicke's area** in the dominant hemisphere usually results in a receptive language deficit with relatively intact speech fluency, whereas damage to **Broca's area** results in the loss of speech fluency manifested as Broca's aphasia.
- Damage to the **arcuate fasciculus** connecting these two regions will result in **conduction aphasia**, and damage to all of these regions will produce **global deficit**.
- **Verbal dyspraxia** may result from damage to Broca's area, but has also been seen with lesions to the supplementary motor area, frontal operculum, and insula.
- **Nondominant hemisphere lesions** often result in a deficit in the **pragmatics**, especially related to monitoring the facial responses of communication partners, information carried in the intonation of speech, and communicative nuance.
- **Frontal lobe lesions** may result in deficits in judgment and in response inhibition, whereas damage to the **hippocampus** will affect short-term memory, especially as it relates to auditory information.

Motor Control for Speech

The production of speech is an extraordinarily complex process. We tend to view area 4 as the "prime mover," but it would be more accurate to view it as the location where the very complex planning, programming, and preparation reach fruition. Movement is initiated at the motor strip, but only after it has been conceived, and after the steps involved for muscle activity have been prepared. To further confound things, control of speech musculature must be precisely coordinated, a process involving afferent input from the muscles. You will want to refer to our discussion of the DIVA model in Chapter 7.

Input to the motor strip arises from the premotor regions that are involved in the preparation of the motor act. The premotor gyrus and supplemental motor area receive input concerning the state of the musculature from the postcentral gyrus, and it appears that the knowledge of articulator position in space is established here. In addition, Broca's area (areas 44 and 45) communicates with the TOP by means of the arcuate fasciculus and is intimately involved in articulatory planning. The supramarginal gyrus of the parietal lobe appears to be involved in phonological processing. The prefrontal association area receives input from diffuse sensory integration regions of the cerebrum, and this information is used to make decisions concerning execution of the motor act (such as inhibiting a response). Prefrontal and premotor regions project to the precentral gyrus, as does Broca's area, so that both immediate planning and cognitive strategies associated with speech influence the output.

The primary motor cortex (MI) receives information concerning the state of muscles, tendons, and tissue through several means. The sensory cortex (SI) receives this information in a well-organized fashion. Area 3 receives muscle afferent information from Group Ia fibers terminating in the thalamus and from mechanoreceptors of the skin that are apparently very important for the speech muscles of the face. Area 1 receives mechanoreceptor input as well, and area 2 receives joint sense. This information is all directed to the MI, either directly or via other SI areas, apparently to modulate the motor command based on current status.

This sensory information obviously is not the only information processed by the MI. The premotor region (lateral area 6) is involved in organization of the motor act for skilled, voluntary movement, and its output is directly routed to the MI in both hemispheres. It receives somatic and visual information and apparently integrates this into its motor plan. The SMA (which is located in superior and medial area 6) appears to be involved in the programming of speech and other sequential movements, as well as in the control of some reflexes. The SMA receives information concerning tactile, auditory, and visual senses. It should be remembered that information from the cerebellum and basal ganglia is exchanged with the MI, SMA, and premotor region as well. Indeed, lesions of the SMA or basal ganglia can result in akinesia (loss of the ability to initiate movement), and lesions of the premotor cortex may result in apraxia (dysfunction in the ability to program movement). Loss of regions of the MI will result in paralysis or weakness of involved muscle groups, reduction in fine motor control, and spasticity arising from the unmodulated reflexes.

Thus, the motor impulse that is initiated by the MI is really the end product of planning and programming (Broca's area, SMA, and premotor area 6), with the strategic formulations arising from areas 8, 9, and 10 of the frontal lobe. The motor areas are influenced by the current state of the musculature of the body via somatosensory afferents to the SI, thalamus, and cerebellum. The afferent information concerning the tissues being acted on will help the MI area modify its output to accommodate fine motor control.

In this way, the motor impulse initiated by the motor strip is the end product of planning and programming, with the strategic formulations arising from the prefrontal region. Remember the executive function of the prefrontal region, and you may think twice about blurting an answer out before it is well formed—and inhibit the response. The motor areas are influenced by the current state of the musculature of the body. Likewise, the executor will carefully examine the propriety of the verbal output in terms of the situation and may be instrumental in revising the content and form to meet specific needs (e.g., your response to your minister's question at church is markedly different from the same question posed by your best friend while at the drive-in).

Clearly, the execution of speech involves extensive interaction of the areas of the brain in a rapidly coordinated fashion. Studies have revealed that we are amazingly versatile at overcoming obstacles to speech production (this is good news for the budding speech-language pathologist). Try this: Say "Sammy is a friend of mine." Now place your pencil between your molars on the side of your mouth, bite down lightly, and say it again a few times. Were you able to produce intelligible speech? Although the pencil interfered with some dental or labial productions, on the whole you were not only intelligible, but accurate. If the program for the individual articulators were "written in stone," you would not have been able to tolerate this aberration (use of a bite block), and your speech would have been unintelligible. Through this sort of examination, we realize that you probably develop an internal standard of what you want your speech to sound like, and then do whatever is necessary to match that standard. Thus, your role as a speech-language pathologist could well include helping your client develop that internal standard. Conditions that alter the internal model will inevitably alter the output.

A bite block is a device used to stabilize the mandible. Often made of hard acrylic or dental impression material, the bite block is used to eliminate the contribution of the mandible to tongue movement for diagnostic and therapeutic purposes. For an excellent discussion on preparation and use of the bite block, see Dworkin (1994).

CHAPTER SUMMARY

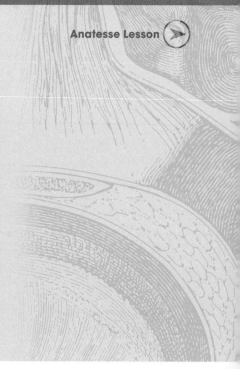

Anatesse Lesson

Communication between neurons of the nervous system occurs at the synapse, and neurotransmitters passing through the synaptic cleft will either excite or inhibit the postsynaptic neuron. When the neuron is sufficiently stimulated, an action potential will be generated, causing membrane depolarization and exchange of ions between the extracellular and intracellular spaces. Ion movement results in a large and predictable change in voltage across the membrane. Resting membrane potential is the relatively stable state of the neuron at rest. The absolutely refractory period, after excitation, is an interval during which the neuron cannot be excited to fire. During the relative refractory period, a neuron may be stimulated to fire, given increased stimulation. Neurons are capable of representing differences in input only through their rate of response. Myelinated fibers conduct the wave of depolarization more rapidly than demyelinated fibers, primarily because of saltatory conduction.

Muscle consists of thick and thin myofilaments that slide across each other during contraction. Activation of a muscle fiber causes the release of calcium into the environment of thick myofilaments,

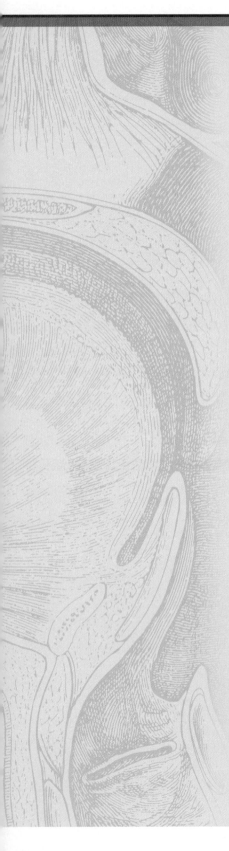

revealing the binding sites on the thin filaments that permit cross-bridging with the thick filaments. Muscle shortening is the product of repeated contraction of the cross-bridges. Slow twitch muscle fibers remain contracted longer than fast twitch fibers, with the former being involved in maintenance of posture and the latter in fine and rapid motor function.

Muscle spindles provide feedback to the neuromotor system about muscle length, tension, motion, and position. Muscle spindles running parallel to the intrafusal muscle fibers are sensors for muscle length, whereas Golgi tendon organs sense muscle tension. Nuclear bag fibers convey information concerning acceleration, and nuclear chain fibers respond to sustained lengthening. When a muscle is passively stretched, a segmental reflex is triggered. Extrafusal muscles paralleling the muscle spindles are activated and the muscle is shortened. Golgi tendon organs apparently respond to the tension of musculature during active contraction.

Higher function of the brain defies a strict localization approach to functional organization. General regions, such as Wernicke's area, can be ascribed broad function, and this view facilitates the examination of brain function and dysfunction. Brain function may be classified into regions of primary, higher-order, and association regions. Primary sensory and motor regions include the primary reception area for somatic sense, primary motor area, primary auditory cortex, and primary region of visual reception. Higher-order areas of processing are apparently responsible for extracting features of the stimulus. Association areas are the regions of highest cognitive processing, integrating sensory information with memory. The prefrontal area appears to be involved in higher function related to motor output, while the temporal-occipital-parietal association area is involved in spoken and written language function. The limbic association area integrates information relating to affect, motivation, emotion, and memory.

Dysarthria is a speech disorder resulting from damage to the motor execution system of the central nervous system; it causes muscular weakness and reduction in motor control. Flaccid dysarthria results from damage to LMNs, whereas UMN lesions result in spastic dysarthria. Ataxic dysarthria arises from cerebellar damage. Hyperkinetic dysarthria is the result of damage to the inhibitory processes of the extrapyramidal system, whereas hypokinetic dysarthria results from lesions to excitatory mechanisms. Apraxia arises from lesions to the regions associated with preparation and planning of the motor act, specifically the insular cortex, Broca's area, and the SMA. Apraxia is a deficit in motor planning, existing without muscular weakness or paralysis.

The hemispheres of the brain display clear functional differences. Language and speech, brief-duration stimuli, and detailed information are processed in the left hemisphere in most individuals. The right hemisphere appears to process information in a more holistic fashion, preferring spatial and tonal information. Lesions in Wernicke's area in the dominant hemisphere result in a receptive language deficit with relatively intact speech fluency, whereas damage to Broca's area results in the loss of speech fluency. Damage to the arcuate fasciculus connecting these two regions will result in conduction aphasia, and damage to all of these regions will produce global deficit. Verbal dyspraxia may result from damage to Broca's area, the supplementary motor area, the frontal operculum, and the insula. Right-hemisphere lesions often result in deficit in pragmatics, misinterpretation of information carried in the speech intonation, and loss of communicative nuance. Frontal lobe lesions often result in impaired judgment and failure to inhibit responses, whereas damage to the hippocampus will affect short-term memory.

Movement is initiated at the motor strip, but a great deal of planning occurs prior to that point. The premotor regions, including Broca's area, are involved in planning for the motor act, and project that plan to the motor strip. The prefrontal association area also provides input to the motor strip concerning the higher cognitive elements of the speech act, and the lowest levels of information (information about muscle stretch and tension) are also fed to the motor strip.

Media Connection

Go to the accompanying online resources at CengageBrain.com and have fun learning! Study with the Anatesse software program, play games, view animations and videos, and take practice tests to help reinforce the key concepts you learned in this chapter.

Study Questions

1. _____ is a change in electrical potential that occurs when a cell membrane is stimulated adequately to permit ion exchange between the intra- and extracellular spaces.

2. The _____ is the time during which the cell membrane cannot be stimulated to depolarize.

3. The _____ is a period during which the membrane may be stimulated to excitation again, but only with greater than typical stimulation.

4. The _____ of the axon myelin promote saltatory conduction.

5. The substance known as _____ is discharged into the synaptic cleft, stimulating the postsynaptic neuron.

6. Activation of a muscle fiber causes the release of calcium into the environment of _____ myofilaments.

7. _____ twitch muscle fibers remain contracted longer than _____ twitch fibers.

8. _____ provide feedback to the neuromotor system about muscle length, tension, motion, and position.

9. Higher cognitive processing occurs generally in _____ areas.

10. The _____ area is involved in language function.

11. _____ dysarthria results from damage to LMNs, whereas UMN lesions result in spastic dysarthria.

12. _____ dysarthria is the result of damage to the inhibitory processes of the extrapyramidal system.

13. _____ arises from cerebellar damage.

14. The _____ area of the cerebrum appears to be involved in higher function related to motor output (such as inhibition of motor function and the ability to change motor responses), whereas the TOP association area is involved in language function.

15. The _____ area integrates information related to motivation, emotion, and memory.

16. The _____ hemisphere in most individuals is dominant for language and speech, processes brief-duration stimuli, and performs detailed analysis.

17. The _____ hemisphere appears to process information in a more holistic fashion, preferring spatial and tonal information.

18. Damage to _____ area in the dominant hemisphere usually results in a receptive language deficit with relatively intact speech fluency.

19. Damage to _____ area in the dominant hemisphere often results in loss of speech fluency manifested as Broca's aphasia.

20. Damage to the _____ fasciculus will result in conduction aphasia.

21. A client of yours had a stroke, and reveals some muscular weakness on the left side of her body. Her speech is precisely articulated but the intonation is flat. She complains that, despite her lack of physical problems, she has noticed that her friends don't call any more. Where is the site of lesion, and where should therapy be directed?

Study Question Answers

1. **ACTION POTENTIAL** is a change in electrical potential that occurs when a cell membrane is stimulated adequately to permit ion exchange between the intra- and extracellular spaces.

2. The **ABSOLUTE REFRACTORY PERIOD** is the time during which the cell membrane cannot be stimulated to depolarize.

3. The **RELATIVE REFRACTORY PERIOD** is a period during which the membrane may be stimulated to excitation again, but only with greater than typical stimulation.

4. The **NODES OF RANVIER** of the axon myelin promote saltatory conduction.

5. The substance known as **NEUROTRANSMITTER** is discharged into the synaptic cleft, stimulating the postsynaptic neuron.

6. Activation of a muscle fiber causes the release of calcium into the environment of **THICK** myofilaments.

7. **SLOW** twitch muscle fibers remain contracted longer than **FAST** twitch fibers.

8. **MUSCLE SPINDLES** provide feedback to the neuromotor system about muscle length, tension, motion, and position.

9. Higher cognitive processing occurs generally in **ASSOCIATION** areas.

10. The **TEMPORO-OCCIPITAL-PARIETAL ASSOCIATION** area is involved in language function.

11. **FLACCID** dysarthria results from damage to LMNs, whereas UMN lesions result in spastic dysarthria.

12. **HYPERKINETIC** dysarthria is the result of damage to the inhibitory processes of the extrapyramidal system.

13. **ATAXIC DYSARTHRIA** arises from cerebellar damage.

14. The **PREFRONTAL** area of the cerebrum appears to be involved in higher function related to motor output (such as inhibition of motor function and the ability to change motor responses), whereas the TOP association area is involved in language function.

15. The **LIMBIC ASSOCIATION** area integrates information related to affect, motivation, and emotion.

16. The **LEFT** hemisphere in most individuals is dominant for language and speech, processes brief-duration stimuli, and performs detailed analysis.

17. The **RIGHT** hemisphere appears to process information in a more holistic fashion, preferring spatial and tonal information.

18. Damage to **WERNICKE'S** area in the dominant hemisphere usually results in a receptive language deficit with relatively intact speech fluency.

19. Damage to **BROCA'S** area in the dominant hemisphere often results in loss of speech fluency manifested as Broca's aphasia.

20. Damage to the **ARCUATE** fasciculus will result in conduction aphasia.

21. This individual suffered frontal lobe damage of the right hemisphere. Speech was unaffected because the left hemisphere dominates speech and many language functions. Nonetheless, she has a reduction in the ability to examine the context of communication (right hemisphere) and may be insensitive to cues that her friends are giving her that would otherwise cause her to change some communication strategy. An important goal of therapy would be to increase her awareness of the pragmatic cues and to develop strategies to increase her sensitivity to context.

Bibliography

Adams, R. D., Victor, M., & Ropper, A. H. (1997). *Principles of neurology* (6th ed.). New York: McGraw-Hill.

Akshoomoff, N.A., & Courchesne, E. (1992). A new role for the cerebellum in cognitive operations. *Behavioral Neuroscience, 106*(5), 731–738.

Albom, M. (1997). *Tuesdays with Morrie*. New York: Broadway Books.

Andermann, M. L., Kerlin, A. M., Roumis, D. K., Glickfeld, L. L., & Reid, R. C. (2012). Functional specialization of mouse visual cortical areas. *Neuron, 72*(6), 1025–1039.

Aronson, A. E. (2000). *Aronson's neurosciences pocket lectures.* San Diego, CA:Singular Publishing Group.

Bach, P., Peelen, M. V., & Tipper, S. P. On the role of object information in action observation: An fMRI study. (2010). *Cerebral Cortex, 20*(12), 2798–2809.

Bear, M. F., Connors, B. W., & Paradiso, M. A. (1996). *Neuroscience: Exploring the brain.* Baltimore, MD: Williams & Wilkins.

Bechera, A., Tranel, D., Damasio, H., Adolphs, R., Rockland, C., & Damasio, A. R. (1995). Double dissociation of conditioning and declarative knowledge relative to the amygdala and hippocampus in humans. *Science, 269,* 1115–1118.

Belmonte, M. K., Allen, G., Beckel-Mitchener, A., Boulanger, L. M., Carper, R. A., & Webb, S. J. (2004). Autism and abnormal development of brain connectivity. *Journal of Neuroscience, 24*(42), 9228–9231.

Berkovitz, B. K. B., & Moxham, B. J. (2002). *Head and neck anatomy.* New York: Taylor & Francis.

Betarbet, R., Sherer, T. B., MacKenzie, G., Garcia-Osuna, G., Panov, A. V., & Greenamyre, J. T. (2000). Systemic pesticide exposure reproduces features of Parkinson's disease. *Nature Neuroscience, 3,* 1301–1306.

Bhatnagar, S. C. (2007). *Neuroscience for the study of communicative disorders* (3rd ed.). Baltimore, MD: Williams & Wilkins.

Blakemore, C., & Cooper, G. F. (1970). Development of brain depends on the visual environment. *Nature, 228,* 477–478.

Bly, L. (1994). *Motor skills acquisition in the first year.* Tucson, AZ: Therapy Skill Builders.

Bowman, J. P. (1971). *The muscle spindle and neural control of the tongue.* Springfield, IL: Charles C. Thomas.

Campbell, N. A. (1987). *Biology.* Menlo Park, CA: Cumming.

Carpenter, M. B. (1978). *Core text of neuroanatomy* (2nd ed.). Baltimore, MD: Williams & Wilkins.

Chun, J., & Schatz, D. G. (1999). Developmental neurobiology: Alternative ends for a familiar story? *Current Biology, 9*(7), R251–R253.

Chusid, J. G. (1979). *Correlative neuroanatomy and functional neurology* (17th ed.). Los Altos, CA: Lange Medical Publications.

Collins, M. J. (1989). Differential diagnosis of aphasic syndromes and apraxia of speech. In Square-Storer (Ed.), *Acquired apraxia of speech in aphasic adults* (pp. 87–114). London: Taylor & Francis.

Corkin, S. (2002). What's new with the amnesic patient H.M.? *Nature Reviews Neuroscience, 3*(2), 153–160.

Cotman, C. W., & McGaugh, J. L. (1980). *Behavioral neuroscience.* New York: Academic Press.

Crary, M. A. (1993). *Developmental motor speech disorders.* San Diego, CA: Singular Publishing Group.

Darley, F. L., Aronson, A. E., & Brown, J. R. (1975). *Motor speech disorders.* Philadelphia, PA: W. B. Saunders.

Dronkers, N. F. (1996). A new brain region for coordinating speech articulation. *Nature, 384,* 159–161.

Duffy, J. R. (2005). *Motor speech disorders* (2nd ed.). St. Louis, MO: Mosby.

Dworkin, J. P. (1994). *Motor speech disorders: A treatment guide.* St. Louis, MO: C. V. Mosby.

Edvinsson, L., & Krause, D. N. (2002). *Cerebral blood flow and metabolism.* Philadelphia, PA: Lippincott/ Williams & Wilkins.

Filskov, S. B., & Boll, T. J. (1981). *Handbook of clinical neuropsychology.* New York: John Wiley & Sons.

Fiorentino, M. R. (1973). *Reflex testing methods for evaluating CNS development.* Springfield, IL; Charles Thomas Publishers.

Ganong, W. F. (1981). *Review of medical physiology.* Los Altos, CA: Lange Medical Publications.

Gelfand, S. A. (1990). *Hearing.* New York: Marcel Dekker.

Gelfand, S. A. (2001). *Essentials of audiology* (2nd ed.). New York: Thieme Medical Publishers.

Ghez, C. (1991). Voluntary movement. In E. R. Kandel, J. H. Schwartz, & T. M. Jessell (Eds.), *Principles of neural science* (3rd ed., pp. 609–625). Norwalk, CT: Appleton &Lange.

Gilman, S., & Winans, S. S. (1982). *Manter and Gatz's essentials of clinical neuroanatomy and neurophysiology.* Philadelphia, PA: F. A. Davis.

Gilroy, J. (2000). *Basic neurology* (3rd ed.). New York: McGraw-Hill.

Gilroy, A. M., MacPherson, B. R., & Ross, L.M. (2012). *Atlas of anatomy* (2nd ed.). New York: Thieme.

Gray, H., Bannister, L. H., Berry, M. M., & Williams, P. L. (Eds.). (1995). *Gray's anatomy.* London: Churchill Livingstone.

Hubel, D. H. (1979). The visual cortex of normal and deprived monkeys. *Scientific American, 67*, 532–543.

Johnson, J. (2009). Late auditory event-related potentials: Children with cochlear implants. *Developmental Neuropsychology, 34*(6), 701–720.

Kandel, E. R. (1991). Brain and behavior. In E. R. Kandel, J. H. Schwartz, & T. M. Jessell (Eds.), *Principles of neural science* (3rd ed., pp. 5–17). Norfolk, CT: Appleton & Lange.

Kandel, E. R., Schwartz, J. H., & Jessell, T. M. (2000). *Principles of neural science* (4th ed.). New York: McGraw-Hill.

Kandel, E. R., Siegelbaum, S. A., & Schwartz, J. H. (1991). Synaptic transmission. In E. R.Kandel, J. H. Schwartz, & T. M. Jessell (Eds.), *Principles of neural science* (3rd ed., pp. 1–1135). Norwalk, CT: Appleton & Lange.

Kandel, E. R., Schwartz, J. H., Jessell, T. M., Siegelbaum, S. A., & Hudspeth, A. J. (2013). *Principles of neural science* (5th ed.). New York: McGraw Hill.

Kanwisher, N., McDermott, J., & Chun, M. M. (1997). The fusiform face area: A module in human extrastriate cortex specialized for face perception. *Journal of Neuroscience, 17*(11), 4302–4311.

Kaufman, D. M. (2000). *Clinical neurology for psychiatrists* (5th ed.). Philadelphia, PA: W. B. Saunders.

Keene, D. L., Whiting, S., & Ventureyra, E. C. (2000). Electrocorticography. *Epileptic Disorders, 2*(1), 57–63.

Kelly, J. P. (1991). *The neural basis of perception and movement*. In E. R.Kandel, J. H. Schwartz, & T. M. Jessell (Eds.), *Principles of neural science* (3rd ed., pp. 792–803). Norwalk, CT: Appleton & Lange.

Kuehn, D. P., Lemme, M. L., & Baumgartner, J. M. (1989). *Neural bases of speech, hearing, and language*. Boston: College-Hill Press.

Kupferman, I. (1991). Localization of higher cognitive and affective functions: The association cortices. In E. R. Kandel, J. H. Schwartz, & T. M. Jessell (Eds.), *Principles of neural science* (3rd ed., pp. 823–838). Norwalk, CT: Appleton & Lange.

Lutz, A., Greischar, L. L., Rawlings, N. B., Ricard, M., & Davidson, R. J. (2004). Long term meditators self-induce high amplitude gamma synchrony during practice. *Proceedings of the National Academy of Science, 101*(46), 16369–16373.

Mackay, L. E., Chapman, P. E., & Morgan, A. S. (1997). *Maximizing brain injury recovery*. Gaithersburg, MD: Aspen Publishers.

Martinez, L. M., Wang, Q., Reid, R. C., Pillai, C., Alonso, J. M., Sommer, F. T., & Hirsch, J. A. (2005). Receptive field structure varies with layer in primary visual cortex. *Nature Neuroscience, 8*(3), 372–379.

Mayeux, R., & Kandel, E. R. (1991). Disorders of language: The aphasias. In E. R. Kandel, J. H. Schwartz, & T. M. Jessell (Eds.), *Principles of neural science* (3rd ed., pp. 839–851). Norwalk, CT: Appleton & Lange.

McKay, L. C., Janczewski, W. A., & Feldman, J. L. (2005). Sleep-disordered breathing after targeted ablation of preBotzinger complex neurons. *Nature Neuroscience, 8*, 1142–1144.

Miller, K J., denNijs, M., Shenoy, P., Miller, J. W., Rao, R. P. N., & Ojemann, J. G. (2007). Real time functional brain mapping using electrocorticogaphy. *Neuroimage, 37*, 504–507.

Møller, A. R. (2003). *Sensory systems: Anatomy and physiology*. New York: Academic Press.

Mueller, S., Kesser, D., Samson, A. C., Kirsch, V., Blautzik, J., Grothe, E., Erat, O., Hegenloh, M., Coates, U., Reiser, M. F., Hennig-Fast, K., & Meindl, T. (2013). Convergent findings of altered functional and structure brain connectivity in individuals with high functioning autism: A multimodal MRI study. *PLoS One, 8*(6), e67329.

Myers, P. (1999). *Right hemisphere damage*. San Diego, CA: Singular Publishing Group.

Naqvi, N. H., Rudrauf, D., Damasio, H., & Bechara, A. (2007). Damage to the insula disrupts addiction to cigarette smoking. *Science, 315*(5811), 531–534.

Netter, F. H. (1983). *The CIBA collection of medical illustrations. Vol. 1. Nervous system. Part I. Anatomy and physiology*. West Caldwell, NJ: CIBA Pharmaceutical.

Netter, F. H. (1983). *The CIBA collection of medical illustrations. Vol. 1. Nervous system. Part II. Neurologic and neuromuscular disorders*. West Caldwell, NJ: CIBA Pharmaceutical Company.

Noback, C. R., Demarest, R. J., & Strominger, N. L. (1991). *The human nervous system*. Philadelphia, PA: Lea & Febiger.

Noback, C. R., Demarest, R. J., & Strominger, N. L. (1991). *The nervous system: Introduction and review*. Philadelphia, PA: Williams & Wilkins.

Nolte, J. (1993). *The human brain*. St. Louis, MO: Mosby Year Book.

Penfield, W., & Roberts, L. (1959). *Speech and brain-mechanisms*. Princeton, NJ: Princeton University Press.

Poritsky, R. (1992). *Neuroanatomy: A functional atlas of parts and pathways*. St. Louis, MO: Mosby Year Book.

Raymond, J. L., Lisberger, S. G., & Mauk, M. D. (1996). The cerebellum: A neuronal learning machine. *Science. 272*, 1126–1131.

Schuell, H., Jenkins, J., & Jiménes-Pabon, E. (1964). *Aphasia in adults: Diagnosis, prognosis, and therapy*. New York: Hoeber.

Schuenke, M., & Ross, L. M., (2010). *Thieme atlas of anatomy*. New York: Thieme.

Square-Storer, P., & Roy, E. A. (1989). The apraxias: Commonalities and distinctions. In P. Square-Storer (Ed.), *Acquired apraxia of speech in aphasic adults* (pp. 20–63). London: Taylor & Francis.

Standring, S. (2008). *Gray's anatomy: The anatomical and clinical basis of practice* (40th ed.). London: Churchill Livingstone.

Sugiura, L., Ojima, S., Matsuba-Kurita, H., Dan, I., Tsuzuki, D., Katura, T., & Hagiwara, H. (2011). Sound to language: Different cortical processing of the first and second language in elementary school children as revealed by a large scale study using fNIRS. *Cerebral Cortex, 21*(10), 2374–2393.

Treadway, M. T., McGarvey, M., Quinn, B. T., Dusek, J. A., Benson, H., Rauch, S. L., et al. (2005). Meditation experience is associated with increased cortical thickness. *NeuroReport, 16*(17), 1893–1897.

Tsao, D. Y., Freiwald, W. A., Tootell, R. B. H., & Livingstone, M. S. (2006). A cortical region consisting entirely of face-selective cells. *Science, 311*, 670–674.

Twietmeyer, A., & McCracken, T. (1992). *Coloring guide to regional human anatomy*. Philadelphia, PA: Lea & Febiger.

Webster, D. B. (1999). *Neuroscience of communication* (2nd ed.). San Diego, CA: Singular Publishing Group.

Whittle, S., Yap, M. B., Yücel, M., Fornito, A., Simmons, J. G., Barrett, A., et al. (2008). Prefrontal and amygdala volumes are related to adolescents' affective behaviors during parent-adolescent interactions. *Proceedings of the National Academy of Science USA, 105*(9), 3652–3657.

Williams, P., & Warrick, R. (1980). *Gray's anatomy* (36th British ed.). Philadelphia, PA: W. B. Saunders.

Winans, S. S., Gilman, S., Manter, J. T., & Gatz, A. J. (2002). *Manter and Gatz's essentials of clinical neuroanatomy and neurophysiology* (10th ed.). Philadelphia, PA: F. A. Davis.

Wood, P. J., & Criss, W. R. (1975). *Normal and abnormal development of the human nervous system*. Hagerstown, MD: Harper & Row.

Yost, W. A., & Nielsen, D. W. (1977). *Fundamentals of hearing*. New York: Holt, Rinehart, and Winston.

Zemlin, W. R. (1998). *Speech and hearing science: Anatomy and physiology* (4th ed.). Needham Heights, MA: Allyn & Bacon.

APPENDIX A

Anatomical Terms

Anatomical position:	Upright, palms forward, eyes directly ahead, feet together
Anterior:	Toward the front of the body or subpart
Asthenia:	Weakness
Bifurcation:	A fork; split into two parts
Caudal:	Toward the tail or coccyx
Central:	Relative to the center of a structure
Cranial:	Toward the head
Deep:	Away from the surface
Distal:	Further from the trunk or thorax; further from the attached end
Dorsal:	Pertaining to the back of the body or the posterior surface
Extension:	Straightening or moving out of the flexed position
External:	Toward the exterior of a body
Flexion:	The act of bending
Frontal plane:	Divides the body into anterior and posterior halves
Horizontal plane:	Divides the body or body part into upper and lower halves
Inferior:	The lower point; nearer the feet
Insertion:	Distal attachment of a muscle; typically the most mobile point of attachment
Internal:	Enclosed or on the interior
Lateral:	Away from the midline of the body or subpart
Medial/mesial:	Toward the midline of the body or subpart
Origin:	Proximal attachment of a muscle; typically the least mobile point of attachment
Palmar:	Pertaining to the palm of the hand
Peripheral:	Relative to the periphery or away from the center
Plantar:	Pertaining to the sole of the foot
Posterior:	Toward the back of the body or subpart
Prone:	Body in horizontal position with face down
Proximal:	Closer to the trunk or thorax; nearer to the attached end
Radial:	Pertaining to the radius bone
Sagittal plane:	Divides the body or body part into right and left halves
Superficial:	Near the surface
Superior:	The upper point; nearer the head
Supine:	Body in horizontal position with face up
Ventral:	Pertaining to the belly or anterior surface

APPENDIX B

Useful Combining Forms

-a-	Without; lack of
ab-	Away from
ad-	Toward
-algia	Pain
amphi-	On both sides
an-	Without; lack of
ana-	Up
angio-	Blood vessels
ante-	Before
antero-	Before
apo-	Away from
arthr-	A joint
bi-	Two
blast-	Germ
brachy-	Short
brady-	Slow
capit-	Head, or toward the head end
-carpal	Wrist
-cele	Tumor
cephalo-	Head, or toward the head end
circum	Around
-cle	Implies something very small
com-	With or together with
con-	With or together with
contra-	Opposite
cor-	Heart
corp-	Body
crus-	Cross; leglike part
crur-	Cross; leglike part
cryo-	Cold
-cule	Implies something very small
-culum	Diminutive form of a noun
-culus	Diminutive form of a noun
-cyte	Cell

de-	Away from
dextro-	Right
-dynia	Pain
dys-	Bad; with difficulty
e-	Out from
ec-	Out of
ecto-	On the outer side; toward the surface
-ectomy	Excision
-emia	Blood
endo-	Toward the interior; within
ento-	Toward the interior; within
ep-	Upon or above something else
epi-	Upon or above something else
etio-	Cause or origin
ex-	Out of, toward the surface
extero-	Aimed outward or nearer to the surface
extra-	Outside
-gen	Producing
-genic	Producing
hemi-	Half
hyper-	Above; increased, or too much of something
hypo-	Below; decreased, or too little of something
idio-	Peculiar
-ilos	Diminutive form of a noun
infra-	Below
inter-	Between
intero-	Aimed inward or farther from the surface
intra-	Within
intro-	Into
ipsi-	Same
iso-	Equal
-itis	Inflammation or irritation
-ium	Diminutive form of a noun
latero-	Side
lepto-	Thick
leuco-	White
levo-	Left
macro-	Large
medio-	Middle
megalo-	Large
meso-	Middle
meta-	After; mounted or built upon

micro-	Small
mono-	Single
morph-	Form
my-	Pertaining to muscle
myelo-	Pertaining to spinal cord
myo-	Pertaining to muscle
naso-	Nose
neo-	New
neuro-	Nerve
oculo-	Eye
-oma	Morbid condition of a part, often a tumor
oro-	Mouth
ortho-	Straight
-osis	Condition
osseo-	A hardened or bony part, but not strictly
osteo-	Bone
pachy-	Thick
palato-	Palate
para	Beside; partial
patho-	Abnormal in some way
-pathy	Disease
ped-	Child
ped-	Foot
-penia	Poverty
per-	Through; passing through; before
peri-	Around
-phage	Eating
-phagia	Eating
-pher-	Bearing or carrying
-plasia	Growth
-plastic	Capable of being molded
-plasty	Molding, forming
-poiesis	Making
poly-	Many
post-	After; behind
postero-	Behind
pre-	Before; in front of
pro-	Before; in front of
proto-	Primitive; simple form
quadra-	Four
quadri-	Four
-raphy	Suturing or stitching

re-	Back or again; curved back
retro-	Backward, toward the rear
-rrhea	A flowing
scirrho-	Hard
sclero-	Hard
-sclerosis	Hardening
scolio-	Curved
semi-	Half
sinistro-	Left
soma-	Pertaining to the body
somato-	Pertaining to the body
steno-	Narrow
strepto-	Swift
sub-	Under
sup-	Under; moderately
super-	Above; excessively
supra-	Above, upon
sym-	With or together
syn-	With or together
tachy-	Swift; fast
-tarsal	Ankle
telo-	Far from, toward the extreme
tetra-	Four
-tomy	Cutting
trans-	Beyond or on the other side
tri-	Three
-trophic	Related to nourishment
-trophy	Growth, usually by expanding
-tropy	Implies seeking or heading for something
uni-	One

APPENDIX C

Muscles of Respiration

THORACIC MUSCLES OF INSPIRATION

Primary Inspiratory Muscle

Muscle:	**Diaphragm** (sternal head, costal head, and vertebral head)
Origin:	Sternal head: Xiphoid process of the sternum; costal head: the inferior margin of the rib cage (ribs 7 through 12); vertebral head: the corpus of L1, and the transverse processes of L1 through L5
Course:	Up and medially
Insertion:	Central tendon of diaphragm
Innervation:	Phrenic nerve arising from cervical plexus of spinal nerves C1, C2, C3 and C4
Function:	Depresses central tendon of diaphragm, enlarges vertical dimension of thorax, distends abdomen

Accessory Thoracic Muscles of Inspiration

Muscle:	**External intercostal**
Origin:	Inferior surface of ribs 1 through 11
Course:	Down and obliquely in
Insertion:	Upper surface of rib immediately below
Innervation:	Intercostal nerves: thoracic intercostal nerves arising from T1 through T6 and thoracoabdominal intercostal nerves from T7 through T11
Function:	Elevates rib

Muscle:	**Internal Intercostal, interchondral portion**
Origin:	Superior margin of ribs 1 through 11
Course:	Up and in
Insertion:	Inferior surface of the rib below
Innervation:	Intercostal nerves: thoracic intercostal nerves arising from T1 through T6 and thoracoabdominal intercostal nerves from T7 through T11
Function:	Elevate ribs 1 through 11

Note that the internal intercostal muscles are considered muscles of expiration, with the exception of the those muscles of the interchondral portion of the rib cage, which pull the rib cage up and are therefore considered accessory muscles of inspiration.

Muscle:	**Levator costarum, brevis**
Origin:	Transverse processes of vertebrae C7 through T11
Course:	Obliquely down and out
Insertion:	Tubercle of the rib below
Innervation:	Dorsal rami (branches) of the intercostal nerves arising from spinal nerves C7 through T11
Function:	Elevates rib cage

Muscle:	**Levator costarum, longis**
Origin:	Transverse processes of C7 through T11
Course:	Down and obliquely out
Insertion:	Bypasses the rib below the point of origin, inserting instead into the next rib
Innervation:	Dorsal rami (branches) of the intercostal nerves arising from spinal nerves C7 through T11
Function:	Elevates rib cage

Muscle:	**Serratus posterior superior**
Origin:	Spinous processes of C7 and T1 through T3
Course:	Down and laterally
Insertion:	Just beyond the angles of ribs 2 through 5
Innervation:	Ventral intercostal portion of spinal nerves T1 through T4 or T5
Function:	Elevates ribs 2 through 5

Erector spinae (sacrospinal muscles). Consists of three major types: lateral (iliocostocervicalis), intermediate (longissimus), and medial (spinalis). Each of these heads is further subdivided.

Lateral (iliocostocervicalis) bundle: Subdivided into iliocostalis lumborum, iliocostalis thoracis, and iliocostalis cervicis.

Muscle:	**Iliocostalis lumborum of the lateral (iliocostocervicalis) bundle**
Origin:	Sacral crest, L1 through L5, T11 through T12
Course:	Up
Insertion:	Angles of ribs 6 through 12
Innervation:	Dorsal rami of lower cervical nerves and thoracic and lumbar nerves
Function:	Stabilizes and moves the vertebral column

Muscle:	**Iliocostalis thoracis of the lateral (iliocostocervicalis) bundle**
Origin:	Ribs 6 through 12
Course:	Up
Insertion:	Ribs 1 through 6 and C7 vertebra
Innervation:	Dorsal rami of lower cervical nerves and thoracic and lumbar nerves
Function:	Stabilizes and moves the vertebral column

Muscle:	**Iliocostalis cervicis of the lateral (iliocostocervicalis) bundle**
Origin:	Ribs 3 through 6
Course:	Up
Insertion:	C4 through C6 vertebrae
Innervation:	Dorsal rami of lower cervical nerves and thoracic and lumbar nerves
Function:	Stabilizes and moves the vertebral column

Intermediate (longissiumus) bundle: Subdivided into longissimus thoracis, longissimus cervicis, and longissimus capitis.

Muscle:	**Longissimus thoracis of the intermediate (longissiumus) bundle**
Origin:	L1 through L5 transverse processes and thoracolumbar fascia
Course:	Up
Insertion:	T1 through T12 vertebrae, transverse processes and ribs 3 through 12
Innervation:	Dorsal rami of lower cervical nerves and thoracic and lumbar nerves
Function:	Stabilizes and moves the vertebral column

Muscle:	**Longissimus cervicis of the intermediate (longissiumus) bundle**
Origin:	T1 through T5 vertebrae
Course:	Up
Insertion:	C2 through C6 vertebrae, transverse processes
Innervation:	Dorsal rami of lower cervical nerves and thoracic and lumbar nerves
Function:	Stabilizes and moves the vertebral column

Muscle:	**Longissimus capitis of the intermediate (longissiumus) bundle**
Origin:	C1 through C5 vertebrae
Course:	Up
Insertion:	Posterior mastoid process of temporal bone
Innervation:	Dorsal rami of lower cervical nerves and thoracic and lumbar nerves
Function:	Stabilizes and moves the vertebral column

Medial (spinalis) bundle: Subdivided into three muscles: Spinalis thoracis, spinalis cervicis, and spinalis capitis.

Muscle:	**Spinalis thoracis of the medial (spinalis) bundle**
Origin:	T11 and T12, L1 through L3 vertebrae
Course:	Up
Insertion:	T1 through T8
Innervation:	Dorsal rami of lower cervical nerves and thoracic and lumbar nerves
Function:	Stabilizes and moves the vertebral column

Muscle:	**Spinalis cervicis of the medial (spinalis) bundle**
Origin:	Nuchal ligament and C7 vertebra
Course:	Up
Insertion:	C2 vertebra
Innervation:	Dorsal rami of lower cervical nerves and thoracic and lumbar nerves
Function:	Stabilizes and moves the vertebral column

Muscle:	**Spinalis capitis of the medial (spinalis) bundle**
Origin:	T1 through T6, C4 through C7
Course:	Up
Insertion:	Nuchal line of skull
Innervation:	Dorsal rami of lower cervical nerves and thoracic and lumbar nerves
Function:	Stabilizes and moves the vertebral column

Accessory Muscles of Neck

Muscle:	**Sternocleidomastoid**
Origin:	Mastoid process of the temporal bone
Course:	Down
Insertion:	Sternal head: Superior manubrium sterni; Clavicular head: clavicle
Innervation:	XI accessory, spinal branch arising from the spinal cord in the regions of C2 through C4 or C5
Function:	Elevates sternum and rib cage

Muscle:	**Scalenus anterior**
Origin:	Transverse processes of vertebrae C3 through C6
Course:	Down
Insertion:	Superior surface of rib 1
Innervation:	C4 through C6
Function:	Elevates rib 1

Muscle:	**Scalenus medius**
Origin:	Transverse processes of vertebrae C2 through C7
Course:	Down
Insertion:	Superior surface of the first rib
Innervation:	Cervical plexus derived from C3 and C4 and spinal nerves C5 through C8
Function:	Elevates rib 1

Muscle:	**Scalenus posterior**
Origin:	Transverse processes of C5 through C7
Course:	Down
Insertion:	Second rib
Innervation:	Spinal nerves C5 through C8
Function:	Elevates rib 2

Muscles of Upper Arm and Shoulder

Muscle:	**Pectoralis major**
Origin:	Sternal head: length of the sternum at costal cartilages; clavicular head: anterior clavicle
Course:	Fans laterally, converging at humerus
Insertion:	Greater tubercle of humerus
Innervation:	Superior branch brachial plexus (spinal nerves C5 through C8 and T1)
Function:	Elevates sternum, and subsequently increases transverse dimension of rib cage

Muscle:	**Pectoralis minor**
Origin:	Anterior surface of ribs 2 through 5 near the chondral margin
Course:	Up and laterally
Insertion:	Coracoid process of scapula
Innervation:	Superior branch of the brachial plexus (spinal nerves C4 through C7 and T1)
Function:	Increases the transverse dimension of the rib cage

Muscle:	**Serratus anterior**
Origin:	Ribs 1 through 9, lateral surface of the thorax
Course:	Up and back
Insertion:	Inner vertebral border of scapula
Innervation:	Brachial plexus, long thoracic nerve from C5 through C7
Function:	Elevates ribs 1 through 9

Muscle:	**Subclavius**
Origin:	Inferior surface of the clavicle
Course:	Oblique and medial
Insertion:	Superior surface of rib 1 at chondral margin
Innervation:	Brachial plexus, lateral branch, from fifth and sixth spinal nerves
Function:	Elevates rib 1

Muscle:	**Levator scapulae**
Origin:	Transverse processes of C1 through C4
Course:	Down
Insertion:	Medial border of scapula
Innervation:	C3 through C5
Function:	Neck support, elevates scapula

Muscle:	**Rhomboideus major**
Origin:	Spinous processes of T2 through T5
Course:	Down and laterally in
Insertion:	Scapula
Innervation:	Spinal C5 from the dorsal scapular nerve of upper root of brachial plexus
Function:	Stabilizes shoulder girdle

Muscle: **Rhomboideus minor**

Origin: Spinous processes of C7 and T1

Course: Down and laterally in

Insertion: Medial border of scapula

Innervation: Spinal C5 from the dorsal scapular nerve of upper root of brachial plexus

Function: Stabilizes shoulder girdle

Muscle: **Trapezius**

Origin: Spinous processes of C2 to T12

Course: Fans laterally

Insertion: Acromion of scapula and superior surface of clavicle

Innervation: XI accessory, spinal branch arising from spinal cord in the regions of C2 through C4 or C5

Function: Elongates neck, controls head

Thoracic Muscles of Expiration

Muscle: **Internal intercostal, interosseous portion**

Origin: Superior margin of ribs 1 through 11

Course: Up and in

Insertion: Inferior surface of rib above

Innervation: Intercostal nerves: thoracic intercostal nerves arising from T2 through T6 and thoracoabdominal intercostal nerves from T7 through T11

Function: Depresses ribs 1 through 11

Note that the interosseous portion of the internal intercostal is a muscle of expiration, although the interchondral portion of the internal intercostal muscle is considered to be a muscle of inspiration.

Muscle: **Innermost intercostal**

Origin: Superior margin of ribs 1 through 11; sparse or absent in superior thorax

Course: Up and in

Insertion: Inferior surface of rib above

Innervation: Intercostal nerves: thoracic intercostal nerves arising from T2 through T6 and thoracoabdominal intercostal nerves from T7 through T11

Function: Depresses ribs 1 through 11

Muscle: **Transversus thoracis**

Origin: Inner thoracic lateral margin of the sternum

Course: Laterally

Insertion: Inner chondral surface of ribs 2 through 6

Innervation: Thoracic intercostal nerves and thoracoabdominal intercostal nerves and subcostal nerves derived from T2 through T6 spinal nerves

Function: Depresses rib cage

Posterior Thoracic Muscles

Muscle:	**Subcostal**
Origin:	Inner posterior thorax; sparse in the upper thorax; from inner surface of rib near angle
Course:	Down and lateral
Insertion:	Inner surface of second or third rib below
Innervation:	Intercostal nerves of thorax, arising from the ventral rami of the spinal nerves
Function:	Depresses thorax

Muscle:	**Serratus posterior inferior**
Origin:	Spinous processes of T11, T12, L1 through L3
Course:	Up and lateral
Insertion:	Lower margin of ribs 7 through 12
Innervation:	Intercostal nerves from T9 through T11 and subcostal nerve from T12
Function:	Contraction tends to pull rib cage down, supporting expiratory effort

ABDOMINAL MUSCLES OF EXPIRATION

Anterolateral Abdominal Muscles

Muscle:	**Transversus abdominis**
Origin:	Posterior abdominal wall at the vertebral column via the thoracolumbar fascia of the abdominal aponeurosis
Course:	Lateral
Insertion:	Transversus abdominis aponeurosis and inner surface of ribs 6 through 12, interdigitating at that point with the fibers of the diaphragm; inferior-most attachment is at the pubis
Innervation:	Thoracic and lumbar nerves from the lower spinal intercostal nerves (derived from T7 to T12) and first lumbar nerve, iliohypogastric and ilioinguinal branches
Function:	Compresses abdomen

Muscle:	**Internal oblique abdominis**
Origin:	Inguinal ligament and iliac crest
Course:	Fans medially
Insertion:	Cartilaginous portion of lower ribs and the portion of the abdominal aponeurosis lateral to the rectus abdominis
Innervation:	Thoracic and lumbar nerves from the lower spinal intercostal nerves (derived from T7 to T12) and first lumbar nerve, iliohypogastric and ilioinguinal branches
Function:	Rotates trunk, flexes trunk, compresses abdomen

Muscle:	**External oblique abdominis**
Origin:	Osseous portion of the lower seven ribs
Course:	Fans downward
Insertion:	Iliac crest, inguinal ligament, and abdominal aponeurosis lateral to rectus abdominis
Innervation:	Thoracoabdominal nerve arising from T7 through T11 and subcostal nerve from T12
Function:	Bilateral contraction flexes vertebral column and compresses abdomen; unilateral contraction results in trunk rotation

Muscle:	**Rectus abdominis**
Origin:	Originates as four or five segments at pubis inferiorly
Course:	Up to segment border
Insertion:	Xiphoid process of sternum and the cartilage of ribs 5 through 7, lower ribs
Innervation:	T7 through T11 intercostal nerves (thoracoabdominal) subcostal nerve from T12 (T7 supplies upper segment, T8 supplies the second, T9 supplies remainder)
Function:	Flexion of vertebral column

Posterior Abdominal Muscles

Muscle:	**Quadratus lumborum**
Origin:	Iliac crest
Course:	Fans up and in
Insertion:	Transverse processes of the lumbar vertebrae and inferior border of rib 12
Innervation:	Thoracic nerve T12 and L1 through L4 lumbar nerves
Function:	Bilateral contraction fixes the abdominal wall in support of abdominal compression

MUSCLES OF UPPER LIMB

Muscle:	**Latissimus dorsi**
Origin:	Lumbar, sacral, and lower thoracic vertebrae
Course:	Fans up
Insertion:	Humerus
Innervation:	Brachial plexus, posterior branch; fibers from the regions C6 through C8 form the long subscapular nerve
Function:	For respiration, stabilizes posterior abdominal wall for expiration

Muscles of Phonation

INTRINSIC LARYNGEAL MUSCLES

Muscle:	**Aryepiglotticus muscle**
Origin:	Continuation of the oblique arytenoid muscle from the arytenoid apex
Course:	Back and up as muscular component of aryepiglottic fold
Insertion:	Lateral epiglottis
Innervation:	X vagus, recurrent laryngeal nerve
Function:	Constricts laryngeal opening
Muscle:	**Lateral cricoarytenoid**
Origin:	Superior-lateral surface of the cricoid cartilage
Course:	Up and back
Insertion:	Muscular process of the arytenoid
Innervation:	X vagus, recurrent laryngeal nerve
Function:	Adducts vocal folds, increases medial compression
Muscle:	**Transverse arytenoid**
Origin:	Lateral margin of the posterior arytenoid
Course:	Laterally on posterior surface of arytenoid
Insertion:	Lateral margin of posterior surface, opposite arytenoid
Innervation:	X vagus, recurrent laryngeal nerve
Function:	Adducts vocal folds
Muscle:	**Oblique arytenoid**
Origin:	Posterior base of the muscular processes
Course:	Obliquely up on posterior surface of arytenoid
Insertion:	Apex of the opposite arytenoid
Innervation:	X vagus, recurrent laryngeal nerve
Function:	Pulls the apex medially, adducts the vocal folds
Muscle:	**Posterior cricoarytenoid**
Origin:	Posterior cricoid lamina
Course:	Superiorly
Insertion:	Posterior aspect of the muscular process of arytenoid cartilage
Innervation:	X vagus, recurrent laryngeal nerve
Function:	Abducts vocal folds

Muscle:	**Cricothyroid**
Origin:	Pars recta: anterior surface of the cricoid cartilage beneath the arch; Pars oblique: cricoid cartilage lateral to the pars recta
Course:	Pars recta: up and out; Pars oblique: obliquely up
Insertion:	Pars recta: lower surface of the thyroid lamina Pars oblique: thyroid cartilage between laminae and inferior horns
Innervation:	External branch of superior laryngeal nerve of X vagus
Function:	Depresses thyroid relative to cricoid, tenses vocal folds

Muscle:	**Thyrovocalis (medial thyroarytenoid)**
Origin:	Inner surface of thyroid cartilage near notch
Course:	Back
Insertion:	Lateral surface of the arytenoid vocal process
Innervation:	X vagus, recurrent laryngeal nerve
Function:	Tenses vocal folds

Muscle:	**Thyromuscularis (lateral thyroarytenoid)**
Origin:	Inner surface of the thyroid cartilage near the notch
Course:	Back
Insertion:	Base of arytenoid cartilage and muscular process
Innervation:	X vagus, recurrent laryngeal nerve
Function:	Relaxes vocal folds

Muscle:	**Superior thyroarytenoid**
Origin:	Inner surface of the thyroid cartilage near the angle
Course:	Back
Insertion:	Muscular process of arytenoid
Innervation:	X vagus, recurrent laryngeal nerve
Function:	Relaxes vocal folds

EXTRINSIC LARYNGEAL, INFRAHYOID, AND SUPRAHYOID MUSCLES

Hyoid and Laryngeal Elevators

Muscle:	**Digastricus, anterior and posterior**
Origin:	Anterior: inner surface of the mandible, near symphysis; Posterior: mastoid process of the temporal bone
Course:	Medial and down
Insertion:	Hyoid, by means of intermediate tendon
Innervation:	Anterior: V trigeminal nerve, mandibular branch, via the mylohyoid branch of the inferior alveolar nerve; Posterior: VII facial nerve, digastric branch
Function:	Anterior belly: draws hyoid up and forward; Posterior belly: draws hyoid up and back; together: elevate hyoid

Muscle: **Stylohyoid**
Origin: Styloid process of the temporal bone
Course: Medially down
Insertion: Corpus hyoid
Innervation: Motor branch of the VII facial nerve
Function: Elevates and retracts hyoid bone

Muscle: **Mylohyoid**
Origin: Mylohyoid line, inner surface of the mandible
Course: Fanlike to median fibrous raphe and hyoid
Insertion: Corpus of hyoid
Innervation: Alveolar nerve, V trigeminal, mandibular branch
Function: Elevates hyoid or depresses mandible

Muscle: **Geniohyoid**
Origin: Mental spines, inner surface of the mandible
Course: Back and down
Insertion: Corpus, hyoid bone
Innervation: XII hypoglossal nerve and C1 spinal nerve
Function: Elevates hyoid bone, depresses mandible

Muscle: **Hyoglossus**
Origin: Hyoid bone, greater cornu, and corpus
Course: Down
Insertion: Side of tongue
Innervation: Motor branch of the XII hypoglossal
Function: Elevates hyoid; depresses tongue

Muscle: **Genioglossus**
Origin: Mental spines, inner surface of mandible
Course: Up, back, and down
Insertion: Tongue and corpus hyoid
Innervation: Motor branch of XII hypoglossal
Function: Elevates hyoid

Muscle: **Thyropharyngeus of inferior pharyngeal constrictor**
Origin: Thyroid lamina and inferior cornu
Course: Up and medially
Insertion: Posterior pharyngeal raphe
Innervation: X vagus, recurrent laryngeal nerve (external laryngeal branch) and superior laryngeal nerve (pharyngeal branch), and XI accessory
Function: Constricts pharynx; elevates larynx

Hyoid and Laryngeal Depressors

Muscle: **Sternohyoid**
Origin: Manubrium sterni and clavicle
Course: Up
Insertion: Inferior margin of hyoid corpus
Innervation: Ansa cervicalis from spinal C1 through C3
Function: Depresses hyoid

Muscle: **Sternothyroid**
Origin: Manubrium sterni and first costal cartilage
Course: Up and out
Insertion: Oblique line, thyroid cartilage
Innervation: XII hypoglossal and spinal nerves C1 and C2
Function: Depresses thyroid cartilage

Muscle: **Thyrohyoid**
Origin: Oblique line, thyroid cartilage
Course: Up
Insertion: Greater cornu, hyoid
Innervation: XII hypoglossal nerve and fibers from spinal C1
Function: Depresses hyoid or elevates larynx

Muscle: **Omohyoid, superior and inferior heads**
Origin: Superior: intermediate tendon; Inferior: upper border, scapula
Course: Superior: down; Inferior: up and medially
Insertion: Superior: lower border, hyoid; Inferior: intermediate tendon
Innervation: Superior belly: superior ramus of ansa cervicalis from C1; Inferior belly: ansa cervicalis, spinal C2 and C3
Function: Depresses hyoid

APPENDIX E

Muscles of Face, Soft Palate, and Pharynx

FACIAL MUSCLES

Muscle: **Risorius**
Origin: The fascia of the masseter
Course: Forward
Insertion: Orbicularis oris at corners of mouth
Innervation: Buccal branch of the VII facial nerve
Function: Retracts lips at the corners

Muscle: **Buccinator**
Origin: Pterygomandibular ligament
Course: Forward
Insertion: Orbicularis oris at corners of mouth
Innervation: Buccal branch of the VII facial nerve
Function: Moves food onto the grinding surfaces of the molars; constricts oropharynx

Muscle: **Levator labii superioris**
Origin: Infraorbital margin of the maxilla
Course: Down and in to the upper lip
Insertion: Mid-lateral region of the upper lip
Innervation: Buccal branches of the VII facial nerve
Function: Elevates upper lip

Muscle: **Levator anguli oris**
Origin: Canine fossa of maxilla
Course: Down
Insertion: Corners of upper and lower lips
Innervation: Superior buccal branches of VII facial nerve
Function: Draws corner of mouth up and medially

Muscle: **Zygomatic minor**
Origin: Facial surface of the zygomatic bone
Course: Downward
Insertion: Mid-lateral region of upper lip
Innervation: Buccal branches of the VII facial nerve
Function: Elevates upper lip

Muscle: **Levator labii alaeque nasi superioris**
Origin: Frontal process of the maxilla
Course: Vertically along the lateral margin of the nose
Insertion: Mid-lateral region of the upper lip
Innervation: Buccal branches of the VII facial nerve
Function: Elevates upper lip

Muscle: **Zygomatic major (zygomaticus)**
Origin: Lateral to the zygomatic minor on the zygomatic bone
Course: Obliquely down
Insertion: Corner of the orbicularis oris
Innervation: Buccal branches of the VII facial nerve
Function: Elevates and retracts angle of mouth

Muscle: **Depressor labii inferioris**
Origin: Mandible at the oblique line
Course: Up and in
Insertion: Lower lip
Innervation: Mandibular marginal branch of facial nerve
Function: Dilates orifice by pulling lip down and out

Muscle: **Depressor anguli oris (triangularis)**
Origin: Lateral margins of mandible on the oblique line
Course: Fans up
Insertion: Orbicularis oris and upper lip at corner
Innervation: Mandibular marginal branch of the facial nerve
Function: Depresses corners of mouth and helps to compress upper lip against lower lip

Muscle: **Mentalis**
Origin: Region of the incisive fossa of the mandible
Course: Down
Insertion: Skin of the chin below
Innervation: Mandibular marginal branch of the facial nerve
Function: Elevates and wrinkles chin and pulls lower lip out

Muscle:	**Orbicularis oris inferior and superior**
Origin:	Corner of lips
Course:	Laterally within lips
Insertion:	Opposite corner of lips
Innervation:	VII facial nerve
Function:	Constricts oral opening

Muscle:	**Platysma**
Origin:	Fascia overlaying pectoralis major and deltoid
Course:	Up
Insertion:	Corner of the mouth, region below the symphysis mente, lower margin of the mandible, and skin near the masseter
Innervation:	Cervical branch of the VII facial nerve
Function:	Depresses mandible

Intrinsic Tongue Muscles

Muscle:	**Superior longitudinal**
Origin:	Fibrous submucous layer near the epiglottis, the hyoid, and from the median fibrous septum
Course:	Fans forward and outward
Insertion:	Lateral margins of the tongue and region of apex
Innervation:	XII hypoglossal nerve
Function:	Elevates, assists in retraction of, or deviates tip of tongue

Muscle:	**Inferior longitudinal**
Origin:	Root of the tongue and corpus hyoid
Course:	Forward
Insertion:	Apex of the tongue
Innervation:	XII hypoglossal nerve
Function:	Pulls tip of the tongue downward, assists in retraction, deviates tongue

Muscle:	**Transverse**
Origin:	Median fibrous septum
Course:	Laterally
Insertion:	Side of the tongue in the submucous tissue
Innervation:	XII hypoglossal nerve
Function:	Narrows tongue

Muscle:	**Vertical**
Origin:	Base of the tongue
Course:	Vertically
Insertion:	Membranous cover
Innervation:	XII hypoglossal nerve
Function:	Pulls tongue down into floor of mouth

Extrinsic Tongue Muscles

Muscle: **Genioglossus**

Origin:	Inner mandibular surface at the symphysis
Course:	Fans up, back, and forward
Insertion:	Tip and dorsum of tongue and corpus hyoid
Innervation:	XII hypoglossal nerve
Function:	Anterior fibers retract tongue; posterior fibers protrude tongue; together, anterior and posterior fibers depress tongue

Muscle: **Hyoglossus**

Origin:	Length of the greater cornu and lateral body of hyoid
Course:	Upward
Insertion:	Sides of tongue between styloglossus and inferior longitudinal muscles
Innervation:	XII hypoglossal nerve
Function:	Pulls sides of tongue down

Muscle: **Styloglossus**

Origin:	Anterolateral margin of the styloid process
Course:	Forward and down
Insertion:	Inferior sides of the tongue
Innervation:	XII hypoglossal nerve
Function:	Draws tongue back and up

Muscle: **Chondroglossus**

Origin:	Lesser cornu hyoid and corpus
Course:	Up
Insertion:	Interdigitates with intrinsic muscles of the tongue medial to the point of insertion of hyoglossus
Innervation:	XII hypoglossal nerve
Function:	Depresses tongue

Muscle: **Palatoglossus (glossopalatine)**

Origin:	Anterolateral palatal aponeurosis
Course:	Down
Insertion:	Sides of posterior tongue
Innervation:	Pharyngeal plexus from the pharyngeal branch of the IX glossoharyngeal, the pharyngeal branch of the X vagus nerves, and perhaps the XI accessory nerve
Function:	Elevates tongue or depresses soft palate

Mandibular Elevators and Depressors

Muscle: **Masseter**
Origin: Zygomatic arch
Course: Down
Insertion: Ramus of the mandible and coronoid process
Innervation: Anterior trunk of mandibular nerve arising from the V trigeminal
Function: Elevates mandible

Muscle: **Temporalis**
Origin: Temporal fossa of the temporal and parietal bones
Course: Converging downward and forward, through the zygomatic arch
Insertion: Coronoid process and ramus
Innervation: Temporal branches arising from the mandibular nerve of V trigeminal
Function: Elevates mandible and draws it back if protruded

Muscle: **Medial pterygoid (internal pterygoid)**
Origin: Medial pterygoid plate and fossa
Course: Down and back
Insertion: Mandibular ramus
Innervation: Mandibular division of the V trigeminal nerve
Function: Elevates mandible

Muscle: **Lateral pterygoid (external pterygoid)**
Origin: Lateral pterygoid plate and greater wing of sphenoid
Course: Back
Insertion: Pterygoid fovea of the mandible
Innervation: Mandibular branch of the V trigeminal nerve
Function: Protrudes mandible

Muscle: **Digastricus, anterior belly**
Origin: Inner surface of mandible at the digastricus fossa, near the symphysis
Course: Medially and down
Insertion: Intermediate tendon to juncture of hyoid corpus and greater cornu
Innervation: Mandibular branch of V trigeminal nerve via the mylohyoid branch of the inferior alveolar nerve
Function: Pulls hyoid forward; depresses mandible if in conjunction with digastricus posterior

Muscle: **Digastricus, posterior belly**
Origin: Mastoid process of the temporal bone
Course: Medially and down
Insertion: Intermediate tendon to juncture of hyoid corpus and greater cornu
Innervation: Digastric branch of the VII facial nerve
Function: Pulls hyoid back; depresses mandible if in conjunction with anterior digastricus

Muscle: **Mylohyoid**

Origin:	Mylohyoid line, inner mandible
Course:	Back and down
Insertion:	Median fibrous raphe inferior to hyoid
Innervation:	Alveolar nerve, arising from the V trigeminal nerve, mandibular branch
Function:	Depresses mandible

Muscle: **Geniohyoid**

Origin:	Mental spines of the mandible
Course:	Medially
Insertion:	Corpus hyoid
Innervation:	XII hypoglossal nerve and C1 spinal nerve
Function:	Depresses mandible

Muscles of The Velum

Muscle: **Levator veli palatini (levator palati)**

Origin:	Apex of the petrous portion of temporal bone and medial wall of the auditory tube cartilage
Course:	Down and forward
Insertion:	Palatal aponeurosis of soft palate, lateral to musculus uvulae
Innervation:	Pharyngeal plexus from the pharyngeal branch of the IX glossoharyngeal, the pharyngeal branch of the X vagus nerves, and perhaps the XI accessory nerve
Function:	Elevates and retracts posterior velum

Muscle: **Musculus uvulae**

Origin:	Posterior nasal spines of the palatine bones and palatal aponeurosis
Course:	Runs the length of soft palate
Insertion:	Mucous membrane cover of the velum
Innervation:	Pharyngeal plexus from the pharyngeal branch of the IX glossoharyngeal, the pharyngeal branch of the X vagus nerves, and perhaps the XI accessory nerve
Function:	Shortens soft palate

Muscle: **Tensor veli palatini (tensor veli palati)**

Origin:	Scaphoid fossa of sphenoid, sphenoid spine, and lateral auditory tube wall
Course:	Down, terminates in tendon that passes around pterygoid hamulus, then is directed medially
Insertion:	Palatal aponeurosis
Innervation:	Mandibular nerve of V trigeminal
Function:	Dilates auditory tube

Muscle:	**Palatoglossus**
Origin:	Anterolateral palatal aponeurosis
Course:	Down
Insertion:	Sides of posterior tongue
Innervation:	Pharyngeal plexus from the pharyngeal branch of the IX glossoharyngeal, the pharyngeal branch of the X vagus nerves, and perhaps the XI accessory nerve
Function:	Elevates tongue or depresses soft palate

Muscle:	**Palatopharyngeus**
Origin:	Anterior hard palate, midline of the soft palate
Course:	Laterally and down
Insertion:	Posterior border of thyroid cartilage
Innervation:	Pharyngeal plexus from the pharyngeal branch of the IX glossoharyngeal, the pharyngeal branch of the X vagus nerves, and perhaps the XI accessory nerve
Function:	Narrows pharynx; lowers soft palate

MUSCLES OF PHARYNX

Muscle:	**Superior pharyngeal constrictor**
Origin:	Pterygomandibular raphe
Course:	Posteriorly
Insertion:	Median raphe of pharyngeal aponeurosis
Innervation:	Pharyngeal plexus from the pharyngeal branch of the IX glossoharyngeal, the pharyngeal branch of the X vagus nerves, and perhaps the XI accessory nerve
Function:	Pulls pharyngeal wall forward and constricts pharyngeal diameter

Muscle:	**Middle pharyngeal constrictor**
Origin:	Horns of the hyoid and stylohyoid ligament
Course:	Up and back
Insertion:	Median pharyngeal raphe
Innervation:	Pharyngeal plexus from the pharyngeal branch of the IX glossoharyngeal, the pharyngeal branch of the X vagus nerves, and perhaps the XI accessory nerve
Function:	Narrows diameter of pharynx

Muscle:	**Inferior pharyngeal constrictor: cricopharyngeus**
Origin:	Cricoid cartilage
Course:	Back
Insertion:	Orifice of esophagus
Innervation:	Pharyngeal plexus from the pharyngeal branch of the IX glossoharyngeal, the pharyngeal branch of the X vagus nerves, and perhaps the XI accessory nerve
Function:	Constricts superior orifice of esophagus: is the muscular component of the upper esophageal sphincter (UES).

Muscle: **Inferior pharyngeal constrictor: thyropharyngeus muscle**

Origin: Oblique line of the thyroid lamina

Course: Up and back

Insertion: Median pharyngeal raphe

Innervation: Pharyngeal plexus from the pharyngeal branch of the IX glossoharyngeal, the pharyngeal branch of the X vagus nerves, and perhaps the XI accessory nerve

Function: Reduces diameter of lower pharynx

Muscle: **Salpingopharyngeus**

Origin: Lower margin of the auditory tube

Course: Down

Insertion: Converges with palatopharyngeus

Innervation: Pharyngeal plexus from the pharyngeal branch of the IX glossoharyngeal, the pharyngeal branch of the X vagus nerves, and perhaps the XI accessory nerve

Function: Elevates lateral pharyngeal wall

Muscle: **Stylopharyngeus**

Origin: Styloid process

Course: Down

Insertion: Pharyngeal constrictors and posterior thyroid cartilage

Innervation: Muscular branch of IX glossophyarngeal nerve

Function: Elevates and opens pharynx

APPENDIX F

Sensors

GENERAL CLASSES

Interoceptors: Monitor events within the body (e.g., distention of stomach, blood pH)

Exteroceptors: Respond to stimuli outside the body (touch, hearing, vision)

Proprioceptors: Monitor change in body position or position of its parts (body position sense) (e.g., muscle and joint sensors, vestibular sensation)

SPECIFIC TYPES

Teloreceptors: Respond to intangible stimuli (hearing, vision)

Contact receptors: Respond to tangible stimuli (e.g., tactile, pain, deep and light pressure, temperature)

Chemoreceptors: Respond to chemical change (smell, taste, pH, etc.)

Photoreceptors: Respond to light changes (vision)

Thermoreceptors: Respond to heat

Mechanoreceptors: Respond to mechanical force (touch, muscle length and tension, auditory, vestibular receptors, etc.)

Nociceptors: Pain sensors

CLASSES OF SENSATION

Somatic sense: Related to pain, temperature, mechanical stimulation of somatic structures (skin, muscles, joints)

Kinesthesia: Sense of motion

Special senses: Senses mediating specific exteroceptive information such as vision, audition, olfaction

APPENDIX G

Cranial Nerves

CLASSES OF CRANIAL NERVES

GSA	**General somatic afferent:**	Related to pain, temperature, mechanical stimulation of somatic structures (skin, muscles, joints)
GSE	**General somatic efferent:**	Innervates skeletal (striated) muscles
GVA	**General visceral afferent:**	From receptors in visceral structures (e.g., digestive tract)
GVE	**General visceral efferent:**	Autonomic efferent fibers
SSA	**Special somatic afferent:**	Special senses—sight, hearing, equilibrium
SVA	**Special visceral afferent:**	Special senses of smell, taste
SVE	**Special visceral efferent:**	Innervation of muscle of branchial arch origin: larynx, pharynx, face

CRANIAL NERVES, SOURCES, AND FUNCTIONS

I. Olfactory

SVA: Sense of smell

Source: Mitral cells of olfactory bulb

II. Optic

SSA: Vision

Source: Rod and cone receptor cells synapse with bipolar interneurons that synapse with the multipolar ganglionic neuron; optic nerve is axon of multipolar ganglionic neurons; nerve becomes myelinated after exiting eye socket and entering cranium; left and right nerves decussate at chiasma and project as optic tract to lateral geniculate body; projects to occipital cortex via optic radiations; left nasal nerve portion and right temporal nerve portion join after chiasma; left temporal nerve portion and right nasal aspect of nerve join after chiasma; visual field result is that left nasal and right temporal visual fields (right portion of image) project to left cerebral cortex; left temporal and right nasal visual fields (left portion of image) project to right cerebral cortex

III. Oculomotor

GSE: All extrinsic ocular muscles except superior oblique and lateral rectus

Source: Oculomotor nucleus

GVE: Light and accommodation reflexes

Source: Edinger-Westphal nucleus

IV. Trochlear

GSE: Superior oblique muscle of eye (turns eye down when eye is adducted)
Source: Trochlear nuclei

V. Trigeminal

GSA: Exteroceptive afferent for pain, thermal, and tactile stimuli from face, forehead, mucous membrane of mouth and nose, teeth cranial dura; proprioceptive (deep pressure, kinesthesis) from teeth, gums, temporomandibular joint, stretch receptors of mastication
Source: Sensory nucleus of trigeminal
SVE: To muscles of mastication, tensor tympani, tensor veli palatini
Source: Motor nucleus of trigeminal

Components of V Trigeminal:

Ophthalmic branch: Sensory only
GSA: From cornea, iris, upper eyelid, external nose, conjunctiva, anteior scalp back to lamdoidal suture.
Maxillary branch: Sensory only
GSA: From lower eyelid, alar portion of nose, palate, upper jaw, cheek, part of temple, upper lip
Mandibular branch: Sensory and motor
GSA: skin of mandible and lower teeth, mucosa, cheeks, temporomandibular joint, anterior two-thirds of tongue, lower lip, part of pinna, part of temple, lower labial gingivae
SVE: To muscles of mastication (internal and external pterygoid, temporalis, masseter), tensor tympani, tensor veli palatine

VI. Abducens

GSE: Lateral rectus muscle for ocular abduction
Source: Abducens nucleus

VII. Facial

SVE: To facial muscles of expression: platysma, buccinator, muscles of pinna, facial muscles around eye and forehead
Source: Motor nucleus of VII
SVA: Taste, anterior two-thirds of tongue
Source: Solitary nucleus
GSA: Cutaneous sense of EAM and skin of ear
Source: Trigeminal nuclei
GVE: Lacrimal gland (tears); sublingual and submandibular salivary glands; mucous membrane of mouth and nose
Source: Superior salivatory and lacrimal nuclei

VIII. Vestibulocochlear

SSA: Vestibular and cochlear sensation

Cochlear (auditory) portion: Sensors are hair cells; cell bodies are in spiral ganglion; axons are of VIII nerve, in auditory portion; input divides so that all frequencies are represented in anteroventral cochlear nucleus (AVCN), posteroventral cochlear nucleus (PVCN) and dorsal cochlear nucleus (DCN); transfer of auditory sensation to central nervous system

Source: Spiral ganglion

Vestibular portion: From semicircular canals, utricle, saccule; project to vestibular nuclei of medulla and subsequently to all levels of brain stem, spinal cord, cerebellum, thalamus, and cerebral cortex; maintenance of extensor tone, antigravity responses, balance, sense of position in space; coordinated eye/head movement through projection to III oculomotor, IV trochlear, VI abducens cranial nerves

Source: Vestibular ganglion

IX. Glossopharyngeal

GVA: Somatic (tactile, thermal, pain sense) from posterior one-third of tongue and pharynx (mediating gag reflex), tonsils, mastoid cells, tonsils

Source: Solitary nucleus

SVA: Taste, posterior one-third of tongue

Source: Inferior salivatory nucleus

GSA: Somatic sense of middle ear, auditory tube, fauces, nasopharynx, uvula

Source: Trigeminal nuclei

SVE: Innervation of stylopharyngeus, superior pharyngeal constrictor

Source: Inferior salivatory nucleus

GVE: Parotid gland

Source: Inferior salivatory nucleus

X. Vagus

GSA: Cutaneous sense from EAM

Source: Trigeminal nuclei

GVA: Sensory from pharynx, larynx, trachea, esophagus, viscera of thorax, abdomen

Source: Solitary nucleus

SVA: Taste buds near epiglottis and valleculae

Source: Solitary nucleus

GVE: To parasympathetic ganglia, thorax, abdomen

Source: Dorsal motor nucleus of X

SVE: Striated muscles of larynx and pharynx

Source: Nucleus ambiguus

XI. Accessory

SVE, cranial portion: Joins with X vagus to form recurrent laryngeal nerve to innervate intrinsic muscles of larynx

SVE, spinal portion: Innervates sternocleidomastoid and trapezius

Source: Cranial portion: nucleus ambiguus of medulla; spinal portion: anterior horn of C1 through C5 spinal nerves; unite and ascend; enter skull via foramen magnum; exit with vagus at jugular foramen

XII. Hypoglossal

GSE: Muscles of tongue

Source: Nucleus of hypoglossal nerve

Clinical Note: Lesion of LMN produces ipsilateral damage (tongue deviates toward side of damage)

APPENDIX H

Pathologies That Affect Speech Production

The following list is far from exhaustive but is rather a sampler of the many speech, language, and hearing problems that can arise from physical sources.

Respiration Subsystem	Impact
Emphysema:	Reduced volumes and capacities and increased respiratory effort result in lower subglottal pressure, reduced phrase length, and reduced vocal intensity.
Spastic paralytic conditions:	Cerebral palsy, acquired spastic paralysis; results in increased tone of muscles of respiration and reduced range of motion, causing reduction in capacities, paradoxical respiratory effort; result is reduced ability to generate high subglottal pressures, reduced phrase length, impaired prosody secondary to inability to generate microbursts of pressure.
Ataxic conditions:	Ataxic dysarthria affecting respiration results in loss of coordination between subsystems, reduction of coordinated effort for inspiration and expiration; result may be inappropriate timing of inspiration and expiration and explosive expiratory bursts.
Muscular dystrophy and other flaccid paralytic conditions:	Loss of ability to generate high subglottal pressure, reduction in capacities, and reduced range of motion of muscles of respiration result in reduced phrase length, impaired prosody, low vocal intensity.
Huntington's disease athetosis, and other hyperkinetic conditions:	Uncontrollable motion overlaid upon voluntary contraction produces unpredictable inspiration and expiration; speech impairment may include explosive bursts, inappropriate termination or pausing of inspiration or expiration, loss of control of vocal intensity, and disrupted prosody.
Parkinson's disease and other conditions resulting in hypokinesias:	The muscular rigidity results in loss of capacities and range of; motion speech result is of extremely low vocal intensity, including loss of subglottal pressure adequate to sustain phonation.
Respiratory insufficiency causing ventilator dependency:	Many diseases result in a dependence on mechanical ventilation, and the result is loss of phonation because the phonatory mechanism is bypassed via tracheostomy. Valving technology exists to circumvent this difficulty for some clients.

Phonatory Subsystem

Vocal fold paralysis: Arises from damage to the X vagus nerve; arises from surgical procedures (surgery on thyroid), or trauma (vehicular accident); results typically in paralysis of adduction if lesion is extracranial, or of abductors if lesion is intracranial. Abductor paralysis results in phonation on both inhalation and exhalation (stridor), whereas adductor paralysis results in loss of ability to adduct vocal folds for phonation.

Space-occupying lesions: Include papilloma, carcinoma, polyps. Lesions that occupy space can cause asymmetrical vibration of the vocal folds (resulting in diplophonia), reduction in fundamental frequency and range of phonation, harsh and hoarse phonation, "popping" sound on inhalation or exhalation but with little other phonatory impact (pedunculated polyps), aphonia, and reduction in vocal intensity.

Spastic paralytic conditions: Includes spasticity arising from cerebrovascular accident or other disease conditions. Speech result is strained and harsh phonation, reduced range of intensity and fundamental frequency, dysprosody secondary to excessive and equal syllabic stress, and sometimes excessively high vocal intensity.

Hormone treatment: Use of male hormones to treat some carcinomas can result in irreversible lowering of fundamental frequency.

Vocal hyperfunction: Functional abuse of vocal mechanism, such as that resulting from excessively loud speech, can cause vocal nodules.

Laryngectomy: Removal of larynx because of carcinoma results in complete loss of phonation.

Flaccid paralytic conditions: Lower motor neuron damage can result in flaccid paralysis of vocal apparatus. Direct damage to recurrent laryngeal nerve or superior laryngeal nerve results in vocal fold paralysis (as seen earlier). More generalized conditions such as muscular dystrophy result in weakened adductory force, reduced ability to abduct vocal folds, reduced range of fundamental frequency, and reduced vocal intensity. Myasthenia gravis (a disease of the myoneural junction) presents a unique constellation of phonatory signs, in that the flaccid condition progresses as a result of exertion, with phonatory ability returning to near-baseline levels following adequate rest.

Ataxic conditions: Conditions causing damage to the cerebellum or pontine nuclei of the brain stem result in discoordination of the phonatory act. Adduction and abduction will be poorly timed, with discoordination of phonation with other subsystems (respiration, articulation), explosive bursts of phonation, inappropriate terminations of phonation, and inadequate control of vocal intensity and fundamental frequency.

Hypokinetic conditions: Predominantly, Parkinson's disease results in muscular rigidity. The phonatory mechanism shows a marked reduction in vocal intensity, as well as a reduced range of vocal intensity and fundamental frequency.

Hyperkinetic conditions:	Huntington's disease, athetosis, dystonia, and other hyperkinesias result in unpredictable muscular contraction overlaid upon voluntary movements. In the case of the phonatory mechanism, hyperkinesias result in uncontrollable increases and decreases in vocal intensity, fluctuations in fundamental frequency, and loss of voicing during normally phonated segments. In spasmodic dysphonia (a type of dystonia), the spasticity may cause uncontrollable abduction or adduction of the vocal folds, causing loss of phonation and harsh phonatory onset.
Dyspraxic conditions:	Dyspraxia is reduction in the ability to voluntarily contract musculature in the absence of muscular weakness or paralysis, and typically with retained involuntary function. Frequent etiology is cerebrovascular accident (CVA), and the result is difficulty initiating phonation voluntarily, but with retained ability to phonate in overlearned situations, as well as normal cough and throat-clearing.
Mixed dysarthria:	Diseases such as amyotrophic lateral sclerosis or Wilson's disease result in mixed dysarthrias. The impact on phonation depends on the type of dysarthria (spastic, flaccid, ataxic, unilateral upper motor neuron, hypokinetic, hyperkinetic).
Cleft palate:	Although cleft palate does not typically directly involve the phonatory mechanism, there is very often an impact on phonation. The child with inadequate mechanical separation of the oral and nasal cavities may resort to vocal hyperfunction, perhaps in an attempt to increase vocal intensity or the high-frequency energy in the acoustic phonatory source (see hyperfunction, mentioned earlier). In addition, the child may resort to vocal hyperfunction in an attempt to increase laryngeal control, as loss of adequate supraglottal (oral) pressure results in excessive transglottal pressure and poor laryngeal control.
Laryngeal web:	Congenital laryngeal web consists of connective tissue above, below, or at the level of the vocal folds. Webs may be life threatening and will compromise phonation.

Articulatory Subsystem

Cleft lip and cleft palate:	Congenital defect of lip and palate that results in inadequate closure of bony or muscular palate in cleft palate, and in alveolar, lip, and premaxillary suture in cleft lip. The impact on speech will be primarily on high-pressure consonants (fricatives, stops, affricates), often resulting in phonological deficiencies arising from compensatory articulations.
Submucous cleft:	Presence of a fistula or cleft of the bony palate that is covered by epithelium so that it is hidden ("occult") to casual examination. The cleft will have a bluish cast to it and will move during palpation. Speech will have a nasal quality despite no apparent communication between the oral and nasal cavities, arising from the acoustical coupling provided by the epithelial lining separating the two cavities.
Palatal insufficiency:	Insufficient muscular tissue of soft palate, or inadequate movement of soft palate arising from muscular weakness, can result in hypernasality or assimilated nasality (nasalization of phonemes that occur before or after nasal sounds).

Maxillary carcinoma:

Surgical removal of the maxilla results in communication between the oral and nasal cavities that must be instrumentally corrected for production of non-nasal speech.

Flaccid paralytic conditions:

Any condition (e.g., muscular dystrophy and myasthenia gravis) that results in muscular weakness to the oral or velar muscles will result in articulatory distortion. Flaccid paralysis may result in loss of accuracy in articulatory contact, weak plosion, weak fricatives or even conversion of fricatives to plosives, hypernasality secondary to inadequate velopharyngeal valving, but with relatively normal diadochokinetic rates.

Spastic paralytic conditions:

Conditions that produce spasticity (e.g., cerebrovascular accident) will result in increased resistance to movement of the articulators. Speech accuracy and rate of speaking are reduced, and signs of spasticity characterized as "gaglike" sounds during articulation can be noted during palatal and velar articulations.

Ataxic dysarthria:

Damage to the cerebellum or nuclei and pathways serving the cerebellum can result in discoordination of the articulatory muscles, as well as loss of intersystem coordination with respiration and phonation. Articulatory inaccuracies will be characterized as inconsistent distortions, explosive articulations, errors in rate, range, and force of motion. Diadochokinesis will be defective.

Hyperkinetic conditions:

Addition of involuntary movements arising from disease states such as Huntington's disease, dystonia, or athetosis will result in inaccurate articulations characterized by distortions.

Hypokinetic conditions:

Primarily arising from Parkinson's disease, the result of progressive muscular rigidity is increasingly reduced range of motion, weak and inadequate articulations, and (paradoxically) rapid diadochokinetic rate resulting from reduced range of motion.

Mixed dysarthrias:

Arising from disease states such as hepatolenticular degeneration, amyotrophic lateral sclerosis, or multiple sclerosis, the impact on speech will be determined by the type of dysarthria involved.

Dental anomalies:

Absent dentition or teeth that are off-axis can cause distortion of fricatives and other articulatory inaccuracies.

Oral myofunctional disorders:

"Tongue thrust" disorder is a common manifestation of oral myofunctional disorders and involves loss of balance of oral/pharyngeal musculature, loss of tone of muscles of mastication and lingual musculature, and increased or decreased tone of labial musculature. The individual with tongue thrust may develop a low-tone, open-mouthed posture that, if uncorrected, may result in a permanently vaulted hard palate and long, narrow face. The uncorrected tongue thrust swallow includes inadequate bolus preparation and propulsion. Speech in tongue thrust is most often characterized by distorted lingual fricatives secondary to the weakened lingual musculature. Speech remediation is frequently inconsequential until the underlying oral myofunctional deficits have been remediated.

Relative macroglossia: When the tongue is excessively large relative to the oral cavity, it is termed *macroglossia*. This condition is often seen in individuals with hypotonic conditions (Down syndrome). Distorted articulation may be due to the relatively large tongue or the flaccid condition.

Ankyloglossia (Tongue tie):   A short lingual frenum results in the inability to make alveolar, palatal, and velar articulations. Surgical release of the frenum can improve speech in cases where frenum is demonstrated to be short.

Hypertrophied adenoids: Hypertrophied adenoidal tissue may result in difficulty breathing through the nose, increased upper respiratory disease, inadequate ventilation of the middle ear by means of the auditory (Eustachian) tube, habitual mouth breathing, and hyponasal speech. Depending on the individual, the result may be facial dysmorphia (mouth breathing), chronic otitis media and hearing loss (auditory tube dysfunction), and substitution of non-nasal consonants for nasals.

Auditory Mechanism

Inflammatory conditions of the external ear: Otitis media externa is the painful inflammation of the outer ear, especially of the external auditory meatus. Pain is particularly acute due to the tight bonding of the epithelial lining to ear cartilage.

Congenital deficiencies of the outer ear: A number of congenital conditions exist that have an impact on external ear structures. The pinna may be congenitally absent (congenital atresia) or dysmorphic. The external auditory meatus may be congenitally absent (atresia) or narrowed (stenosis). Preauricular pits and ear tags are of no clinical significance but signal the potential presence of genetic conditions such as branchio-oto-renal syndrome. Low-set auricles are characteristics for a number of genetic syndromes (e.g., Apert syndrome), and posteriorly rotated auricles are one component of fetal alcohol syndrome.

Inflammatory middle ear disease   Chronic otitis media frequently arises from inadequate ventilation of the middle ear space or from bacterial infection. The result is conductive hearing loss that appears to have a significant impact on speech and language development.

Trauma to middle ear: Disarticulation of the ossicles can occur as a result of temporal bone trauma or from high-intensity acoustic shock, such as that experienced during explosions. Fracture of the temporal bone can occur as a result of head trauma and can result in cerebrospinal fluid otorrhea (drainage of cerebrospinal fluid from the cranial space into the middle ear space), which, of course, can be a life-threatening condition considering the potential for bacterial infection of the meninges.

Neoplasm of middle ear: Glomus jugulare tumors can be mistaken for a host of otologic conditions. If the tumor contacts the tympanic membrane, it will provide objective, pulsatile movement of the ear drum; if it contacts the ossicles, it can cause what appears to be otosclerosis. The degree of hearing impairment is typically related to the degree to which structures of the middle ear conduction mechanism are involved.

Otosclerosis: This disease condition involves fixation of the stapes in the oval window, resulting in a conductive hearing loss.

Diseases of inner ear: Viral or bacterial infection may cause labyrinthitis, an inflammation of the inner ear. The effects of labyrinthitis include dizziness, balance problems, and tinnitus, potentially remitting at the end of the infection course. Other problems include perilymph fistula, in which one of the cochlear membranes (typically Reissner's) is torn so that perilymph and endolymph mix, producing a relatively localized sensorineural loss. Endolymphatic hydrops is a disease characterized by increased endolymph and perilymph pressure, resulting in permanent damage to vestibular and cochlear sensing mechanisms, with symptoms ranging from tinnitus to vestibular disturbances. Head trauma can fracture the temporal bone, causing sensorineural hearing loss.

Neurological Conditions

Cerebrovascular accident: Cerebrovascular accidents include conditions in which obstruction of blood flow results in damage to neuronal tissue. Because of the centrality of the brain to speech function, the impact on speech can range from none to complete loss of motor, cognitive, and linguistic function.

Degenerative conditions: A number of disease conditions result in the degeneration of nervous tissue. Cerebellar degeneration arises from a number of conditions but results in the loss of coordination of motor function. Frontal lobe degeneration in Huntington's disease results in the loss of cognitive function, while substantia nigra degeneration in Parkinson's disease results in loss of the ability to initiate movement. Generally, the focal nature of a given lesion will define the nature of the deficit experienced, with diseases having a broader impact (e.g., multiple sclerosis) showing more diverse symptomatology.

Trauma: Head trauma can have a widespread impact on speech, language, and cognitive functions. The degree and type of impairment depend in large part on the location of the trauma, the magnitude and type of trauma, and the speed with which treatment was implemented. Frontal lobe damage is common in vehicular trauma and may result in memory, cognitive, motor, and expressive language deficits. Missile trauma (e.g., gunshot wounds and shrapnel) may affect any portion of the brain but will have more focal effects. Rotatory trauma can produce devastating damage to the brain stem and projection fibers of the tracts of the brain.

GLOSSARY

3rd ventricle Cerebral ventricle residing between the paired thalami

4th ventricle Cerebral ventricle residing between the brain stem and the cerebellum

VI abducens nerve a.k.a. abducent nerve; nerve mediating abduction of eyeball

VII hypoglossal nerve Cranial nerve serving muscles of the tongue

IX glossopharyngeal nerve Cranial nerve associated with sensation of tongue and pharynx; this is a critical nerve for swallowing function

X vagus nerve Cranial nerve involved with vocal fold action, as well as numerous autonomic functions

XI accessory nerve Cranial nerve working in conjunction with IX glossopharyngeal and X vagus to innervate muscles of pharynx and velum

A band Region of overlap between thin and thick filaments

-a- Without; lack of

-ab- Away from

Abdomen /ˈæbdəmən/ Region of the body between the thorax and pelvis

Abdominal aponeurosis The aponeurotic complex of the anterior abdominal wall that forms points of origination for abdominal musculature

Abdominal fixation Process of impounding air within the lungs through inhalation and forceful vocal fold adduction that results in increased intra-abdominal pressure

Abdominal viscera /æbˈdamənlˈvɪsɚə/ Organs of the abdominal region

Abduction /æbˈdʌkʃən/ To draw a structure away from midline

Abductor paralysis Paralysis of the muscles of abduction, specifically posterior cricoarytenoid muscles

Absolute refractory period Phase of depolarization during which a neuron cannot be stimulated to discharge

Accessory cuneate nucleus of medulla Nucleus mediating kinesthetic sense, muscle stretch, and proprioceptive sense arrives from the lower body

Acetylcholine /əˈsitlkolin/ Neurotransmitter involved in communication among several classes of neurons and between nerve and muscle

Acoustic reflex a.k.a. stapedial reflex. Contraction of stapedius muscle in response to auditory stimulation

Acoustic stria Brain stem auditory pathways arising from the cochlear nucleus

Actin One of two muscle proteins

Action potential Electrical potential arising from depolarization of a cell membrane

Active expiration Expiration arising from muscular activity

ad- Combining form meaning toward

Adduct /æˈdʌkt/ to draw two structures closer together or to move toward midline

Adduction Process of drawing two structures closer together or moving a structure toward midline

Adductor paralysis Paralysis of the muscles of adduction of the vocal folds

Adenoids /ˈædnɔɪdz/ Lymphoid tissue within the nasopharynx

Adequate stimulus Stimulation of sufficient intensity or frequency to cause a response

Adipose /ˈædəpos/ Connective tissue impregnated with fat cells

Aditus to the mastoid antrum Entry way to the epitympanic recess from the middle ear

Aeration /ɛreɪʃən/ The process of introducing air into a space or cavity

Aerodynamic theory For phonation through the lawful interplay of tissue mass, elasticity, and aerodynamic principles

Afferent Carrying toward a central location; generally, sensory nerve impulses

Agonists Muscle contracted for the purpose of a specific motor act (as contrasted to the antagonist)

Ala /ēɪlə/ winglike structure

-algia Combining form meaning pain

Alpha motor neuron fibers Those axons with high conduction velocity, between 50 and 120 m/sec and that innervate skeletal muscle

Alveolar arch Surface of mandible with dental alveoli

Alveolar pressure /æl ˈvilɚ/ Air pressure measured at the level of the alveolus in the lung

Alveolar process Process of maxilla in which dental alveoli reside

Alveolus /ælvi ˈoləs/ Small cavity; as in alveolus of lung, the air sac wherein gas exchange occurs

Ambulation Walking

amphi- On both sides

Amphiarthrodial /æmfiar ˈθrodiəl/ bony articulation in which bones are connected by cartilage

Ampulla /ˈæmpulə/ dilation of structure

Amygdala Structure of the subcortex involved in emotional processing and fear responses

an- Without; lack of

Ana Up

Anastomoses /ænæstə ˈmosəs/ Communication between two vessels or structures

Anatomical Space within the conducting passageway of the respiratory system that is not

Anatomical dead space a.k.a., physiological dead space; space within the airway system that can never participate in gas exchange, such as mouth and trachea;

Anatomical position Erect body, with palms, arms, and hands facing forward

Anatomy The study of structure of an organism

Aneurysm /ˈænjɚɪzm/ abnormal dilation or ballooning of a blood vessel (typically an artery)

angio- /ˈændʒio/ Blood vessels

Angiology /ændʒiˈalədʒi/ Science dealing with blood vessels and the lymphatic system

Angle of mandible Point at which mandible angles upward, joining the ramus and corpus

Angle of rib The portion of the rib between the head and shaft, at which the direction of the rib takes an acute turn

Angular gyrus Gyrus of the posterior parietal lobe associated with written visual information

Annular /ˈænjulɚ/ Ringlike

Annular ligament Ligament binding footplate of stapes into oval window

Anomia /əˈnomiə/ Inability to remember names of objects

Anotia Absence of pinna

Ansa /ænsə/ Structure that forms a loop or arc

Antagonist A muscle that opposes the contraction of another muscle (the agonist)

ante- Before

Anterior cerebral arteries Major arteries arising from the internal carotid arteries, and serving the medial surface of the cerebrum and other structures

Anterior cerebral artery of cerebrovascular supply Artery arising from internal carotid artery, serving anterior cerebrum

Anterior clinoid process of sphenoid bone Projection from lesser wing of sphenoid, under which optic nerve passes within cranial vault

Anterior commissure of brain Anterior portion of corpus callosum, conveying olfactory information between hemispheres, as well as information from middle and inferior temporal gyri

Anterior commissure of larynx Anterior-most opening posterior to the angle of the thyroid cartilage

Anterior communicating artery of cerebrovascular supply Artery connecting left and right anterior cerebral arteries

Anterior corticospinal tract Anterior differentiation of the corticospinal tract arising from the decussation of the corticospinal tract at the pyramids in the medulla

Anterior crus of stapes Anterior pillar of the stapes arch

Anterior faucial pillars Band of tissue in posterior oral cavity separating oral and pharyngeal spaces, and overlying palatoglossus muscle

Anterior gray column of spinal cord Cell bodies of the anterior spinal cord

Anterior horn of lateral ventricle Anterior aspect of the lateral ventricle, residing within the frontal lobes

Anterior inferior cerebellar artery of cerebrovascular supply Artery arising from basilar artery serving the cerebellum

Anterior lateral sulcus of spinal cord Sulcus of spinal cord lateral to anterior median fissure

Anterior ligament of malleus Ligament binding the neck of the malleus to temporal bone, arising from the anterior malleolar process

Anterior limb of internal capsule Anterior aspect of the internal capsule, separating the caudate nucleus and putamen

Anterior lobe of cerebellum a.k.a. superior lobe. Anterior-most lobe of cerebellum

Anterior malleolar fold Region of tympanic membrane anterior to the pars flaccida

Anterior median fissure of spinal cord Deep longitudinal groove on surface of anterior spinal cord

Anterior nasal spine of maxilla a.k.a. nasal crest. Midline prominence of maxilla in anterior nasal cavity

Anterior process of malleus Process of malleus on anterior surface, providing attachment for the anterior malleolar ligament

Anterior process of manubrium /mə´nubriəm/ Anterior prominence of manubrium, providing point of

Anterior semicircular canal a.k.a. anterior vertical semicircular canal; superior semicircular canal. Anteriorly placed semicircular canal of vestibular mechanism

Anterior spinal artery of cerebrovascular supply Artery descending spinal cord in anterior aspect

Anterior spinocerebellar tract Crossed pathway passing afferent information from GTO to cerebellum

Anterior spinothalamic tract Tract within spinal cord conveying information concerning light touch from spinal cord to thalamus

Anterior white commissure of the spine Point of union between left and right halves of spinal cord

Anterior, posterior, lateral semicircular canals The three semicircular canals of the vestibular system, responsible for sensing position of the body in space

Anterior In front of; before

antero- Before

Anthelix Fold of tissue on helix marking the entrance to concha

Antitragus /ænt´ɪrēɪgəs/ Region posterior and inferior to the tragus

Antrum /´æntrəm/ An incompletely closed cavity

Apertures Openings

Apex Peak; extremity

Aphasia /ə´fēɪʒə/ Acquired language disorder, typically arising from cerebrovascular accident

Apical Referring to the apex of a structure

Apical pleurae Parietal pleural linings covering the lung superior aspect

apo- Away from

Aponeurosis /´æpanjɚosəs/ Sheetlike tendon

Appendicular skeleton /´æpəndɪkjulɚ/ The skeleton including upper and lower extremities

Applied anatomy Application of anatomical study for the diagnosis and treatment of disease, particularly as it relates to surgical procedures

Approximate To bring closer together

Apraxia A deficit in the programming of musculature for voluntary movement with an absence of any muscular weakness or paralysis

Arachnoid mater Meningeal lining located between dura and pia mater, consisting of lacey, spiderlike fibers

Arcuate fasciculus Long association fibers connecting superior and middle frontal gyri with temporal, parietal an occipital lobes

Areolar /ɛri ´olar/ Loose connective tissue

Arm The upper extremity including the region from the elbow to the shoulder

arthr- A joint

Arthrology /ar´θralodʒi/ The study of joints

Articulation The point of union between two structures

Articulators In speech production, the moveable and immobile structures used to produce the sounds of speech

Articulatory goals In the motor plan, this is the abstract goal of a motor act

Articulatory system In speech science, the system of structures involved in shaping the oral cavity for production of the sounds of speech

Aryepiglottic muscle Muscle coursing from the lateral epiglottis to the apex of arytenoid cartilage as a continuation of the oblique arytenoid muscle, inserting into the lateral epiglottis, and forming the upper margin of the quadrangular membranes and aryepiglottic folds

Aryepliglottic folds Sheet of connective tissue between arytenoid cartilages and epiglottis, within which the corniculate cartilages and arytenoid cartilages of the larynx reside

Arytenoid gliding During adduction, abduction, or tensing of the vocal folds, movement of the arytenoid along the arytenoid facet in a postero-medial or antero-lateral direction, functionally tensing the vocal folds

Arytenoid rocking During adduction or abduction, tilting medially or laterally along the vertical axis

Arytenoid rotation During adduction or abduction, turning of the arytenoid upon the vertical axis. This action is the least likely of the adductory or abductory movements of the arytenoids

Ascending pathways Sensory pathways of the nervous system

Associated chain theory Learning theory that views the learning process as developing linkages among the sequential steps of an act

Association area Major region of integration of the cerebral cortex

Association areas of the of cerebral cortex Areas that take primary and higher order information from specific modalities (e.g., audition) and combine them with other modalities (e.g., vision)

Association fibers Neurons that transmit information between two regions of the same cerebral hemisphere

Association nuclei of thalamus Nuclei of thalamus involved in communication with association areas of the cortex

Asthenia /əsˈθinjə/ Weakness

Astrocytes /ˈæstrosa͞uts/ A form of neuroglial cell

Ataxia Deficit in motor coordination

Ataxic dysarthria Dysarthria arising from damage to the cerebellum or cerebellar pathways, resulting in dyscoordination of motor function, articulatory imprecision, dysmetria, and often hypotonia

Athetosis Slow, writhing movements of the extremities, including the head

Atlas The first cervical vertebra

Atmospheric pressure Pressure of the atmosphere generated by its weight; approximately 760 mm Hg

Attrition /əˈtrɪʃən/ Wearing away

Audition Hearing

Auditory brain stem responses (ABR) Electrophysiological responses of the brain stem, typically measured cutaneously

Auditory evoked potentials Those auditory potentials that are generated through presentation of an auditory stimulus and subsequently averaging responses to eliminate neural noise and to reveal the auditory pathway response

Auditory information Information that has been transducted from acoustic information by the auditory system

Auditory nerve a.k.a., acoustic branch; auditory branch of the vestibulocochlear nerve

Auditory radiation a.k.a. geniculotemporal radiation. Fibers from medial geniculate body of the thalamus that terminate at Heschl's gyrus of the temporal lobe

Auditory tube Eustachian tube; aerating tube connecting nasopharynx and middle ear

Auricular cartilage The cartilaginous structure of the pinna

Auricular malformation Malformation of the pinna

Auricular tubercle /oˈrɪkjulɚ ˈtubɚkl/ Bulge on superior-posterior aspect of helix

Automaticity The development of patterns of responses that no longer require highly specific motor control but rather are relegated to automated patterns

Autonomic Portion of nervous system controlling involuntary bodily functions

Average (mean) fundamental frequency The average frequency of vibration for a given passage or utterance, for a given period of time; this is typically calculated instrumentally

Axial skeleton Portion of the skeleton including the trunk, head, and neck

Axis Imaginary line representing the point around which a body pivots

Axoaxonic synapses /ˈæksoæk ˈsanɪk/ Synapses between two axons

Axodendritic synapses /ˈæksodɛnˈdrɪtɪk/ Synapses involving axon and dendrite

Axon The process of a neuron that conducts information away from the soma or body

Axon hillock The juncture of the axon with the soma of a neuron

Axosomatic synapse Synapse of axon of one neuron with the soma of another, which is typically inhibitory

Babinski reflex /bəˈbɪnskɪ/ Dorsiflexion of the great toe and spreading of other toes upon stimulation of the ventral surface of the foot

Background activity Muscular contraction that supports action or movement, providing the form against which voluntary movement is placed

Ballism Hyperkinetic disorder arising from lesion to subthalamus that involves uncontrolled flailing of arms and legs

Baroreceptors Pressure sensors

Basal ganglia Nuclei deep within the cerebral hemispheres, involved in movement initiation and termination, and including the caudate nucleus, lentiform nucleus, amygdala, and claustrum

Basal sulcus of pons Prominent anterior landmark of pons marking the course of the basilar artery

Base The lower or supporting portion of a structure

Basement membrane The tissue that underlies the epithelium, which is made predominantly of collagen. See **baseplate**

Baseplate The tissue that underlies the epithelium, which is made predominantly of collagen. See **basement membrane**

Basilar artery of cerebrovascular supply Artery forming as product of anastomosing of the left and right vertebral arteries

Basilar membrane Portion of cochlear duct upon which organ of Corti is attached

Basilar part of occipital bone Portion of occipital bone articulating with the corpus sphenoid

Basilar portion of pons Anterior portion of pons

Basket cells of cerebellum Cells in cerebellum that communicate with Purkinje cells

Bellies The fleshy portions of a muscle

Bernoulli effect /bɚˈnuli/ The effect dictating that, given a constant volume flow of air or fluid, at a point of constriction there will be a decrease in air or fluid pressure perpendicular to the flow and an increase in velocity of the flow

Best frequency Frequency of sound stimulation to which a neuron responds most vigorously

bi- Two

Bifurcate /ˈbaɪfɚˌkeɪt/ Two-forked; to split into two parts or channels

Bilateral Two sides affected

Bipolar neuron Neuron with two processes

Bite block A structure used experimentally or clinically to eliminate movement of the mandible during articulatory tasks

blast- Germ

Blood Connective tissue comprised of plasma and blood cells suspended in this plasma matrix

Body of corpus callosum a.k.a. trunk; the major, central portion of the corpus callosum

Body of incus The largest portion of the incus

Body of sphenoid of sphenoid bone Bulk of the sphenoid bone

Body of the vocal folds The structure of the vocal folds consisting of the third layer of the lamina propria and the thyroarytenoid muscle of the vocal folds

Bolus /ˈboləs/ A ball or lump of masticated food ready to swallow

Bone The hardest of the connective tissues is the hardest of the connective tissues. The characteristic hardness of bone arises from inorganic salts that make up a large portion of bone. Bone is generally classified as being compact or spongy

Bony labyrinth The bony cochlear structure

Boyle's law The law stating that, given a gas of constant temperature, an increase in the volume of the chamber in which the gas is contained will cause a decrease in air pressure

Brachy- Short

Brady- Slow

Brain mapping Procedure of identifying functional regions of the cerebral cortex by electrical stimulation during speech, reading, or other tasks

Breathy Vocal characteristic arising from inadequate adduction of the vocal folds

Breathy phonation Phonation that is produced with escape of air during the closed phase of vibration, resulting from either behavioral, structural or neurological causes

Breathy voice Perception of phonation produced by excessive air loss through the adducted vocal folds

Brevis /ˈbrɛvəs/ Short; brief

Bridging arm In sliding filament model of muscle contraction, arms which bridge the gap between actin and myosin molecules, pulling the myofibrils closer together

Broca's aphasia Aphasia characterized by loss of fluency and paucity of vocabulary, usually arising from lesion to Brodmann areas 44 and 45 of the dominant cerebral hemisphere (Broca's area)

Broca's area Brodmann areas 44 and 45 of the dominant cerebral hemisphere, responsible for motor planning for speech and components of expressive language

Brodmann areas Regions of the cerebral hemisphere, identified by numeric characterization based upon functional and anatomical organization

Bronchi /ˈbrankaɪ/ The two major branches from the trachea leading to right and left lungs

Bronchial tree /ˈbrankijl̩/ Network of bronchi and bronchial tubes

Bronchial tubes Another name for main stem bronchi, the cartilaginous tubes connecting the trachea to the lungs

Bronchioles /ˈbrankijl̩z/ Small divisions of the bronchial tree

Buccal cavity Cavity lateral to the teeth, bounded by the cheek

Buccal surface of tooth Surface of tooth adjacent to cheek region

Buccal /ˈbʌkl̩/ Pertaining to the cheek

Buildup neurons Those neurons in the auditory pathway that show a pattern of slow increase in firing rate through the initial stages of discharge

Bulb Pertaining to the brain stem

Bulbar /ˈbəlbar/ Pertaining to the brain stem

Bundle Processing of a signal in noise

Calcarine sulcus In the occipital lobe of the brain, the site of primary visual reception

Canal of the tensor tympani Canal in anterior wall of middle ear that houses the tensor tympani muscle

Canine eminence Prominence of maxilla formed by the alveolus of the canine (cuspid)

Capacities Combinations of respiratory volumes that express physiological limits

Capillary Minute blood vessel

capit- /ˈkæpət/ Combining form meaning head, or toward the head end

Caput /ˈkæpət/ The head

Cardiac muscle Muscle of the heart, composed of cells that interconnect in a net-like fashion

Caries /ˈkɛriz/ Decay of soft or bony tissue

Carotid body Chemosensor within carotid artery that senses carbon dioxide and oxygen levels within blood

Carotid division of cerebrovascular supply Division of cerebrovascular supply arising from the internal carotid artery

-carpal Combining form meaning wrist

Cartilage Connective tissue embedded in matrix, capable of withstanding significant compressive and tensile forces

Cartilaginous Constructed of cartilage

Cartilaginous glottis Portion of the glottis adjacent to the arytenoid cartilages

Cartilaginous joints Joint in which cartilage serves to connect two bones

Cauda equine of spinal cord Tail-like region inferior to filum terminale of spinal cord in which not spinal cord segments are found

Caudal /ˈkɔdl̩/ Toward the tail or coccyx

Caudate nucleus Major nucleus of basal ganglia, including head, body, and tail

Cavum conchae /ˈkævəm ˈkaŋkēī/ Deep portion of the concha

-cele Combining form meaning tumor

Cementum /səˈmɛntəm/ Thin layer of bone joining tooth and alveolus

Central canal of spinal cord Center space within spinal cord, continuous with 4th ventricle

Central incisors Anterior-most teeth of dental arch

Central nervous system Brain and spinal cord components

Central portion of lateral ventricles Portion of lateral ventricles residing within the parietal lobe, including the region between the interventricular foramen of Monro and the splenium

Central sulcus of insula Insula between anterior short gyrus and posterior long insular gyrus

Central sulcus a.k.a. Rolandic fissure. Sulcus dividing frontal and parietal lobes

Central tendon Large aponeurosis making up the central portion of the diaphragm

Central Relative to the center of a structure

cephalo- /ˈsɛfəlo/ Combining form meaning head, or toward the head end

Cephalocaudally Development that moves from head to tail

Cerebellar fossa Fossa of occipital bone within which cerebellum resides

Cerebellopontine angle of pons Space created by the juncture of the cerebellum, the middle cerebellar peduncle, and the medulla oblongata

Cerebellum Structure of brain responsible for coordination of motor function and integration of sensory information with motor plan

Cerebral aqueduct Narrow tube connecting the 4th ventricle with the 3rd ventricle

Cerebral cortex a.k.a. cerebrum; the largest portion of the human brain, containing neural components and structures responsible for voluntary and conscious function

Cerebral fossa Fossa of occipital bone within which occipital lobe resides

Cerebral hemispheres Paired structures of the central nervous system, consisting of the frontal, parietal, occipital, temporal and insular lobes

Cerebral longitudinal fissure a.k.a. superior longitudinal fissure; interhemispheric fissure; the fissure that completely separates left and right cerebral hemispheres

Cerebral peduncle The major set of neural pathways leading to and from the cerebral cortex

Cerebrospinal fluid /səˈribroˈspaɪnl̩ ˈfluəd/ Fluid originating in the choroid plexuses of the ventricles, and providing a cushion to brain structures

Cerebrovascular accident (CVA) Event that cause cessation of blood flow (**ischemia**) to neural tissue, either through hemorrhaging (rupturing of a blood vessel), thrombosis (closure of a blood vessel by means of a foreign object, such as a blood clot), or embolism (closure of a blood vessel by a floating clot)

Cerebrovascular system Vascular system serving the nervous system

Cerebrum a.k.a. cerebral cortex; the largest portion of the human brain, containing neural components and structures responsible for voluntary and conscious function

Cerumen /sə´rumən/ The waxy secretion within the external auditory meatus

Cervical plexus Group of nerves that anastomoses from the spinal nerves c1, c2, c3, and c4

Cervical vertebra Vertebra of the cervical spinal column

Cervicofacial division of VII facial nerve Branch of VII facial nerve giving rise to buccal, lingual marginal mandibular and cervical branches

Channel proteins Specialized proteins in cell membrane that allow specific ions to pass through the membrane

Characteristic delay The property of a neuron in the auditory pathway wherein the neuron detects delay in signal arrival time between left and right ears

Characteristic frequency Frequency of sound stimulation to which a neuron responds most vigorously

Checking action The use of muscles of inspiration to impede the outward flow of air during respiration for speech

Chemoreceptors /´kimorı´sɛptəˑz/ Sensory organ that is sensitive to properties of specific chemicals

Chiasmatic grove of sphenoid bone Groove in sphenoid bone accommodating the optic chiasm

Chondral /´kandrl̩/ Pertaining to cartilage

Chondrogenesis Embryonic development of cartilage

Chopper response Neural responses characterized by periodic, chopped temporal pattern that is present throughout stimulation

Chorda tympani of VII facial nerve Portion of VII facial nerve that enters middle ear cavity and serves the sense of taste

Choreiform movements Extraneous, writhing movements of the body, often arising from Huntington's disease

Choroid plexus Aggregate of tissue within the cerebral ventricles that secretes cerebrospinal fluid

Cilia /´sılia/ Hairlike processes

Cingulate gyrus Major structure of the limbic system within the medial surface of the cerebral cortex

Cingulum Cingulate gyrus

Circle of Willis of cerebrovascular supply Arterial Portion of cerebrovascular supply that encircles the optic chiasm

Circular sulcus of insula Sulcus surrounding insular cortex

Circum /´sɚkəm/ Around

Class I malocclusion Malocclusion in which there is normal orientation of the molars, but an abnormal orientation of the incisors

Class I occlusion Relationship between upper and lower dental arches in which the first molar of the mandibular arch is one-half tooth advanced beyond the maxillary molar

Class II malocclusion Relationship between upper and lower dental arches in which the first mandibular molars are retracted at least one tooth from the first maxillary molars

Class III malocclusion Relationship between upper and lower dental arches in which the first mandibular molar is advanced farther than one tooth beyond the first maxillary molar

Clava of medulla a.k.a. gracilis tubercle: bulge in posterior medulla caused by nucleus gracilis

-cle Combining form that implies something very small

Clinical anatomy Application of anatomical study for the diagnosis and treatment of disease, particularly as it relates to surgical procedures

Clinical eruption Eruption of the teeth into the oral cavity

Clinker A mass of noncombustible material identified by a master engineer

Clivus of sphenoid bone Union of occipital bone and sphenoid bone that forms foramen magnum

Closed stage of phonation In the cycle of phonation, the stage in which the vibrating vocal folds are in the closed position

Closing stage of phonation In the cycle of phonation, the stage in which the vibrating vocal folds are returning to the closed position

cm Centimeter

Coarticulation The overlapping effect of one sound upon another

Coccygeal ligament of spinal cord Dural attachment of spinal cord to coccyx

Coccygeal vertebra Vestigial vertebral components of the coccyx

Cochlea Structure of inner ear responsible for mediating sense of sound

Cochlear aqueduct /´koklia ́akwədəkt/ Small opening between the scala vestibuli and the subarachnoid space of the cranial cavity

Cochlear canaliculus a.k.a. ochlear acqueduct. Opening between the scala tympani in the region of the round window and the subarachnoid space of the cranial cavity

Cochlear duct The membranous cochlear labyrinth, housing the sensory organs of the inner ear

Cochlear microphonic Stimulus-related auditory potential, being a direct electrical analog of the stimulus

Cochlear nucleus Initial brain stem nucleus of the auditory pathway, found within the pons, and subdivided into anteroventral, posteroventral, and dorsal cochlear nuclei

Cochlear recess Communication between the vestibule and the basal end of the cochlear duct

Cochleariform process a.k.a. trochlear process. Bony outcropping around which courses the tendon of tensor tympani

Cognition Processes involved in higher mental function, including attention, memory, visuospatial processes and linguistic processes

Collagenous fibers Connective fibers containing collagen

Columella a.k.a. columella nasi; paired columns of tissue connecting upper lip and nares

com- Combining form meaning with or together with

Combined sensation Sensation produced as result of integration of multiple types of sensors

Commissural fibers /ˈkamiʃɚl ˈfaɪbɚz/ Neural fibers that run from one location on a hemisphere to the corresponding location on the other hemisphere

Compact bone Bone characterized microscopically by its lamellar or sheet-like structure

Comparative anatomy Study of homologous structures of different animals

Compound action potential a.k.a. whole nerve action potential. Action potential arising directly from stimulation of a large number of hair cells simultaneously, eliciting nearly simultaneous individual action potentials in the viii nerve

Compressive strength The ability to withstand crushing forces

con- Combining form meaning with or together with

Concentration gradient Gradient in which there is a greater concentration of ions on one side of a membrane than another

Concha /ˈkaɴkə/ Entrance to the ear canal

Concha auriculae a.k.a. concha; entrance to the ear canal

Conduction aphasia Aphasia due to lesion of the arcuate fasciculus

Conduction velocity Rate of conduction of impulse through a neuron

Condylar process of mandible Process that forms the mandibular component of the temporomandibular joint

Condyle /ˈkandaɪl/ Rounded prominence of a bone

Condyles of occipital bone Prominences of occipital upon which first cervical vertebrae rests

Cone of light Bright region of tympanic membrane on inferior-anterior aspect, arising from tautness of the membrane

Congenital mandibular hypoplasia Congenital condition in which mandible is under-developed

Consciousness A condition of awareness arising from heightened levels of arousal of the brain

Constrictor muscle Pharyngeal muscles that constrict the pharyngeal space

contra- Combining form meaning opposite

Contracture Permanent contraction of a muscle

Contralateral Originating on the opposite side

Contralateral innervation Innervation of musculature or sensation on one side of the body by neurons of the opposite side

Contralateral stimulation That pattern of stimulation wherein stimulation of a structure in the auditory nervous system arises from stimulus being received in the ear on the side of the body opposite that of the structure

Conus elasticus a.k.a. cricovocal membrane or cricothyroid ligament; membranous lining below the level of the vocal folds, lining the subglottal region, and attaching to the thyroid, cricoid, and arytenoid cartilages

Conus medullaris of spinal cord Lower, cone-shaped projection of spinal cord

Convergence Coming together toward a common point

Convolutions Turns; infoldings

Coordinative structures In motor theory these are functionally defined muscle groups that, when activated, contribute to achieving the goal at the terminal effector

cor- Combining form meaning heart

Corniculate cartilages Cartilages positioned at the apex of the arytenoid cartilages

Cornu /kor ˈnu/ Horn

Corona radiata Mass of projection fibers running from and to the cerebral cortex

Coronal section A section dividing the body into front and back halves

Coronoid process of mandible Process to which the temporalis muscle attaches

corp- Combining form meaning body

Corpora quadrigemina The superior and inferior colliculi of midbrain

Corpus /ˈkorpəs/ Body

Corpus striatum Combination of striatum (putamen and caudate nuclei) and globus pallidus

Cortex Outer covering

Corticopontine projection Feedback system for the control of voluntary movement in the cerebellum: projections from parietal, occipital, temporal, and frontal lobes synapse on the pontine nuclei, projecting via pontocerebellar fibers to the opposite cerebellar cortex, allowing the command for voluntary movement to be modified relative to body position, muscle tension, and muscle movement

Corticopontine tract of pons Tract making up the middle cerebellar peduncle

Cotylica The cup-like portion of a bone into which the head of a bone inserts

Cough Forceful evacuation through the respiratory passageway, entailing deep inhalation through widely abducted vocal folds, tensing and tight adduction of the vocal folds, and elevation of the larynx, followed by forceful expiration

Cover of vocal folds a.k.a., vocal ligament; upper edge of the conus elasticus, between the vocal process of the arytenoid cartilages and the angle of the thyroid cartilage, giving stiffness to vocal folds, and consisting of the second and third layers of the lamina propria. Technically, the cover is considered to be the first and second layers of the lamina propria, while the vocal ligament is considered to be the second and third layers

Cranial Toward the head

Cranial nerves The 12 pairs of nerves arising from the brain

Craniosacral system a.k.a. parasympathetic nervous system. The portion of the autonomic nervous that functions to conserve energy

Craniostosis /krenɪoˈstosəs/ Premature ossification of cranial sutures

Craniosynostosis Premature closure of articulation of cranial bones by means of ossification of a suture

Cranium /ˈkrenɪəm/ The portion of the skull containing the brain

Cribriform plates of ethmoid bone The perforated plate through which the olfactory sensors pass into the nasal cavity

Cricoarytenoid joint The articulation formed between the cricoid and arytenoid cartilages, forming a synovial joint that permits rocking, gliding, and minimal rotation

Cricopharyngeus muscle a.k.a. cricopharyngeus. Portion of inferior constrictor muscle responsible for constricting the upper opening of the esophagus

Cricothyroid joint Diarthrodial, pivoting joint between cricoid and thyroid cartilages that permits the rotation of the two articulating structures

Cricothyroid muscle Muscle coursing from the lateral cricoid cartilage to the inferior thyroid lamina, divided into pars recta and oblique, and serving the function of changing the fundamental frequency of vibration of the vocal folds

Cricotracheal ligament Ligament between the cricoid cartilage of the larynx and tracheal cartilages

Crista ampularis /ˈkristə æmpjəˈlɛrəs/ Thickened region of semicircular canal lining containing sensory cells

Crista galli of ethmoid bone Superior prominence of ethmoid bone that protrudes into cranial vault and forms the anterior attachment for the falx cerebri component of the dura mater

Crossed olivocochlear bundle (COCB) Efferent fibers arising from superior olive of brain stem that decussate, serving efferent function of cochlea by action on the outer hair cells

Crown The highest point of a structure

crur-, crus Combining form meaning cross; leglike part

Crura anthelicis /ˈkrɚˈɔæntɛˈlikəs/ Auricle landmark produced by bifurcation of the antihelix

Crus cerebri Cerebral peduncles, which are the communicating pathways leading to and from the cerebrum

Crus commune Aperture opening into vestibule from anterior and posterior semicircular canals

Crux /krus/ Cross

cryo- Combining form meaning cold

Cryptotia Congential atresia of upper portion of ear

-cule Combining form that implies something very small

-culum, -culus Combining form that gives diminutive form of a noun

Cuneate tubercle of medulla Bulge in posterior medulla caused by terminal of fasciculus cuneatus

Cuneocerebellar tract Communicates sensation of temperature, proprioception (muscle spindle), and touch from the arms to the ipsilateral cerebellum

Cupid's bow Upper surface of upper lip

Cupola Prominence overlying the crista ampularis of the vestibular mechanism

Cuspid a.k.a. canine tooth, eye tooth. Tooth distal to lateral incisors with single cusp

Cycle In acoustics, the point at which an oscillation begins to repeat itself, marking the periodicity of the oscillation

Cycle of respiration Completion of both inspiration and expiration phases of respiration

Cycle of vibration Point in a vibratory cycle at which the function begins to repeat itself

Cymba concha Anterior extension of the helix marking the anterior entrance to the concha

-cyte Combining form meaning cell

Cytology /saɪ ˈtalodʒi/ Science dealing with structure of cells

Darwin's tubercle a.k.a. auricular tubercle; bulge on posterior-superior aspect of helix

de- Away from

Dead space Involved in exchange of gasses

Dead space air The air within the conducting passageways that cannot be involved in gas exchange

Decibel The logarithmic expression of the ratio of two sound pressures or powers to express acoustic level

Deciduous /dəˈsɪdjuəs/ Shedding

Deciduous dental arch The dental arch containing the 10 temporary teeth

Decussate /ˈdɛkəseɪt/ To cross over the midline

Decussation of the pyramids Pyramidal decussation of the medulla

Deep Farther from the surface

Deep sensation Sensation of the deep tissue of the body

Defecation /ˈdɛfəkeɪʃən/ Evacuation of bowels

Deformation Changes in form of a structure

Deglutition /diˈglutɪʃən/ Swallowing

Demyelination Pathological destruction of myelin of the axon

Dendrite The process of a neuron that transmits information to the cell body

Dendrodendritic Synapse between two dendrites

Dental alveoli Small sacs or holes into which teeth insert within the mandible and maxilla

Dentate /ˈdɛnteɪt/ Referring to tooth; notched; toothlike

Dentate gyrus a.k.a. dentate fascia; region between fibria of hippocampus and parahippocampal gyrus

Dentate nucleus of cerebellum Central nucleus of cerebellum; projections from the dentate nucleus synapse in the ventrolateral nucleus of the thalamus and from there ascend to the cerebral cortex by means of thalamocortical fibers

Dentatothalamic The neural pathways that arise in the dentate nucleus and terminate in the thalamus

Denticulate ligaments Connective fibers arising from the pia mater and serving to attach the spinal cord to the vertebral column

Dentin /ˈdɛnt ɪn/ Osseous portion of the tooth

Dentothalamic fibers Fibers arise from the dentate nucleus and synapsing in the opposite red nucleus and thalamus

Depolarization Neutralizing of polarity difference between two structures

Depressor anguli oris muscle a.k.a. triangularis; muscle originating along lateral margins of mandible on the oblique line and inserting into corner of upper lip and orbicularis oris superior

Depressor labii inferioris muscle Counterpart to levator labii superioris, originating at the oblique line of mandible, coursing up and in to insert into the lower lip

Dermatome /ˈdɚmətom/ Region of body innervated by a given spinal nerve

Descending pathways Motor pathways of the central nervous system

Descriptive anatomy The description of individual parts of the body without reference to disease conditions

Developmental Study of anatomy with reference to growth and development from birth

dextro- Right

Diaphragm The primary, unpaired muscle of respiration that completely separates abdomen and thorax

Diaphragma sella Dura mater separation between the pituitary gland and the hypothalamus

Diaphragmatic pleurae Parietal pleural lining covering the diaphragm

Diencephalon Subcortical structures involved in motor control and sensory processing, including the thalamus, hypothalamus, pituitary gland, and optic tract

Diffusion Migration or mixing of one material (e.g., liquid) through another

Digastricus anterior Anterior belly of digastricus muscle, coursing from inner surface of mandible to the hyoid intermediate tendon

Digastricus muscle One of the laryngeal elevators

Digastricus posterior Posterior belly of digastricus muscle, coursing from mastoid process of temporal bone to hyoid intermediate tendon

Digastricus posterior muscle Portion of the digastricus muscle that pulls the hyoid superiorly and back

Digastricus superior muscle Portion of digastricus muscle that pulls the hyoid superiorly and forward

Digestive system The system of organs and glands involved in digestion of food and liquids

Dilate /ˈdaɪleɪt/ To open or expand an orifice

Dissection The process of separating tissues of a cadaveric specimen

Distal Away from the midline

Distal surface of tooth Surface directed away from midpoint between central incisors, along dental arch

Distoverted /ˈdɪstovɚtəd/ Tilted away from midline

Divergence /daɪˈvɚdʒəns/ To become progressively farther apart

Dorsal /ˈdorsl̩/ Pertaining to the back of the body or distal

Dorsal cochlear nucleus (DCN) Component of the first brainstem nucleus in the auditory pathway

Dorsal funiculus Posterior column of spinal cord

Dorsal rami of spinal cord Division of spinal nerve serving posterior part of body

Dorsal root fiber Motor fibers of the spinal cord

Dorsal root ganglia of spinal cord Cell bodies of afferent spinal nerves

Dorsal spinocerebellar tract Tract communicating sensation of temperature, proprioception (muscle spindle), and touch from the lower body and legs to the ipsilateral cerebellum

Dorsal trunk The region commonly referred to as the back of the body

Dorsolateral sulcus of medulla The groove from which the XI accessory, X vagus, and IX glossopharyngeal nerves exit the medulla

Dorsum /ˈdorsəm/ Posterior side of a structure

Dorsum sellae of sphenoid bone Posterior aspect of sella turcica

Ductus reuniens Communication duct between cochlea and saccule of vestibular mechanism

Dural tube of spinal cord Tube of dura mater surrounding spinal cord

Dynamic models of motor function Models of motor function that take into account the physical properties of the motor system, such as elasticity or stiffness

-dynia Pain

dys- Bad; with difficulty

Dysarthria Speech disorder arising from paralysis, muscular weakness, and dyscoordination of speech musculature

Dysdiadochokinesia Deficit in the ability to make repetitive movements

Dysmetria /dɪsˈmɛtriə/ Deficit in control of the range of movement of a structure, such as a limb or the tongue

Dysprosody Deficit in maintenance of intonation and linguistic stress of speech

Dystonia Involuntary movement to a posture, with the posture being briefly held

e- Out from

Ear drum The membranous separation between the outer and middle ear, responsible for initiating the mechanical impedance-matching process of the middle ear

ec- Out of

ecto- On the outer side; toward the surface

-ectomy Excision

Edema Swelling

Edinger–Westphal nucleus Nucleus of midbrain involved in accommodation to light by the iris

Effector system In motor function, the system responsible for execution of the motor act

Efferent /ˈɛfərənt/ Carrying away from a central point

Elastic cartilage Cartilaginous connective tissue that has reduced collagen and increased numbers of elastic fibers. See yellow cartilage

Elastic fibers Connective fiber that returns to its original shape after being deformed

Elasticity The quality of a material that causes it to return to its original position after being distended

Electron Negatively charged particle

Electrophysiological techniques Those techniques that measure the electrical activity of single cells or groups of cells, including muscle and nervous system tissues

Electrophysiology The study of electrical phenomena associated with cellular physiology

Ellipsoid /iˈlipsɔɪd/ Shaped like a spindle

Elliptical recess Perforated portion of vestibule, providing communication between the utricle and the ampullae of the superior and lateral semicircular canals

Emboliform nucleus of cerebellum Central nucleus projecting to the red nucleus

Embolism Obstruction of blood flow caused by an embolus

Embolus Floating blood clot or thrombus

Embryonic In humans, the stage between the second and eighth weeks of gestation

-emia Referring to blood

Emotional lability Excessive and uncontrollable emotional response not necessarily related to the stimulus

En passant /an pə'san/ In passing

Enamel The hard outer surface of the tooth

Encephalon /ɛn'sɛfəlan/ The brain

End effector a.k.a. terminal device; in motor function, the articulator responsible for completion of the motor act

endo- Toward the interior; within

Endocochlear /ɛndo'koklɪɚ/ The constant positive potential difference between the scala

Endocochlear potential Positive electrical potential difference between the scala tympani and scala vestibule, arising from passive osmosis active and active ion pumping by the stria vascularis

Endocrine system The system involved in production and dissemination of hormones

Endolymph The fluid found in the scala media

Endolymphatic duct Duct arising from the saccule of the vestibule, terminating blindly in the petrous portion of the temporal bone

Ensiform /'ɛnsɪform/ Swordlike

ento- Toward the interior; within

Entrance to the auditory tube In anterior wall of middle ear space, the opening leading the auditory tube

ep-, epi- Upon or above something else

Epidural space Space superficial to the dura mater

Epiglottis Unpaired cartilage between the tongue and thyroid cartilage whose functional significance is that it drops down to cover the laryngeal opening during swallowing

Epimysium /ɛpə'mɪziəm/ Sheath of connective tissue around skeletal muscle

Epithelial tissue The superficial (outer) layer of mucous membranes and the cells constituting the skin, as well as the linings of major body cavities and all of the "tubes" that pass into, out of, and through the body

Equatorial region of intrafusal muscle Region near the midpoint of a fiber

Equilibrium A condition of balance

Equipotentialists a.k.a. spiritualists; theoreticians who view brain function as being distributed broadly, with very little or no localization of function

Esophageal reflux /ɛ'safədʒil/ Introduction of gastric juices into the pharyngeal region through the esophagus

Esophagus The tube connecting the laryngopharynx with the stomach, through which food passes during swallowing

etio- Pertaining to cause or origin

Eustachian tube /'justēɪʃən/ Also known as the *auditory tube*, coursing from the middle ear space to the nasopharynx; responsible for aeration of the middle ear

Eversion /i'vɚʒən/ Turning outward

ex- Out of, toward the surface

Excitation Stimulation that causes an increase of activity of the tissue being stimulated

Excitatory effects of neurotransmitters Effect of neurotransmitter that increases the probability that a neuron will discharge

Excitatory postsynaptic potential (EPSP) Depolarization of a neuron membrane potential

Executive function The function of the cerebral cortex that controls cognitive functions in order to complete tasks, including complex planning sequences, memory retrieval and manipulation, goal setting, and self-monitoring (to name a few)

Expectoration Elimination of phlegm from the respiratory passageway

Expiration Process of evacuating air from the lungs during respiration

Expulsive reflex Reflexes designed to remove contents of the stomach (e.g., vomit and retch)

Extension Straightening or moving out of the flexed position

External Toward the exterior of a body

External auditory meatus a.k.a. ear canal, external ear canal; canal terminating at the tympanic membrane

External occipital protuberance Midline prominence of the occipital bone

extero- Aimed outward or nearer to exteroceptors

Exteroceptors Sensory receptors that respond to stimuli from outside the body

extra- Outside

Extrafusal muscle Striated muscle fiber

Extrafusal muscle fibers Skeletal muscle fibers

Extrapyramidal system a.k.a., indirect system; portion of motor control of the nervous system that arises from the cerebral cortex and that is responsible for the background tone and movement supporting the primary acts. It projects to the basal ganglia and reticular formation

Extrinsic laryngeal muscles Muscles whose attachments include one attachment to a laryngeal structure and one attachment to a structure outside of the larynx, including sternothyroid, thyrohyoid, and thyropharyngeus muscles

Extrinsic muscles of the tongue Muscles of the tongue that have one attachment within the tongue and one attachment outside of the tongue

Eye tooth Cuspid

Facet A small surface

Facial colliculus of pons The prominence on the pons marking the location of the nucleus of the VI abducens nerve

Facial part The part of the skull that houses the mouth, pharynx, nasal cavity, and structures related to the upper airway and mastication

Facies Facial presentation

False rib a.k.a. vertebrochondral ribs, consisting of those ribs making indirect attachment with the sternum (ribs 8, 9 and 10)

False vocal folds a.k.a. ventricular folds, vestibular folds. The upper folds of the larynx, separated from the true vocal folds by the ventricle of the larynx

Falsetto The mode of phonation characterized lengthened vocal folds with thin and "reed-like" physical characteristics. The folds vibrate along the tensed, bowed margins, reduced. The posterior portion of the vocal folds tends to be damped, so that the length of the vibrating surface is decreased to a narrow opening. This mode provides the highest frequency of vibration of the vocal folds, with the possible exception of the laryngeal whistle (which is not really a mode of vibration)

Falx cerebelli The dural structure separating the two cerebellar hemispheres

Falx cerebri Dura mater structure completely separating the cerebral hemispheres

Fasciculations Twitching movements of small muscle groups

Fasciculus Tract of white matter

Fasciculus cuneatus Tract conveying sense of touch pressure, vibration and kinesthetic sense from upper limbs

Fasciculus gracilis Tract conveying sense of touch pressure, vibration and kinesthetic sense from lower limbs

Fastigial nucleus of cerebellum Central nucleus communicating with vestibular nuclei, reticular formation and inferior olive of brain stem

Faucial pillars Bands of tissue in posterior oral cavity separating oral and pharyngeal spaces

Feature detectors Neurons that respond to specific characteristics of a stimulus

Feedback theories Motor theories that require feedback from sensory systems to help control movement and learning of motor sequences

Feeding center Region of hypothalamus that regulates desire for food

Fenestra cochlea The round window

Fenestra ovalis Oval window

Fenestra rotundum a.k.a., foramen rotundum; round window

Fenestra vestibule Oval window

Fenestra vestibuli The oval window

Fiber Term generally referring to the axon of a neuron

Fibroblasts Tissue elements able to synthesize and secrete protein

Fibrocartilage Connective tissue fibers that contain collagen, providing a cushioning for structures

Fibroelastic membrane Membranous cover of the larynx consisting of the quadrangular membrane, aryepiglottic folds, conus elasticus, and vocal ligament

Fibrous tissue Tissue that binds structures together and that may contain combinations of fiber types

Filum terminale of spinal cord Fibrous end portion of spinal cord

Final common pathway The lower motor neuron serving a muscle or a muscle bundle

First bicuspid In adult arch, tooth distal to cuspid, with two cusps

First molar Tooth distal to second bicuspid in adult arch and distal to cuspid in deciduous arch

Fissure /ˈfɪʃɚ/ A relatively deep groove

Fixator Muscle responsible for stabilizing a structure

Flaccid dysarthria Dysarthria arising from lower motor neuron lesion, resulting in muscular weakness, flaccidity, and reduced reflexes

Flexion /ˈflɛkʃən/ The act of bending, often upon the ventral surfaces

Floating rib Those ribs that do not articulate with the sternum (ribs 11 and 12)

Flocculi Lateral posterior structure of the cerebellum, being one component of the flocculonodular lobe

Flocculonodular lobe of cerebellum Lobe of cerebellum comprised of left and right floccule and nodulus

Flocculus of cerebellum Region of anterior cerebellum, making up part of the flocculonodular lobe

Footplate of stapes Stapes component inserted within oval window

Foramen /ˈforēīmən/ An opening or passageway

Foramen cecum Deep recess in center of terminal sulcus

Foramen magnum Foramen through which spinal cord passes as it enters the braincase

Foramen ovale of sphenoid bone Canal within sphenoid bone through which mandibular nerve of V trigeminal passes

Foramen rotundum of sphenoid bone Canal of the sphenoid through which the III oculumotor nerve passes

Foramina of Luschka Drainage of the ventricle system of the CNS

Forced inspiration Inspiration that involves both diaphragm and accessory muscles of inspiration

Fossa /ˈfasə/ A depression, groove, or furrow

Fossa triangularis a.k.a. triangular fossa. Region between the crura anthelicis

Fovea /ˈfoviə/ A pit

Frenulum /ˈfrɛnjuləm/ A small frenum; often synonymous with frenum

Frenum /ˈfrinəm/ A small band of tissue connecting two structures, one of which is mobile

Frequency Number of cycles of vibration per second

Frequency perturbation a.k.a. vocal jitter; a measure of cycle-by-cycle variability in phonation

Frequency specificity The ability of the cochlea to differentiate different spectral components of a signal

Frontal Anterior; pertaining to the front

Frontal operculum a.k.a. pars opercularis; region of the frontal lobe overlying the insula

Frontal plane Divides body into anterior and posterior

Frontal process of maxilla Process of maxilla abutting the frontal bone

Frontal process of zygomatic bone Process of zygomatic bone that articulates with frontal bone

Fronto-parietal operculum Portion of parietal lobe overlying the insula

Frontopontine tract of midbrain Fibers from frontal lobe terminating in the pons

Function The process or action of a structure

Functional unity Structures that demonstrate similarities in function

Functional view View of a structure or system with reference to its function in the body

Fundamental frequency The lowest frequency of vibration of the vocal folds or of a harmonic series

Funiculus /fəˈnɪkjuləs/ Small, cordlike structure

Gag reflex Reflex elicited by tactile stimulation of the faucial pillars, posterior pharyngeal wall, or posterior tongue near the lingual tonsils, with the result being elevation of the velum, protrusion of the tongue, and closure of the larynx

Gamma motor neurons a.k.a. fusimotor efferent fibers; fibers innervating intrafusal muscle

Ganglia Group of cell bodies having functional unity and lying outside of the CNS

Ganglion /ˈgæŋgliən/ Mass of nerve cell bodies lying outside of the central nervous system

-gen Producing

General somatic afferent Sensory nerves that communicate sensory information, such as pain, temperature, mechanical stimulation of skin, length and tension of muscle, and movement and position of joints, from skin, muscles, and joints

General visceral afferent Nerves that transmit sensory information from receptors in visceral structures, such as the digestive tract

-genic Producing

Geniculotemporal radiation a.k.a. auditory radiation. Fibers from medial geniculate body of the thalamus that terminate at Heschl's gyrus of the temporal lobe

Genioglossus muscle Muscle making up the bulk of the tongue, arising from inner mandibular surface at symphysis and coursing to tip and dorsum

Geniohyoid muscle Muscle originating at mental spines of mandible and projecting to corpus hyoid

Genu /ˈdʒēīnu/ Knee

Genu of internal capsule Point of union between posterior and anterior limbs of internal capsule, containing corticobulbar tract

Gingiva /ˈdʒɪndʒɪvə/ Gum tissue

Glia Support tissue of the brain

Glial cells Neural tissue with a wide variety of functions in the nervous system, including recycling of neurotransmitter, waste removal, and encapsulation of damaged areas of tissue. They are also involved in long-term memory function

Global aphasia Severe aphasia that includes significant deficits in both expression and comprehension

Globose nuclei Afferent nucleus of the cerebellum

Globose nucleus of cerebellum Central nucleus projecting to the red nucleus

Globus pallidus Most superficial nucleus of basal ganglia, involved in regulation of muscle tone

Glomerulus In the olfactory bulb, the collection of axons converging on a single olfactory neuron

Glosso-epiglottic fold Epithelial covering of the lateral and medial glossoepiglottic ligaments, which produces the prominent valleculae between the tongue and epiglottis

Glottal Referring to the glottis

Glottal fry Phonatory mode characterized by low fundamental frequency and syncopated beat

Glottis /ˈglatəs/ The space between the true vocal folds

Golgi cells of cerebellum Cells projecting dendrites into the molecular layer and axons into the granular layer of the cerebellum. Their soma receive input from both climbing fibers and Purkinje cells, and the axons synapse with granule cell dendrites

Golgi tendon organs Tension sensors within tendons

Gooseflesh, goosebumps Autonomic skin response resulting in erection of skin papillae

Granular layer of cerebellum Deepest cell layer of cerebellum

Gray matter Cell bodies and dendrites of neurons

Greater cornu a.k.a., greater horn. The larger of the two cornu or horns of the hyoid bone, projecting posteriorly

Greater wing of sphenoid of sphenoid bone Processes of sphenoid bone arising from the posterior corpus sphenoid, making up part of the eye socket

Gross anatomy Study of the body and its parts as visible without the aid of microscopy

Group Ia primary afferent fibers Means by which nuclear bag fibers transmit information to spinal cord

Gustation /gəsteɪʃən/ Sense of taste

Gustation The sense of taste

Gyri Plural of gyrus; significant prominence or outfolding of tissue

Gyrus Outfolding of tissue in cerebral cortex

H zone Center of sarcomere with only thick filament

Habenular nuclei of epithalamus Nuclei of epithalamus that receive input from the septum, hypothalamus, brain stem, raphe nuclei, and ventral tegmental area via the habenulopeduncular tract and stria medullaris

Habitual pitch The perceptual correlate of vocal fundamental frequency habitually used by an individual

Hamulus /ˈhæmjuləs/ Hook

Hard glottal attack Glottal attack that uses excessive muscular force, potentially damaging phonatory anatomy

Hard palate The bony portion of the roof of the mouth, made up of the palatal processes of the maxillae and the horizontal plates of the palatine bones

Head Proximal portion of a bone

Head of caudate nucleus Anterior-most portion of caudate nucleus

Head of the caudate nucleus Anterior portion of the caudate nucleus

Hearing The process of receiving and transducing acoustic information as sensation

Helicotrema /ˈhɛlɪkotrimə/ Hooklike region of the cochlea, forming the minute union of the scala vestibuli and scala tympani

hemi- Half

Hemiballism /hɛmiˈbalɪzm/ Hyperkinetic condition involving involuntary and uncontrollable flailing of extremities of the right or left half of the body

Hemispheric specialization The concept that one cerebral hemisphere is more highly specialized for a particular function than that seen in the opposite hemisphere

Hertz Cycles per second

Heschl's gyrus Primary reception area of the temporal lobe, BA 41

Hg Mercury

Hiatus /ˈhaɪeɪtəs/ Opening

High spontaneous rate Auditory nerve fibers demonstrating a high rate of spontaneous discharge and low threshold of stimulation

Higher order processing area for vision (VII) of cerebral cortex The regions involved in higher order feature extraction for vision, including BA 20 and 21 of the temporal lobe, BA 19 of the occipital lobe, and BA 7 of the parietal lobe

Higher order processing area of the of cerebral cortex Areas of the cortex that receive primary activity information and process it further, such as extraction of features

High-level reflexes Those reflexes mediated at the level of the brain stem

Hippocampus Structure of limbic lobe involved in memory

Histogram Display of data arrayed with reference to its frequency of occurrence

Histology Study of tissue through microscopy

Homunculus /ho ˈmʌnkjuləs/ Literally, "little man"; referring to the spatiotopic array of fiber distribution along the central sulcus, representing body parts served by the cortical region

Horizontal plane Divides body or part into upper and lower portions

Horizontal plate of palatine bone Plate of palatine bone that makes up posterior ¼ of hard palate

Hyaline cartilage /ˈhaɪəlɪn/ Smooth cartilage covering the ends of bones at articulations

Hyoepiglottic ligament Ligament coursing from corpus of the hyoid bone to the epiglottis

Hyoglossus muscle Muscle coursing from greater cornu and lateral body of hyoid to sides of tongue

Hyoid bone The bone shared by tongue and larynx, and the only unpaired bone of the body

hyper- Above; increased, or too much of something

Hyperextension Extreme extension

Hyperkinetic dysarthria Dysarthria in which the dominant characteristic is the addition of unintended movements during speech, typically arising from damage to the basal ganglia

Hyperpolarization The condition wherein the threshold for depolarization is elevated, requiring increased stimulation to discharge

Hyperreflexia Hyperfunction of reflexes

Hypertonia Excessive muscle tone

Hypertrophy Increase in size, mass, or volume

hypo- Below; decreased, or too little of something

Hypoglossal nucleus of medulla Nucleus giving rise to the XII hypoglossal nerve

Hypoglossal trigone of medulla Bulge in posterior medulla caused by XII hypoglossal nucleus

Hypokinetic dysarthria Dysarthria characterized by paucity of movement, such as that found in Parkinson's disease

Hypophyseal fossa of sphenoid bone a.k.a. pituitary fossa, sella turcica. Inferior space of sphenoid in which pituitary gland resides

Hypophysis a.k.a., pituitary gland. Structure of central nervous system involved in autonomic regulation

Hypotonia /haɪpoˈtoniə/ Low muscle tone

Hypoxic /ha ˈpaksɪk/ Oxygen deficiency

Ideation Concept development

idio- Peculiar

Ilium One of the bones of the pelvic girdle

-ilos Diminutive form of a noun

Impedance Resistance to flow of energy

Incisive foramen Foramen in hard palate that marks the union of the premaxilla and the palatine processes

Incisors Anterior four teeth of dental arch

Incudostapedial joint /ɪnkjudostəpidɪjəl/ Point of union of incus and stapes

Incus Middle bone of ossicular chain of middle ear

Indirect system Extrapyramidal system of central nervous system, responsible for control of background movement, equilibrium, and muscle tone

Indusium griseum Extension of dentate gyrus, overlying the corpus callosum and continuing as the cingulate gyrus

Inertia /ɪˈnɚʃə/ The tendency for a body at rest to remain at rest, and for a body in motion to remain in motion

Inferior The lower point; nearer the feet

Inferior cerebellar peduncle Inferior pathway for information to and from cerebellum

Inferior colliculus /ɪnˈfɪriɚ koˈlɪkjuləs/ Nuclear relay of brain stem apparently involved in localization of sound in space

Inferior cornu of thyroid Inferior-most processes of the thyroid cartilage, providing the point of articulation between cricoid and thyroid cartilages

Inferior frontal gyrus Gyrus inferior to middle frontal gyrus, which includes the pars opercularis, also known as the frontal operculum

Inferior horn of lateral ventricles Portion of lateral ventricles extending into the temporal lobe

Inferior longitudinal muscle of tongue Muscle originating at root of tongue and corpus hyoid coursing to apex of tongue

Inferior medullary velum of pons Pontine surface providing inferior border of 4th ventricle

Inferior nasal conchae a.k.a. inferior turbinate. Small, scroll-like bones located on the lateral surface of the nasal cavity

Inferior olivary complex of medulla Nucleus serving cerebellum via the inferior cerebellar peduncle

Inferior olivary nuclear complex of medulla Complex of nuclei serving localization of sound in space

Inferior parietal lobules Portion of parietal lobe that includes supramarginal gyrus

Inferior petrosal ganglion Ganglion of IX glossopharyngeal nerve

Inferior pharyngeal constrictor Inferior pharyngeal musculature

Inferior pharyngeal constrictor muscle Inferior-most constrictor muscle of the pharynx

Inferior pontine sulcus Location from which VI abducens emerges in pons

Inferior turbinate a.k.a. inferior nasal conchae. Small, scroll-like bones located on the lateral surface of the nasal cavity

Inferior vestibular nucleus of medulla Nucleus associated with vestibular function

infra- Below

Infrahyoid muscles Muscles attached to the hyoid bone and a structure inferior to the hyoid bone

Infraorbital foramen Foramen of maxilla through which V trigeminal nerve emerges to serve facial sensation

Infraverted /ɪnˈfrəvɚtd/ In dentition, an inadequately erupted tooth

Inhalatory stridor Laryngeal stridor produced during inhalation as result of some form of obstruction of the airway

Inhibition In nervous system function, the process of reducing the ability of a neuron to discharge through synaptic action

Inhibitory postsynaptic potential (IPSP) Inhibition of a neuron membrane potential

Inhibitory synapse Synapse in which result of activation is reduction in probability of excitation of neuron

Inner hair cells The inner row of hair cells of the cochlea, numbering approximately 3500, maintaining the primary role of auditory signal transduction

Inner layer of tympanic membrane a.k.a. mucous layer of tympanic membrane. Deepest layer of the tympanic membrane, continuous with mucous covering of the middle ear space

Innervation Stimulation of a muscle, gland or structure by means of a nerve

Insertion The relatively mobile point of attachment of a muscle

Inspiration Inhalation; drawing air into the respiratory system

Inspiratory capacity The maximum inspiratory volume possible after tidal expiration

Inspiratory reserve The volume of air that can be inhaled after a tidal inspiration

Insular cortex a.k.a., island of Reil. Region located deep to the cerebral operculum

Integration of sensory information The process of combining different types of sensory information to generate a unique percept

Intensity Magnitude of sound, expressed as the relationship between two pressures

inter- Between

Interaural intensity The difference between signal intensity arriving at left and right ears of a listener

Interaural phase The difference in arrival time of an auditory signal arriving at left and right

Interchondral /ɪntɚˈkandrl̩/ The region between the cartilaginous portions of the anterior rib cage

Intercostal Between the ribs

Interhemispheric fissure a.k.a. cerebral longitudinal fissure; superior longitudinal fissure; the fissure that completely separates left and right cerebral hemispheres

Intermaxillary suture a.k.a. median palatine suture. Suture joining palatal processes of the maxilla

Intermediate (fibrous) layer Support layer of the tympanic membrane

Intermediate acoustic stria Auditory pathway arising from cochlear nucleus and terminating in superior olivary complex

Intermediate layer of tympanic membrane a.k.a. fibrous layer of tympanic membrane: middle layer of tympanic membrane consisting of radiating fibers and circular fibers

Intermediate tendon In digastricus muscle, the tendon that forms the attachment for the posterior and anterior digastricus to the hyoid bone

Internal Within the body

Internal auditory meatus Canal through which auditory nerve passes into cranial vault

Internal capsule Region of cerebral projection fibers immediately superior to the cerebral peduncles of the midbrain, at the level of the basal ganglia and thalamus

Internal carotid arteries Major vascular supply to the cerebral cortex, giving rise to the anterior and middle cerebral arteries

Internal carotid artery of cerebrovascular supply Artery arising from common carotid artery, serving of cerebrovascular system

Interneurons Neurons that provide communication between two neurons in a chain

intero- Aimed inward or farther from the surface

Interoceptor /ɪntɚoˈsɛptɚ/ Sensory receptor activated by stimuli from within the body (as opposed to exteroceptor)

Interpeduncular fossa Indentation between the cerebral peduncles from which iii oculomotor nerve exits

Interspike interval Neural response histogram providing detail of the timing between individual neural discharges

Interstitial /ɪntɚ'stɪʃəl/ Space between cells or organs

Interthalamic adhesion Connection between left and right thalamus

Intertragic incisure /ɪntɚ'treɪdʒɪk ɪn'saɪzɚ/ Region between tragus and antitragus

Interventricular foramen of Monro Passageway connecting the lateral and 3rd ventricles

Intervertebral foramen Foramen through which spinal nerve exits and/or enters spinal cord

Intonation The melody of speech, provided by variation of fundamental frequency during speech

intra- Within

Intracellular Within the cell

Intracellular resting potential Electrical potential within hair cells, being –70 mV relative to the endolymph

Intracellular space Space within individual cells

Intrafusal muscle fibers /ɪntrə'fuzl̩/ Muscle to which the muscle spindle is attached

Intraoral /ɪntrə'orl̩/ Within the mouth

Intraosseous eruption Eruption of tooth through bone

Intraparietal sulcus Significant superior-lateral sulcus of parietal lobe, involved in body perception relative to guided movement of hand, making up part of the "where" visual stream

Intrapleural pressure /ɪntrə'plɚəl/ Pressure measured within the pleural linings of the lungs

Intrinsic laryngeal ligaments Ligaments within the larynx that bind the cartilages of the larynx together

Intrinsic laryngeal muscles Muscles whose attachments are to other structures within the larynx, including lateral cricoarytenoid, posterior cricoarytenoid, transverse arytenoid, oblique arytenoid, cricothyroid, thyroarytenoid (thyrovocalis and thyrmomuscularis), thyroepiglottic, aryepiglottic and superior thyroarytenoid muscles

Intrinsic muscles of the tongue Muscles of the tongue that have both attachments within the tongue

intro- Into

Ion A particle carrying positive or negative charge

Ion transport Movement of ions across a membrane

ipsi- Same

Ipsilateral Same side

Ipsilateral stimulation That pattern of stimulation wherein stimulation of a structure in the auditory nervous system arises from stimulus being received in the ear on the same side of the body as the structure

Ipsilaterally Nerve fibers coursing and termination on the same site as origin of the fiber

Ischemia Cessation of blood flow

iso- Equal

Isometric Muscle action that does not result in movement

Isthmus /'ɪsməs/ A narrow passageway between cavities

-itis Inflammation or irritation

-ium Diminutive form of a noun

Joint Articulation

Jugum of sphenoid bone Anterior aspect of body of sphenoid

Kinesthesia /kɪnɛs'θiʒə/ Including sense of range, direction, and weight

Kinesthetic sense Sense of movement

Kinocilium /kaɪno 'sɪliəm/ Unitary cilium found on each hair cell of vestibular mechanism

Labioverted /'leɪbiovɚtd/ Tilted toward the lip

Labyrinth Maze

Labyrinthine hair receptors Mechanoreceptors within the vestibular mechanism that sense body movement

Lacrimal gland Tear gland

Lamdoidal suture of parietal bones Suture uniting the parietal and occipital bones

Lamina /'læmənə/ A flat membrane or layer

Laminae Layers

Laryngeal depressors Muscles that lower the larynx

Laryngeal elevators Muscles that raise the larynx

Laryngeal saccule Pouch of anterior laryngeal ventricle that contains mucus-producing secreting epithelia

Laryngeal stridor Harsh sound produced during respiration as a result of turbulence at the level of the vocal folds or within the respiratory passageway

Laryngeal ventricle See **ventricle of larynx**

Laryngectomee Person undergoing laryngectomy surgery

Laryngectromy Partial or total removal of the larynx

Laryngitis Inflammation of vocal folds

Laryngologist /lɛrɪn'galodʒɪst/ Specialist in the study of vocal pathology

Laryngopharynx a.k.a. hypopharynx; space bounded anteriorly by epiglottis and inferiorly by esophagus

Laryngoscope /lɛˊrɪŋoskop/ Instrument of visualization of the larynx and associated structures

larynx Structure housing the vocal folds and other phonation-related structures

Lateral Toward the side

Lateral apertures a.k.a. foramena of Luschka; left and right openings, lateral to median aperture, connecting the fourth ventricle and the cerebrospinal space outside of the cerebellum

Lateral corticospinal tract Lateral differentiation of the corticospinal tract arising from the decussation of the corticospinal tract at the pyramids in the medulla

Lateral cricoarytenoid muscle Muscle coursing from the muscular process of the arytenoid to superior surface of the cricoid cartilage, serving as the primary adductor of the vocal folds

Lateral funiculus Lateral column of spinal cord

Lateral geniculate body (LGB) Nucleus of thalamus involved in visual function

Lateral glossoepiglottic ligament Lateral ligament binding the tongue to the epiglottis, forming the lateral aspects of the valleculae

Lateral incisors Incisors lateral to central incisors

Lateral ligament of malleus Ligament binding malleus to temporal bone, arising from the lateral process of the malleus

Lateral process of malleus Process of malleus on lateral surface, providing attachment for the lateral malleolar ligament

Lateral pterygoid muscle a.k.a. external pterygoid muscle; muscle arising from the lateral pterygoid plate of sphenoid bone and coursing back to insert into the pterygoid fossa of mandible

Lateral pterygoid plate of sphenoid bone Laterally placed posterior prominence of sphenoid bone

Lateral semicircular canal a.k.a. horizontal semicircular canal; sensory component of vestibular mechanism that senses movement roughly in the transverse plane of the body

Lateral spinothalamic tract Tract conveying pain and thermal sense within spinal cord

Lateral sulcus a.k.a. Sylvian fissure; fissure dividing temporal lobe from frontal and anterior parietal lobes

Lateral superior olive Nuclear aggregate of superior olivary complex involved in processing interaural intensity differences

Lateral thyrohyoid ligament Ligament that runs from the superior cornu of the thyroid to the posterior tip of the greater cornu of the hyoid bone

Lateral ventricles Paired spaces within the cerebral cortex

latero- Side

Leg 1. The lower anatomical extremity, particularly the region between the knee and ankle. 2. A device used for raising grain from ground level to the top of a bin, consisting of a continuous flexible belt with a series of metal buckets or scoops

Lemniscal pathway Pathway cord from medial lemniscus to thalamus

Lentiform nucleus a.k.a., lentiform nucleus; combination of globus pallidus and putamen

lepto- Thick

Lesion /ˈliʒən/ A region of damaged tissue or a wound

Lesser cornu a.k.a., lesser horn; the smaller of the two cornu or horns of the hyoid bone, projecting superiorly from the corpus or the hyoid

Lesser wing of sphenoid of sphenoid bone Processes arising from corpus and clinoid processes of sphenoid bone, partially covering the optic canal

leuco- White

Levator anguli oris muscle Muscle arising from canine fossa of maxilla and coursing to insert into upper and lower lips

Levator labii superioris alaeque nasi muscle Muscle coursing vertically along lateral margin of nose, arising from frontal process of maxilla

Levator labii superioris muscle Muscle originating from infraorbital margin of maxilla, coursing down and in to the upper lip

Levator veli palatini a.k.a. levator veli palate, levator veli paltine; palatal elevator, making up bulk of velum

Lever advantage The benefit derived through reduction of the length of the long process of stapes relative to the manubrium malli

levo- Left

Ligaments Fibrous connective tissue connecting bones or cartilage

Limb apraxia The inability to perform volitional gestures using the limbs

Limbic association cortex The cortical association areas that include ba 23, 24, 38, 28, and 11, the parahippocampal gyrus and temporal pole, cingulate gyri of the parietal and frontal lobes, and orbital surfaces of the inferior frontal lobe. The limbic system is involved with motivation, emotion, and memory, making it an ideal association area

Limbic system The central nervous system structures responsible for mediation of motivation and arousal, including the hippocampus, amygdala, dentate gyrus, cingulate gyrus, and fornix

Lingual frenulum a.k.a. lingual frenum; bands of connective tissue joining inferior tongue with mandible

Lingual nerve of V trigeminal nerve Portion of V trigeminal that mediates somatic sensation of anterior 2/3 of tongue and floor of mouth

Lingual papillae Prominences on posterior surface of tongue

Lingual surface of tooth Surface of tooth adjacent to tongue

Lingual tonsils Lymphoid tissue on palatine surface of tongue

Lingual Referring to the tongue

Linguaverted /ˈlɪŋgwəvɚtd/ Tilted toward the tongue

Literal paraphasias Phoneme substitutions found in aphasia (note that "literal" is an old medical reference to "letters," preceding our concepts of phonemes being the units of speech)

Lobar bronchi Bronchial passageways connecting the main stem bronchi with individual lobes of the lungs

Lobe Major portion of a structure (e.g., frontal lobe of brain; superior lobe of lung)

Localization The process of identification of a sound source presented in free field

Localizationist a.k.a. materialists; theoreticians who view the brain as having very specific regions with clearly identified roles

Long association fibers Association fibers of cerebral cortex that connect lobes of the same hemisphere

Long process of incus Process of incus that runs approximately parallel to the manubrium malli

Loudness The psychological correlate of sound intensity

Low spontaneous rate Auditory nerve fibers with low rate of spontaneous discharge and relatively high threshold of stimulation

Lower extremity Portion of the body made up of the thigh, leg, ankle, and foot

Lower motor neuron Final neuron in a neuron chain that terminates on a muscle fiber

Lower motor neuron The final common neurological pathway leading to the muscle, including the anterior horn cell of the spinal cord, nerve roots, and nerves

Lumbar puncture Insertion of aspiration needle into subarachnoid region of spinal cord, usually below L4

Lumbar vertebra Vertebra of the lumbar spinal column

Lymphoid tissue /ˈlɪmfɔɪd/ Tissue comprising lymphatic organs, including tonsils and adenoids

macro- Large

Macula /ˈmækjələ/ Sensory organ of saccule and utricle

Macula cribrosa media Perforations in spherical recess of vestibule through which vestibular nerve passes to the saccule of the membranous labyrinth

Malleolar facet Point of union between malleus and incus

Malleus /ˈmæliəs/ Initial bone of the ossicular chain

Mandible Lower jaw, including dental arch

Mandibular foramen Opening on posterior inner surface of the mandible through which V trigeminal enters mandible to serve teeth and gums

Mandibular fossa of temporal bone Fossa of temporal bone with which condyle of mandible articulates

Mandibular nerve of the V trigeminal Lowest branch of the V trigeminal nerve

Mandibular notch Notch between condylar and coronoid process of mandible

Manometer Device for measuring air pressure differences

Manubrium /məˈnubriəm/ Process of malleus forming the major attachment to the tympanic membrane

Manubrium Is attached, forming the anterior and posterior malleolar folds and the pars flaccida of the tympanic membrane

Manubrosternal angle The point of articulation of manubrium sterni and corpus sterni

Mass The characteristic of matter that gives it inertia

Masseter muscle Most superficial of muscles of mastication, running from the zygomatic arch to the ramus of the mandible

Mastication Chewing

Mastoid air cells Cells comprising much of the mastoid process and extending to the floor of the middle ear cavity

Mastoid portion of temporal bone Posterior portion of temporal bone

Mastoid process of temporal bone Bony process posterior to external auditory meatus

Maxilla Upper jaw

Maxillary nerve of the V trigeminal Intermediate branch of the V trigeminal nerve

Maxillary process of zygomatic bone Process of zygomatic bone that articulates with maxilla

Maxillary sinus Largest of the sinuses of the maxilla

Maximum phonation time The duration an individual is capable of sustaining a phonation

Meatal atresia Developmental absence of external auditory meatus

Meatus /mi´ēɪtəs/ Passageway

Meatus acousticus externus Outer ear canal; external auditory meatus

Mechanoreceptors Sensory receptors sensitive to mechanical stimulation such as pressure upon the skin

Medial Toward the midline of the body or subpart (syn. mesial)

Medial compression The degree of force that may be applied by the vocal folds at their point of contact

Medial geniculate body (MGB) Nucleus of thalamus involved in auditory function

Medial lemniscus of pons Somatic sense pathway within pons

Medial longitudinal fasciculus (MLF) Group of fiber tracts within spinal cord that includes the rubrospinal tract

Medial pterygoid muscle a.k.a. internal pterygoid muscle; muscle arising from medial pterygoid plate and fossa of the sphenoid and inserting into the inner surface of the ramus of the mandible

Medial pterygoid plate of sphenoid bone Medially placed posterior prominence of sphenoid bone

Medial superior olive Nuclear aggregate of superior olivary complex involved in processing interaural time (phase) differences

Medial surface of tooth a.k.a. mesial; surface directed toward midpoint between central incisors, along dental arch

Medial vestibular nucleus of medulla Nucleus associated with vestibular function

Median Middle

Median aperture a.k.a., foramen of Magendie; midline opening connecting the fourth ventricle and the cerebrospinal space outside of the cerebellum

Median fibrous septum of tongue Dividing wall between right and left halves of tongue that serves as the point of origin for the transverse muscle of the tongue

Median glossoepiglottic ligament Middle ligament binding the tongue to the epiglottis, structurally dividing the left and right valleculae

Median palatine suture a.k.a. intermaxillary suture; suture joining palatal processes of the maxilla

Median pharyngeal raphe Midline connective tissue that forms union of left and right pharyngeal musculature

Median raphe of hard palate Division point between left and right halves of hard palate

Median raphe of medulla Point of decussation of fibers from the principal inferior olivary nucleus

Median sulcus of tongue Midline sulcus dividing tongue into left and right halves

Median thyrohyoid ligament Ligament coursing from the anterior corpus hyoid to the upper border of the anterior thyroid

Mediastinal /midɪ´ə stāɪnḷ/ Referring to the middle space; in respiration, referring to the organs separating the lungs

Mediastinal pleurae Parietal pleural lining covering the mediastinum

medio-, medius Middle

Medulla oblongata a.k.a., medulla; the inferiormost segment of the brain stem

Medullary reticulospinal tract Tract arising from the medulla and descending through the lateral lemniscus of the spinal cord, supporting postural control of lower limb muscles

megalo- Large

Melogenesis imperfeca Congenital condition in which enamel of tooth is thin or missing

Membranous glottis /mɛm´brēɪnəs ´glatəs/ The anterior three-fifths of the vocal fold margin; the soft tissue of the vocal folds (note that the term *glottis* is loosely used here, because glottis is actually the space between the vocal folds)

Membranous labyrinth /mɛm´brēɪnəs ´læbɪrɪnθ/ Membranous sac housed within bony labyrinth of inner ear, holding the receptor organs of hearing and vestibular sense

Meningeal infection /mə´nɪndʒɪəl/ Infection of the meningeal linings of the brain and spinal cord

Meningeal linings a.k.a., meninges. Connective tissue linings of the brain, including dura mater, arachnoid mater, and pia mater

Meninges /mə´nɪndʒiz/ The membranous linings of the brain and spinal cord

Mentalis muscle Muscle arising from region of incisive fossa of the mandible, coursing down to insert into the skin of the chin below

Mesencephalon /mɛsɛn´sɛfəlan/ The midbrain

Mesial /´mi ziəl/ Toward the midline of the body or subpart (syn. medial)

Mesioverted /misio´vɚtd/ Tilted toward the midline

Meso- Middle

Meta- After; mounted or built upon

Metencephalon /mɛtɛnˈsɛfələn/ Embryonic portion of brain from which cerebellum and pons originate

Micro- Small

Microdontia Abnormally small tooth size

Microglia Glial cells responsible for phagocytosis, or scavenging of necrotic tissue in the nervous system

Micron One-thousandth of a millimeter; one-millionth of a meter

Micropotential a.k.a. miniature postsynaptic potential (MPSP) depolarization of a small portion of a neuron membrane

Microscopic anatomy Study of structure of the body by means of microscopy

Microtia Small auricle

Middle cerebellar peduncle a.k.a. brachia pontis; middle pathway for information to and from cerebellum

Middle cerebral arteries Major arteries arising from internal carotid artery, and responsible for serving the entire speech and language regions of the cerebral cortex

Middle ear effusion Secretion of fluid into the middle ear

Middle frontal gyrus Gyrus immediately inferior to superior frontal gyrus

Middle nasal conchae Medially placed process of ethmoid bone, found in nasal cavity

Middle pharyngeal constrictor Middle constrictor muscle of pharynx

Middle temporal gyrus Middle gyrus of the temporal lobe

Mid-sagittal section An anatomical section that divides the body into left and right halves in the median plane

Miniature end plate potential (MEPP) Depolarization of a small portion of a skeletal muscle fiber arising from neurotransmitter action

Minimum driving pressure Minimum air pressure to drive the vocal folds into phonation, approximately 3–5 cm H_2O for healthy vocal folds

Minute volume The volume of air exchanged by an organism in one minute

Mitochondria /maɪtoˈkandriə/ Microscopic cellular structures that provide the energy source for a cell

Mixed dysarthrias Dysarthrias arising from a combination on other forms of dysarthria

Mixed hypokinetic-ataxic-spastic dysarthria Dysarthria with the characteristics of hypokinetic, ataxic and spastic dysarthria, such as is found in Wilson's disease (hepatolenticular degeneration)

Mixed spastic-ataxic dysarthria Dysarthria with the characteristics of both spastic and ataxic dysarthria, such as is found in multiple sclerosis

Mixed spastic-flaccid dysarthria Dysarthria with the characteristics of both spastic and flaccid dysarthria, such as is found in amyotrophic lateral sclerosis

ml Milliliters; one-thousandth of a liter, equal to one centimeter

mm Millimeter; one-thousandth of a meter

Modal register /ˈmodl̩/ The vocal register used during normal conversation (i.e., that vocal register used most frequently)

Mode of vibration Of the vocal folds during sustained phonation, the pattern of activity that the vocal folds undergo during a cycle of vibration

Modiolus /moˈdaɪoləs/ The structure of the bony labyrinth forming the central core of the cochlea

Molars /ˈmolɚz/ The posterior three teeth of the mature dental arch, used for grinding

mono- Single

Monoloud Without variation in vocal loudness (the perception of vocal intensity)

Monopitch Without variation in vocal pitch (the perception of frequency)

Monopolar neuron a.k.a. unipolar neuron; neuron with a single, bifurcating process arising from the soma

morph- Form

Morphology /morˈfalədʒɪ/ Study of the form of a structure without regard to function

Motor endplate Synaptic union of muscle fiber and nerve

Motor function The processes of planning, programming, and activation of the sequence of muscle firings required to complete a desired act

Motor neurons Neurons that innervate muscle

Motor planning Process of planning for the motor act

Motor strip a.k.a., precentral gyrus; the region immediately anterior to the central sulcus and considered to be the primary activation region for muscles

Motor unit The lower motor neuron and muscle fibers it innervates

Mucosal lining of vocal folds Epithelial lining and first layer of the lamina propria

Mucous /ˈmjukəs/ Tissue that secretes mucus

Mucus /ˈmjukəs/ Viscous fluid secreted by mucous tissue and glands

Multiple motor unit summation Use of many motor neurons to activate a muscle

Multipolar neurons Neurons possessing more than two processes

Muscle spindles Structures found within specific muscles that are responsible for monitoring and maintaining tonic muscle length

Muscle Contractile tissue

Muscle tone The perception of resistance to the passive movement of stretching

Muscular processes Lateral processes of the arytenoid cartilages to which the lateral cricoarytenoid and posterior cricoarytenoid muscles attach

Musculus uvulae Muscular portion of uvula

my- Pertaining to muscle

Myelencephalon /ˈmaɪɛlɛnsɛfəlan/ Portion of embryonic brain giving rise to the medulla oblongata

Myelin Fatty sheath surrounding axons of some nerves

myelo- Pertaining to spinal cord

Mylohyoid line Prominence on inner surface of mandible to which mylohyoid muscle attaches

Mylohyoid muscle Muscle originating at underside of mandible and coursing to corpus hyoid

myo- Pertaining to muscle

myoelastic- /maɪoəˈlæstɪk-ɛrodaɪˈnæmɪk/ Theory of vocal fold function that accounts

Myofibrils Components making up muscle fiber

Myology /maɪalədʒɪ/ The study of muscles and their parts

Nares Nostrils

Naris /ˈnerɪs/ Nostril (plural, nares)

Nasal assimilation The unintended overlapping coarticulatory effect of nasal consonants upon adjacent phonemes arising from altered timing of the velopharyngeal mechanism

Nasal choanae Posterior portals connecting the nasal cavities and nasopharynx

Nasal crest Within nasal cavity, the midline ridge of the palatal bone

Nasal notch Notch formed on either side of anterior nasal spine in anterior nasal cavity

Nasal portion of frontal bone Process of frontal bone that articulates with the nasal bone

Nasal septum Dividing plate between left and right nasal cavities, made up of the vertical component of

the vomer, perpendicular plate of ethmoid, and the septal cartilage

naso- Nose

Nasopharynx /nezoˈfɛrɪŋks/ The region of the pharynx posterior to the nasal cavity and superior to the velum

Neck Constricted portion of a structure

Negative pressure Air pressure that is less than atmospheric pressure

neo- New

Neocerebellum a.k.a. pontocerebellum; posterior lobe and intermediate vermis of cerebellum

Neologism /ni ˈoləldʒɪzm/ New word; in pathology, novel word coined by individual, but without meaning shared with listener

Nerve Bundle of nerve fibers outside the central nervous system that has functional unity

Nervous system System of neural tissue that serves as the control mechanism for motor function as well as the integration center for sensory information

Nervous tissue Highly specialized communicative tissue consisting of neurons or nerve cells

Nervus intermedius Nerve arising from salivatory nucleus, serving salivation

Neuraxis /nɚˈæksɪs/ The axis of the nervous system, representing the embryonic brain axis

neuro- Nerve

Neurogenic Of neurological origin

Neurology Neurology study of the diseases of the nervous system

Neuromotor dysfunction Neurological condition in motor ability arising from lesion within the nervous system or at the neuromotor junction

Neuromuscular junction The point of contact between a muscle fiber and the nerve innervating it

Neurons Nerve cell tissue whose function is to transmit information from one neuron to another, from neurons to muscles, or from sensory receptors to other neural structures

Neurotransmitters Substance that is released into synaptic cleft upon excitation of a neuron

Neutroclusion /ˈnutrokluʒən/ Normal molar relationship between upper and lower dental arches

Nodes of Ranvier /ˈnodz ʌv ˈranviēi/ Regions of myelinated fibers in which there is no myelin

Nodulus of cerebellum Central region of the anterior cerebellum, making up part of the flocculonodular lobe

Non-pyramidal cells Small neurons involved in sensory function or intercommunication between brain regions

Nuclear bag fibers Stretch receptors clustered at the equatorial region of the intrafusal muscle fiber

Nuclear chain fibers Row of stretch sensors at the equatorial region of the intrafusal muscle fiber. Bags surrounding nuclear chain fibers may have either primary Ia or group II secondary afferent fibers

Nucleus /ˈnukliəs/ An aggregate of neuron cell bodies within the central nervous system

Nucleus ambiguus Nucleus giving rise to the IX glossopharyngeal, X vagus, and XI accessory nerves

Nucleus cuneatus Nucleus of fasciculus cuneatus

Nucleus interpositus of cerebellum Combination of embliform and globose nuclei of cerebellum

Nucleus solitarius of medulla Nucleus of the X vagus nerve

Oblique Diagonal

Oblique arytenoid muscle a.k.a. oblique interarytenoid muscles; muscle coursing from the posterior apex of one arytenoid to the posterior base of the other arytenoid, serving as adductor of the vocal folds

Oblique interarytenoid muscle a.k.a. oblique arytenoid muscles; muscle coursing from the posterior apex of one arytenoid to the posterior base of the other arytenoid, serving as adductor of the vocal folds

Oblique line of thyroid Point of attachment on the thyroid cartilage of the thyrohyoid and sternothyroid muscles

Occipitomastoid suture of temporal bone Suture joining mastoid region with occipital bone

Occlusal surface /əˈkluzl̩/ The surfaces of teeth within opposing dental arches that make contact

Occlusion Process of bringing upper and lower teeth into contact

oculo- Eye

Olfaction The sense of smell

Olfactory bulb Nuclei of the olfactory nerve

Olfactory sulcus Sulcus on inferior surface of the frontal lobe along which optic tract passes

Oligodendrocytes Glial cells that are instrumental in production of myelin in the central nervous system

Olive of medulla Bulge between the ventrolateral and dorsolateral sulci, caused by the inferior olivary nuclear complex, which consists of nuclei serving to localize sound in space

Olivocerebellar fibers Fibers that arise from the inferior olivary and medial accessory olivary nucleus

of the medulla and project to the contralateral cerebellum, terminating as climbing fibers

Olivocochlear bundle /ˌalɪ voˈkokliɚ/ Collective term for crossed and uncrossed olivocochlear bundles, the efferent auditory nerve fibers involved in processing auditory signal in noise

-oma Morbid condition of a part, often a tumor

Omohyoid muscle Laryngeal depressor with two bellies; the inferior belly arises from the scapula and inserts into an intermediate tendon; the superior belly arises from the intermediate tendon and inserts into the hyoid; together, the two bellies depress the hyoid

Onset response Neural response in which there is an initial burst of activity related to the onset of a stimulus, followed by silence

Opening stage of phonation In the cycle of phonation, the stage in which the vibrating vocal folds are opening up

Ophthalmic nerve of the V trigeminal Superior branch of the V trigeminal nerve

Optic canal of sphenoid bone Canal within sphenoid through which optic nerve passes

Optic chiasm Decussation point for optic nerve

Optic radiation Portion of the visual pathway projecting from lateral geniculate body of thalamus

Optic tracts Extension of the optic nerve coursing around the crus cerebri following the decussation at the optic chiasm

Optimal pitch The perceptual characteristic representing the ideal or most efficient frequency of vibration of the vocal folds or powers

Oral apraxia Difficulty using the facial and lingual muscles for nonspeech acts in absence of muscular weakness or paralysis

Oral cavity The region extending from the orifice of the mouth in the anterior, and bounded laterally by the dental arches and posteriorly by the fauces

Oral diadochokinesis /ˈdaɪədokokɪ ˈnisɪs/ A task involving repetition of movements requiring alternating contraction of antagonist muscles associated with speech (lips, mandible, tongue)

Oral surface of tongue a.k.a. palatine surface of tongue; superior surface of the portion of the tongue within the oral cavity

Oral-peripheral examination a.k.a., oral mechanism examination; procedure for examining structure and function of the oral mechanism with particular interest in functionality related to speech

Orbicularis oris inferior muscle Muscle underlying lower lip of oral cavity

Orbicularis oris muscle Muscle underlying lips of oral cavity

Orbicularis oris superior muscle Muscle underlying upper lip of oral cavity

Orbital margin of zygomatic bone Portion of zygomatic bone that contributes to eye socket

Orbital plates of ethmoid bone The ethmoid component of the eye socket

Orbital portion of frontal bone Process of the frontal bone that makes up a portion of the eye socket

Orbital process of palatine bone Process making up the lower portion of eye socket

Orbital region a.k.a., pars orbitale. Region of inferior frontal lobe overlying the eyes

Orbital surface On inferior surface of the frontal lobe, region overlying the eyes

Organ of Corti Sensory organ of hearing within inner ear

Organelles Specialized structures of a cell (e.g., mitochondria)

Organs Aggregates of tissues with functional unity

Orienting reflex Reflex elicited by touching the side of a newborn's tongue, with the result being that the infant's tongue moves in the direction of the stimulus

Orifice Mouth or opening

Origin Proximal attachment of a muscle; point of attachment of a muscle with relatively little movement

oro- Mouth

Orofacial myofunctional therapy a.k.a. oromyofunctional therapy; therapy directed toward remediating problems of muscular imbalance related to oral stage swallowing or habitual oral patterns related to oral stage swallowing

Oropharynx /oro'fɛrɪŋks/ The region of the pharynx bounded posteriorly by the faucial pillars, superiorly by the velum, and inferiorly by the epiglottis

ortho Straight

Oscillation /asɪ'leɪʃən/ Predictably repetitive movement

-osis Condition

osseo- A hardened or bony part

Osseous labyrinth /asiəs/ The bony cavities of the inner ear

Osseous spiral lamina Bony shelf on modiolus of cochlea, forming the point of attachment for the scala media

Ossicles The three bones of the middle ear

Ossicular chain /a'sɪkjulɚ/ Collective term for malleus, incus, and stapes

Ossified The process of tissue turning into bone

Osteo- Bone

Osteology Study of the structure and function of bones

Otitis externa Inflammation of the outer ear

Otolithic membrane /oto'lɪθɪk/ Membranous covering over the utricular macula

Otoliths Crystals within otolithic membrane of macula

Outer hair cells Outer three rows of hair cells of the organ of Corti, numbering approximately 12,000

Outer layer of typmpanic membrane a.k.a. cuticular layer of tympanic membrane; layer of tympanic membrane that is a continuation of the epithelial lining of the ear canal

Oval window The opening into the scala vestibuli to which the footplate of stapes is attached

Overbite The vertical overlap of maxillary incisors over the mandibular incisors when molars are occluded

Overjet Vertical overlap of maxillary incisors over mandibular incisors

Overshoot In motor function, failure to integrate sensory information that results in failure to apprehend a target by going beyond the target

pachy- Thick

Pacinian corpuscles Pressure sensors that respond to rapid deep pressure to the outer epithelium

Pain withdrawal reflex Withdrawal of a limb or body part in response to a painful stimulus

Palatal aponeurosis Mid-front portion of soft palate, serving as extension of aponeurosis arising from tensor veli palatini

Palatal lift prosthesis Prosthetic device designed to elevate the velum in order to achieve velopharyngeal closure

Palatine process Paired processes of the maxilla that form the anterior hard palate

Palatine tonsils /pælətaɪn/ Lymphoid tissue between the fauces

palato- Palate

Palatoglossus muscle a.k.a. glossopalatine muscle. Muscle coursing from the sides of posterior tongue to velum

Palatopharyngeus muscle Palatal depressor coursing from velum to pharyngeal wall and making up posterior faucial pillar

Palmar grasp reflex That reflex elicited by lightly stimulating the palm of the hand, causing the flexed fingers to grasp

Palmar /ˈpalmɚ/ Pertaining to the palm of the hand

Palpate /ˈpælpeɪt/ To examine by touch

Para Beside; partial

Paracentral lobule In the medial surface of the cerebral cortex, superior aspect of medial cortex, marking the union of precentral and postcentral gyrus of frontal and parietal lobes

Parahippocampal gyrus Gyrus of inferior frontal lobe in which hippocampus resides

Paralysis Loss of voluntary motor function

Parasympathetic nervous system a.k.a. craniosacral system; the portion of the autonomic nervous that functions to conserve energy

Paresis Muscular weakness

Parietal pleurae Pleural linings of the thoracic cavity

Parieto-occipital sulcus Sulcus on superior surface of cerebrum, marking the boundary between parietal and occipital lobes

Pars Part

Pars flaccida /ˈparz ˈflæsɪdə/ A flaccid portion of the tympanic membrane in the superior region

Pars oblique More posterior aspect of the cricothyroid muscle

Pars opercularis a.k.a. frontal operculum; region of the frontal lobe overlying the insula

Pars orbitale a.k.a., orbital region; region of inferior frontal lobe overlying the eyes

Pars recta Portion of the cricothyroid muscle most active during change of fundamental frequency

Passavant's pad Pad of muscle at posterior pharyngeal wall that forms landing pad for velum

Passive expiration Expiration arising from passive forces of muscular tissue elasticity

patho- Abnormal in some way

Pathological anatomy Study of parts of the body with respect to the pathological entity

-pathy Disease

Pauser neurons Those neurons in the auditory pathway that show a pattern of discharge, followed by cessation of discharge, and then return to discharge

Pauser response /ˈpazɚ/ Nerve response characterized by an initial on-response followed by silence, and subsequent low-level firing rate throughout stimulation

ped- Foot; child

Pedicle Foot

Pelvic girdle The area comprised of the ilium, sacrum, pubic bone, and ischium

Pelvis The area formed by the sacrum, coccyx, and innominate bones of the body

-penia Poverty

Per Through; passing through; before

Perfusion Migration of fluid through a barrier

Peri Around

Periaqueductal nucleus a.k.a. central gray. Region in the midbrain housing the nucleus of IV trochlear nerve

Pericardium /pɛrəˈkardiəm/ The membranous sac surrounding the heart

Perilymph /ˈpɛrəlɪmf/ Fluid of the scala vestibuli and scala tympani

Perimysium /pɛrəˈmisiəm/ The sheath surrounding muscle bundles

Period The time required to complete one cycle of vibration or movement

Period histogram Display of neuron firing rate based upon the point in the cycle of vibration at which firing occurs

Periodic Having predictable repetition

Periodontal ligament Suspensory ligament for tooth

Peripheral Relative to the periphery or away from

Peripheral nervous That portion of the nervous system including spinal and cranial nerves

Permanent teeth Teeth of the adult dental arch

Permeability /pɚmiəˈbɪlətɪ/ The quality of penetrability

Permeable Property of a membrane that determines the ease with which ions may pass through a membrane

Persistent closed bite The condition wherein supraversion of the anterior dental arch prohibits the posterior teeth from occlusion

Persistent open bite The condition wherein the incisors of upper and lower dental arches show a vertical gap due to malocclusion of the posterior arch that prohibits anterior contact

Perturbation Sudden, unexpected force applied to an articulator

Pes A footlike structure

Petrous portion of temporal bone Portion of temporal bone including cochlea and semicircular canals

-phage, phagia Eating

Pharyngeal branch of X vagus Branch mediating taste and visceral sensation from base of tongue and upper pharynx, as well as innervation of superior and middle pharyngeal constrictors

Pharyngeal cavity a.k.a. pharynx; space posterior to oral and nasal cavities, including oropharynx, nasopharynx, and laryngopharynx

Pharyngeal portion of tongue a.k.a base of tongue; portion of tongue that resides in the oropharynx

Pharyngeal recesses In swallowing literature, the combined valleculae and pyriform sinuses

Pharyngeal tonsil /fɛˈrɪndʒɪəl/ The mass of lymphatic tissue within the nasopharynx; a.k.a. *adenoids*

Pharyngotympanic tube a.k.a. auditory tube, Eustachian tube

Pharynx /ˈfɛrɪŋks/ The respiratory passageway from the larynx to the oral and nasal cavities

Phase-locking The tendency of a neuron to respond to a particular phase of an acoustic signal

Phasic lengthening of muscle spindle Condition in which muscle length undergoes lengthening

-pher- Bearing or carrying

Philtrum Space between columella nasi

Phonation The voiced tone produced by the vibrating vocal folds

Phonatory sign Objective evidence of pathology of the phonatory mechanism

Phonatory system The system including the laryngeal structures through which phonation is achieved

Phonological system System of sounds relevant to language

Photoreceptors Sensory receptors for visual stimulation

Phrenic nerve The nerve arising from the cervical plexus that innervates muscular activity of the diaphragm

Phrenology Historically early analytic process that posited the ability to infer characteristics of a person based upon head shape and conformation

Physiological dead space Volume of air that cannot undergo gas exchange as a result of physiological limits

Physiology /fɪziˈalədʒɪ/ The study of function of the body and its components

Pillar cells of Corti Supportive cells of the organ of Corti

Pinna /pɪnə/ Auricle, making up the readily visible portion of the outer ear

Pitch The psychological (perceptual) correlate of frequency of vibration

Pitch range The perceptual correlate of the range of fundamental frequency variation possible for an individual

Pituitary fossa a.k.a sella turcica, hypophyseal fossa; inferior space of sphenoid in which pituitary gland resides

Place theory of hearing Theory of hearing stating that frequency processing of the cochlea arises

Planning Identification of steps of an action

Plantar /ˈplæntɚ/ Pertaining to the sole of the foot

Plantar grasp reflex Grasping by the toes upon light stimulation of the sole of the foot

-plasia Growth

-plastic Capable of being molded

-plasty Molding, forming

Pleural /ˈplɝˌl/ Pertaining to the pleurae of the lungs

Pleurisy /plɝˈəsɪ/ Inflammation of the pleural linings of the lungs

Plexus /ˈplɛksəs/ A network of nerves

poly- Many

Polyotia Portion of auricle that is duplicated in development

Pontine nuclei of pons Nuclei receiving input from cerebrum and spinal cord, relaying that information to the cerebellum

Pontine reticulospinal tract Extrapyramidal tract arising from nuclei in the medial tegmentum of the pons and descends near the MLF in the spinal cord, and terminating in the spinal cord, supporting postural control of lower limb muscles

Pontine tegmentum Continuation of reticular formation of medulla within pons

Pontocerebellar fibers Fibers providing input to the cerebellum that ascend through the middle cerebellar peduncle and terminate as mossy fibers

Pontocerebellar tract Prominent band of transverse fibers visible in the posterior pons that provide communication between the cerebellum and the pons

Positive pressure Air pressure that exceeds atmospheric pressure

post- After; behind

Postcentral gyrus Gyrus of parietal lobe that is the primary site of sensory reception in the cerebral cortex

Postcentral sulcus Sulcus of parietal lobe separating postcentral gyrus from the central sulcus

Posterior Toward the rear

Posterior cerebral arteries of cerebrovascular supply Arteries arising from the basilar artery to serve the posterior cerebral cortex

Posterior commissure Region between the arytenoid cartilages

Posterior communicating artery of cerebrovascular supply Artery connecting left and right posterior cerebral arteries

Posterior cricoarytenoid muscle Muscle coursing from the lateral process of the arytenoid cartilage to the posterior cricoid cartilage, serving as the only abductor of the vocal folds

Posterior crus of stapes Posterior pillar of the stapes arch

Posterior faucial pillars Band of tissue in posterior oral cavity separating oral and pharyngeal spaces, and overlying palatopharyngeus muscle

Posterior gray column of spinal cord a.k.a., posterior horn. Cell bodies of dorsal spinal cord

Posterior horn of lateral ventricles a.k.a. occipital horn of lateral ventricles. Portion of lateral ventricles extending into the occipital lobe

Posterior inferior cerebellar artery of cerebrovascular supply Artery arising from vertebral artery serving the cerebellum

Posterior intermediate sulcus of spinal cord Sulcus lateral to posterior median sulcus of spinal cord

Posterior ligament of incus Ligament binding incus to temporal bone, arising from the short process of the incus

Posterior limb of internal capsule Portion of internal capsule that includes the optic radiation and thalamic portion of internal capsule

Posterior malleolar fold Region of the tympanic membrane posterior to the pars flaccida

Posterior median sulcus of spinal cord Sulcus on posterior surface of spinal cord

Posterior nasal spines Prominence in posterior aspect of nasal cavity formed by union of left and right palatine bones

Posterior quadrate lamina Posterior aspect of cricoid cartilage; superior surface of posterior quadrate lamina includes facets for arytenoid articulation

Posterior semicircular canal a.k.a. posterior vertical semicircular canal; posteriorly placed semicircular canal of vestibular mechanism

Posterior spinal arteries cerebrovascular supply Arteries descending spinal cord in posterior aspect

Posterior spinocerebellar tract Uncrossed spinal cord tract conveying afferent information from GTOs and muscle spindle stretch receptors to the cerebellum

postero- Behind

Postsynaptic neuron The neuron receiving input

Potential energy Energy that may be expended

Pre-auricular tags Prominences that form prenatally anterior to pinna

Precentral gyrus a.k.a., motor strip; the region immediately anterior to the central sulcus and considered to be the primary activation region for muscles

Precuneus Region posterior to paracentral lobule in the medial surface of the cerebrum

Prefrontal association area Major association area of the cerebral cortex involved in cognitive function

Prefrontal association cortex The cortical regions anterior to BA 6 that are involved with the integration of information in preparation for the motor act, as well as higher-level cognitive processes, including executive function, planning and initiating motor acts, and emotional regulation

Premature sagittal synostosis Premature closure of sagittal suture

Premaxilla Anterior-most portion of hard palate, marked by the premaxillary suture dividing the region of the cuspids and lateral incisors, and terminating in the incisive foramen

Premaxillary suture Suture joining premaxilla with palatine processes

Premotor area The region of the cerebral cortex anterior to the precentral gyrus (area 6)

Premotor region of the of cerebral cortex Generally considered to be BA 6, the premotor gyrus, but also including the supplementary motor area

Preoccipital notch Sulcus on lateral surface of cerebrum, marking the boundary between parietal and occipital lobes

Pressed phonation Mode of vibration of the vocal folds in which medial compression is greatly increased, producing a perception of stridency or harsh quality of the voice

Pressure The derived measure representing force expended over an area

Presynaptic neurons Neurons in a chain that precede (are upstream of) the synapse

Primary activity of cortical region The specific function identified for a cortical region, such as primary receptive area for vision, primary receptive area for audition, etc.

Primary dyspraxia Deficit in ability to program articulators for speech production in absence of muscular weakness or paralysis

Primary fissure of cerebellum Fissure that separates cerebellar cortex into two lobes

Primary oral apraxia /əˈpræksiə/ Deficit in planning the nonspeech act, resulting in difficulty with imitating or producing voluntary nonspeech oral gestures, but in the absence of muscular weakness or paralysis

Primary oral dyspraxia Deficit in ability to program articulators for non-speech production in absence of muscular weakness or paralysis

Primary reception area for vision (VI) of cerebral cortex The region of the occipital lobe that receives the visual information provided by the visual sensation system

Primary verbal apraxia /əˈpræksiə/ Deficit in planning the speech act, resulting in inconsistent phonemic distortions and substitutions with oral groping behaviors for voluntary verbal motor acts, but in the absence of muscular weakness or paralysis

Primary-like response Neural response patterns of brain stem fibers that have characteristics similar to those of the auditory nerve

Prime mover Agonist; this is the muscle responsible for the primary or desired movement

Principle inferior olivary nucleus of medulla major nucleus of inferior olivary complex

pro- Before; in front of

Process A prominence of an anatomical structure

Projection fibers Neural tracts running to and from the cerebral cortex connecting it with distant locations

Prominence of facial nerve In medial wall of middle ear space, prominence through which facial nerve passes

Prominence of stapedial pyramid a.k.a. pyramidal eminence; outcropping in posterior wall

of middle ear space from which stapedial tendon arises

Prominence of the facial nerve Bulge on brain stem marking location of the nucleus of facial nerve

Promontory Bulge in medial wall of middle ear created by lateral semicircular canal

Pronate /ˈproneɪt/ To place in the prone position

Prone /ˈpron/ Body in horizontal position with face down

Propagation Spreading effect of wave action

Proprioception /proprioˈsɛpʃən/ The awareness of weight, posture, movement, and position in space

Proprioceptive sense Sense of body position in space

Proprioceptors Sensors that monitor change in body's position or the position of its parts, including muscle and joint sensors, muscle spindles, and Golgi tendon organs

Prosencephalon /prasɛnˈsɛfəlan/ In embryology, the forebrain, from which the telencephalon and diencephalon will arise

proto- Primitive; simple form

Protuberance /protubəˈəns/ A bulge or prominence above a structure's surface

Proximal /ˈpraksəml/ Closer to the trunk or thorax; nearer to the pubic bone

Proximodistally Development that moves from medial structures to distal structures

Psychoacousticians Researchers involved in study of the psychological correlate of auditory stimulus parameters

Puberphonia a.k.a. mutational voice; disorder in which pre-pubescent voice characteristics are retained past the age of puberty

Pubic symphysis Joint between the paired pubic bones

Pulp of tooth Portion of tooth in which nerves resides

Pulse register Glottal fry; the vocal register characterized by low fundamental frequency, with syncopated vibration of vocal folds

Pulvinar Nucleus of thalamus involved in language function

Purkinje cells of cerebellum Large neurons forming the boundary between the molecular and granular layers of the cortex; excitation of a Purkinje cell causes inhibition of the nucleus with which it communicates

Purkinje layer of cerebellum Intermediate cell layer of cerebellum

Pyramidal cells Large, pyramid-shaped cells typically within the cerebral cortex, and that are involved in motor function

Pyramidal decussation of medulla Point within the medulla at which fibers of the corticospinal tract cross from one side to the other

Pyramidal eminence a.k.a. prominence of stapedial pyramid: outcropping in posterior wall of middle ear space from which stapedial tendon arises

Pyramidal pathway Motor pathway arising from frontal lobe of cerebral cortex, consisting of corticospinal and corticobulbar tracts

Pyramidal system Motor portion of the nervous system arising predominantly from the precentral gyrus of the cerebral cortex, and comprised of the pyramidal tracts (corticospinal and corticobulbar tracts)

Pyriform lobe Lobe composed of the uncus and lateral olfactory stria

Pyriform sinuses a.k.a. piriform sinuses; spaces created by the epithelia overlying the arytenoid and superficial surface of the thyroid cartilages, through which the swallowed bolus passes on its way to the cricopharyngeal sphincter and subsequent esophagus

Quadra-, quadri Four

Quadrangular membranes Connective tissue running from the arytenoids to the epiglottis and thyroid cartilage and forming the false vocal folds

Quiet inspiration Inspiration that involves minimal muscular activity, primarily that of the diaphragm

Quiet tidal respiration Respiration that occurs during periods of low respiratory activity and that is periodic in nature

Quiet tidal volume Tidal volume at rest, approximately 525 cc for male and female adults combined

Radial Pertaining to the radius bone

Radicular arteries of cerebrovascular supply arteries serving the anterior spinal cord and anterior funiculus

Ramus /ˈreɪməs/ A branch or division

-raphy Suturing or stitching

Rapidly adapting sensors Those sensors that respond briefly and then cease responding after change has occurred, such as vibration sensors

Rate of discharge Of a neuron, the rate at which the neuron depolarizes

Rate of flow A measure of airflow that is measured in cubic centimeters of air moving into or out of lungs per second or minute

re- Back or again; curved back

Reciprocal Interchangeable

Recurrent laryngeal nerve (RLN) of X vagus Branch of X vagus nerve serving adductors, tensors and relaxers of vocal folds, as well as cricopharyngeus

Red nucleus Nucleus in midbrain that gives rise to rubrospinal tract

Reflex Motor acts that are involuntary responses to stimulation

Reflex arc The system of basic spinal reflexes involving a muscle spindle, afferent output from the spindle, and a motor nucleus and fiber that respond to the stimulus by causing muscle contraction

Refractory period Will not result in further depolarization

Regional equipotentiality Theoretical stance that takes the middle ground between equipotentialist and localizationist stance, stating that areas of the brain have functional unity, but the degree of functional loss a person suffers from trauma is also related to the volume of damage

Reissner's membrane /ˈraɪznɚz/ Membranous separation between scala vestibuli and scala media

Relative micrognathia /maɪkrəˈnæθiə/ The hypoplasia of the mandible relative to the maxilla

Relative refractory period Period during which the membrane may be stimulated to excitation again, but only with greater than typical stimulation

Reproductive system The system of the body involved in reproduction

Residual volume In respiration, the volume of air remaining after a maximum exhalation

Resonant frequency Frequency of stimulation to which a resonant system responds most vigorously

Resonatory system The portion of the vocal tract through which the acoustical product of vocal fold vibration resonates (usually the oral, pharyngeal, and nasal cavities combined; sometimes referring only to the nasal cavities and nasopharynx)

Respiration The process of exchange of gas between an organism and its environment

Respiratory capacities See **Capacities**

Respiratory physiology The study of function in respiration

Respiratory system The physical system involved in respiration, including the lungs, bronchial passageway, trachea, larynx, pharynx, and oral and nasal cavities

Resting lung volume The volume of air remaining within the lungs after quiet tidal expiration (a.k.a. *expiratory reserve volume*)

Resting membrane potential (RMP) Electrical potential difference between inside and outside of a cell

Resting potential Voltage potential differences that can be measured from the cochlea at rest

Retching Involuntary attempt at vomiting

Reticular activating system (RAS) a.k.a., anterior reticular activating system. System including reticular formation of the brain stem and intralaminar nuclei of thalamus, involved in regulation of cortical arousal

Reticular fibers Extremely fine connective fibers

Reticular formation Posterior aspect of brain stem

retro- Backward, toward the rear

Rhinorrhea /raɪnəˈriə/ Liquid discharge from the nose

Rhombencephalon /rambənˈsɛfəlan/ Embryonic division of the brain from which the pons, cerebellum, and medulla oblongata ultimately arise

Rima glottidis /ˈraɪmə glaˈtidɪs/ Space between the vocal folds; glottis

Rima vestibuli /ˈraɪmə vɛˈstɪbjulɪ/ The space between the false (ventricular) vocal folds

Risorius muscle Most superficial of cheek muscles

Rolandic fissure a.k.a. central sulcus. Sulcus dividing frontal and parietal lobes

Root The part of an organ hidden within other tissues

Rooting reflex Reflex elicited by tactile contact with the mouth region, with the result being that the individual orients toward the direction of the contact

Rostral spinocerebellar tract Transmits proprioception information (GTOs) and pain sense from the upper trunk and arms to the ipsilateral cerebellar cortex

Rostrum /ˈrastrəm/ A beaked or hooked structure

Round window The opening between the scala tympani of the inner ear and the middle ear space

-rrhea A flowing

Rubrospinal tract Extrapyramidal pathway of the CNS running from the red nucleus of the midbrain to the spinal core

Ruga, rugae /ˈrugə/ /ˈrugeɪ/ Folds or creases of tissue

Saccule The smaller of the vestibular sensory mechanisms housed within the vestibule of the inner ear

Sacral vertebra Vertebral components of the sacrum

Sagittal plane /ˈsædʒɪtəl/ Divides body or body part into right and left

Salivatory nucleus Nucleus of pons mediating salivation

Salivatory nucleus of pons Nucleus for VII facial nerve GVE component

Salpingopharygneal fold Ridge of tissue coursing down from the orifice of auditory tube within nasopharynx and overlying the salpingopharyngeal muscle

Salpingopharyngeus muscle Muscle coursing from lower margin of auditory tube to lateral pharynx

Saltatory conduction Neural conduction of an action potential passing from node to node

Sarcomere Bundle of striated muscle myofibrils

Satiety center Region of the hypothalamus that regulates perception of satiation

Scala media /ˈskeɪlə/ The middle space of the cochlea created by the membranous labyrinth, containing the sensory organ of hearing

Scala tympani /ˈtɪmpənɪ/ The peripheral cavity of the cochlea that communicates with the middle ear via the round window

Scala vestibuli /ˈskeɪlə vɛˈstɪbjulɪ/ The peripheral cavity of the cochlea that communicates with the middle ear via the vestibule and oval window

Scaphoid fossa /ˈskæfɔɪd ˈfasə/ The region between the helix and antihelix

Scaphoid fossa of sphenoid bone Space between medial and lateral pterygoid plates

Scapula The major structure of the pectoral girdle

Schwann cells Glial cells that are instrumental in production of myelin in the peripheral nervous system

scirrho-, sclero Hard

-sclerosis /sklæˈosɪs/ Hardening

scolio- Curved

Second bicuspid In adult arch, tooth distal to first bicuspid, with two cusps

Second molar Tooth distal to first molar in adult arch

Secondary tympanic membrane a.k.a., round window

Segmental Divided into segments

Segmental spinal arc reflex Reflex system arising at the spinal cord level, which is involved in reflexive contraction of skeletal muscle as result of passive stretching

Selective enhancement Relative benefit of auditory signal arising from resonance of the auditory mechanism

Sella turcica of sphenoid bone a.k.a. pituitary fossa of sphenoid bone, hypophyseal fossa; inferior space of sphenoid in which pituitary gland resides

Sellar /ˈsɛlɚ/ Saddlelike

semi- Half

Semicircular canals Canals of the vestibular system, responsible for sensation of movement of the head in space

Sensation Awareness of body conditions

Septal cartilage Anterior cartilaginous component of the nasal septum

Septum /ˈsɛptəm/ A divider

Serous Pale, yellow body fluid

Shaft of rib The long, relatively straight component of a rib, between the neck and the angle of the rib

Shearing action The bending action of the hair cells arising from the relative movement of the basilar membrane and tectorial membrane during auditory stimulation

Shedding teeth a.k.a. deciduous teeth, milk teeth; teeth within the deciduous arch that are shed during development

Short association fibers Association fibers of cerebral cortex that connect gyri of the same hemisphere

Short process of incus Posteriorly projecting process of incus

Shoulder girdle Another term for pectoral girdle

Single neuron response Measurement of response of a single neuron

sinistro- Left

Sinus A cavity or passageway

Skeletal muscle Striated or voluntary muscle

Sliding filament model of muscle contraction Process in which cross-bridges connect actin and myosin of parallel myofilaments, pulling the fibers closer together

Slow twitch fibers Fibers that a slow acting and remain contracted longer than fast twitch fibers, typically found in postural muscles

Slowly adapting sensors Those sensors that continue responding once stimulated, such as pain sensors

Smooth muscle Sheet-like muscle with spindle-shaped cells; this makes up the muscular tissue of the digestive tract and blood vessels

Sodium inactivation Closure of sodium channels in cell wall, prohibiting transport of sodium

Sodium–potassium pump Biological mechanism by which sodium and potassium are actively moved through a cell wall

Soft palate The musculotendinous structure separating the oropharynx and nasopharynx; a.k.a. *velum*

Solitary tract nucleus Nucleus of brain stem; inner portion includes axons from the VII facial, IX glossopharyngeal, X vagus cranial nerves

Soma A cell body

Somatic muscle Skeletal muscle; striated muscle

Somatic nervous system The voluntary component of the nervous system

Somatic sense Body sense

somato- Pertaining to the body

Somatosomatic synapse Synapse of the soma of one neuron with the soma of another

Somesthetic /soməsˈθætɪk/ Pertaining to awareness of body sensation

Somesthetic Body sense

Sound Audible disturbance in a medium

Sound wave The acoustical manifestation of physical disturbance in a medium

Source-filter theory The theory of vowel production that states that a voicing source is generated by the vocal folds and routed through the vocal tract where it is shaped into the sounds of speech

Spastic dysarthria Dysarthria arising from upper motor neuron lesion, resulting in spasticity, hypertonicity, hyperreflexia reflexes, and muscular weakness

Spatial orientation Knowledge of body position in space

Spatial summation Phenomenon of many near-simultaneous synaptic activations, representing many points of contact arrayed over the surface of the neuron

Spatiotopic /speɪʃioˈtɑpɪk/ The physical array of many of the regions of the cerebral cortex that defines the specific region of the body represented (e.g., the pre- and postcentral gyri)

Special senses Olfaction, audition, gustation, and vision

Special somatic afferent Cranial nerves that serve the special body senses such as vision and hearing

Special visceral efferent Cranial nerves that innervate striated muscle of branchial arch origin, including the larynx, pharynx, soft palate, face, and muscles of mastication

Specialization Given task or function (e.g., language) than the other hemisphere

Spectral analysis Analysis of an acoustical signal to determine the relative contribution of individual frequency components

Speculum /ˈspɛkjuləm/ Instrument used to examine orifices and canals

Sphenoid sinuses Air-filled sinuses in sphenoid bone

Spherical recess of vestibule Recess in inner ear vestibule that contains perforations through which vestibular nerve passes to the saccule of the membranous labyrinth

Spheroid /ˈsfirōīd/ Shaped like a sphere

Spike rate Rate of discharge of a neuron

Spinal column The vertebral column

Spinal cord The nerve tracts and cell bodies within the spinal column

Spinal cord segment A segment of the spinal cord corresponding to a vertebral region

Spinal meningeal linings Meningeal linings of the spinal cord

Spinal nerves Nerves arising from the spinal cord

Spinal tract nucleus of V trigeminal Sensory nucleus of V trigeminal served by input from IX glossopharyngeal nerve

Spinocerebellum a.k.a. paleocerebellum. Portion of cerebellum made up of anterior lobe of cerebellum and posterior lobe related to arm and leg

Spinous process Posterior-most process of vertebra

Spiral ligament Region of scala media to which stria vascularis is attached

Spiral limbus Region of scala media from which the tectorial membrane arises

Spirometer /spāīrˈamətər/ Device used to measure respiratory volume

Splenium of corpus callosum The posterior portion of the corpus callosum through which information for the temporal and occipital lobes passes

Spongy bone Bone that contains the marrow that produces red and white blood cells as well as the blood plasma matrix

Squamosal suture of parietal bones Suture uniting parietal and temporal bones

Squamous portion of temporal bone Fan-shaped portion of temporal bone

S-segment Lateral superior olive of superior olivary complex

Stahl's ear Pointy, elfin-shaped ears

Stapedius /stəˈpidiəs/ Muscle of middle ear that acts on the stapes

Stapes /ˈstēīpiz/ The final bone of the ossicular chain

Stellate cells of cerebellum Cells in cerebellum that communicate with Purkinje cells

steno- Narrow

Stereocilia /stɛrioˈsɪliə/ Minute cilia protruding from the surface of hair cells

Stereognosis /ˈstɛriagnosəs/ Ability to recognize objects through tactile sensation

Sternal notch a.k.a. suprasternal notch; the notch on the superior aspect of the manubrium sterni

Sternohyoid muscle Hyoid depressor coursing from the sternum to the hyoid bone

Sternothyroid muscle Muscle arising from the sternum and inserting into the thyroid cartilage and depressing the thyroid cartilage and larynx

Stiffness The strength of the forces within a given material that restore it to its original shape on being distended

Stoma Mouth of an opening; in larygectomee, stoma is short for tracheostoma

strepto- Swift

Stress In speech, the product of relative increase in fundamental frequency, vocal intensity, and duration

Stria vascularis /ˈstriə væskjuˈlɛrɪs/ Vascularized tissue arising from the spiral ligament of the scala media

Striated Striped

Striatum Combination of putamen and caudate nucleus of basal ganglia

Strohbass Glottal fry; pulse register

Styloglossus muscle Muscle arising from Styloid process of temporal bone and inserting into inferior sides of tongue

Stylohyoid ligament Ligament attaching Styloid muscle with hyoid bone

Stylohyoid muscle Muscle coursing from styloid process of mandible to hyoid bone

Styloid process of temporal bone Process protruding beneath the external auditory meatus and medial to the mastoid process

Stylopharyngeus Muscle arising from Styloid process of temporal bone and inserting into pharyngeal constrictors and thyroid cartilage

sub- Under

Subcortical nuclei Nuclei of thalamus with no direct communication with the cerebral cortex

Subdural hematoma Release of blood through hemorrhage beneath the dura mater

Subglottal /sʌbˈglatl̩/ Beneath the glottis

Subglottal pressure Air pressure generated by the respiratory system beneath the level of the vocal folds

Sublingual fold Fold on lower surface of tongue that marks salivary glands

Sublingual gland Salivary gland beneath tongue

Submandibular gland Salivary gland posterior to sublingual gland

Substantia nigra Dopamine-producing cells within cerebral peduncles, critical for function of the basal ganglia

Subthalamic nucleus Nucleus on inner surface of internal capsule that receives input from globus pallidus and motor cortex and is involved in control of striated muscle

Successional tooth Tooth in adult dental arch that replaces a homologous deciduous tooth

Sulci Plural of sulcus; significant in-folding of tissue

Sulcus /ˈsʌlkəs/ A groove

Summating potential A sustained, direct current (DC) shift in the endocochlear potential that occurs when the organ of Corti is stimulated by sound

sup- Under; moderately

super- Above; excessively

Superadded tooth Tooth in adult dental arch not represented in deciduous arch

Superficial Near the surface

Superficial sensation Sensation of the surface tissue of the body

Superior The upper point; nearer the head

Superior cerebellar artery of cerebrovascular supply Artery arising from basilar artery, serving cerebellum

Superior cerebellar peduncle a.k.a., brachia conjunctiva; superior pathway for information to and from cerebellum

Superior colliculus Midbrain relay for visual stimuli

Superior cornu of thyroid Superior-most processes of the thyroid cartilage, providing the point of articulation between the greater cornu of the hyoid bone and thyroid cartilages

Superior frontal gyrus Gyrus bordering the longitudinal fissure in superior aspect of frontal lobe

Superior laryngeal nerve (SLN) of X vagus Branch of X vagus innervating cricothyroid muscle for laryngeal pitch change

Superior ligament of incus Ligament binding incus to temporal bone, arising from the superior surface of the incus and coursing to the epitympanic recess

Superior ligament of malleus Ligament binding malleus to temporal bone, arising from the head of the malleus

Superior longitudinal fissure a.k.a., cerebral longitudinal fissure; interhemispheric fissure; the fissure that completely separates left and right cerebral hemispheres

Superior longitudinal muscle of tongue Superior-most muscle on surface of tongue, coursing from median fibrous sulcus to lateral surface

Superior medullary velum Pontine surface providing superior border of 4th ventricle

Superior nasal conchae Superiorly placed process of ethmoid bone, found in nasal cavity

Superior olivary complex in pons Important auditory nuclear complex within the pons, responsible for localization of sound in space

Superior orbital fissure of sphenoid bone Canal of the sphenoid bone through which the IV trochlear nerve passes

Superior parietal lobule Superior-most gyrus of the parietal lobe

Superior petrosal ganglion Ganglion of IX glossopharyngeal nerve

Superior pharyngeal constrictor muscle Muscle coursing fro pterygomandibular raphe to median pharyngeal raphe

Superior temporal gyrus Superior-most gyrus of the temporal lobe

Superior temporal sulcus Sulcus separating superior and middle temporal gyri

Superior thyroarytenoid muscle Auxiliary intrinsic musculature of larynx that is inconsistently present, arising from the inner angle of the thyroid cartilage and coursing to the muscular process of the arytenoid, and being an extension of the thyroarytenoid (thyromuscularis)

Supernumerary teeth Teeth in addition to the normal number

Supination /supɪˈneɪʃən/ Placement in the supine position

Supine /ˈsupaɪn/ Body in horizontal position with face up

Supplementary motor area (SMA) Upper and medial portions of Brodmann area 6, involved in aspects of motor planning

Supplementary motor area of cerebral cortex (SMA) The superior and medial portions of BA 6, which is involved in complex motor acts, including rehearsal and initiation of motor function

supra- Above, upon

Suprahyoid muscles Muscles attached to the hyoid bone and a structure superior to the hyoid bone

Supramarginal gyrus Portion of inferior parietal lobule

Suprasternal notch a.k.a. sternal notch. The notch on the superior aspect of the manubrium sterni

Supraverted /suprə ˈvɚtɪd/ Turning up

Surface anatomy Study of the body and its surface markings, as related to underlying structures

Surfactant /sɚˈfæktənt/ A chemical agent that reduces surface tension

Suture /ˈsutʃɚ/ The demarcation of union between two structures through immobile articulation

Sylvian fissure a.k.a. lateral sulcus; fissure dividing temporal lobe from frontal and anterior parietal lobes

sym- With or together

Sympathetic nervous system a.k.a. thoracolumbar system: the portion of the autonomic nervous system that responds to stimulation through energy expenditure

Sympathetic trunk ganglia Collection of cell bodies coursing parallel to the vertebral column

Symphysis /sɪmfɪsɪs/ A type of union of two structures that were separated in early development, resulting in an immobile articulation

Symphysis menti a.k.a. mental symphysis; the juncture of the fused paired bones of the mandible

syn- With or together

Synapse /ˈsɪnæps/ The junction between two communicating neurons

Synaptic cleft The region between two communicating neurons into which neurotransmitter is released

Synaptic vesicles /sɪˈnæptɪk ˈvɛsəklz/ The saccules within the end bouton of an axon, containing neurotransmitter substance

Synergist /ˈsɪnɚdʒɪst/ A muscle in conjunction with another muscle to facilitate movement

Synostosis Articulation of adjacent bones by means of ossification of a suture

Synostosis Ossification of a suture

Synovial fluid /sɪnoviəl/ The fluid within a synovial joint

System A functionally defined group of organs

Systematic anatomy Descriptive anatomy

Systemic anatomy The description of individual parts of the body without reference to disease conditions

tachy- Swift; fast

Tactile Referring to the sense of touch

Tactile sense The specific sense of touch, mediated by sensors within the epithelial lining

Tail of caudate nucleus Posterior-most portion of caudate nucleus

-tarsal Ankle

Tectorial membrane /tɛkˈtoriəl/ The membranous structure overlying the hair cells of the cochlea

Tectospinal tract Tract arising in superior colliculus of midbrain that terminates in the cervical spinal cord, mediating visual orientation by head turning

Tectum Portion of posterior midbrain behind the cerebral aqueduct

Tegmen tympani of temporal bone Thin plate of bone above tympanic antrum

Tegmentum of pons Posterior portion of pons

Teleceptors /ˈtɛlɛsɛptɚz/ Sensory receptors responsive to stimuli originating outside the body

Telencephalon /tɛlɛnˈsɛfəlan/ Embryonic structure from which cerebral hemispheres and rhinencephalon develop

telo- Far from, toward the extreme

Telodendria /tɛlodɛnˈdriə/ The terminal arborization of an axon

Temporal fossa of temporal bone Indentation of external temporal bone to which temporalis muscle attaches

Temporal operculum Portion of temporal lobe overlying insula

Temporal process of zygomatic bone Process of zygomatic bone that articulates with the temporal bone

Temporal summation Phenomenon in which small number of regions depolarize virtually simultaneously

Temporalis muscle Muscle deep to masseter arising from temporal fossa and inserting into the coronoid process of mandible

Temporal-occipital-parietal association cortex (TOP) The cortical association area that includes portions of the temporal, parietal, and occipital lobes (BA 39 and 40; and portions of 19, 21, 22, and 37), and that is involved in integration of auditory, visual, and somatosensory information into language function

Temporofacial division of VII facial nerve Branch of VII facial giving rise to temporal and zygomatic branches

Tendon /ˈtɛndən/ Connective tissue attaching muscle to bone or cartilage

Tensile strength The quality of a material that provides resistance to destructive pulling forces

Tensor tympani /ˈtɛnsɚ ˈtɪmpənɪ/ Middle ear muscle acting on the malleus

Tensor veli palatini a.k.a., tensor veli palti, tensor veli paltine. Dilator of auditory tube coursing from scaffoid fossa and medial and lateral pterygoid plates of sphenoid bone to lateral auditory tube

Tentorium cerebelli Dura mater structure separating the cerebral cortex from the cerebellum

Teratogen /tɛˈrætodʒən/ An agent that causes abnormal embryonic development

Terminal device a.k.a. end effector; in motor function, the articulator responsible for completion of the motor act

Terminal end bouton Terminal portion of axon, notably housing synaptic vesicles

Terminal endplate Terminal component of an axon that is exciting a muscle fiber

Terminal respiratory bronchioles The last bronchioles in the respiratory tree, connecting the respiratory tree to the alveoli

Terminal sulcus Terminal sulcus on posterior tongue separating the oral surface of the tongue from the palatine surface

Termination of phonation Completion of the period during which vocal folds are vibrating for a given segment

tetra- Four

Thalamus Major sensory relay, and dominant component of diencephalon

Thermoreceptors Sensors responsive to temperature

Thick myofilaments Myosin component making up myofibril

Thin myofilaments Component making up myofibril

Thoracic vertebra Vertebra of the thoracic spinal column

Thoracolumbar system a.k.a. sympathetic nervous system. The portion of the autonomic nervous system that responds to stimulation through energy expenditure

Thorax The part of the body between the diaphragm and the seventh cervical vertebra

Thrombosis Obstruction caused by thrombus

Thrombus Foreign body, such as a blood clot or bubble of air, that obstructs a blood vessel

Thyroarytenoid muscle Muscle coursing from the thyroid cartilage, just below the thyroid notch, to the vocal process of the arytenoid cartilage. This muscle is further divided into thyrovocalis and thyrmuscularis muscles by speech and hearing scientists

Thyroepiglottic ligament Ligament coursing from the inner surface of the thyroid cartilage to the epiglottis

Thyroepiglottic muscle Auxiliary intrinsic musculature of larynx, coursing from posterior attachment of the thyrovocalis muscles to the lateral epiglottic cartilage

Thyrohyoid membrane The membranous laryngeal spanning the space between the greater cornu of the hyoid bone and the lateral thyroid

Thyrohyoid muscle Muscle arising from the thyroid cartilage and inserting into the hyoid bone, which elevates the thyroid cartilage or depresses the hyoid bone

Thyroid angle Point of articulation of the paired thyroid laminae

Thyroid cartilage The major cartilage of the larynx

Thyroid notch Superior-most point of thyroid angle

Thyromuscularis muscle Lateral-most muscle of the thyroarytenoid muscle, responsible for relaxation of the vocal folds

Thyropharyngeus Muscle component of cricopharyngeal muscle arising from oblique line of thyroid lamina and coursing to median pharyngeal raphe

Thyropharyngeus muscle Muscle coursing from thyroid and cricoid cartilages to insert into the posterior pharyngeal raphe

Thyrovocalis muscle Medial most muscle of the thyroarytenoid muscle, responsible for tension of the vocal folds

Tidal volume The volume inspired and expired during normal, quiet respiration

Tip of tongue a.k.a. apex; anterior most portion of tongue

Tissue recoil The property of tissue that causes it to return to its original form after distention and release

-tomy Cutting

Tongue Primary articulatory structure of speech, made up primarily of genioglossus muscle but also including numerous other extrinsic and intrinsic muscles

Tongue thrust Anterior protrusion of tongue during swallow

Tongue tie a.k.a. ankyloglossia; condition in which lingual frenulum is short, restraining movement of tongue

Tonic Pertaining to muscular contraction

Tonic lengthening of muscle spindle Condition wherein muscle spindle length is held constant after change

Tonicity Partial contraction of musculature to maintain muscle tone

Tonotopic arrangement /tonə´tapɪk/ The arrangement of auditory nerve fibers such that fibers innervating the apex process low-frequency information, while fibers in the basal region process high-frequency information

Tonotopicity Characteristic of cochlea wherein sensitivity to the frequency spectrum is arrayed with higher frequencies near base of cochlea and lower frequencies near apex

Torque Rotary twisting

Torsiversion /torsə´vɚʒən/ Rotating a tooth about its long axis

Torso The trunk of the body

Torus tubarius Ridge of tissue encircling the orifice of the auditory tube

Total lung capacity Sum of tidal volume, inspiratory reserve volume, expiratory reserve volume, and residual volume

Tracheostoma Opening placed surgically in the trachea

Tracheostomy Process of surgically placing an opening in trachea

Tracts A bundle of nerve fibers in the central nervous system

Tragus /´treɪgəs/ Flaplike landmark of auricle approximating the concha

Trajectories Predicted or actual movement paths for an articulator

trans- Beyond or on the other side

Transduce To change from one form of energy to another

Transducer Mechanism for converting energy from one form to another

Transport stage Stage of deglutition in which bolus is moved from oral to pharyngeal space

Transverse At right angles to the long axis

Transverse arytenoid muscle a.k.a. transverse interarytenoid muscle. Muscle coursing from lateral posterior aspect of one arytenoid to the lateral posterior aspect of the other arytenoid, serving as adductor of the vocal folds

Transverse dimension of thorax expansion The antero-posterior and lateral dimensional expansion of the thorax generated by contraction of the accessory muscles of inspiration

Transverse interarytenoid muscle a.k.a. transverse arytenoid muscle; muscle coursing from lateral posterior aspect of one arytenoid to the lateral posterior aspect of the other arytenoid, serving as adductor of the vocal folds

Transverse muscle of tongue Muscles originating at median fibrous septum of tongue and coursing laterally to insert into the side of the tongue

Transverse process Lateral process of vertebra

Trapezoid body of pons Pons level relay within the auditory pathway

Traveling wave The wavelike action of the basilar membrane arising from stimulation of the perilymph of the vestibule

Tremor Minute, involuntary repetitive movements

tri- Three

Triangular fossa /´truɪæŋgjulɚ fasə/ Region between the crura anthelicis

Trifurcate /´traɪfɚkeɪt/ To divide into three parts

Triticeal cartilage a.k.a., tritiate cartilage; variably present cartilage between the superior horn of the thyroid cartilage and the greater horn of the hyoid bone

Trochleariform process /trakli´arəform ´prasɛs/ Bony outcropping of middle ear from which the tendon for the tensor tympani arises

-trophic Related to nourishment

-trophy Growth, usually by expanding

-tropy Implies seeking or heading for something

True rib a.k.a. vertebrosternal ribs, consisting of those ribs making direct attachment with the sternum (ribs 1 through 7)

Trunk The body excluding head and limbs

Tubercle /´tubɚkl/ A small rounded prominence on bone

Tunnel of Corti Region of the organ of Corti produced by articulation of the rods of Corti

Turbulence Disturbance within fluid or gas caused by irregularity in its passage

Tympanic antrum of temporal bone Portion of petrous portion of temporal bone that communicates with the mastoid portion

Tympanic membrane The membranous separation between the outer and middle ear, responsible for initiating the mechanical impedance-matching process of the middle ear

Tympanic portion of temporal bone Portion of temporal bone including the anterior and inferior walls of the external auditory meatus

Tympanic sulcus Groove in external auditory meatus portion of temporal bone into which fits the fibrocartilaginous of the tympanic membrane

Type Ia sensory fibers Primary afferent fibers from the muscle spindle

Type Ib sensory fibers Primary afferent fibers from Golgi tendon organs

Type III sensory fibers Sensory fibers conducting pain, pressure touch and coolness sensation

Umbo /ˈʌmbo/ The most distal point of attachment of the inner tympanic membrane to the malleus

Uncrossed olivocochlear bundle (UCOB) efferent fibers arising from superior olive of brain stem that remain ipsilateral, serving efferent function of cochlea through action on the inner hair cells

Uncus Gyrus of the inferior cortex, within which the amygdala resides

uni- One

Unilateral One side affected

Unilateral upper motor neuron dysarthria (UUMN) Dysarthria with signs of spastic dysarthria presented unilaterally, and typically with less severity than bilateral spastic dysarthria

Upper extremity The arm, the forearm, wrist, and hand

Upper motor neurons Any motor neuron in a neuron chain that does not terminate on a muscle

Urinary system The system of the body involved in elimination of waste through urination

Utricle /ˈjutrɪkl̩/ Regions of vestibule housing the otolithic organs of the vestibular system

Uvula Midline structure of velum or soft palate, consisting of the musculus uvulae

Vagal trigone of medulla Bulge in posterior medulla caused by nucleus of X vagus

Vagus nerve X cranial nerve; vagus means "wanderer" in Latin

Vascularized /ˈvæskjulɚ͞aɪzd/ To become vascular

Vasoconstriction /væsoˈkənstrɪkʃən/ Decrease in diameter of blood vessel

Velar hypoplasia Inadequate velum tissue to achieve velopharyngeal closure

Velopharyngeal port Space connecting oropharynx and nasopharynx

Velum /ˈviləm/ Soft palate

Venous system of cerebrovascular supply Drainage system of veins for blood supply of the brain

Ventilation Air inhaled per unit time

Ventral Pertaining to the belly or anterior surface

Ventral acoustic stria Auditory pathway arising from cochlear nucleus and terminating in superior olivary nucleus

Ventral cochlear nucleus (VCN) Component of the first brain stem nucleus in the auditory pathway

Ventral funiculus Anterior column of spinal cord

Ventral rami of spinal cord Division of spinal nerve serving anterior part of body

Ventral spinocerebellar tract Tract transmitting proprioception information (GTOs) and pain sense from the legs and lower trunk to the ipsilateral cerebellar cortex

Ventricle of the larynx a.k.a. rima vestibule, vestibular sinus; space between the true and false vocal folds

Ventricles of the brain /vɛnˈtrɪkjulɚ/ System of cavities and passageways of the brain and spinal cord through which cerebrospinal fluid passes

Ventricular folds a.k.a. vestibular folds, false vocal folds; the upper folds of the larynx, separated from the true vocal folds by the ventricle of the larynx

Ventrolateral sulcus of medulla Lateral margin of the pyramid and the groove from which the XII hypoglossal nerve exits the medulla

Venules /ˈvɛnulz/ A minute vein

Verbal apraxia Deficit in planning the motor act and programming the articulators for speech sound production

Verbal paraphasias Word substitutions found in aphasia

Vertebra Bony segment of the vertebral (spinal) column

Vertebral division of cerebrovascular supply Division of cerebrovascular supply arising from vertebral arteries

Vertebral foramen Foramen of vertebral segment through which spinal cord passes

Vertical dimension of thoracic expansion The superior-inferior dimension of thorax movement, generated by contraction of the diaphragm

Vertical mode of vibration The mode of vibration of the vocal folds in which they open from inferior to superior (bottom to top) and also close from inferior to superior

Vertical muscle of tongue Muscles perpendicular to transverse muscles of the tongue, coursing from the base of the tongue to the membranous cover

Vestibular folds a.k.a. ventricular folds, false vocal folds. The upper folds of the larynx, separated from the true vocal folds by the ventricle of the larynx

Vestibular ganglion Ganglion giving rise to vestibular branch of VIII vestibulocochlear nerve

Vestibular ligament Structural element of ventricular folds

Vestibule /ˈvɛstəbjul/ Entryway

Vestibulocerebellar tract Tract providing tract provides input from the vestibular nuclei to the flocculonodular lobe via the inferior cerebellar peduncles

Vestibulocerebellum of cerebellum a.k.a. archicerebellum; portion of cerebellum made up of flocculonodular lobe

Vestibulospinal tract Tract arising from lateral vestibular nucleus of pons and medulla and descending ipsilaterally through the spinal cord, facilitating spinal reflexes and muscle tone of extensor muscles

Viscera /ˈvisɚə/ Internal organs within a cavity

Visceral /ˈvisɚəl/ Pertaining to internal organs

Visceral pleurae Pleural lining encasing the lungs

Visual sense The physical sensation associated with reception and processing of visual stimuli

Vital capacity The total volume of air that can be inspired after a maximal expiration

Vocal attack The process of bringing vocal folds together to begin phonation

Vocal fundamental Primary frequency of vibration of the vocal folds

Vocal hyperfunction Use of excessive adductory force in phonation

Vocal intensity Sound pressure level associated with a given speech production

Vocal jitter Cycle-by-cycle variation in fundamental frequency of vibration

Vocal ligament Upper edge of the conus elasticus, between the vocal process of the arytenoid cartilages and the angle of the thyroid cartilage, giving stiffness to vocal folds

Vocal nodules Aggregates of tissue on vocal folds, typically arising from vocal abuse

Vocal processes Medial processes of the arytenoid cartilages to which the vocal folds attach

Vocal registers Perceptual vocal variations defined by differential modes of vibration of the vocal folds

Vocal tract The tract consisting of the mouth (oral cavity), the region behind the mouth (pharynx), and the nasal cavity

Voiced Speech produced using the vibrating vocal folds

Voiceless phonemes Phonemes produced without the use of vocal folds

Voltage-sensitive proteins Proteins that respond to the presence of an electrical current in the environment

Volume A measure of three-dimensional space

Volume of air Amount of air within lungs, measured in cubic centimeters, liters, milliliters, or cubic inches

Vomiting a.k.a. emesis. The oral expulsion of gastrointestinal contents

Waveform Graphic depiction of change in amplitude of vibration over time

Wernicke's aphasia A fluent aphasia typically caused by damage to Wernicke's area and the region of the superior temporal sulcus and middle temporal gyrus inferior to Wernicke's area, and resulting in fluent speech with reduced content

Wernicke's area Language center of the posterior superior temporal gyrus of the temporal lobe, posterior BA 22

Wet spirometer /spaɪrˈamətɚ/ Device used for measurement of respiratory volumes

Whispering Whispering is not a true phonatory mode, because no voicing occurs; whispering is produced by partially adducted and tensed vocal folds that develop turbulence in the airstream as airflow crosses the tensed vocal fold margins; the arytenoid cartilages are rotated slightly in but are separated posteriorly, so that there is an enlarged "chink" in the cartilaginous larynx

Whistle register Not a true mode of vibration of the vocal folds, since the vocal folds are not set into vibration. Whistle register is the product of turbulence on the edge of the vocal fold and occurs at frequencies as high as 2,500 Hz, typically in females, and sounds very much like a whistle

White fibrous tissue Tissue that is strong, dense, and highly organized; it has a white cast to it

White matter Myelinated fibers

Whole nerve action potential a.k.a. compound action potential; action potential arising directly from stimulation of a large number of hair cells simultaneously, eliciting nearly simultaneous individual action potentials in the VIII nerve

Wisdom tooth Third molar, in adult arch

Wormian bones of parietal bones Irregular bones created by bifurcations of the lambdoidal suture

Xerostomia a.k.a., dry mouth; reduced sensation of salivary output

Yellow cartilage Cartilaginous connective tissue that has reduced collagen and increased numbers of elastic fibers. See elastic cartilage

Yellow elastic tissue Tissue that is found in locations where connective tissue must return to its original shape after being distended

Z-line Margin of sarcomere

Zygomatic arch Arch consisting of the temporal process of zygomatic bone and zygomatic process of temporal bone, and to which masseter attaches and through which temporalis passes

Zygomatic major muscle Muscle arising lateral to zygomatic minor on zygomatic bone that courses obliquely down to insert into the corner of the orbibularis oris

Zygomatic minor muscle Muscle coursing down from facial surface of zygomatic bone, inserting into upper lip

Zygomatic process of frontal bone Process of frontal bone that articulates with the zygomatic bone

Zygomatic process of maxilla The maxillary process abutting the zygomatic bone

INDEX

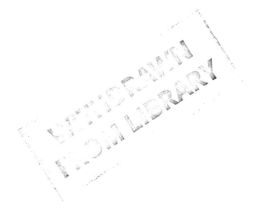